Selected Topics in Cataract Surgery

Selected Topics in Cataract Surgery

Edited by **Ray George**

hayle medical

New York

Published by Hayle Medical,
30 West, 37th Street, Suite 612,
New York, NY 10018, USA
www.haylemedical.com

Selected Topics in Cataract Surgery
Edited by Ray George

International Standard Book Number: 978-1-63241-351-2 (Hardback)

Printed in China.

Contents

Preface

The main aim of this book is to educate learners and enhance their research focus by presenting diverse topics covering this vast field. This is an advanced book which compiles significant studies by distinguished experts in the area of analysis. This book addresses successive solutions to the challenges arising in the area of application, along with it; the book provides scope for future developments.

This book provides information regarding the selected topics related to the field of cataract surgery. Cataract is one of the most common causes of blindness among people and is conventionally treated with surgery. This book has been compiled with the contributions of international experts discussing about fundamentals of the subject and intensive description of some essential topics related to cataract. Some of the topics discussed in the book are: preoperative measures, cataract surgery and its history, common complications and surgeries in special situation. This is an innovative, comprehensive and impactful read on various facets of cataract and cataract surgery. This book is not just for the doctors and researchers but also for general readers who are interested in reading about cataract.

It was a great honour to edit this book, though there were challenges, as it involved a lot of communication and networking between me and the editorial team. However, the end result was this all-inclusive book covering diverse themes in the field.

Finally, it is important to acknowledge the efforts of the contributors for their excellent chapters, through which a wide variety of issues have been addressed. I would also like to thank my colleagues for their valuable feedback during the making of this book.

Editor

Section 1

Pre-Operative Care

1

Pre-Operative Evaluation

Mammie Motiang
University of Limpopo (Medunsa Campus)
South Africa

1. Introduction

Cataracts are the most prevalent cause of visual loss around the world. Their only effective treatment is surgery; which has fortunately become one of the safest, most successful, and most frequently performed outpatient surgeries.

Most cataract patients tend to be elderly and to have serious coexisting illnesses; which puts them at a higher risk for peri-operative complications (Lira et al., 2001). The eye procedure is however, minimally invasive and considered low risk. A thorough pre-operative evaluation by the anaesthesiologist should therefore be performed before these patients can be considered eligible for surgery.

Pre-operative preparation is the first stage in the enhanced recovery process of modern day cataract surgery. If it goes wrong it will adversely impact on the peri- and post-operative stages of enhanced recovery. If done well it enables enhanced recovery (Swart and Houghton, 2010).

According to Hepner (2009), the goals of pre-operative evaluation are the following:

1. To evaluate patient readiness for anaesthesia and surgery;
2. To optimize the patient's health before surgery;
3. To enhance the quality of peri-operative care;
4. To reduce surgical morbidity and length of hospital stay;
5. To answer all questions and obtain informed consent.

This chapter discusses the steps in management and reasons behind them that should be followed in the pre-operative evaluation by the anaesthesiologist before patients can be considered eligible for surgery. It will focus on the following topics: (1) history, (2) physical examination, (3) investigations, (4) fasting guidelines, (5) functional classification, (6) pre-medication. The chapter concludes by recommending that there is an argument for all patients receiving a pre-operative anaesthetic assessment before cataract surgery as the anaesthesiologist is in many centres the final physician who questions and determines the patient's appropriateness and stability for surgery.

2. The pre-operative assessment clinic

The pre-operative assessment clinic or evaluation centre provides the opportunity for anaesthesiologists to see those patients who have been identified by screening and assessment as presenting potential anaesthetic problems. The clinic tends to be cost-effective, as it keeps consultations and redundant provider interviews to a minimum, encourages more targeting of tests, reduces unnecessary laboratory testing, and help avoid last-minute operating room delays and cancellations. It is also associated with increased patient satisfaction, because patients get to meet the surgical team and have risks, side effects and possibility of post-operative intensive care admission explained to them.

3. Pre-operative assessment

3.1 History

3.1.1 Medical history

3.1.1.1 Hypertension

Hypertension is one of the most common diseases in the world and it is clear that its prevalence increases with aging. Most of the patients undergoing cataract surgery are over 60 years old, the group most affected by hypertension. In the study by Motiang and Rantloane (2009) they found a positive correlation between an increase in systolic blood pressure and intraocular pressure. This increase in intraocular pressure may force the intraocular contents towards the surgical incision. The iris, lens or vitreous may prolapse either immediately or when the surgeon attempts to move the lens (Motiang and Rantloane, 2009). Lira et al. (2010) confirmed that hypertensive patients, even those with a history of good blood pressure control, are at increased risk for rise in blood pressure in the peri-operative period (Lira et al., 2010).

Hypertension should be well controlled before the patient is scheduled for surgery and should not be lowered immediately prior to surgery. It is generally recommended that elective surgery be delayed for severe hypertension until the blood pressure is below 180/110mmHg.

3.1.1.2 Diabetes mellitus

Diabetic patients should have their blood sugar controlled pre-operatively. Those with longstanding disease should be assessed in conjunction with a Physician because they have an increased incidence of associated renal and cardiac disease. If the patient is required to fast after midnight on the day of surgery, oral hypoglycaemic agents should be withheld on the day of surgery. Insulin-dependant patients should have their usual insulin dose adjusted. All diabetic patients should have intravenous access peri-operatively in order to treat a potential hypoglycaemic reaction (American Academy of Ophthalmology, 2008-2009). If surgery is planned under local anaesthesia, they should have their usual medication and oral intake.

3.1.1.3 Coronary artery disease

Patients with myocardial infarction should not have surgery within three months of the infarct. Angina should be controlled by the patient's usual medication.

3.1.1.4 Chronic obstructive pulmonary disease (COPD)

COPD patients should have their pulmonary function assessed and maximized pre-operatively. They should be encouraged to bring their inhalers into the operating room. These patients may have increased venous pressure, which may increase intraocular pressure and make the surgery riskier.

Monitored local anaesthesia is preferred in these patients. General anaesthesia can be considered if the patient can tolerate it but cannot endure the required operating table position due to inability to lie flat. Those with severe pulmonary disease may require long term oxygen therapy, which may increase the risk of peri-operative endophthalmitis (American Academy of Ophthalmology, 2008-2009).

All efforts should be made to ensure that the patient does not cough peri-operatively.

The choice of topical, local or general anaesthesia will be influenced by factors limiting the patient's ability to co-operate in the operating room table, which include:

- Arthritis - patients with severe arthritis may be less able to co-operate during surgery because of discomfort. The patient's position on the operating table may have to be adjusted to optimize comfort, but that may create technical difficulties for the surgeon such as not being able to access the patient's eye. A compromise position should be found to allow the patient to lie still and give the surgeon adequate access to the eye. General anaesthesia should be considered if such a compromise cannot be reached.
- Claustrophobia - all patients should be questioned pre-operatively about their ability to tolerate having their face covered during surgery. These patients are better done under general anaesthesia.
- Cognitive function - the patient's caregiver should be questioned about whether the patient can co-operate if local anaesthesia is used. Sedating a patient with a mental disability may cause confusion and increased agitation. General anaesthesia should be used if the patient cannot co-operate but is otherwise in good health. Regression in mental status following general anaesthesia is not uncommon in patients with dementia.
- Hearing loss - good communication with the patient is a definitive advantage if local anaesthesia is planned. Patients with a hearing loss should be reminded to wear a hearing aid into the operating room. An interpreter or family member can be brought into the operating room if the patient and the surgeon do not speak the same language.

3.2 Previous anaesthetics and operations

The patient should be questioned regarding any difficulties with previous anaesthetics. This should include checking records of previous anaesthetics to rule out problems like difficult intubation, drug allergy or adverse reactions, e.g malignant hyperthermia. Details of previous operations like cardiac surgery, may reveal potential anaesthetic problems.

3.3 Family history

Patients should be questioned about any inherited diseases in the family, e.g. porphyria. Family members' experiences with anaesthesia should also be documented. An unexplained death suggests malignant hyperthermia and a history of prolonged apnea suggests butyrylcholinesterase deficiency.

3.4 Drug history

3.4.1 Prescription drugs

Information regarding the patient's medication should be obtained. This will not only provide insight regarding their medical status, but may also alert the anaesthesiologist to possible drug interactions as well as helping to determine which drugs to withhold pre-operatively.

There is normally very little reason to discontinue medications for cardiovascular disease, except for diuretics to minimize need for micturition.

Antihypertensive drugs can potentiate the hypotensive influences of sedatives and anaesthetics, but there is even greater risk of acute rebound hypertensive episodes, if long term medications are withheld. This may pose a risk of an increase in intraocular pressure.

All chronically prescribed psychoactive agents should be continued pre-operatively. The use of meperidine is contraindicated in patients taking monoamine oxidase inhibitors because their interaction can precipitate a seizure and a hypertensive crisis.

In the case of corticosteroids, supplementation should be considered in patients who received more than 10mg prednisone (or equivalent) per day in the last three months.These patients present a potentially impaired stress response due to hypothalamic-pituitary-adrenal (HPA) suppression. They should take their usual prednisone dosage on the morning of surgery, or 25mg hydrocortisone intravenously at induction.

The use of anticoagulation therapy is not associated with an additional risk of peri-operative bleeding in the eye, but can potentiate bleeding should it occur.

Patients on warfarin should have their international normalized ratio (INR) checked to ensure that it is within the desired therapeutic range. There are potential systemic risks of stopping anticoagulation, the decision should therefore be done in conjunction with the primary care physician. Retrobulbar and peribulbar anaesthetic injections carry an increased risk of retrobulbar haemorrhage in these patients. Either a sub-Tenon's or topical anaesthesia is recommended in them. If the surgeon is not comfortable or experienced with these techniques, he should consider referring the patient to an appropriately qualified surgeon.

Aspirin is generally not discontinued prior to cataract surgery.

The Ophthalmologist should specifically enquire about tamsulosin hydrochloride (Flomax). Tamsulosin is used to treat benign prostatic hypertrophy in men and urinary retention in women. This drug, together with other α_{1A} - antagonists, is strongly associated with iris complications during phacoemulsification known as intraoperative floppy iris syndrome (IFIS), as well as with fluctuations in pupil size during cataract surgery. This syndrome is manifested by a pupil that may not dilate fully and may constrict intraoperatively. The iris may billow and prolapse through the incision. Tamsulosin binds to postsynaptic nerve endings of the iris dilator muscle for a prolonged period, causing excessive iris mobility. It should be discontinued two weeks prior to surgery, (Malhotra, 2008) though this practice is not felt to be effective by all surgeons since the effects may be chronic.

3.4.2 Non-prescription drugs

Drugs with anticholinergic properties, such as diphenhydramine, are likely to increase the risk of peri-operative delirium and should be withheld. Women and patients in the age range of 40 to 60 years are more likely to use herbal medicine. The most highly used compounds, include echinecea, Gingko biloba, St.John's wort, garlic and gingseng.

The most common potential adverse effects of herbal medicines in the peri-operative period include impaired coagulation, cardiovascular side effects, electrolyte disturbances, and prolongation of the effects of anaesthetic agents. Of concern is that unless specifically questioned, patients may not report the use of these non-prescription drugs. The American Society of Anaesthesiologists (ASA) recommends discontinuation of all alternative therapies 2 weeks before elective procedures, although there are no definitive data supporting this recommendation (Fischer et al., 2010).

3.5 Allergies

Patients should be questioned with regard to the history of allergy to drugs such as antibiotics, nonsteroidal anti inflammatory drugs, and for those undergoing local anaesthesia, ester local anaesthetics. Esters are preserved in para-aminobenzoic acid, which is responsible for the allergic reaction. Anaphylactic reactions to amide local anaesthetics are extremely rare. Muscle relaxants account for a high incidence of true anaphylactic and anaphylactoid reactions, followed by latex and antibiotics.

Latex is a milky-white sap obtained from rubber trees (Hevea brasiliensis) and is used in more than 40,000 medical products. Adverse reactions to rubber products should be sought for because a number of IgE-mediated reactions to latex have been confirmed, including anaphylaxis and death (Becker, 2009).

Any report of allergy should be further questioned to clarify that signs and symptoms were consistent with hypersensitivity reactions (eg. rash, pruritus, urticaria, severe hypotension, airway compromise). It is not uncommon for patients to label any adverse drug experience as an 'allergic reaction'.

3.6 Social history

3.6.1 Smoking

Patients who smoke are prone to hyper-reactive airways and bothersome episodes of coughing, which poses a problem post-operatively with the risk of lens extrusion. Coughing greatly increases the venous pressure and raises the intraocular pressure as much as 40mmHg or more (McGoldrick and Gayer, 2009). Heavy smokers have a reduction in oxygen binding sites on haemoglobin due to the presence of carbon monoxide. It is therefore wise to oxygenate them to maintain the saturation above 95% due to the leftward shift of the oxyhaemoglobin dissociation curve. Nicotine stimulates the sympathetic nervous system, causing tachycardia and hypertension. If smoking is stopped for 8 weeks it improves the airways and reduces the rate of post-operative pulmonary complications; for 2 weeks reduces irritability; and for as little as 24hrs pre-operatively decreases carboxyhaemoglobin levels, abolish nicotine effects and improve mucous clearance (Gwinnut, 2004). Because smokers often show increased airway reactivity, administering a bronchodilator pre-operatively may also be useful, especially when a general anaesthetic is planned.

4. Examination

4.1 Airway assessment

The airway should be examined and the modified Mallampati classification noted, which has become the standard for assessing the relationship of the tongue size relative to the oral cavity, although it has a low positive predictive value in identifying patients who are difficult to intubate (Hata and Moyers, 2009). This is an essential component of the pre-operative assessment since airway management forms the most important aspect of patient care during sedation or general anaesthesia.

With the patient sitting upright, he is asked to open his mouth and maximally protrude his tongue. The view of the pharyngeal structures is noted and scored class I-IV. Those who have a visible epiglottis on mouth opening are scored class zero. Patients who have class III and IV airways are more difficult to intubate, more likely to obstruct, and more difficult to manually ventilate, should this become necessary.

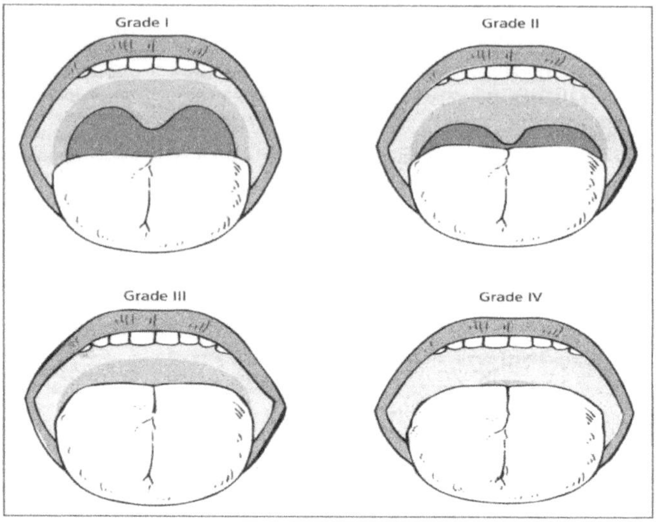

Fig. 1. The pharyngeal structures seen during the Mallampati assessment (Gwinnut 2004)

There are other simple bedside tests which include the following:

- Thyromental distance - with the head fully extended on the neck, the distance between the bony point of the chin and the prominence of the thyroid cartilage is measured. A distance of less than 7cm suggests difficult intubation.
- Wilson score - increasing weight, a reduction in head and neck movement, reduced mouth opening, and the presence of a receding mandible or buck-teeth all predispose to increased difficulty with intubation.
- Calder test - the patient is asked to protrude the mandible as far as possible. The lower incisors will lie anterior to, aligned with or posterior to the upper incisors. The latter two suggest reduced view at laryngoscopy.

Additional factors that warn of difficulty in attaining a good mask seal for positive pressure ventilation include those who are fully bearded or edentulous, and those with a large neck circumference.

Patients with severe rheumatoid arthritis should also have their cervical spine assessed.

None of these tests, alone or in combination, predicts all difficult intubations. If problems are anticipated, anaesthesia should be planned accordingly. If intubation proves difficult, it must be recorded in a prominent place in the patient's notes and the patient be informed.

4.2 Cardiovascular system

The physical examination can be altered by age and disease. For example, a systolic ejection murmur suggesting aortic stenosis may represent aortic valve sclerosis rather than a haemodynamically significant valvular stenosis.

Examination should focus on signs of hypertension, arrhythmias, heart failure and valvular heart disease. Diabetics should be examined for signs of autonomic neuropathy, which is the best predictor of silent ischemia.

Also inspect the peripheral veins to identify any potential problems with intravenous access.

4.3 Respiratory system

Auscultate for additional or added breath sounds and look for signs of collapse, consolidation, pleural effusion and respiratory failure.

4.4 Other systems

Examination of other systems should be guided by problems that are relevant to anaesthesia that are identified in the history.

Since most of the cataract patients are elderly, any evidence of dementia should be documented as it will be useful in evaluating any concerns regarding residual influences of sedatives or anaesthetic agents post-operatively. A discussion with family members should be sought if clinical data is unclear, cognitive impairment is profound, or the responses are misleading.

5. Investigations

Routine investigations have been found to be unnecessary as they do not increase the safety of cataract procedures. They should only be done if medical history or physical examination reveal a new or worsening medical disease. According to Fleisher, pre-operative testing should only be performed if it will actually be used to modify care (Fleischer, 2001). They have also been found to be important as baseline information if problems develop.

Most abnormalities in laboratory values can be predicted from the patient's history and findings on physical examination; moreover, laboratory abnormalities, when discovered, rarely lead to changes in peri-operative treatment. A study by Schein et al. (2000) demonstrates that peri-operative morbidity and mortality are not reduced by routine use of commonly ordered pre-operative medical tests. These tests have been shown to be of no benefit in either predicting patients liable to suffer peri-operative complications or in lowering operative risk. All tests should be interpreted within the context of the clinical situation.

Except for the electrocardiogram (ECG), banks of pathology tests and radiology examinations can be avoided (MacPherson, 2004). The resting 12-lead ECG is however not appropriate for identifying patients with an increased peri-operative cardiac risk scheduled for low-risk surgery. In cataract surgery it is recommended only for those patients with recent episodes of chest pain and asymptomatic patients with long standing diabetes mellitus. (Kubitz and Motsch, 2003).

The ASA issued the following guideline for general principles for avoiding unnecessary pre-operative testing:

- Routine laboratory tests are not good screening devices and should not be used to screen for disease.
- Repetition should be avoided: there is no need to repeat a recent test.
- Healthy patients may not need testing.
- Patients undergoing minimally invasive procedures may not need testing.
- A test should be ordered only if its results will influence management.

Four criteria for making an educated decision about whether a pre-operative test is indicated have been listed (Table1). A test that meets only one or none of the four criteria is probably not a good test, and if it meets three or four of the criteria, it is a very good test (Hepner, 2009).

Diagnostic efficacy	Does the test correctly identify abnormalities?
Diagnostic effectiveness	Would the test change your diagnosis?
Therapeutic efficacy	Would the test change your management?
Therapeutic effectiveness	Would the test change the patient's outcome?

*Adapted from Hepner (Hepner, 2009)

Table 1. Criteria for determining whether a pre-operative test is indicated

6. Fasting guidelines

The purpose of fasting is to reduce the risk of anaesthesia-related pulmonary aspiration of gastric contents and the consequent risk of aspiration pneumonia.

The Canadian Anesthesiologists' Society's Guidelines to the Practice of Anesthesia (Lindley,2009) states that fasting policies should vary to take into account age and pre-existing medical conditions and should apply to all forms of anesthesia, including monitored anesthesia care. However, the ophthalmological Society in Canada states that fasting is not necessary if topical anesthesia, without intravenous opiate or sedative, is administered for cataract surgery. In 2004, the Royal College of Ophthalmologists decided that it is unnecessary to fast patients for local anesthetic cataract surgery (Lindley, 2009).

General fasting guidelines for normal patients undergoing elective surgery, as published by the ASA are as follows:

- 2 hours for clear non-particulate and non-carbonated fluids. The volume of the liquid ingested is less important than the type of liquid ingested.
- 6 hours after a light meal.
- 8 hours after a meal that includes fried or fatty food.

7. Functional classification – American society of anaesthesiologists (ASA)

This classification was the first attempt to quantify the risk associated with anaesthesia and surgery (Table 2). The system attempts to give a subjective and relative risk based only on the patient's pre-operative medical history (i.e no consideration of diagnostic studies). Its limitation is that it cannot be used as a tool to communicate meaningful expectations to patients and other caregivers.

ASA 1	A normal healthy patient
ASA 2	A patient with mild systemic disease
ASA 3	A patient with significant or severe systemic disease
ASA 4	A patient with severe disease that is a constant threat to life
ASA 5	A moribund patient who is equally likely to die in the next 24 hours with or without surgery
ASA 6	A brain – dead organ donor

"E" added to the classification indicates emergency surgery

*Adapted from Fisher,Bader,Sweitzer (Fisher,Bader,Sweitzer,2010)

Table 2. American Society of Anaesthesiologists Physical Status Classification

8. Premedication

Premedication is useful to control anxiety, post-operative pain, nausea, vomiting and hypnosis. Specific pharmacologic actions should be kept in mind when these drugs are administered before operation, and they should be tailored to the needs of each patient. Patients should also be advised on which chronic medication to withhold pre-operatively.

No consensus exists on the choice of pre-operative medications, but there is general agreement that most patients should enter the theatre after anxiolysis, without undue sedation, has been accomplished. The patients' physical status, age, surgical procedure and its duration should be considered in selecting the appropriate drugs for pre-operative medication (Hata and Moyers, 2009).

Although historically many classes of drugs (eg.barbiturates, antihistamines) have been used to reduce anxiety and induce sedation, benzodiazepines are currently the drugs most commonly used. Even though oral diazepam has been found to be useful in controlling anxiety in adult patients, either the day before surgery or on the day of surgery; midazolam is the benzodiazepine most commonly used pre-operatively. At proper doses, neither midazolam nor diazepam place patients at any additional risk for cardiovascular and respiratory depression (Lichtor, 2009).

Melatonin is a hormone secreted by the pineal gland. In their study, Ismael and Mowafi concluded that oral premedication with melatonin provided anxiolytic effects, improved peri-operative analgesia, decreased intraocular pressure with better operating conditions, and stabilized the hemodynamic variables during cataract surgery under topical anesthesia (Ismael and Mowafi, 2009).

Possible interaction between drugs used to dilate the pupil pre-operatively and those used in premedication and anaesthesia should be considered. The commonly used mydriatics are tropicamide and phenylephrine.

Phenylephrine eye drops are α_1 agonists used as vasoconstrictors and mydriatics. Care should be taken when using them in patients on monoamine oxidase inhibitors as they exaggerate the adrenergic response. They also increase the possibility of hypertension and cardiac dysrhythmias in other patients.

9. Conclusion

The anaesthesiologist is often in many centres the final physician who questions and determines the patient's appropriateness and stability for surgery.

A satisfactory pre-operative preparation and medication facilitate an uneventful peri-operative course. Poor preparation may begin a series of problems and misadventures. All patients should receive a pre-operative anaesthetic assessment (Hata and Moyers, 2009).

10. References

American Academy of Ophthalmology (2008-2009).Basic and Clinical Science Course:Lens and Cataract, San Francisco

Becker, D.(2009).Preoperative Medical Evaluation: Part 1: General Principles and Cardiovascular Considerations. Anesthesia Progress, 56(3): 92-103

Fischer, S., Bader, A., & Sweitzer, B. (2010).Preoperative Evaluation, In Anesthesia, Miller, R, pp 1001-1066, Churchill Livingstone, ISBN 978-0-443-06959-8, Philadelphia

Fleisher, L.(2001).Routine Laboratory Testing in the Elderly: Is it indicated ? Anesthesia and Analgesia, 93: 249-250

Fong, K., Malhotra, R.(2008).Assessment of the patient with cataract, In: Cataract (eye essentials), Malhotra, R, pp 18-32, Elsevier, ISBN 978-0-08-044977-7, USA

Gwinnut, C.(2004).Clinical Anaesthesia (2nd ed), Blackwell, ISBN 978-1-4051-1552-0, Massachusets

Hata, T., Moyers, J.(2009).Preoperative patient assessment and management, In: Clinical Anesthesia, Barash, P, pp 569-597, Lippincott Williams & Wilkins, ISBN 978-0-7817-8763-5, Philadelphia

Hepner, D. (2009). The role of testing in the preoperative evaluation. *Cleveland* Clinic Journal of Medicine, 76(4): S22-27

Ismael, S., Mowafi, H.(2009).Melatonin provides anxiolysis, enhances analgesia, decreases intraocular pressure, and promotes better operating conditions during cataract surgery under topical anesthesia. Anaesthesia and Analgesia, 108(4):1058-1061

Kubitz, J., Motsch, J.(2003).Eye surgery in the elderly. Best Practice and Research clinical Anaesthesiology, 17(2): 245-257

Lichtor, J.(2009).Ambulatory Anesthesia, In: Clinical Anesthesia, Barash, P, pp 833-846, Lippincott Williams & Wilkins, ISBN 978-0-7817-8763-5, Philadelphia

Lindley, S.(2009).Is fasting required before cataract surgery? Canadian Journal of Ophthalmology, 44(6): 645-647

Lira, R., Nascimento, M. & Moreira-Filho, D.(2001).Are routine preoperative medical tests needed with cataract surgery? Pan American Journal of Public Health, 10(1):13-17

Lira, R.Nascimento, M., & Arieta, C.(2010). Incidence of preoperative high blood pressure in cataract surgery among hypertensive and normotensive patients. Indian Journal of Ophthalmology, 58(6): 493-495

MacPherson, R.(2004).Structured assessment tool to evaluate patient suitability for cataract surgery under local anaesthesia. British Journal of Anaesthesia, 93(4): 521-524

McGoldrick, K., Gayer, S.(2009).Anesthesia for ophthalmologic surgery, In: Clinical Anesthesia, Barash, P, 1321-1345, Lippincott Williams & Wilkins, ISBN 978-0-7817-8763-5, Philadelphia

Motiang, M., Rantloane, J.(2009).Intraocular pressure changes in patients undergoing cataract extraction and lens implantation: laryngeal mask airway versus endotracheal tube. Southern African Journal of Anaesthesia and Analgesia, 15(2): 23-27, ISSN-1027-9148

Schein, O., Katz, J. & Bass, E.(2000).The value of routine preoperative medical testing before cataract surgery. The New England Journal of Medicine, 342: 168-175

Swart, M., Houghton, K.(2010).Preoperative preparation: Essential elements for delivering enhanced recovery pathways. Current Anaesthesia & Critical Care, 21:142-147

2

Pathophysiology and Pre-Operative Evaluation of Patients at Risk for Intraoperative Floppy Iris Syndrome (IFIS)

Matthew A. Cantrell[1], Heather R. Bream-Rouwenhorst[1], Christopher Watts[2] and Thomas A. Oetting[2]
[1]University of Iowa College of Pharmacy, Department of Pharmacy Practice and Science, Iowa City, Iowa
[2]University of Iowa Carver College of Medicine, Iowa City, Iowa
USA

1. Introduction

Intraoperative Floppy Iris Syndrome (IFIS) has received a significant amount of attention and subsequent research since it was first reported in 2005 (Bell et al., 2009; Blouin et al., 2007; Chang & Campbell, 2005; Chang et al., 2007; Oshika et al., 2007; Srinivasan et al., 2007; Takmaz & Can, 2007). Current and former uses of alpha-1 adrenergic receptor (α_1AR) antagonists—most notably tamsulosin—appear to be at the highest risk for this surgical complication (Chang & Campbell, 2005). IFIS is characterized by loss of muscle tone in the iris, thereby preventing mydriasis and involves a triad of pupil constriction, fluttering and billowing of the iris stroma, and propensity for iris prolapse during cataract surgery (Chang & Campbell, 2005). While α_1AR antagonists are often used for various urological conditions, they also block α_1AR receptors in the iris dilator muscle and may worsen muscle tone and lead to the iris billowing sometimes seen in cataract surgery. Without adequate pupil dilation, IFIS reduces visualization of the surgical field, including the cataract itself. This impairs removal and can lead to other complications including rupture of the posterior capsule, which further increases the risk of other vision-threatening complications of cataract surgery (Schwinn & Afshari, 2006).

2. Use of alpha-1 adrenergic receptor (AR) antagonists

Since there is a significant association between α_1AR antagonist use and IFIS, a brief review of the indications of α_1AR antagonists is necessary to identify the at-risk population. The principal indication is treatment of benign prostatic hyperplasia (BPH). This urological disorder shares risk factors with cataract development, with advanced age being the most significant (Congdon et al., 2004). If left untreated, BPH increases risk for significant complications including acute urinary retention, recurrent urinary tract infections, and urinary incontinence (Crawford et al., 2006). In patients with mild BPH as indicated by an American Urological Association (AUA) scores of 8 or less, pharmacotherapy may not be indicated as lower urinary tract symptoms (LUTS) often improve spontaneously. Identifying suitable candidates for this strategy, often called "watchful waiting," is critical to reduce unnecessary exposure to α_1AR therapy and is recommended by the AUA to invariably reduce risk for IFIS (American Urological Association [AUA], 2010). Pharmacotherapy for BPH is indicated in patients with moderate to severe disease and includes the 5-alpha reductase inhibitors (5ARI) and α_1AR receptor antagonists. The 5ARI finasteride and dutasteride inhibit conversion of testosterone to dihydrotesterone, thereby shrinking the prostate; the α_1AR antagonists reduce bladder outlet obstruction by relaxing prostatic smooth muscle tissue surrounding the urethra. The currently available agents include terazosin, doxazosin, alfuzosin, tamsulosin, and silodosin. They have comparable effects in symptom reduction (Djavan et al., 2004; Marks et al., 2009). While terazosin and doxazosin were originally developed for treatment of hypertension, their use for this indication has waned largely due to publication of the ALLHAT trial which demonstrated a higher incidence of hospitalization for congestive heart failure (CHF) in the doxazosin arm relative to chorthalidone (ALLHAT, 2000). Subsequent "uroselective" agents that target the α_{1A} AR have been developed including tamsulosin, and most recently silodosin. (Package insert Flomax 2007; Package insert Rapaflo 2008). Alfuzosin's improved tolerability is largely attributable to its extended-release formulation, which prevents peaks in serum concentrations (Roehrborn et al., 2000)

Aside from the robust data demonstrating benefit in men with BPH, these agents have an emerging role in other areas of urology including facilitating the passage of urinary caliculi, as an adjunctive treatment for chronic prostatitis, following ureteral stent placement, and also improving symptoms of overactive bladder in select patients (Anothaisintawee et al., 2011; Kaplan et al., 2006; Navanimitkul & Lojanapiwat, 2010; Singh et al., 2007). Use of α_1AR is limited outside the urological arena; however, some patients are undoubtedly still taking them for treatment refractory hypertension. Finally, data suggests that prazosin—an agent no longer endorsed by the AUA for treatment of BPH due to its unfavorable adverse effect and pharmacokinetic profile—has been shown to be effective in reducing nightmares secondary to post-traumatic stress disorder (PTSD) (Dierks et al., 2007; Raskind et al., 2003). It is imperative that ophthalmologists recognize the various indications for α_1AR therapy to identify those at risk for IFIS. While men are at higher risk based on their respective use of α_1AR for treatment of BPH, physicians should recognize that that some women may be taking these agents for other indications as well.

3. Pathophysiology of IFIS

The α_1ARs are G-protein coupled receptors and subdivided into α_{1A}AR, α_{1B}AR, and α_{1D}AR subtypes. Stimulation of α_1AR elicits contraction of cardiac and most innervated vascular smooth muscle throughout the body (Biaggioni & Robertson, 2009). Like the iris dilator muscle, the prostate contains a significant volume of smooth muscle rich in ARs. BPH and its associated LUTS involve the prostate, urethra, bladder, and spinal cord. The α_{1A} and α_{1D}AR predominate in these organs, but α_{1B}AR are also present. As the prostate grows in BPH, there is upregulation of α_1AR expression, with studies demonstrating that expression of α_{1A}ARs increases up to 9-fold and α_{1D}ARs by 3-fold. This upregulation, especially of α_{1A}AR, is thought to be responsible for the disproportionate increase in smooth muscle contraction and worsening of LUTS in patients with BPH (Thiyagarajan, 2002). Therefore, α_1AR antagonists are useful in ameliorating symptoms associated with BPH by decreasing prostatic urethral resistance although this blockade may influence iris behavior (Shapiro et al., 1992). Specifically, use of α_1AR antagonists for BPH relieves straining and hesitancy, improves bladder emptying, and increases the force of the urinary stream.

Commonly used second-generation α_1AR antagonists include doxazosin and terazosin, although patient tolerability to these agents is variable, with the most vexing clinical problems being orthostatic hypotension and dizziness (McNaughton-Collins & Barry, 2005). Frail geriatric patients often suffer from gait problems, and the addition of a medication that could increase the potential of a fall is undesirable. The increased α_{1A}AR selectivity of the third-generation "uroselective" agents tamsulosin and silodosin is postulated to provide additional relief of LUTS in patients with BPH without increasing the rate of serious adverse cardiovascular effects due to systemic αAR antagonism. (Cantrell et al., 2008; Cantrell et al., 2010)

α_1AR antagonists not only therapeutically inhibit prostatic α_1AR but may also selectively antagonize these receptors in the iris dilator muscle. In the iris, α_{1A}AR mediate iris dilator smooth muscle contraction whereas iris arteriolar contraction is mediated via α_{1B}AR. Blockade of this muscle's α_1AR is hypothesized to lead to poor muscle tone and the subsequent iris billowing sometimes seen in cataract surgery (Schwinn & Afshari, 2006). Figure 1 illustrates the clinical dilemma of IFIS and the subsequent potential for surgical complications.

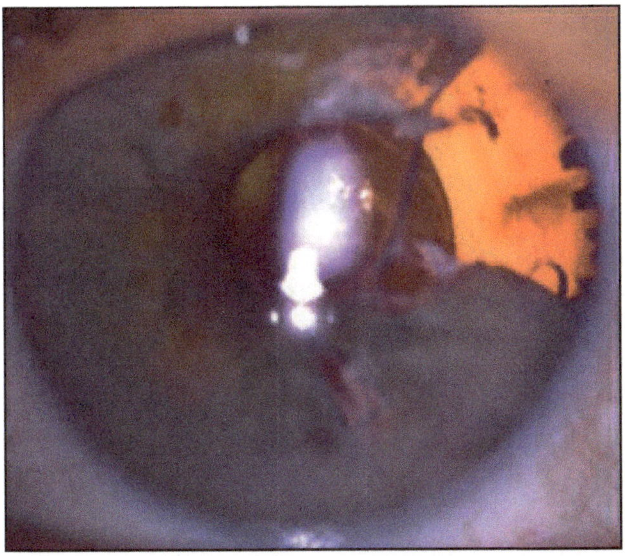

Fig. 1. Iris damage following cataract surgery in a patient taking tamsulosin

Although Chang and Campbell first associated IFIS with tamsulosin in 2005, other available α_1AR antagonists were subsequently linked to IFIS as well (Dhingra et al., 2007; Herd, 2007; Package insert Rapaflo, 2008; Settas & Fitt, 2006; Venkatesh et al., 2007).

Potentially, the high α_{1A}AR-specific antagonism of tamsulosin made the association easier to identify. In rabbits, tamsulosin was more effective than the non-specific α_1AR antagonist alfuzosin at blocking adrenergic-mediated iris dilator contraction (Palea et al., 2008). Interestingly, functional studies assessing the affinity of different ARs as measured by pKi (negative logarithm of the equilibrium dissociation constant) reflect higher affinity of silodosin for α_{1A}AR compared to older agents; when compared to other currently available α_1AR antagonists, silodosin is 1400 times more specific in terms of α_{1A}AR versus α_{1B}AR binding than doxazosin and terazosin and 40 times greater compared to tamsulosin (Thiyagarajan, 2002). It remains to be seen if silodosin has a greater likelihood to cause IFIS than the other available agents.

In a rabbit study, Palea et al. suggested an additional unrecognized receptor may be involved in contraction of the iris dilator muscle as α_1AR blockade with tamsulosin and alfuzosin was less prominent in the iris than the prostate (Palea et al., 2008). While α_{1A}AR are commonly reported as the predominant subtype in the iris dilator muscle in animal studies (Suzuki et al., 2002; Yu & Koss, 2003), Flach pointed out that assuming α_{1A}AR predominate in the human iris dilator muscle based off rabbit studies may be misleading (Flach, 2009). Nevertheless, human immunohistochemical analysis has shown α_{1A}ARs to localize to iris arteriolar muscularis and the iris dilator muscle (Panagis et al., 2010).

4. Risk factors for IFIS

The most comprehensive assessment of risk factors for IFIS was recently published. This meta-analysis included seventeen studies totaling 17,588 eyes (Chatziralli & Sergentanis, 2010). It assessed current use of α_1AR antagonist therapy as well as the effect of co-variates hypertension and diabetes. Current tamsulosin use was associated with the highest risk among the groups studied. Current use of alfuzosin and terazosin was associated with lower risk relative to tamsulosin but remained statistically significant. The pooled analysis of doxazosin did not reach statistical significance; however, the authors cautioned that more studies are needed to gain statistical power. Of the covariates tested, only current hypertension increased risk for IFIS. Despite mixed results in various studies, diabetes did not emerge as a significant risk factor for IFIS. The authors concluded that, consistent with previous reports, it appears that tamsulosin use is associated with the highest risk of IFIS relative to other agents.

There is limited information regarding doxazosin, prazosin and the most recently approved agent silodosin. However, as the latter's pharmacology most resembles tamsulosin and because of its high affinity for the α_{1A}AR, it should be presumed that there is an inherent risk with silodosin until data suggests otherwise. A complete list of medications medications associated with IFIS is described in Table 1.

5. Literature review

IFIS was originally reported in a retrospective study of 511 patients who underwent cataract surgery (Chang & Campbell, 2005). Twenty-seven patients (5.3%) totaling 40 eyes had preoperative exposure to α_1AR antagonists. Ten of sixteen (62.5%) patients who received tamsulosin prior to surgery developed IFIS. In the remaining eleven patients on other α_1AR antagonists, there were no documented cases of IFIS. However, the authors reported that all twenty-seven patients had "poor or moderately poor dilation." A complete list of studies assessing incidence of IFIS as well as studies assessing rates of surgical complications in patients prescribed α_1AR antagonists are described in Table 2

Alpha-1 adrenergic receptor (AR) antagonists	Miscellaneous medications
tamsulosin	finasteride
terazosin	saw palmetto
doxazosin	donepezil
alfuzosin	risperidone
prazosin	chlorpromazine
silodosin	

Table 1. Medications associated with IFIS

In a prospective analysis of 900 consecutive cataract surgeries among 741 patients, IFIS was observed in sixteen patients (2.2%), fourteen of whom had documented concomitant use of tamsulosin (Chang & Campbell, 2005). In the two remaining patients, one had discontinued tamsulosin three years prior to surgery, and one had no history of tamsulosin exposure. Furthermore, IFIS was reported in both eyes of the five patients taking tamsulosin that required bilateral cataract surgery.

Despite the authors' initial identification of a potentially serious complication of cataract surgery, reported limitations of the study include lack of covariate data and the modest reported use of α_1AR antagonists at 1.9% (Chang & Campbell, 2005; Schwinn & Afshari, 2006). As stated above, patients with BPH may not always require pharmacologic treatment, specifically in patients with mild American Urological Association (AUA) symptom scores (AUA, 2010). This may partially explain the relatively low percentage of tamsulosin use in a population with a historically high prevalence of BPH.

In a recent study assessing incidence, IFIS was reported to be 1.6% among 774 patients (Takmaz & Can, 2007). IFIS was documented in 14 of 18 patients (77.8%) taking tamsulosin, and consistent with the original report by Chang and Campbell, tamsulosin use overall was observed in 2.2% of patients. Duration of tamsulosin use—although increased among patients diagnosed with IFIS—was not statistically significant relative to those without IFIS.

A recent study directly compared the incidence of IFIS attributable to tamsulosin with an active comparator group. (Blouin et al., 2007). In this retrospective study of 64 men totaling 92 eyes, there was an increased risk of IFIS in patients exposed to tamsulosin (86.4%) when compared to alfuzosin (15.4%). The adjusted odds ratio for IFIS in patients taking tamsulosin when compared to alfuzosin was 32.15 (95% confidence interval, 2.74-377.41). Furthermore, a five-fold increase in surgical complication rates was observed in patients diagnosed with IFIS, highlighting its clinical significance.

Reference	Design	Objective	Population	Overall Prevalence or Incidence of IFIS (%)	Exposure to Systemic α_1AR Antagonist (%)	Prevalence or Incidence of IFIS in Tamsulosin-Treated Patients (%)	Comments
Chang & Campbell, 2005	Clinical study 1: retrospective chart review	Assess incidence and possible causative factors of IFIS	511 patients; 706 eyes	10/511 patients (2.0)	27/511 patients (5.3)	10/16 patients (62.5)	
	Clinical study 2: prospective case series		741 patients; 900 eyes	16/741 patients (2.2)	Not available	15/16 patients (93.8)	
Chang et al., 2007	Prospective, multicenter, nonrandomized observational series	Evaluate surgical outcomes and rate of complications when ophthalmologist knew patient was taking tamsulosin	135 patients; 167 eyes	No IFIS: 10% of eyes; mild: 17% of eyes; moderate – severe: 73% of eyes	135/135 patients (100)	150/167 eyes (89.8)	
Blouin et al., 2007	Retrospective chart review	Compare IFIS risk in men taking tamsulosin vs. alfuzosin	332 patients; 461 eyes	61/461 eyes (13.2)	64/332 patients (19.3)	19/22 patients (86.4)	IFIS in 2/13 (15.4%) patients exposed to alfuzosin
Srinivasan et al., 2007	Retrospective chart review	Determine occurrence of IFIS in those exposed to systemic α_1AR antagonists	1298 patients; 1612 eyes	13/1298 patients (1.0)	65/1298 patients (5.0)	10/13 patients (76.9)	IFIS in 2 patients exposed to terazosin and 1 patient exposed to doxazosin
Takmaz & Can, 2007	Prospective, nonrandomized observational study	Evaluate complication rates, effect of intracameral adrenaline, and incidence of IFIS in patients taking tamsulosin	774 patients; 858 eyes	16/858 eyes (1.9)	24/858 eyes (2.8)	14/18 eyes (77.8)	IFIS in 1 of 4 eyes exposed to terazosin and 1 of 2 eyes exposed to alfuzosin
Oshika et al., 2007	Prospective, interventional case series	Compare incidence of IFIS with topical vs. systemic α_1AR antagonists	1968 patients; 2643 eyes	29/2643 eyes (1.1)	134/2643 eyes (5.1)	25/58 eyes (43.1)	No IFIS in bunazosin (topical a1AR antagonist which is not a1AAR-specific) group

Reference	Design	Objective	Population	Overall Prevalence or Incidence of IFIS (%)	Exposure to Systemic α_1AR Antagonist (%)	Prevalence or Incidence of IFIS in Tamsulosin-Treated Patients (%)	Comments
Amin et al. (2008)	Prospective observational study	Assess incidence of IFIS associated with tamsulosin	1267 patients; 1462 eyes	Not available	Not available	13/23 eyes (56.5)	
Keklikci et al. (2009)	Prospective, nonrandomized observational study	Assess incidence of IFIS associated with tamsulosin	579 patients; 594 eyes	15/579 eyes (2.6)	Not available	12/23 patients (52.2)	
Chen et al. (2010)	Retrospective cohort study	Determine incidence of IFIS in patients taking tamsulosin, effect of prophylactic measures	1163 eyes	Not available	Not available	24/81 eyes (29.6)	
Horvath & Vultur (2011)	Prospective, nonrandomized observational study	Report incidence, etiology and management of IFIS	438 patients; 439 eyes	37/439 eyes (8.4)[a]	15/439 eyes (3.4)	Not available	Incidence of IFIS in patients treated w/α_1AR = 86.7%

[a] Includes patients that experienced an IFI-like syndrome

Table 2. Incidence and prevalence of IFIS in selected studies

Following the original report suggesting a stronger link between tamsulosin and IFIS relative to other α_1AR antagonists, subsequent case reports of IFIS have been published in men taking alfuzosin, doxazosin, and terazosin (Dhingra et al., 2007; Herd, 2007; Settas & Fitt, 2006; Venkatesh et al., 2007).

Aside from IFIS, α_1AR antagonist therapy prior to cataract surgery has been shown to predispose patients to complications following cataract surgery (Bell et al., 2009). A nested case control study examined health care records of 96,128 Canadian men aged 66 years or older who had undergone cataract surgery over a 5 year period. Post-operative complications that were examined included retinal detachment, lost lens or lens fragment, or endophalmitis. Overall, 3.7% had a history of exposure to tamsulosin, and 7.7% had recently taken other alpha blockers. Cases—that is men with a history of complications—were matched to control patients. The authors identified complications in 280 patients (0.3%). These cases were randomly matched to control patients based on age, surgeon, and year of procedure. Complications were more common among current users of tamsulosin. This risk was not significantly increased with exposure to other α_1AR antagonists or to previous exposure to tamsulosin or other α_1AR antagonists. However, tamsulosin use within 14 days of cataract surgery increased the risk for complications.

Currently, risk of IFIS has only been associated with systemic use of α_1AR antagonists. In a study comparing the incidence of IFIS between topical and systemic administration, no cases were observed in patients taking bunazosin, a topical, non-selective, α_1AR antagonist which is not currently available in the United States (Oshika et al., 2007). In the tamsulosin comparator group, the incidence of IFIS was 1.1%. Notably, results may have differed had the topical agent used also been specific for the α_{1A}AR subtype.

In response to multiple reports of an increased risk of IFIS, the package labeling of tamsulosin and other α_1AR antagonists has been updated to reflect this potential risk. The labeling further acknowledges that benefits of stopping an α_1AR antagonist prior to cataract surgery remains unknown (Package insert Flomax, 2007).

The 5ARI finasteride and the extract of saw palmetto (*Serona repens*) a type of palm plant utilized largely as alternative medicine for treatment of BPH have been linked to IFIS (Issa & Dagres, 2007; Yeu & Grostern, 2007). The patients in the aforementioned cases were specifically stated to not have received α_1AR antagonists prior to cataract surgery; however, the possibility exists that the patients may have received an unrecognized α_1AR antagonist either currently or in the past. No mechanism for how these agents may cause IFIS has been postulated, and the effect of how 5ARIs interact with the iris has not been studied. While confounders common to patients taking either 5ARIs or α_1AR antagonists such as increased age or male gender cannot be ruled out, certainly the strongest evidence of a link between medication and IFIS is with α_1AR antagonists and not 5ARIs.

Aside from α_1AR antagonists, IFIS has been associated with other medications as well. Lending credence to the theory that α_1AR antagonism is heavily responsible for IFIS, the antipsychotics chlorpromazine and risperidone, both mild α_1AR antagonists, have been linked to IFIS in patients not previously haven received conventional α_1-AR antagonists (Ford et al., 2011; Unal et al., 2007). Labetalol, a dual α_1- and β-AR antagonist, has also been associated with IFIS (Calotti & Steen, 2007).

One case of acetylcholinesterase-inhibitor-associated IFIS with donepezil has been reported. The authors hypothesized that through enhancement of cholinergic activity on the pupil sphincter, the pharmacological effect of the preoperative dilating drops was overcome (Papadopoulos & Bachariou, 2007). The patient reportedly had never received an α_1AR antagonist. However, a complete medication list was not documented in the case, and receipt of other α_1AR antagonists cannot be ruled out.

6. Pre-operative evaluation

The relationship of α_1AR antagonists to IFIS has changed the preoperative process for cataract surgeons. The pre-operative evaluation is particularly difficult as there is currently no reliable way to predict which patients will demonstrate IFIS. Furthermore as IFIS can present unilaterally the absence in one eye does not preclude the other eye from demonstrating features of IFIS in a subsequent surgery (Issa et al., 2008). During the pre operative visit, there are a number of questions and observations which may highlight for the surgeon any patients at potential risk for IFIS.

Most importantly is to ask all patients about current or former use of α_1AR antagonists. Simply reviewing the current medication list is not sufficient. Many patients are unable to recall specific medication names or classes they are currently taking, much less a medication they took previously and since discontinued. Because of this, often times asking a patient or an accompanying family member if they have ever been treated for an enlarged prostate or

for difficulty emptying their bladder will help elicit a more accurate history. If a patient does have a history of α_1AR antagonists it is also important to counsel them on the associated increased risk of IFIS and subsequent risk of complications postoperatively.
The most reliable preoperative predictive feature of IFIS in a patient with a history of α_1AR antagonists is poor pupillary dilation (Oetting, 2009). This can and should be noted during the office pre-operative cataract surgery evaluation, and not just on the day of surgery. When the pupil does not dilate well, the surgeon should be wary of IFIS during surgery. Although poor dilation can also be a harbinger of other intra ocular conditions such as pseudoexfoliation and trauma, recognition will help the surgeon prepare for and adapt intra operative management strategies for all possible complications (Altan-Yaycioglu. et al., 2007).

7. Conclusion

Recognizing patients at risk for IFIS is paramount to management. Without adequate preparation and management IFIS and subsequent postoperative complications are possible. A detailed pre-operative evaluation including recognizing those at risk for IFIS will ensure the best outcome.

8. References

Altan-Yaycioglu, R. Yaycioglu, & O. Gul, U. et al. (2007). The effects of two systemic alpha-1 adrenergic blockers on pupil diameter: a prospective single blind study. *Arch Pharmacol,* (2007). Vol. 375, No.3 (May 2007), pp. 199-203.

Amin, K.; Fong, K. & Horgan, SE. (2008). Incidence of intra-operative floppy iris syndrome in a U.K. district general hospital and implications for future workload. Surgeon. Vol. 6, No. 4, (August 2008), pp. 207-209.

Anothaisintawee, T.; Attia, J. & Nickel, JC. et al. (2011). Management of chronic prostatitis/chronic pelvic pain syndrome: a systematic review and network meta-analysis. *JAMA*, Vol.305, No.1, (January 2011), pp. 78-86.

Bell, CM.; Hatch, WV. & Fischer, HD. et al. (2009). Association between tamsulosin and serious ophthalmic adverse events in older men following cataract surgery. *JAMA*, Vol.301, No.19, (May 2009), pp. 1991-1996.

Biaggioni, I., & Robertson, D. (2009). Adrenoceptor Agonists & Sympathomimetic Drug, In: *Basic & Clinical Pharmacology*, Katzung, BG., Masters, SB. & Trevor, AJ. The McGraw-Hill Companies, Inc., Retrieved from http://www.accesspharmacy.com.proxy.lib.uiowa.edu/content.aspx?aid=4520412

Blouin, MC.; Blouin, J. & Perreault, S. et al. (2007). Intraoperative floppy-iris syndrome associated with alpha1 adrenoreceptors: comparison of tamsulosin and alfuzosin. *J Cataract Refract Surg*, Vol.33, No.7, (July 2007),pp. 1227-1234.

Calotti, F. & Steen, D. (2007). Labetalol causing intraoperative floppy-iris syndrome. *J Cataract Refract Surg*, Vol.33,No.1, (January 2007), pp. 170-171.

Cantrell, MA.; Bream-Rouwenhorst, HR. & Steffensmeier, A. et al. (2008). Intraoperative floppy iris syndrome associated with α1-adrenergic receptor antagonists. *Ann Pharmacother*, Vol. 42, No. 4, (April 2008), pp. 558-563.

Cantrell, MA.; Bream-Rouwenhorst, HR. & Hemerson, P. et al. (2010). Silodosin for benign prostatic hyperplasia. *Ann Pharmacother*, Vol.44, No.2, (February 2010), pp. 302-310.

Chang, DF. & Campbell, JR. (2005). Intraoperative floppy iris syndrome associated with tamsulosin. *J Cataract Refract Surg,* Vol.31, No.4, (April 2005), pp. 664-673.

Chang, DF.; Osher, RH. & Wang, L. et al. (2007). Prospective multicenter evaluation of cataract surgery in patients taking tamsulosin (Flomax). *Ophthalmology.* Vol.114, No.5, (May 2007), pp. 957-964.

Chatziralli, IP. & Sergentanis, TN. (2010). Risk Factors for Intraoperative Floppy Iris Syndrome: A Meta-Analysis. *Ophthalmology,* (December 2010). [Epub ahead of print].

Chen, AA.; Kelly, JP. & Bhandari, A. et al. (2010). Pharmacologic prophylaxis and risk factors for intraoperative floppy-iris syndrome in phacoemulsification performed by resident physicians. J Cataract Refract Surg. Vol. 36, No. 6, (June 2010), pp. 898-905.

Congdon, N.; Vingerling, JR. & Klein, BE. et al. (2004). Prevalence of cataract and pseudophakia/aphakia among adults in the United States. *Arch Ophthalmol,* Vol.122, No.4, (April 2004), pp. 487-494.

Crawford, ED.; Wilson, SS. & McConnell, JD. et al. (2006). Baseline factors as predictors of clinical progression of benign prostatic hyperplasia in men treated with placebo. *J Urol,* Vol.175, No.4, (April 2006), pp. 1422-1426;discussion 1426-1427.

Dhingra, N.; Rajkumar, KN. & Kumar, V. (2007). Intraoperative floppy iris syndrome with doxazosin. *Eye,* Vol.21,No.5, (May 2007), pp. 678-679.

Dierks, MR.; Jordan, JK. & Sheehan, AH. (2007). Prazosin treatment of nightmares related to posttraumatic stress disorder. Ann Pharmacother, Vol.41, No.6, pp. 1917-1918.

Djavan, B.; Chapple, C. & Milani, S. et al. (2004). State of the art on the efficacy and tolerability of alpha1 adrenoceptor antagonists in patients with lower urinary tract symptoms suggestive of benign prostatic hyperplasia. *Urology,* Vol.64, No.6, (December 2004), pp. 1081-1088.

Flach AJ. (2009). Intraoperative floppy iris syndrome: pathophysiology, prevention, and treatment. Trans Am Ophthalmol Soc, Vol.107, (December 2009), pp. 234-239.

Ford, RL.; Sallam, A. & Towler, HM. (2011). Intraoperative floppy iris syndrome associated with risperidone intake. *Eur Ophthalmol,* Vol.21, No.22, (March-April 2011), pp. 210-211.

Herd, MK. Intraoperative floppy-iris syndrome with doxazosin (letter). (2007). *J Cataract Refract Surg,* Vol.33, No.4, (April 2007), p. 562.

Horvath, K. & Vultur, F. (2011). Correlation between urological alpha1-AR antagonist medication and changed intraoperative iris behavior. Int Ophthalmol. Vol. 31, No. 2, (April 2011), pp. 99-104.

Issa, SA. & Dagres, E. (2007). Intraoperative floppy-iris syndrome and finasteride intake. *J Cataract Refract Surg,* Vol.33, No.12, (December 2007), pp. 2142-2143.

Issa, S. Hadid, OH. & Baylis, O.et al. (2008). Alpha antagonists and intraoperative floppy iris syndrome: A spectrum. Clinical Ophthalmology, Vol.2, No.4, (December 2008). pp. 735-741.

Kaplan, SA.; Roehrborn, CG. & Rovner, ES. et al. (2006). Tolterodine and tamsulosin for treatment of men with lower urinary tract symptoms and overactive bladder: a randomized controlled trial. *JAMA,*Vol.296,No.19, (November 2006), pp. 2319-2328.

Keklikci, U.; Isen, K. & Unlu, K. et al. (2009). Incidence, clinical findings and management of intraoperative floppy iris syndrome associated with tamsulosin. Acta Ophthalmol. Vol. 87, No. 3, (May 2009), pp. 306-309.

Major cardiovascular events in hypertensive patients randomized to doxazosin vs chlorthalidone: the antihypertensive and lipid-lowering treatment to prevent heart attack trial (ALLHAT) ALLHAT collaborative research group. *JAMA*, (2000). Vol. 283, No.15, (April 2000), pp. 1967-1975.

Mc Vary, K. Roehrborn, C. & Avins, A. et al. (2010). American Urological Association. Clinical Guideline: Management of benign prostatic hyperplasia (BPH). http://www.auanet.org/content/guidelines-and-quality-care/clinical-guidelines.cfm. Accessed March 25, 2011.

Marks, LS. Gittelman MC. & Hill, LA. et al. (2009). Rapid efficacy of the highly selective alpha(1A) adrenoceptor antagonist silodosin in men with signs and symptoms of benign prostatic hyperplasia: pooled results of 2 phase 3studies. *J Urol.* Vol.181, No.6, (June 2009), pp. 2634-2640.

McNaughton-Collins, M. & Barry, MJ. (2005). Managing patients with lower urinary tract symptoms. *Am J Med,* Vol. 118, No.12, (December 2005), pp. 1331-1339.

Navanimitkul, N. & Lojanapiwat, B. (2010). Efficacy of tamsulosin 0.4 mg/day in relieving double-J stent-related symptoms: a randomized controlled study. *J Int Med Res,* Vol.38, No 4, (July-August 2010), pp. 1436-1441.

Oetting, TA. (2009) Advances in the Management of Intraoperative Floppy Iris Sydnrome (IFIS). *Refractive EyeCare.* http://www.refractiveeyecare.com/articles/advances-in-the-management-of-intraoperative-floppy-iris-syndrome-ifis-301.html. Accessed March 26, 2011.

Oshika, T.; Ohashi, Y. & Inamura M. et al. (2007). Incidence of intraoperative floppy iris syndrome in patients on either systemic or topical alpha(1)-adrenoceptor antagonist. *Am J Ophthalmol.* Vol.143, No.1, (January 2007), pp. 150-151.

Package insert. Flomax (tamsulosin hydrochloride). Ridgefield, CT: Boehringer Ingelheim, February 2007.

Palea, S.; Chang, DF. & Rekik, M. et al. (2008). Comparative effect of alfuzosin and tamsulosin on the contractile response of isolated rabbit prostatic and iris dilator smooth muscles: possible model for intraoperative floppy-iris syndrome. *J Cataract Refract Surg,* Vol.34, No.3, (March 2008), pp. 489-496.

Panagis, L.; Basile, M. & Friedman, AH. et al. (2010). Intraoperative floppy iris syndrome: report of a case and histopathologic analysis. *Arch Ophthalmol,* Vol.128, No.11 (November 2010), pp. 1437-1441.

Papadopoulos, R. & Bachariou, A. (2007). Intraoperative floppy-iris syndrome associated with chronic intake of donepezil. *J Cataract Refract Surg,* Vol.33, No.11, (November 2007), pp. 1997-1998.

Product information. Rapaflo (silodosin). Corona, CA: Watson Pharmaceuticals, Inc., October 2008.

Raskind, MA.; Peskind, PR. & Kanter, ED. et al. (2003). Reduction of nightmares and other PTSD symptoms in combat veterans by prazosin: a placebo-controlled study. *Am J Psychiatry,* Vol.160, No.2, (February 2003), pp. 371-373.

Roehrborn, CG.; for the ALFUS STUDY GROUP. (2001). Efficacy and safety of once-daily alfuzosin in the treatment of lower urinary tract symptoms and clinical benign prostatic hyperplasia: a randomized, placebo-controlled trial. *Urology*, Vol.58, No. 6, (December 2001), pp. 953-959.

Schwinn, DA. & Afshari, NA. (2006). alpha(1)-Adrenergic receptor antagonists and the iris: new mechanistic insights into floppy iris syndrome. *Surv Ophthalmol*, Vol.51, No.5, (September-October 2006), pp. 501-512.

Settas, G. & Fitt, AW. (2006). Intraoperative floppy iris syndrome in a patient taking alfuzosin for benign prostatic hypertrophy. *Eye*, Vol.20, No.12, (December 2006), pp. 1431-1432.

Shapiro, E.; Hartanto, V. & Lepor, H. (1992). Quantifying the smooth muscle content of the prostate using double immuno-enzymatic staining and color assisted image analysis. *J Urol*, Vol.147, No.4, (April 1992), pp. 1167-1170.

Singh, A.; Alter, HJ. & Littlepage, A. (2007). A systematic review of medical therapy to facilitate passage of ureteral calculi. Ann Emerg Med, Vol. 50, No. 5, (November 2007), pp. 552-563.

Srinivasan, S.; Radomski, S. & Chung, J. et al. (2007). Intraoperative floppy-iris syndrome during cataract surgery in men using alpha-blockers for benign prostatic hypertrophy. *J Cataract Refract Surg*, Vol.33, No.10, (October 2007), pp. 1826-1827.

Suzuki, F.; Taniguchi, T. & Nakamura, S. et al. (2002). Distribution of alpha-1 adrenoceptor subtypes in RNA and protein in rabbit eyes. *Br J Pharmacol*, Vol.135, No.3, (February 2002), pp. 600–608.

Takmaz, T. & Can, I. (2007). Clinical features, complications, and incidence of intraoperative floppy iris syndrome in patients taking tamsulosin. *Eur J Ophthalmol*, Vol. 17, No.6, (November-December 2007), pp. 909-913.

Thiyagarajan, M. (2002). α-Adrenoceptor antagonists in the treatment of benign prostate hyperplasia. *Pharmacology*, Vol.65, No.3, (July 2002), pp. 119-128.

Unal, M.; Yucel, I. & Tenlik, A. (2007). Intraoperative floppy-iris syndrome associated with chronic use of chlorpromazine. *Eye*, Vol.21, No.9, (September 2007), pp. 1241-1242.

Venkatesh R.; Veena, K. & Gupta, S. et al. (2007). Intraoperative floppy iris syndrome associated with terazosin. *Indian J Ophthalmol*, Vol.55 No.5, (September-October 2007), pp. 395-396.

Yeu, E. & Grostern, R. (2007). Saw palmetto and intraoperative floppy-iris syndrome. *J Cataract Refract Surg*, Vol.33,No.5, (May 2007), pp. 927-928.

Yu, Y. & Koss, MC. (2003). Studies of alpha adrenoceptor antagonists on sympathetic mydriasis in rabbits. *J Ocul Pharmacol Ther*, Vol.19, No.3, (June 2003), pp. 255–263.

3

Prevention and Management of Intraoperative Floppy Iris Syndrome

James A. Davison
Wolfe Eye Clinic, Iowa,
USA

1. Introduction

Other than using it to attach the IOL optic in McCannel suture procedures, the iris, in any amount, only causes problems for the cataract surgeon. In its extreme, there are no iris related complications in aniridia patients, other than not having an iris. Even in normal cases, there are always some disturbances of iris tissue as evidenced by postoperative inflammation, pigment dispersion, and sometimes iris transillumination.

One of the keys then to successful cataract surgery is to reduce the effect that the iris has on the intra and postoperative course of events. So during cataract surgery, the iris needs to be minimized and isolated. We dilate the pupil as much as we can which gives us better visualization and less iris to influence either directly by touching or indirectly through hydraulic means. The key is to make the iris as inconsequential as it can be by reducing its area pharmacologically or physically. If the iris area presentation is large to start with, there will be more of it to be caught in the flow of BSS and it may become floppy in the fluidic turbulence. If it is dilated and contracted, there will be less presentation of tissue to BSS flow and less muscle reaction to the buffeting of turbulence.

2. Planning

The axiom "the pupil never gets larger during surgery" needs to be a critical part of the surgery planning process. Whatever the pupil diameter is at the start of a case, it will only stay the same or get smaller as the case goes on. We have a good estimate of surgical pupil size when we see patients in the office so we can plan ahead. Sometimes the pupil gets larger before surgery vs. the clinic because of the stronger drops used in surgery rather than in the examination lane. My general rule is that I want at least a 4.5 - 5.0 mm. pupil at the outset of surgery so that I can get an additional 0.5 mm. dilation with viscoelastic anterior chamber pressurization and I can create the tremendously important capsulorhexis in a diameter of approximately 5.0 - 5.5 mm. in ideal circumstances but at least 4.5 mm. at a minimum. But clinical circumstances may appear to require an even larger pupil because of lens and/or zonule character. So a 4.5 mm. pupil in a normal eye with an average character cataract of LOCS III NO 3.7 NC 3.7, (Chylack 1993) will likely be maintained because surgery should be routine, brief, and uneventful. But that same pupil size may not be maintainable during a longer more difficult case such as if the cataract is very soft, very hard, or if it is accompanied by an inherently loose zonule as in pseudoexfoliation, or if the iris is unusually flaccid. A pupil of 6.0 mm. is desirable at the outset of these types of difficult cases.

If the pupil is smaller than 4.5 mm. and I can't create a capsulorhexis of that diameter, I employ a mechanical device to physically enlarge it prior to performing capsulorhexis. That rule has yielded an overall rate of mechanical pupil enlargement for me of 10 % but an iris related complication rate (significant iris aspiration or prolapse or an associated posterior capsule rupture) of zero (unpublished data, JAD 2008-2011). This utilization may seem high, but the risks of problems and the significance of the problems created by a small pupil are more important to the outcome of these cases than the time and expense it takes to temporarily physically enlarge the pupil and accomplish them in normal fashion

3. Pharmacologic pupil dilation

A topical non-steroidal preparation is used 3 days prior to surgery in the hopes of reducing inflammation and maybe assisting in dilating the pupil. There are numerous ways to accomplish the instillation but, Cyclogyl 1% and NeoSynephrine 2.5% are longtime key ingredients for dilating the eye starting about 45 minutes prior to surgery. Lidocaine 1% preservative free is injected into the anterior chamber just after the normal clear corneal primary and paracentesis incisions are created. This substance also assists with initiating and maintaining pupil dilation. Epinephrine 1:10,000 (1 ml.) is used in 500 cc in the continuous irrigation of BSS

Epi-Shugarcaine (Shugar 2006), a mixture of preservative free lidocaine and epinephrine has been shown by Joel Shugar, MD to be an effective supplementary agent in maintaining pupil dilation just before phacoemulsification and again before cortex aspiration as well. Intraoperative unpreserved epinephrine preceded by topical atropine has also been demonstrated to achieve and maintain larger pupil sizes and help reduce the incidence of IFIS (Masket 2007).

4. Mechanical pupil dilation

Viscoelastic anterior chamber pressurization prior to performing capsulorhexis will generally yield 0.5 mm. diameter additional pupil dilation. I use a DuoVisc (Alcon Surgical) strategy injecting enough Viscoat (Alcon Surgical) to fill approximately 40 % of the anterior chamber and following with ProVisc (Alcon Surgical) underneath to the point that some is just refluxing out the incision as it's being injected. If I can achieve a 4.5 mm pupil, I'll generally proceed with capsulorhexis but if I can't I will mechanically dilate the pupil with one of two devices.

I employ the Graether Pupil Expander (EagleVision) which was invented by John Graether, MD in 1991 (Graether 1996) and use it part of the time i.e. in normal eyes with small pupils. Its advantages are the average time it takes to accomplish the insertion, about 30 - 60 seconds, removal in about 10 seconds, and the fact that no additional incisions are needed.

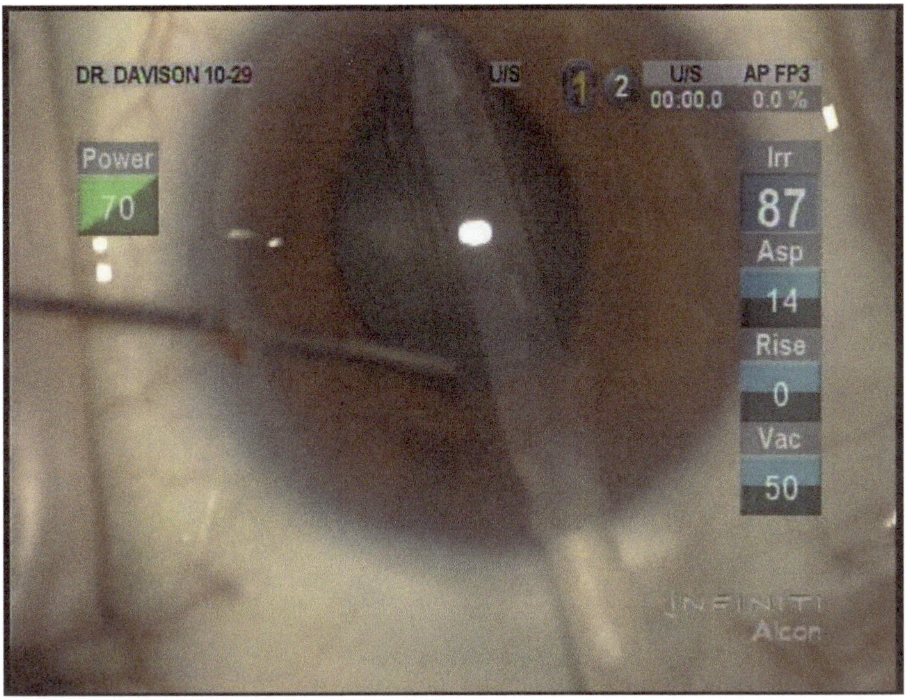

Fig. 1. The expander is draped over its insertion rod and has engaged the distal pupillary iris

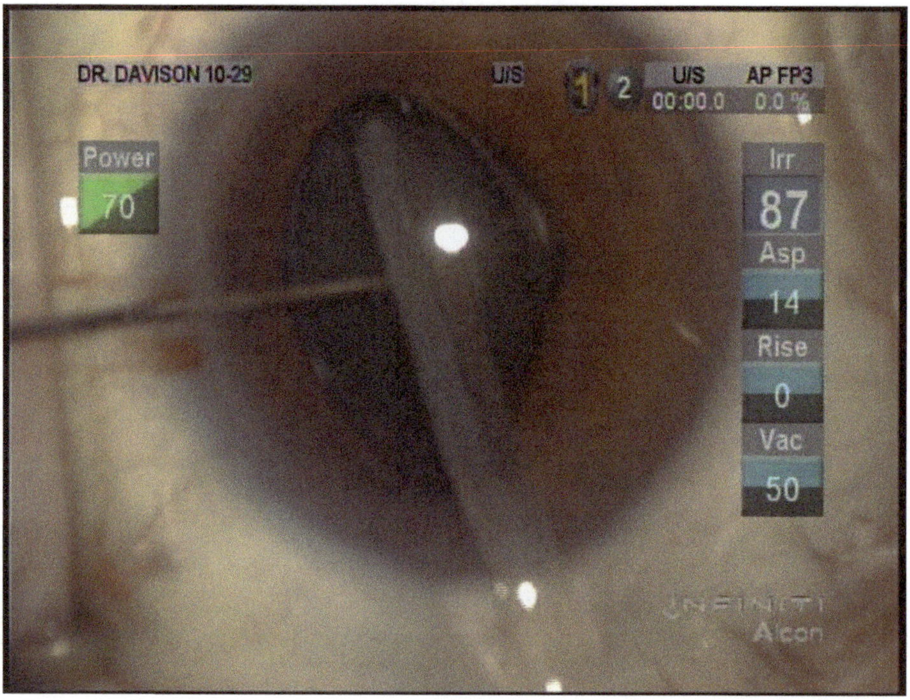

Fig. 2. As the insertion rod is withdrawn, the expander is engaged distally and on the left side but has missed engaging the pupil on the right side.

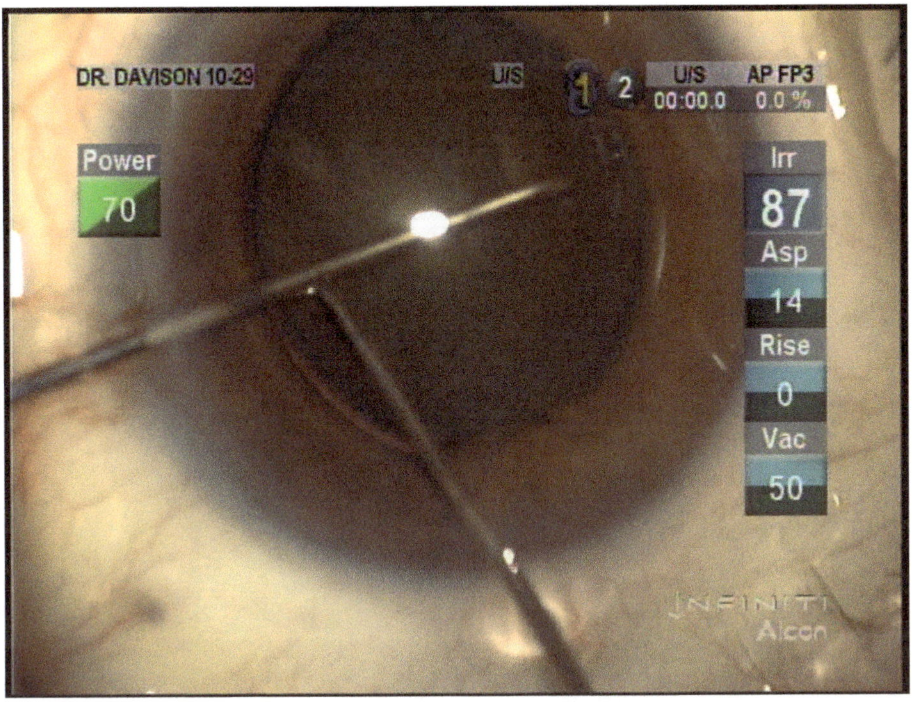

Fig. 3. The Lester hook and side port manipulator have just completed a kind of cross handed stretching maneuver and are about to be withdrawn. The expander is fully engaged and the pupil size will be maintained throughout the entire case. The Lester hook will engage the small proximal strap and easily withdraw the expander at the conclusion of the case

Interestingly, it is easier to insert in smaller pupils rather than medium sized ones because the pupillary iris tissue more tightly grabs the attachment points if the pupil is smaller rather than if it is larger where it tends to fall off. But, I worry that, at least in my hands, the downward pressure required to place the device may have a tendency to create some zonular fiber disruption in some cases. This has never been clinically significant to me but I still tend not to use it in patients with pseudoexfoliation or trauma cases which have an already loose zonule propensity.

In those patients with pseudoexfoliation and a potentially weak zonule, medium size pupils or eyes with very compact anterior segment anatomy, I generally employ Grieshaber iris retractors (Alcon Surgical). Their disadvantage is that they require 4 additional incisions and take about 2 minutes to place and maybe 30 seconds to remove. I orient them in a square pattern by creating incisions with a 22,5 degree blade. I create all four of the incisions first, and then create the paracentesis incision for my left hand and 2.4 mm keratome primary incision before introducing intracameral lidocaine or viscoelastic.

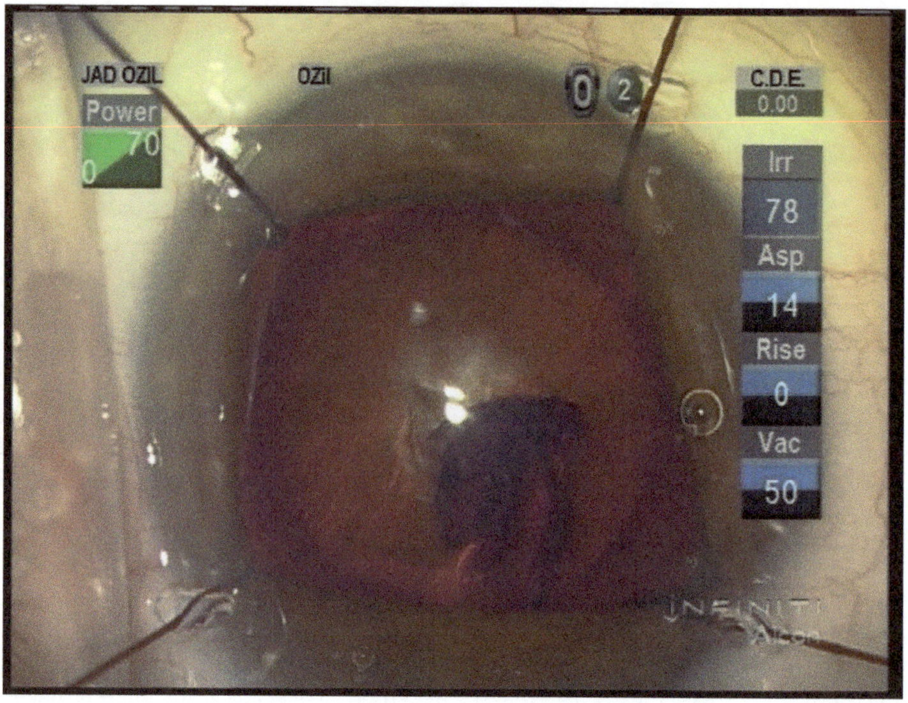

Fig. 4. The capsulorhexis has just been completed using Trypan blue dye. The retractors have been placed in each quadrant and fairly fully retracted to expose the anterior capsule for CCC creation and hydrodissection.

Prior to introducing the phacoemulsification tip, I loosen the proximal retractors so that the iris falls posterior and will not be rubbed by the phaco tip and sleeve during emulsification of the lens.

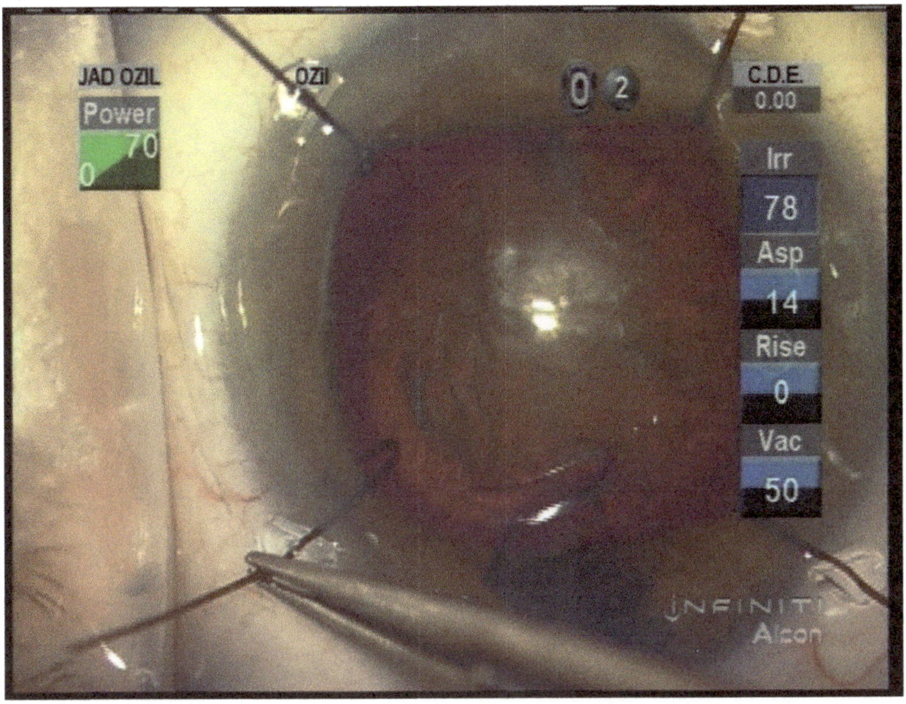

Fig. 5. The retractor on the lower left is being pushed into the anterior chamber with a tying forceps for a length of about 1.0 mm. The iris will hug the retractor in its new position within a second just as it already has the retractor on the lower right. Just that much less retraction under the phacoemulsification tip allows the iris to fall away from it and not suffer damage from its vibration.

5. Physically dampening hydraulic shock and minimizing turbulence

During the sculpting phase of contemporary in situ fracture phacoemulsification there is a balanced and continuous inflow and outflow of BSS. This equilibrium exists because of the advantages of modern cataract surgery equipment and technique. Only a small volume controlled leakage of BSS is observed to leak around the infusion sleeve. A similar amount of leakage occurs during the quadrant removal phase of the surgery as well. Unnecessary surgeon generated motions are eliminated as are extremes and consequent substantial changes in vacuum and occlusion levels.

Most machines can create this scenario to varying degrees. I use the Alcon Infiniti (Alcon Surgical) micro-coaxial system. In this system, all of the components are matched to each other in order to minimize imprecision and maximize efficiency, reproducibility, and safety. The 2.4 mm. keratome is capable of creating a perfect 2.4 mm. width with a 1.8 mm. length shelf incision before the introduction of viscoelastic. This can be accomplished while the 22.5 degree angle paracentesis blade stabilizes the globe.

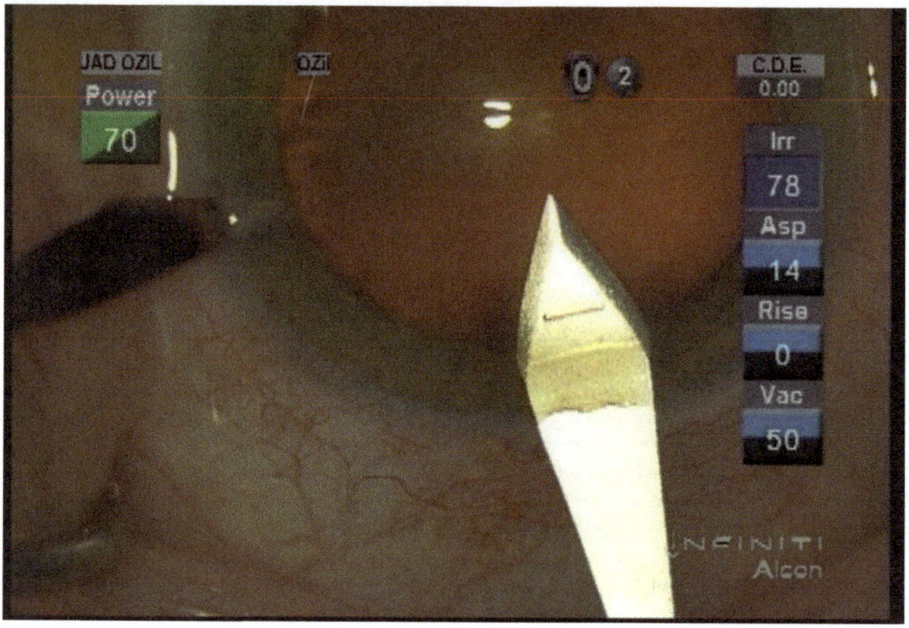

Fig. 6. The 22.5 degree angle paracentesis blade stabilizes the globe by pulled slightly upward and toward the surgeon while the 2.4 mm keratome is used to create the primary incision.)

The Ultra infusion sleeve is specifically designed to use within that incision surrounding the 0.9 mm. outside diameter shaft phacoemulsification tip (12 degree shaft bend mini-flare, 45 degree aperture angle, ABS featured).

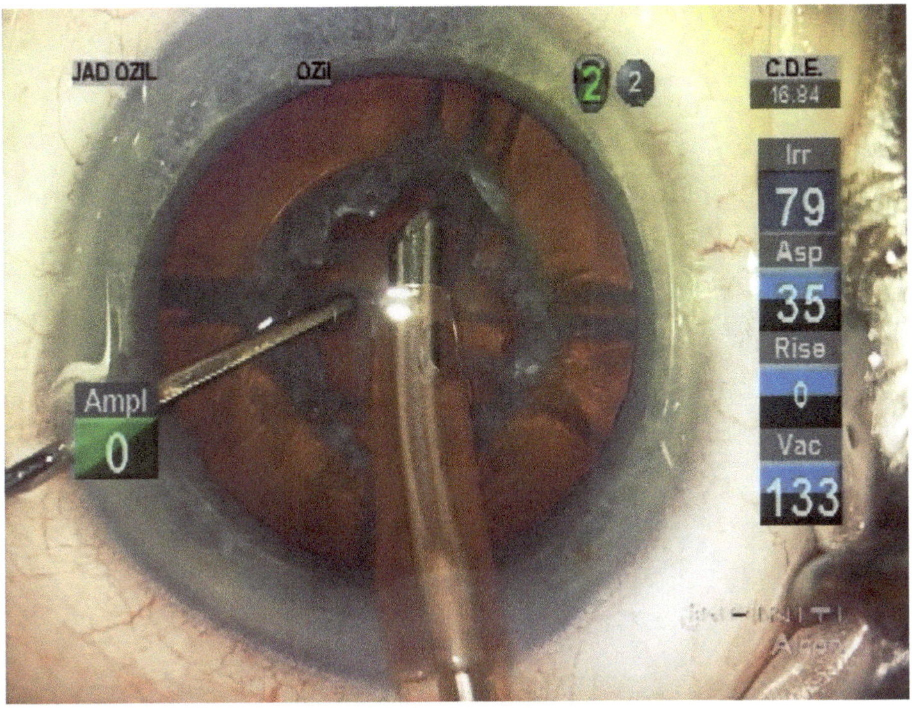

Fig. 7. The 0.9 mm. outside diameter 12 degree shaft bend tip is surrounded by the Ultra infusion sleeve through a 2.4 mm. clear corneal incision in the micro-coaxial system.

For sculpting, I use relatively low settings featuring a bottle height of 78 cms, surgeon control of continuous longitudinal phacoemulsification maximum 90%, vacuum of 50 mmHg., and AFR of 14 cc./min. I use enough power as necessary to efficiently sculpt to a level without displacing the lens that will create circumstances that yield four equal nuclear fragments after cracking. If the lens is hard, I'll use the tip on its side in sculpt mode to reduce the size of the quadrants by buzzing off their internal corners thus rendering them a relatively two-dimensional plate.

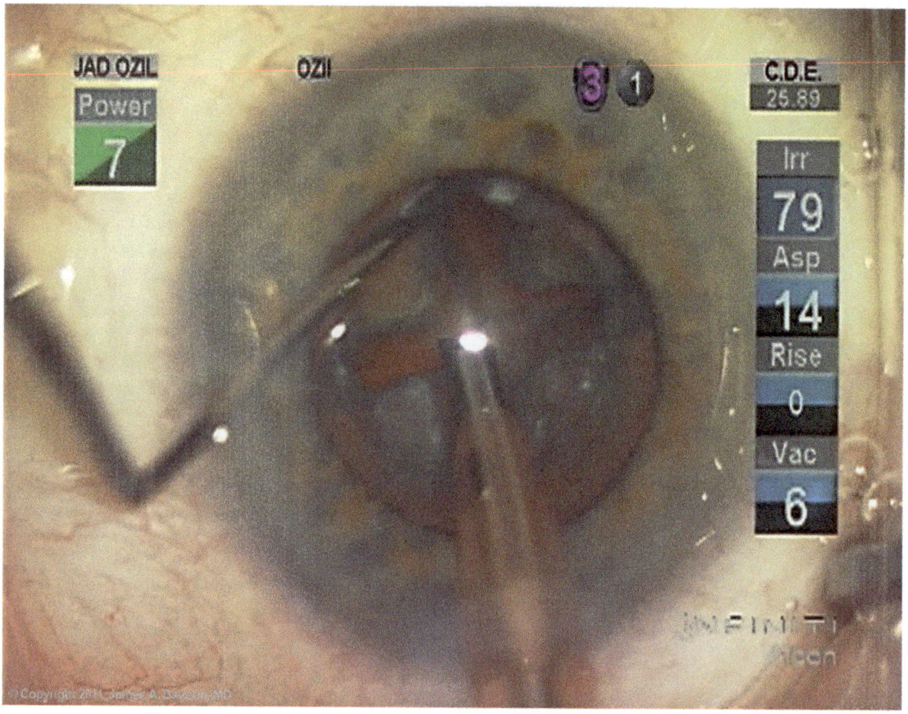

Fig. 8. Moderate width grooves have been sculpted through the nucleus creating 4 quadrants to be removed.

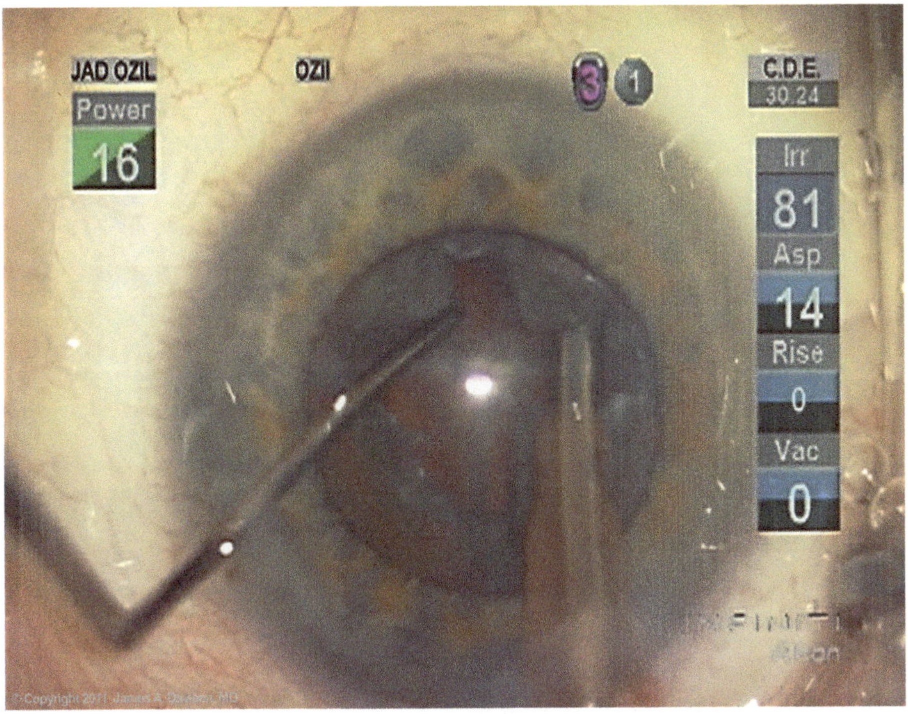

Fig. 9. The lower left quadrant has been de-bulked and the upper right one is about to be shaved in similar fashion.

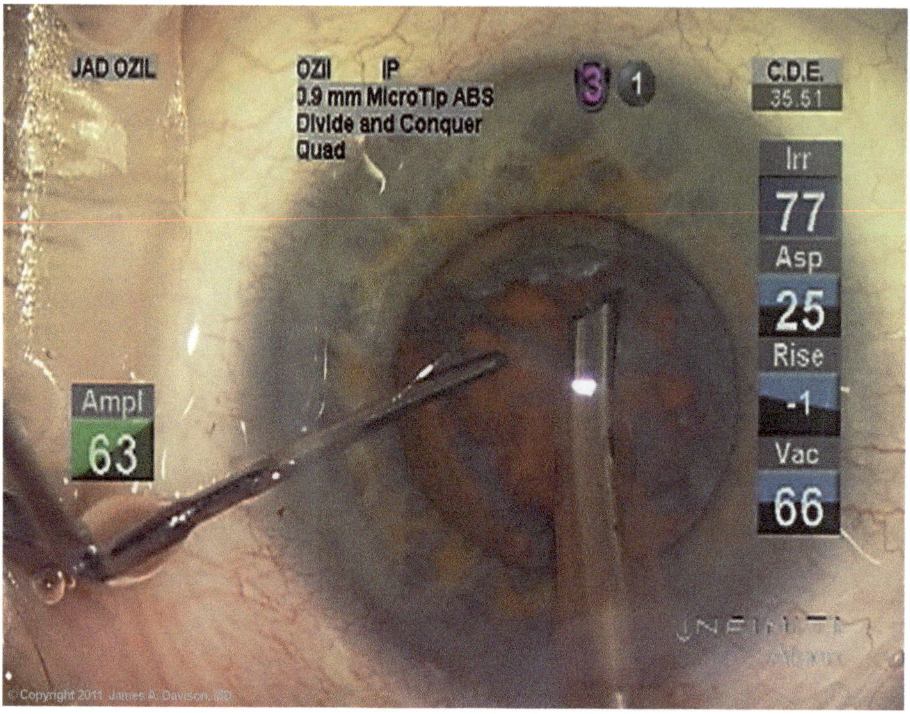

Fig. 10. All four quadrants have been debulked of the most firm central nuclear material leaving the more soft shell to be centralized and aspirated during quadrant removal.

In normal cases with normal size pupils, the quadrant removal settings are increased to a still fairly modest bottle height of 85 cms., vacuum of 400 mm. Hg and AFR 35 cc. /min. maintaining a rise time of -1 but changing to a torsional motion with vacuum triggered interjected longitudinal ultrasonic tip motion (I.P., Alcon Surgical) (Vacuum Trigger = 90% of 400 mm. Hg, On Time = 7 msec, Longitudinal/Torsional ratio = 1.0). Continuous longitudinal ultrasound may be needed in extremely hard lenses in which I also use a rise time of -1 on the Infiniti to slow the rate of vacuum accumulation. In cases with borderline pupils, I reduce the aspiration flow rate to 25 cc/min in either IP or longitudinal to reduce flow, turbulence, iris fluttering, and miosis. This is extremely effective in maintaining pupil size.

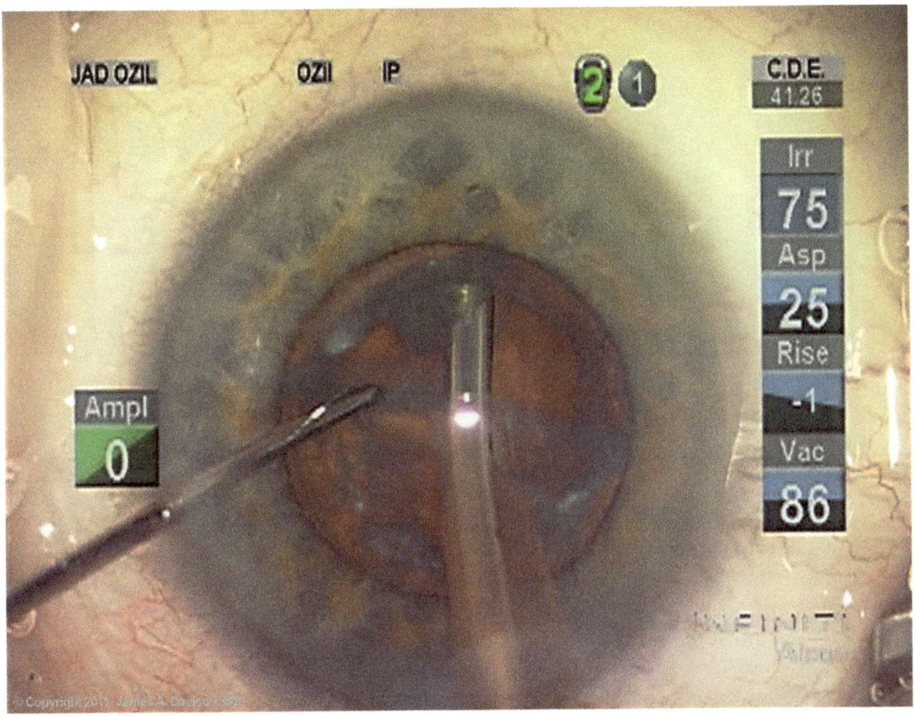

Fig. 11. The second quadrant is about to be engaged by the tip aperture which has been turned on its side for safer and easier access.

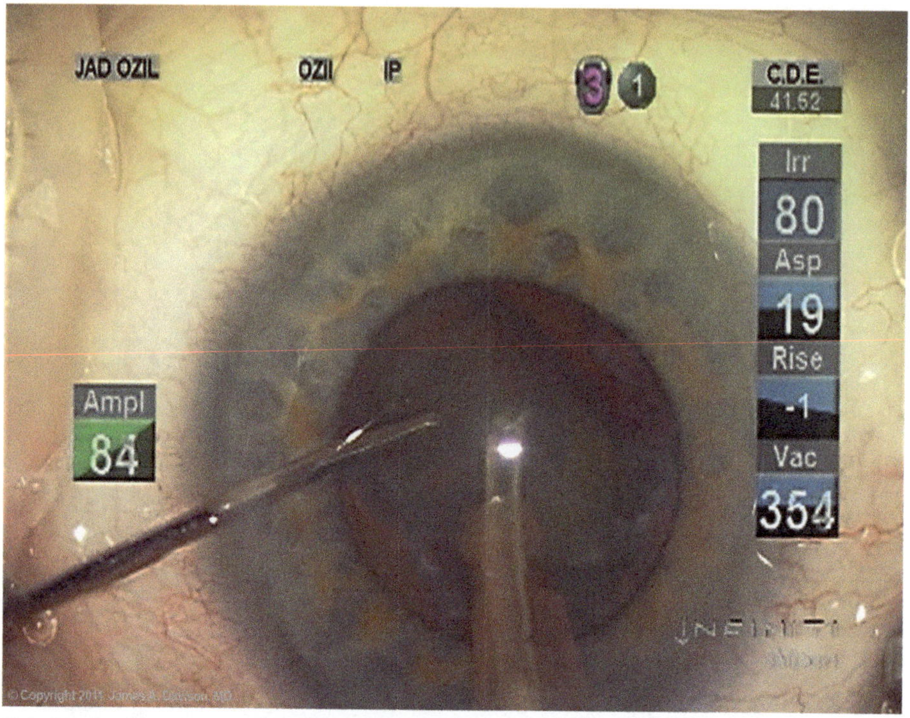

Fig. 12. The second quadrant has been centralized and the tip is oriented obliquely for best visualization and separation from the posterior capsule during its aspiration.

This reduction in flow creates a very quiet and stable anterior chamber and virtually eliminates any iris fluttering and consequent pupil size reduction. I'll usually shave the corners away during sculpting in these cases too, even if the nucleus is average firmness or soft so that the volume of material that is removed during this phase of surgery will be less. An additional measure which can be helpful is the injection of some additional Viscoat into the anterior chamber, especially preceding removal of the last quadrant. This protects the cornea, posterior capsule, and creates some additional dampening of hydraulic shock to the iris. To prevent thermal effects of the moving phacoemulsification tip at the incision, it's important to re-establish outflow by applying vacuum in foot position 2 prior to engaging phacoemulsification energy in foot position 3.

Modern machines like the Infiniti have minimized post-occlusion surge but there are still some shock waves transmitted to the iris by the quick oscillations of IOP secondary to the varying degrees of occlusion and pressure changes associated with aspiration of nuclear fragments in the quadrant removal mode. These pulsations are reduced by reducing the AFR to 25 while efficient removal of firm fragments is still possible using proportionally greater ultrasonic and vacuum contributions. It is most efficient to create a dynamic and continuous balance of ultrasonic energy, vacuum, and outflow during this phase of phacoemulsification. That way the extremes in pressure and flow are minimized and their secondary effects on the iris are minimized as well. In extremely hard nuclei, it may be sometimes necessary to use longitudinal phacoemulsification during the occlusion mode of quadrant removal to create this smooth balance.

6. Prevention

Preventing a floppy iris is much easier than managing it. By definition, an iris with or without a baseline flaccid tone only becomes floppy because of the turbulence it experiences once surgery has begun and BSS is flowing around it. Prevention is the key:

1. Use maximal pharmacologic dilation.
2. Create perfect incisions.
3. If the pupil size is small and there is too much iris surface area to start with, the pupil should be mechanically dilated i.e. the iris area should be made smaller. In normal circumstances, a 4.5 mm. pupil and capsulorhexis diameter will be the minimum considered. Because of the affects of capsule contraction syndrome, it is particularly important to create at least a 5.0 mm. diameter capsulorhexis in patients with pseudoexfoliation (Davison 1993).
4. Reduce nucleus bulk during sculpting with low vacuum and AFR
5. Use a longer rise time to reach maximum vacuum (-1 for me on the Infiniti).
6. A huge reduction in turbulence can be accomplished by using a low bottle height and aspiration flow rate during quadrant removal. Reducing the AFR to 25 cc/min. and maintaining a BSS bottle height of 78 cm. creates a quiet chamber, minimal turbulence, and virtually no iris fluttering and pupil diameter reduction.
7. If the iris does becomes floppy but the pupil size is still reasonable to continue phacoemulsification (depending on where in the process one is), additional Viscoat may tamponade turbulence effects on the iris, keep the pupil from becoming even smaller, and allow the case to be finished safely.
8. Whether the iris is floppy or not, if the pupil comes down to a level that makes the surgeon uncomfortable with the adequacy of visualization and the ability to execute surgical maneuvers, things can get difficult. That is, it's not so much about discovering if the iris will become floppy; it's more about the initial size of the pupil and attempting to maintain it by exercising smooth surgical technique through controlled hydrodynamics. If visualization becomes compromised because of pupil reduction or if iris is aspirated, iris retractors can still be placed at any stage during phacoemulsification, or even during the cortex aspiration stage if necessary. It's always better to stop and take a few moments to improve the situation and finish in an orderly fashion rather than to continue on an unnecessarily higher risk course.

7. Opinions on floppy iris syndrome

David Chang M.D. and John R. Campbell M. D. made an important discovery of an association of intraoperative complications caused by irises which appeared to be floppy during phacoemulsification in patients who were shown to be taking Tamsulosin (Flomax). (Chang 2005) Ever since then ophthalmic surgeons have been concerned about "Flomax patients" and iris related complications during cataract surgery. Even in television commercials for the product, patients are advised to reveal to their eye surgeons if they are on the medication.

The author feels that the relationships between Flomax and floppy iris complications are in fact a statistical one. Almost all of the floppy iris cases of in their series were on Flomax but only about 60% of the patients who were on Flomax developed intraoperative floppy iris syndrome IFIS (Chang 2005). Mechanical stretching of the iris to make the pupil larger seemed to make the iris even more exposed to increased floppiness.

Even if patients are not on alpha 1 adrenergic antagonist, often patients with medium size pupils seem to have irises which suddenly flutter within the turbulence of BSS flow within the anterior chamber and behind the iris during phacoemulsification. Many times in these cases, the very first fluttering seems to initiate an almost immediate pupil constriction thus beginning the cascade to smaller and smaller pupil size because of increasing iris area and consequent increased capture of fluidic turbulence and more iris fluttering, just like a sailboat's larger jib catches more wind.

8. References

Chang DF, Campbell JR. Intraoperative floppy iris syndrome associated with tamsulosin. J Cataract Refract Surg. 2005; 31:664-673.

Chylack LT. The lens opacities classification system III. Arch Ophthalmol. June 1993; 111: 831-836.

Davison JA. Capsule Contraction Syndrome. J Cataract Refract Surg 1993; 19: 582-589.

Graether JM. Graether pupil expander for managing the small pupil during surgery. J Cataract Refract Surg 1996; 22:530-535.

Masket S, Belani S. Combined preoperative topical atropine sulfate 1% and intracameral nonpreserved epinephrine hydrochloride 1:2500 for management of intraoperative floppy-iris syndrome. J Cataract Refract Surg 2007; 33:580-582.

Shugar JK. Use of epinephrine for IFIS prophylaxis. J Cataract Refract Surg. July 2006; 32: 1074-1075.

4

Anaesthetic Management in Cataract Surgery

Alparslan Apan
Department of Anaesthesiology and Reanimation,
Kırıkkale University Faculty of Medicine,
Turkey

1. Introduction

Cataract surgery is one of the most commonly performed surgical procedures in our ageing world. The majority of patients have concurrent disorders including hypertension, diabetes mellitus and coronary artery disease. The anaesthetic management varies between topical anaesthetic applications, regional blocks to general anaesthesia. The patients' medical/mental condition and current medications are of prime importance in terms of their implications for anaesthesia. It is also prudent to define and prevent drug interactions of ocular medication that are required during the perioperative or postoperative period. The type of intervention and skill of the surgeon are variables that influence the selection of the anaesthetic regimen. Preoperative evaluation is therefore as important as anaesthetic care for this surgical population.

Cataract surgery performed in the setting of an office-based, day case surgical set-up is considered in this chapter. Unsutured incisions and less invasive techniques are increasingly popular. Extraocular muscle akinesia is important for an optimum operating field.

Topical anaesthesia includes local anaesthetic applied to the cornea as drops or ointment. Benoxinate, tetracaine, ametocaine, lignocaine, and bupivacaine are common ester and amide types of local anaesthetic used for this purpose. Lack of ocular akinesia and insufficient analgesia are considered as disadvantages of topical methods.

Retrobulbar block was one of the most frequently implemented techniques. It is performed via introduction of a needle at the infero-lateral rim of the lower eyelid passing through the muscle cone with advancement in a medial and superior direction at about 10° and injecting 4-8 mL of local anaesthetic / hyaluronidase mixture behind the globe. Maintaining a short advancement distance and use of blunt-tipped needles are advised for this practice. Besides the advantages, including obtaining ocular akinesia and sufficient analgesia, the procedure can for this reason still be considered and useful where other procedures are unsuitable, though this is rare. There is a risk of damage to surrounding structures including globe perforation, as well as penetration into the cerebrospinal fluid and vascular structures behind the eye, causing respiratory depression and cardiovascular collapse. While rare these are significant and limit its use in practice, especially in view of newer 'blunt needle' techniques.

Peribulbar block is performed as a retrobulbar block with straight advancement of a short needle from the infero-lateral border of the lower eyelid. This technique is infrequently utilized due to the disadvantages such as high rate of chemosis, lower quality of akinesia, increased local anaesthetic requirements and longer latent period requirement for akinesia.

Sub-Tenon's block (a type of 'blunt needle' block) is performed by introducing a cannula between the conjunctiva and Tenon's capsule after delicate but mainly blind dissection of the sub-Tenon's space. Advantages are reduction of complication rates especially in myopic eyes and it offers the option of re-injections to top up the anaesthetic during surgery. Local anaesthetic leakage, need for dissection and possible need for sutures are limitations.

Gentle pressure application on the globe for local anaesthetic spread after regional blocks are useful for avoiding the oculocardiac reflex. Local anaesthetic infiltration for facial nerve branches might be indicated for eyelid akinesia.Sedation and analgesia may be required during topical anaesthesia or regional blocks. In continuum and during surgery verbal contact between the anaesthetist and the surgeon is important for reducing complications at an early a stage as possible. Depending on the operation it might be preferable to use sedatives/hypnotics or opioid analgesics with a shorter half-life. In the case of repeated drug administrations, accumulating drugs should be avoided and/or a specific antidote should be given if necessary. It is not always possible to approximate additive effects of drug combinations in elderly patients and patients with co-morbidities, and using the lower doses might be important for preventing unforeseen complications though must be balanced with the need to prevent pain or awareness of surgery. Midazolam, propofol and dexmedetomidine, might be frequently used alone as a bolus or infusion, or in combination with fentanyl or remifentanil.

General anaesthesia might be preferred in patients with limited co-operation or advanced co-existing disorders. With a few exceptions, all general anaesthetics decrease intraocular pressure. Laryngeal mask insertion with a smooth induction using etomidate, propofol or thiopentone with or without a non-depolarizing muscle relaxant is frequently chosen. Propofol infusion with fentanyl or remifentanil might be delivered alone or with volatile anaesthetics. Besides the anti-emetic effects of propofol, the emetic and depressive effects of opioids should be remembered in the postoperative period. General anaesthesia may offer almost motionless optimal surgical conditions (though the Bell's reflex can persist at lower doses), allows bilateral surgery (rarely needed in intraocular surgery) and possesses virtually no major complication risk related to the injection. On the other hand it needs anaesthetic staff and equipment during administration and is increasingly expensive.

Analgesics and anti-inflammatory drugs might be combined with topical local anaesthetic during the postoperative period. It is important to ensure patients are free from side-effects or residual drug effects of medications to prevent further complications and re-hospitalisation.

Cataract surgery is one of the most common interventions made in day-case surgery (Cullen et al., 2009). Although lens opacification is generally a time-related process, it can be observed at an earlier period of life such as in newborns related to congenital metabolic errors and in all age groups due to trauma. The majority of the patients have concurrent disorders including hypertension, diabetes, rheumatoid arthritis, coronary artery or chronic pulmonary disease and take medication. Pre-operative evaluation, including anaesthetic and surgical planning should be performed as per the demands of co-morbidities. Cataract surgery is major surgery as it is intra-ocular surgery, technically challenging, with abundant scope for devastating complications like loss of sight, but it is from an anaesthetic perspective limited in terms of stress to the body overall. Advances in techniques including phacoemulsification and intraocular foldable silicone lens implantation through suture-less mini incisions decrease the surgical recovery period with lower complication rates and improved surgical outcomes.

2. Preoperative evaluation

The responsibility of the anaesthetist is to ensure that the patient is in an optimal condition before undergoing surgery. Pre-operative interview with anaesthetic and surgical staff may reduce anxiety and stress concerning the operation. Patients may also be informed about unexpected visual experiences during anaesthesia and surgery in order to prevent undesirable outcomes (Tan et al., 2006).

The pre-operative visit includes determinations concerning the patient's history, habits, current disease with medications, complete systemic physical evaluation, and occult disease if not diagnosed. Patients may be referred to other physicians when concurrent pathology is not stable. Potential airway problems with a difficult airway must be evaluated and an anaesthetic plan should also be explained with informed consent. Patients may be categorized according to the American Society of Anesthesiologists (ASA) Physical Classification System that is shown in Table 1 to document their status before surgery (Davenport et al., 2006). Mild asthma or well controlled hypertension are examples of ASA Class II patients that are unlikely to have an impact on anaesthesia and surgery. More advanced disease such as renal failure on dialysis or class II congestive heart failure indicates ASA class III patients and is likely to have an impact on anaesthesia and surgery. Patients are classified as ASA class IV if disease requires special medical care e.g., acute myocardial infarction, and respiratory failure that requires mechanical ventilation with major impact on anaesthesia and surgery. The physical condition of patient over ASA III generally requires hospitalization even when performing surgery with otherwise comparatively limited potential for major systemic stress like cataract surgery.

Class	Description
I	Healthy patient without organic, biochemical, or psychiatric disease.
II	A patient with mild systemic disease. No significant impact on daily activity.
III	Significant or severe systemic disease that limits normal activity. Significant impact on daily activity.
IV	Severe disease that is a constant threat to life or requires intensive therapy. Serious limitation of daily activity.
V	Moribund patient who is likely to die without surgery.
VI	Brain-dead organ donor.

Table 1. American Society of Anaesthesiologists physical status (ASA PS) classification

The history of the patient may include social habits, cigarette and alcohol consumption, illicit drug use, allergies, past medical history including operations with enquiries about possible adverse outcomes, current medications, and questioning relatives on whether there is a family history of attack from malignant hyperthermia - thus halogenated volatile anaesthetic agents, which may trigger malignant hyperthermia, may be avoided.

Systemic evaluation must include careful examination for a difficult airway, including jaw and neck movements, mouth opening, and intra-oral pathology. Special precautions or devices must be prepared to be used for patients who are likely to have an airway problem. Patients, especially with increased body mass index, must also be questioned about snoring during their sleep and evaluated for possible sleep apnoea syndrome. The physical capacity of patients can be determined with simple questions on for instance being able to do daily activities, climbing stairs, swimming or other sports.

Physicians may require symptom-oriented laboratory investigations instead of ordering a battery of tests (Schein et al., 2000). Laboratory results and an electrocardiogram (ECG) performed within 6 months is sufficient to determine the gravity of most cardiac conditions. The consensus is to obtain an ECG from all elderly patients to determine the baseline cardiac condition. Haemoglobin levels may also be necessary to exclude anaemia that can precipitate cardiac events. Levels under 7 g/dL require transfusion therapy.

Chronic medical conditions such as congestive heart failure or chronic obstructive pulmonary disease must be optimized before surgery. Patients with a recent attack of angina, arrhythmia, ischemia or infarction must be identified and elective cataract surgery may be postponed for month(s). A recent cerebrovascular attack or exacerbation of a chronic cerebral disorder e.g. multiple sclerosis is also a reason for postponing elective surgery. For patients with chronic renal failure it is necessary to determine the status of the ECG, plasma electrolytes, blood urea nitrogen (BUN) and creatinine levels. In the case of acute hepatitis or its exacerbation, surgery must be postponed until return to systemic baseline levels, requiring monitoring using a liver enzyme profile.

Hypertension must be controlled and blood pressure must be decreased to the acceptable levels, 140/90 mmHg if possible. Blood pressure of 200/110 mmHg or more before the operation requires postponement of elective surgery.

It is not usually necessary to discontinue current medication but herbal medicines should be withdrawn due to possible drug interference or due to the possibility of postoperative complications at least 1 week beforehand. Patients on anticoagulation therapy may also continue their medication as the risk of cessation of treatment outweighs the risk of bleeding (Hirschman & Morby, 2006) though clotting needs to be checked before surgery to ensure patients are not over-anticoagulated. Patients receiving aspirin, clopidogrel or warfarin may switch to low molecular weight or regular heparin should they be felt to be at risk of deep vein thrombosis during prolonged general anaesthesia.

Patient who are unable to lie flat due to their disorder, musculoskeletal disease such as kyphoscoliosis, paediatric patients, those with claustrophobia, altered cognitive function or orientation such as in Alzheimer's Disease, deafness, language problems that affect co-operation and abnormal movements or tremor such as in Parkinson's Disease are often unable to undergo surgery under local or regional anaesthesia.

Most physicians seem to allow eating or drinking ad libitum before cataract surgery under topical and regional blocks (Steeds & Mather, 2001). However many wisely prefer to limit this. Nausea and vomiting may occur with serious consequences such as aspiration into the airways. Therefore, the safe way is to perform the surgery on an empty stomach even with local or regional anaesthesia, and it may be necessary for some units to change their anaesthetic plan in view of this danger. Patient undergoing general anaesthesia must follow instructions about fasting regimens, which are simply allowing clear fluids up to two hours before induction, light meals up to four hours before, and regular meals up to six hours before induction. However, this may not guarantee an empty stomach in certain patients such as those with diabetes mellitus, oesophageal hernia and obstruction of the gastrointestinal passages. Metoclopramide 0.07 mg/kg intravenously (IV) can be administered in such patients at least 10 min before the operation to facilitate gastric passage. Placing and securing an intravenous line and intravenous premedication instead of painful intramuscular injections is preferred. Patients with dentures are allowed to wear them in order to decrease stress and not to interfere with communication during topical or regional block, but they may be removed in the case of general anaesthesia.

The anaesthetic options and possible complications must be explained in detail to the patient or to their relatives. Question sheets, consent forms and physical examination cards are a simple and efficient method for documentation. Physician must prescribe a short acting benzodiazepine such as lorazepam to the anxious patient, which may be recommended before and on the day of the surgery.

2.1 Monitored anaesthesia care

Monitored anaesthesia care (MAC) defines patients who require sedation and analgesia under the care of anaesthesia personnel with a monitor and oxygen supplementation in the operating theatre or in remote locations. Cataract surgery performed under local or regional anaesthesia is one of the classical examples of MAC that necessitates an anaesthetist who is familiar with the procedure. Equipment must be available in the case of airway emergencies and drugs should be prepared and ready for use in the case of hemodynamic consequences such as lignocaine, ephedrine, epinephrine, and atropine. The American Society of Anesthesiologists (ASA) determined the minimum requirements of monitoring during MAC that indicates the ECG, pulse oximetry, non-invasive blood pressure, temperature, end-tidal CO_2, and monitoring respiratory rate (Standards for Basic Anesthetic Monitoring). Oxygen must be administered with a face mask or nasal cannula at a rate of at least 6 L/min. One side of the sterile drapes may be raised in order to observe the patient, prevent CO_2 retention and claustrophobia, instead of a tight closure of the drapes. Continuous assessment of the level of sedation is mandatory in order to maintain contact with the patient and to prevent respiratory or hemodynamic side effects. The level can commonly be determined by using the Ramsay sedation score (Ramsay et al., 1974) categorized as:
Patient awake, anxious/restless, or both
Patient awake, cooperative, oriented and tranquil
Patient awake, responds to commands only
Patient asleep, brisk response to light glabellar tap or loud auditory stimulus
Patient asleep, sluggish response to light glabellar tap or loud auditory stimulus
Patient asleep, no response to light glabellar tap or loud auditory stimulus
The Observer's Assessment of Alertness/Sedation Scale (OAA/S) shown in Table 2 is used to determine the change of consciousness during the procedure, which may help to avoid deeper levels of sedation and their probable consequences (Chernik et al., 1990).

Subscore	Responsiveness	Speech
5	Responds readily to name in normal tone	Normal
4	Lethargic response to name spoken loudly repeatedly	Mild slowing or thickening
3	Responds only after name spoken loudly or repeatedly	Slurring or slowing
2	Responds after mild padding or shaking	Few recognized words
1	Does not respond to mild padding or shaking	

Table 2. Observer's Assessment of Alertness/Sedation Scale

Midazolam, a short acting and water soluble form of benzodiazepine is frequently used during premedication and for the maintenance of sedation. Mini bolus doses such as 0.5 mg in increments are frequently administered to maintain co-operation and to prevent adverse effects on respiration. Continuous infusion can also be used with success.

Propofol in lipid emulsion is a shorter acting hypnotic, sedative with anti-emetic properties. Bolus doses such as 20-30 mg are usually sufficient for the majority of patients. Propofol is unique for infusion with its context-sensitive half-life, longer metabolism and lack of residual effects. It can also be administered carefully and in certain surroundings by patients themselves in patient controlled sedation (PCS). However a danger is the level of sedation cannot be ascertained despite computerized systems in use even in healthy volunteers let alone patients (Murdoch et al., 2000).

Fentanyl, a semi-synthetic opioid derivative is frequently needed for premedication or during surgery in cases of insufficient analgesia, either on its own or in combination with sedatives or hypnotics. Co-administration with a sedative or hypnotic has additive depressive effects on respiration and hemodynamic variables, which requires dose adjustments. The half-life of fentanyl is longer and accumulation may ensue especially when repeated doses are administered, requiring attention before discharging the patient. The emetic potential and effects on other systems should also be kept in mind for special circumstances such as gallbladder stones or prostate hypertrophy. Doses of 25 to 50 μg repeated in the case of pain are usually sufficient for the majority of patients (Aydin et al., 2002).

Alfentanil and promazine in combination produce a superior quality of sedation, operating conditions and a milder side effect profile when compared with meperidine-promazine (el-Bassiouny et al., 1992). Remifentanil, a shorter acting opioid derivate, which undergoes metabolism by plasma esterase can be used solely or as a complementary drug. Lower doses of 0.25-0.5 μg/kg may be advised as needed (Rewari et al., 2002). Piritramide is another analgesic available in certain countries that has been found to be efficient against retrobulbar block-induced pain, hemodynamic changes and stress responses (Reinhardt et al., 2002).

A combination of fentanyl with a major tranquilizing drug droperidol, which is available commercially as Innovar, induces anaesthesia/analgesia without complications when concurrently used with topical anaesthesia and facial nerve block in a large number of patients (Hodgkins et al., 1992). Droperidol is also a potent anti-emetic. However this technique is no longer used due to the longer period of cognitive impairment and limitations in patients such as those with Parkinson's disease (Chung et al., 1989).

A low dose of ketamine (0.3 mg/kg) for sedation does not increase intraocular pressure and reduces pain from injection when combined with diazepam and droperidol (Cugini et al., 1997). Clonidine, an alpha-2 agonist, has sedative, anxiolytic, and analgesic properties through spinal and cortical pathways. It has been used during premedication and has been demonstrated to decrease preoperative anxiety, intraocular pressure, and neuroendocrine responses, but the potential of reducing heart rate and blood pressure limits its widespread use (Weindler et al., 2000). Dexmedetomidine, another alpha-2 agonist, is an optic isomer of medetomidine with a shorter elimination half-life and requires infusion during maintenance. It is also used with success (Apan et al., 2009).

Elderly patients require careful titration of lower doses of sedatives, hypnotics and opioids because these drugs can frequently produce over-sedation, apnoea, hypoxia, hypotension and bradycardia. The sedation level that allows communication with the patient is usually appropriate. Benzodiazepines, opioids and alpha-2 agonists have special antagonists that may increase their safety profile. These drugs may be required in the case of slower metabolism or unexpected delay in recovery.

A large proportion of patient requires sedative and analgesics during the regional block. Frequently it is not possible to identify the apprehensive patient till after they have entered the operating area. Hypnotics or sedatives alone usually augment excitement with disappearing cortical suppression and combination with an opioid is usually necessary to manage such patients with extremes of fear during surgery. This is frequently encountered in patients with coronary artery disease. The sedation requirement in cataract surgery is demonstrated to be lower and similar between patients receiving either topical anaesthesia or retrobulbar block when using patient-controlled sedation devices (Balkan et al., 2004). On the other hand, sedative and analgesic supplementation may be associated with adverse outcomes and the clinician should weigh the risks and benefits for individual patients (Katz et al., 2001).

2.2 Local anaesthetics and adjuvants

Local anaesthetic drugs act by producing reversible conduction block in exposed nerves by acting on sodium channels. A benzene ring is connected to another molecular group comprising a carbon chain with an ester or amide which thereby creates the two diverse groups of local anaesthetic agents. These different molecular structures also give rise to the main diversity in the metabolism of local anaesthetic agents. The amide group of local anaesthetics undergo metabolism in the liver, but the ester group of local anaesthetics are degraded by plasma esterase. Ester local anaesthetics have increased allergic potential due to para-aminobenzoic acid-like constituents in their molecules and their half-life is commonly brief when compared with the amide group. Interest has focussed on optical and stereo-isomers with reduced severity of side effects. Local anaesthetics can be used alone or combined with another local anaesthetic in order to produce a faster onset of action and longer duration of anaesthesia in ophthalmic practice. Lidocaine is the most commonly used local anaesthetic, and ropivacaine and levobupivacaine may be added instead of the older agent bupivacaine. The characteristics of local anaesthetics commonly used in ophthalmic surgery are shown in Table 3. Local anaesthetics with prolonged effect can also produce long lasting muscle paralysis that can distress the patient and clinician (Cass, 2006).

Agent	Duration of onset	Potency	Toxicity	Duration
Amide local anaesthetics				
Bupivacaine	Intermediate	High	High	Long
Levobupivacaine	Intermediate	High	Intermediate	Long
Etidocaine	Fast	High	High	Long
Lidocaine	Fast	Intermediate	Low	Intermediate
Mepivacaine	Fast	Intermediate	Low	Intermediate
Prilocaine	Fast	Intermediate	Low	Intermediate
Ropivacaine	Intermediate	Intermediate	Intermediate	Long
Esther local anaesthetics				
Cocaine	Slow	High	Very high	Long
Amethocaine	Slow	Intermediate	Intermediate	Intermediate
Procaine	Slow	Low	Low	Short

Table 3. Clinical properties of local anaesthetics

Hyaluronidase is commonly added to the local anaesthetic solution to decrease the time to onset and to perform homogenous dispersion. It is also believed to increase local anaesthetic metabolism or spread and thereby also decreases the period of contact with muscles hence decreasing paresis, which is otherwise increased when local anaesthetics are used solely. 15-30 U per mL is commonly added to the local anaesthetic solution but some authors advocate using as low as 1 U/mL in order to reduce the cost (Fanning, 2006). Within reason the more given the better the effects, though manufacture from animal sources gives rise to concerns about the possibility of non-infectious encephalopathy (Ripart et al., 2005).

Epinephrine use is controversial. In local anaesthetics, it is believed to increase the non-ionic form by increasing pH, therefore decreasing the duration between injection and onset of effect and also enhances penetration into nerves. It also decreases metabolism of local anaesthetics by performing vasoconstriction and delaying systemic uptake and degradation. However, it seems unwise to use it for regional blocks for cataract surgery because of long-acting local anaesthetics which are commercially available. Further, addition to the local anaesthetic mixture has been demonstrated to increase the myotoxicity in experimental models. In addition to the pressure effect of the local anaesthetic mixture, which arrests circulation to the eye namely pulsatile ocular blood flow for a brief period, epinephrine may further reduce blood flow due to vasoconstriction, which may be harmful in susceptible individuals. Addition of epinephrine may not increase the duration of anaesthesia and if indicated it should be avoided in a concentration of more than 1: 200 000 (Hamilton, 1996).

Clonidine, an alpha-2 agonist, has been mixed with local anaesthetics at the dose of 1 µg/kg in order to increase duration of analgesia (Madan et al., 2001). Vecuronium, a non-depolarizing muscle relaxant has also been added to the local anaesthetic solution (Reah et al., 1998). However, the latter drugs have increased potential for serious systemic adverse effects and injection into the orbit generally constitutes a non-retrieval route of administration, which may be dangerous.

The myotoxicity of local anaesthetics is controversial. It is suggested that they occur with long term exposure of the extra-ocular muscles to local anaesthetics when they are administered in a closed intra-orbital environment. Local anaesthetic injection into the muscle belly produces damage probably through needle trauma or pressure effect. Injection must not be performed when resistance is felt and if may be necessary to change needle position. Local anaesthetic may be administered slowly and incrementally with gentle aspirations after checking for possible vessel entry.

3. Topical anaesthesia

Topical anaesthesia of the eye, as demonstrated by the anaesthetic effect of cocaine on the cornea and its initiation of use in ophthalmic surgery, started with Karl Koller as early as 1886. Its popularity declined after initial enthusiasm according to the addiction potential and side effects of cocaine that complicated the surgery (Bacon, 2006). Topical anaesthesia regained popularity, this time without cocaine, since it removed complications from regional anaesthesia, increasing confidence and patient safety owing to improvements in monitored anaesthesia care and short-acting anaesthetic use (Chandradeva et al., 2010). It can be performed using local anaesthetic drops, gels or sponges that are applied to the conjunctival sac and gentle pressure applied to prevent loss from the nasolacrimal duct (Page & Fraunfelder, 2009). Benoxinate, ametocaine, lignocaine, and bupivacaine are examples of commercially available local anaesthetics. It has been demonstrated that intraocular pressure (IOP) can decrease after instillation (Almubrad & Ogbuehi, 2007). Topical anaesthesia may be insufficient to obtain complete analgesia. Supplemental blocks including intracameral injection of 0.1-0.5 mL of preservative-free 1% lignocaine or 0.5% bupivacaine in 1:100 000 epinephrine mixture, may cause sensory blockade of the iris and ciliary body and increase comfort during intraocular lens placement. It may also dilate the pupil. Subconjunctival and eyelid infiltrations are other blocks that can be used to increase the quality of analgesia.

The duration of the anaesthesia is brief and usually requires repeat drops after 0.5 hours. Toxic potential is questioned during long term use. Topical anaesthesia is increasingly used - it is convenient. However pain during the surgery is frequently encountered and therefore opioid administration may be required in these patients. It requires close co-operation with the patient during the operation (Weindler et al., 2004).

4. Regional anaesthesia

Regional anaesthesia is preferred in ophthalmic surgery - it allows day-case procedures, facilitates co-operation by the patient and has fewer systemic effects especially in geriatric patients with accompanying disease. The optimum size of needle including its diameter is one of the debated issues. Serious complications such as perforation of the globe and intra-orbital haemorrhage may occur due to use of very fine needles during retrobulbar and peribulbar block, related to the lower potential for sensation to be felt from a very fine needle during inadvertent insertion into the globe. On the other hand, use of blunt and larger calliper needles was criticized owing to potentially increased pain and trauma during insertion. It was also speculated that vessel trauma, if encountered, would easily be managed from a fine bore needle (Hamilton et al., 1988). The majority of complications are believed to be prevented by using a fine (27-30 G) and short (32 mm) needle. Warm local anaesthetic use and slow administration could greatly decrease the pain. Light sedation or analgesia may frequently be necessary, especially in anxious patients before giving the block.

A pressure device such as a Honan's cuff or gentle finger compression of the globe is advisable and should be applied for at least few minutes in order to obtain uniform dispersion of anaesthetic and to decrease intraocular pressure after performing the regional block.

4.1 Retrobulbar block

Retrobulbar block is a widely accepted regional technique for globe anaesthesia that was re-introduced to ocular surgery by Atkinson in 1936 (Atkinson, 1936). The aim of the block was to inject local anaesthetic into connective tissue inside the extra-ocular muscle cone behind the globe. Conic structure formed by the muscles around the eye surrounded by a loose connective tissue allows the dispersion of local anaesthetic agents (Ripart et al., 2001).

Insertion of the needle is onto the inferior orbital rim, two-thirds lateral from the inner canthus since it is free from vascular and neural components. A skin wheal is made with a 30 G needle on the lower eyelid at the temporal border of the inferior rim. 'Atkinson gaze' or an up and inner deviation of the globe is no longer used because of the risk of advancing the optic nerve and vascular supply into the path of the needle. Therefore, the eye must be kept in the neutral position. The globe may be displaced nasally with the finger of the free hand. The needle is advanced directly then angulated about 10° medially and superiorly. It is generally advisable not to introduce the needle more than 25 mm in order to prevent complications. A local anaesthetic volume of 2-4 mL is usually sufficient but this may be increased up to 8 mL. The analgesia and akinesia of the globe is higher than with other techniques and the technique is considered to be efficient for cataract surgery. Figure 1 depicts the needle direction in the orbit (See Figure 1 and Figure 3).

Pain from the injection is a common complaint that may be reduced by using fine needles. Rare but serious complications may be observed during the block including globe perforation, ipsilateral or contralateral vision loss due to retrograde spread of local anaesthetic solution, palsies, and cardiac or respiratory arrest (Ramsay & Knobloch 1978, Freidberg & Kline, 1986). Amaurosis and panophthalmia may occur after injecting the local anaesthetic solution into the eye (Ramsay & Knobloch 1978). The use of atraumatic, very fine needles (26-30 G) during performing the block, may be a possible reason for patients not feeling perforation. The incidence of perforation can increase with necessity of re-injection in the case of insufficient anaesthesia (Ripart et al., 2000). Constitutional increase in axial curvature in myopia (> 27 mm) and relatively thinner sclera with weak scleral tissue (staphylomata) behind the globe increase risk of perforation (Vohra & Good, 2000, Kallio et al., 2000), emphasizing the importance of careful evaluation of such eyes. The dural sac around the optic nerve is accepted as a path for retrograde leakage (Nicoll et al., 1987). Complications related to local anaesthetic mixing with the cerebrospinal fluid may occur within minutes and it is advised to keep patient for up to 10 min close to emergency equipment and drugs (Hamilton et al., 1988). Persistent diplopia is a rare but serious complication encountered predominantly after retrobulbar block and it can occur with a direct injury to the inferior rectus muscle and to a lesser extent to the inferior oblique muscle (Gómez -Arnau et al., 2003).

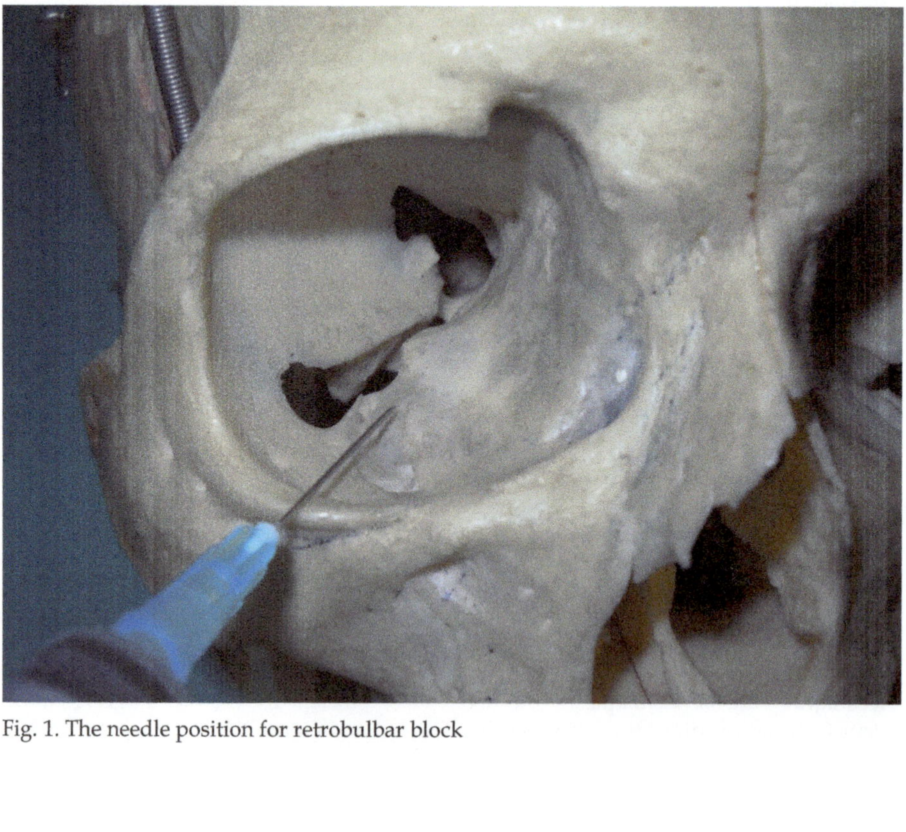

Fig. 1. The needle position for retrobulbar block

4.2 Peribulbar block

The peribulbar technique is another widely employed block that has been introduced in ocular anaesthetic practice more recently (Fry & Henderson, 1989). This technique involves the injection of local anaesthetic mixture externally to the muscle cone - hence it is also called the 'extraconal' block.

The needle entry point is the same as that of retrobulbar block, which is from two-thirds lateral to the inferior rim of the lower conjunctiva. The needle may be advanced from the lower lid with a skin wheal or through the conjunctiva after topical anaesthetic drops have been applied. The needle is introduced directly and is shorter than in the former technique. It is advised to use 26 G 25 mm needles (See Figure 2 and Figure 3).

The complication rate of the peribulbar block is considered to be lower than that of the retrobulbar technique. A larger volume of local anaesthetic solution is required compared to the other regional blocks. A longer duration of onset and repeated need for re-injection are other limitations (Frow et al., 2000). Efficient and satisfactory blocks can be performed even using lower volumes (Rizzo et al., 2005). A modified peribulbar technique was described with injection with a more superficial needle placement, which decreased the incidence of

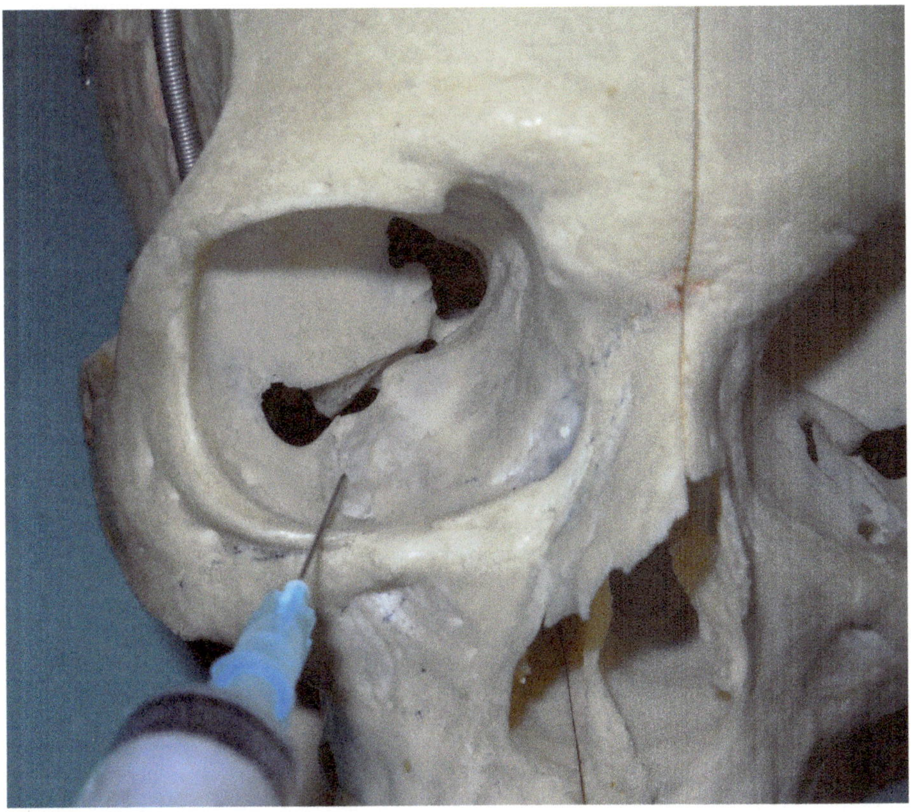

Fig. 2. The needle position for peribulbar block

re-injection but with a higher degree of subconjunctival haemorrhage (Mahfouz & Kalberi, 2007). Rare but serious complications including brainstem anaesthesia may also occur during the block (Gomez et al., 1997). Aside the important issue of safety there are no other advantages over retrobulbar block as complete anaesthesia and further injections are needed; an increased rate of subconjunctival haemorrhage instead of lid haematoma with retrobulbar block was observed in a large scale of review (Alhassan et al., 2008).

4.3 Sub-Tenon's block

Sub-Tenon's block is defined as a local anaesthetic injection into the tissues of the episcleral area under the Tenon's sheath. It was established in ocular surgery in about the mid-1950s (Swan, 1956). Tenon's fascia covers the globe and envelopes the ocular muscles from attaching sites to the sclera. More recently the technique was re-established as a sole anaesthetic block for eye surgery (Stevens, 1992). It was the most popular and commonly performed technique in the UK (Chandradeva et al., 2010).

The block can be performed with a surgical manipulation to reach the Tenon's sheath. Local anaesthetic drops or ointment are placed on the conjunctiva and the eye must be prepared by cleansing with povidone-iodine solution. The patient is asked to look upward and outward. The technique requires making a little hole in the conjunctiva, positioned 3-5 mm infero-nasally away from the limbus. Blunt Westcott scissors are required during careful dissection. Various types of metal and plastic curved or blunt tipped cannulas are in use for injection. A volume of local anaesthetic solution of 3-5 mL is generally sufficient for globe anaesthesia, but larger volumes may be required for akinesia. Many other techniques have been described in different sites of the globe, including a medial canthus episcleral technique from Ripart and colleagues (Ripart et al., 2000), which requires needle insertion. The patient is instructed to look inwards and downward during insertion of the needle through slightly shifting medially and advancing strictly to the posterior. The globe is changed to the neutral position after a small loss of resistance is felt. The needle is advanced 10-15 mm and up to 10 mL of local anaesthetic may be injected (See Figure 3).

The incidence of pain during the injection is higher. Loss of local anaesthetic during injection is frequent. Chemosis is increased with short needle use and incomplete akinesia and other limitations of this block are commonly encountered. In this 'blunt needle technique' complications from sharp needle techniques are reduced. However in addition to the complications occurring with retrobulbar block such as retrobulbar haemorrhage, cardiorespiratory arrest related to central spread, scleral perforation was observed in a patient who had previously undergone retinal surgery (Kumar et al., 2005).

All regional techniques produce cosmetic complications such as local bruising, haemorrhage, oedema and subconjunctival ecchymosis near the needle entry site and long-acting muscle paresis that distress the patient. Comparative studies show no benefit over each other. There is a lower requirement for sedation in the retrobulbar anaesthesia group but patient satisfaction is greatest with sub-Tenon's block (Ryu et al., 2009). It is convenient to perform blocks at the lower half of the globe in order to decrease complications. Owing to the thin lamina papyracea of the orbit care must be exercised when a medial approach is used. The incidence of nausea and vomiting are lower with phacoemulsification performed under topical or retrobulbar anaesthesia and no technique-related difference has been found (Chan et al., 2002). However, in spite of defined limitations, a survey indicated that in general patients predominantly prefer scenarios using blocks to topical anaesthesia and oral sedation regimens instead of IV medications (Friedman et al., 2004).

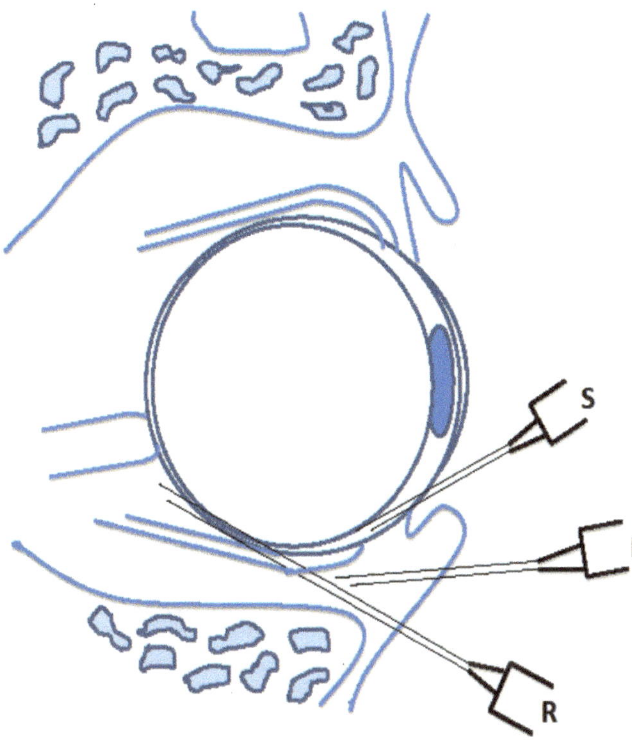

Fig. 3. Schematic drawing for regional anaesthetic techniques of the eye, R: retrobulbar, P: peribulbar, and S: sub Tenon's block

4.4 Oculocardiac reflex

The oculocardiac reflex is a trigeminovagal reflex response initiated by pain, compression or traction of eye muscles. The afferent pathway starts in the ciliary nerves, ciliary body and Gasserian ganglion through the ophthalmic division of the trigeminal nerve to reach the nucleus of the trigeminal nerve at the floor of the fourth ventricle. The efferent pathways are cardiac vagal nerves that induce hypotension and bradycardia. Nausea and vomiting may also be induced with decrease in the blood pressure. Surgical manipulation or stretching of muscles must be stopped when it is observed during an operation. Atropine or IV glycopyrrolate are effective for the treatment (Feldman & Patel, 2010).

4.5 Post-cataract ptosis

Ptosis after cataract surgery is observed with an incidence as high as 13%. Multiple factors have been implicated in the aetiology, including local anaesthetic injection to the upper eyelid to obtain akinesia, sutures and traction of the upper components of the eye, retrobulbar injection, peribulbar anaesthesia through the upper eyelid at the 12 o'clock position, excessive ocular compression, placement of the eyelid speculum, performing large conjunctival flaps, eyelid oedema, and tight or long term patching in the postoperative

period. Local anaesthetic injection cannot be accepted per se as the primary source, because this complication is also observed after general anaesthesia (McGoldrick & Gayer, 2006).
The measures that possibly decrease such complications are limiting the local anaesthetic volume to 6 mL during regional block, avoiding injection to the upper eyelid or muscles, and gentle tractions when necessary.

5. General anaesthesia

General anaesthesia offers motionless optimal surgical conditions including ocular akinesia with decreased intraocular pressure. Standard anaesthetic care including ECG on V5 or D II derivation, peripheral oxygen saturation, non-invasive arterial blood pressure, end-tidal CO_2 and temperature measurement is implemented to all patients as performed in monitored anaesthesia care. End tidal inspired anaesthetic gas concentrations may be estimated to assess the depth and timing during the anaesthesia. Venous access is mandatory and usually found on the dorsum of the hand.
Congenital cataract can be detected at earlier periods of life, even in the intrauterine period in pregnancies at risk of the condition which may be screened. Controversies exist on the optimal timing for congenital cataract surgery. Intervention before four weeks was associated with increasing glaucoma and secondary membrane formation, on the other hand incidences of nystagmus and diplopia were increased after this period (Birch et al., 2009). Therefore surgery for congenital cataract is advised to be performed between 5-8 weeks of life or before the 10th week to ensure optimal visual acuity (Lambert et al., 2006).
Deep sedation or general anaesthesia is required for patients in the paediatric age group. Mask induction can be achieved with sevoflurane starting from 8-7% and the anaesthetic concentration may be slowly decreased to the desired level. Flavoured masks such as those smelling of strawberry or banana may facilitate the procedure. This may be sufficient for short procedures such as examination, diagnosis or foreign body removal. Airway control with endotracheal intubation is a safe alternative for babies who already have venous access. On the other hand laryngeal mask use is also performed with success in this surgical subpopulation. A eutectic mixture of local anaesthetic (EMLA) cream that is applied on the dorsum of the hand about one hour before the procedure can facilitate painless venous puncture in infants and toddlers. In addition to the usual anaesthetic care temperature monitoring and heating or measures undertaken to prevent heat loss are especially important for patients under 1 year in age. Although intramuscular ketamine injection is another option the nystagmus which it causes may preclude eye examination. In congenital cataract surgery, a sub-Tenon's block performed during general anaesthesia has been demonstrated to be superior to fentanyl in terms of postoperative pain relief, reducing anxiety and helping induce calmer behaviour in patients in recovery, and a lower incidence of the oculocardiac reflex during surgery (Ghai et al., 2009).
All general anaesthetics except ketamine and succinylcholine decrease intraocular pressure. Propofol may be desirable for day case surgery during induction and maintenance of anaesthesia owing to advantages including faster onset and offset time, no residual effect, and reduction in nausea and vomiting. Etomidate can require a stable hemodynamic circulation during induction. In the case of neuromuscular blocking agents, concurrent disorders should be borne in mind. Cisatracurium can be used safely in patients with renal insufficiency. Rocuronium bromide may be indicated in emergence situations and facilitates endotracheal intubation as fast as succinylcholine. Having ready access to sugammadex, an

inactivation substrate that is specific for rocuronium, is another advantage in the case of residual neuromuscular blockade – the drug is available in many countries (Chambers et al., 2010). Lignocaine and beta blockers such as esmolol may be preferred to opioids for decreasing neuroendocrine responses to endotracheal intubation because of potential to increase postoperative nausea and vomiting. However, remifentanil, an opioid of shorter half-life can be used for this purpose. Laryngeal mask insertion may decrease possible complications related to endotracheal intubation. Propofol and opioid infusions or bolus doses may be administered during the maintenance- namely for total intravenous anaesthesia. The modern inhalation anaesthetics including sevoflurane or desflurane, have a comparable recovery period that can also be chosen. Recovery from anaesthesia must be as smooth as induction. The agents that are administered during induction may be repeated during recovery to prevent complications related to a sudden increase in blood pressure that can increase the risk of intra-ocular complications. Postoperative keratitis may be prevented by closing the opposite eye with a tape to prevent dehydration of the tear film such as with petroleum-based ointments in patients in whom the expected surgery exceeds one hour. An air-oxygen mixture may be preferred instead of nitrous oxide, a volatile anaesthetic agent that has emetic properties.

General anaesthesia provides optimal surgical conditions including an immobile eye and patient. The Bell's reflex can be present during light anaesthesia. Patients who refuse or have extreme fear of regional blocks require general anaesthesia. It also indicated in patients with allergy to local anaesthetic agents and in patients unable to control their movements such as those with Parkinson's Disease, those who cannot lie supine, or those with advanced concurrent disease. Other advantages are in offering bilateral surgery to patients in vulnerable conditions at a single session and refraining from complications due to needle insertion during regional anaesthesia.

Loss of communication with the patient during surgery and the requirement for an anaesthesia team, delay in recovery, and increasing expense, are disadvantages. Patients with advanced concurrent disorders under general anaesthesia should be managed as inpatients in order to stabilize their systemic pathologies.

5.1 Postoperative care

A patient may be discharged when regaining full consciousness - in the presence of stable vital signs in a calm patient who has no complaints. Patients should be observed carefully for residual drug effects and possible adverse outcomes should be explained to them. Pain is usually minimal and can be managed easily with non-steroidal anti-inflammatory (NSAID) drugs which also have topical ophthalmic solutions for use. These drugs are also efficient against intraocular inflammation after surgery and long-term complications such as cystoid macular oedema (Kim et al., 2010). On the other hand, drugs should be withheld in susceptible individuals such as patients with asthma. Eye drops containing corticosteroids can be used efficiently for the same purpose. Local anaesthetic solutions may also be combined for postoperative pain originating from causes like oedema or chemosis. While injection of intracameral antibiotic may decrease the risk of endophtalmitis, the benefit of perioperative NSAIDs over corticosteroids and the efficacy of combination in short or long term use remains to be demonstrated (DeCroos & Afshari, 2008). Patients with increased IOP preoperatively have been shown to be at risk of postoperative IOP spikes, which some authors feel makes it necessary to recommend surgery in the earlier period of the day so there is follow-up prior to discharge of at least a few hours (O'Brien et al., 2007).

6. Conclusion

Cataract surgery is increasingly becoming safer, faster and non-invasive. There is an increasing trend toward utilizing topical anaesthesia. Decisions on the type of anaesthesia to be used depend largely on the patient, the expected duration of the operation and preferences of the surgeon. For patients on anticoagulation therapy and who have previously had ocular surgery it is best to avoid needle trauma. General anaesthesia may be reserved only for special circumstances. Thorough knowledge including of drugs, anatomy of the orbit, and techniques are fundamental for implementing sound regional anaesthetic practice. Meticulous patient selection, careful pre-operative evaluation, selecting the anaesthetic technique properly and with care, along with increasing knowledge and skill may decrease peri- and postoperative complications and improve patient experience. The success of intervention may also be increased by optimizing collaboration between the surgical and anaesthetic team.

7. References

Alhassan, M.B., Kyari, F., Ejere, H.O. (2008) Peribulbar versus retrobulbar anaesthetsia for cataract surgery. *Cochrane Database of Systematic Reviews,* 16, No.3, CD004083. ISSN 1469-493X.

Almubrad, T.M., Ogbuehi, K.C. (2007) Clinical investigation of the effects of topical anesthesia on intraocular pressure. *Clinical Ophtalmology,* V.1, pp.305-9. ISSN 1177-5467.

Apan, A., Doganci, N., Ergan, A., Buyukkocak, U. Bispectral index-guided intra-operative sedation with dexmedetomidine and midazolam in outpatient cataract surgery. *Minerva Anestesiologica,* 2009; 75(5): 239-244. ISSN 0026-4717.

Atkinson, W.S. (1936) Retrobulbar injection of anesthetic within the muscular cone. *The Archieves of Ophtalmology,* V.16, pp.494-503. ISSN 0003-9950.

Aydin, O.N., Kir, E., Ozkan, S.B., Gürsoy, F. (2002) Patient-controlled analgesia and sedation with fentanyl in phacoemulsification. *Journal of Cataract & Refractive Surgery,* V.28, No.11, pp.1968-72. ISSN 0886-3350.

Bacon, D.R. (2006) Seeing an anesthetic revolution: ocular anesthesia in history. In Ocular Anesthesia, Moster MR, Azuara-Blanco A, eds. *Ophtalmology Clinics of North America,* V.19, No.2, pp.151-4. ISSN 0896-1549.

Balkan, B.K., İyilikçii L., Günenç, F., Uzümlü, H., Kara, H.C., Celik, L., Durak, I., Gökel, E. (2004) Comparison of sedation requiremenst for cataract surgery under topical anesthesia. *European Journal of Ophtalmology,* V.14, No.6, pp.473-7. ISSN1468-2079

Basic anesthetic monitoring standards. American Society of Anesthesiologists http://www.asahq.org/publictionsAndServices.

Birch, E.E., Cheng, C., Stager, D.R.Jr, Weakley, D.R., Stager D.R.Sr. (2009) The critical period for surgical treatment of dense congenital bilateral cataracts. *Journal of American Association for Pediatric Ophtalmology and Strabismus, V.*13, No.1, pp.67-71. ISSN 1091-8531.

Cass, G.D. (2006) Choices of local anesthetics for ocular surgery in Ocular Anesthesia, Moster MR, Azuara-Blanco A, eds. *Ophtalmology Clinics of North America,* V.19, No.2, pp.203-7. ISSN 0896-1549.

Chambers, D., Paulden, M., Paten, F., Heirs, M., Duffy, S., Hunter, J.M., Sculpher, M., Woolacott, N. (2010) Sugammaedx for reversal of neuromuscular block after rapid sequence intubation a systematic review and economic assessment. *British Journal of Anaesthesia,* V.105, No.5, pp.568-75. ISSN 0007-0912.

Chan, J.C., Lai, J.S., Lam, D.S. (2002) Nausea and vomiting after phacoemolsification using topical or retrobulbar anesthesia. *Journal of Cataract & Refractive Surgery,* V.28, No.11, pp.1973-6. ISSN 0886-3350.

Chandradeva, K., Nangalia, V., Hugkulstone, C.E. (2010) Role of the anaesthetist during cataract surgery under local anaesthesia in the UK: a national survey. *British Journal of Anaesthesia,* V.104, No.5, pp.577-81. ISSN 0007-0912.

Chernik, D.A., Gillings, D., Laine, H., Hendler, J., Silver, J.M., Davidson, A.B., Schwam, E.M., Siegel, J.L. (1990) Validity and reliability of the Observer's assessment of Awareness/Sedation Scale: study with intravenous midazolam. *Journal of Clinical Psychopharmacology,* V.10, No.4, pp.244-51. ISSN 0271-0749.

Chung, F., Lavalle, P.A., McDonald, S., Chung, A., McDonald, N.J. (1989) Cognitive impairement after neuroleptanalgesia in cataract surgery. *Anesthesia & Analgesia,* V.68, No.5, pp.614-8. ISSN 0003-2999.

Cugini, U., Lanzetta, P., Nadbath, P., Menchini, U. (1997) Sedation with ketamine during cataract surgery. *Journal of Cataract & Refractive Surgery,* V.23, No.5, pp.784-6. ISSN 0886-3350.

Cullen, K.A., Hall, M.J., Golosinskiy, A. (2009) Ambulatory surgery in the United States, 2006. *National Health Statistics Report,* Vol.28, No.11, pp.1-25. ISSN

Davenport, D.L., Bowe, E.A., Henderson, W.G., Khuri, S.F., Mentzer, R.M,. (2006) National surgical quality improvement program (NSQIP) risk factors can be used to validate American Society of Anesthesiologists physical status (ASA PS) levels. *Annals of Surgery,* V.243, No.5, pp.636-44. ISSN 0003-4932.

DeCroos, F.C. & Afshari, N.A. (2008) Perioperative antibiotics and anti-inflammatory agents in cataract surgery. *Current Opinion in Ophtalmology,* 19: No.1, pp.22-6. ISSN 1040-8738.

el-Bassiouny, O., el-Taher EM, el-Din ABD, el-Ghaffar ME. (1992) Alfentanil/promazine versus meperidine/promazine as a sedative regimens during local analgesia for cataract operation. *Documenta Ophtalmologica,* V.82, No.3, pp.201-10. ISSN 0012-4486.

Fanning, G.L. (2006) Orbital regional anesthesia. In Ocular Anesthesia, Moster MR, Azuara-Blanco A, eds. *Ophtalmology Clinics of North America,* V.19, No.2, pp.221-32. ISSN 0896-1549.

Feldman, M.A., Patel, A. (2010) Anesthesia for eye, ear, nose, and throat surgery In *Miller's Anesthesia* Miller RD ed Churchill-Livingstone (7th ed.) pp.2189-10. ISBN 978-0-44306959-8, Philadelphia,

Freidberg, H.L., Kline, O.R. (1986) Contralateral amaurosis after retrobulbar injection. *American Journal of Ophtalmology,* V.101, No.6, pp.688-90. ISSN 0002-9394.

Friedman, D.S., Reeves, S.W., Bass, E.B., Lubomski, L.H., Fleisher, L.A., Schein, O.D. (2004) Patient preferences for anesthesia management during cataract surgery. *British Journal of Ophtalmology,* V.88, No.3, pp.333-5. ISSN 1468-2079.

Frow, M.W., Miranda-Caraballo, J.I., Akhtar, T.M., Huigkulstone, C.E. (2000) Single injection peribulbar anaesthesia. *Anaesthesia,* V.55, No.3, pp.750-6. ISSN 1365-2044.

Fry, R.A., Henderson, J. (1990) Local anesthesia for eye surgery. the periocular technique. *Anaesthesia,* 45, No.1, pp.14-7. ISSN 1365-2044.

Ghai, B, Ram, J., Makkar, J.K., Wig, J., Kaushik, S. (2009) Subtenon block compared to intravenous fentanyl for perioperative analgesia in pediatric cataract surgery. *Anesthesia & Analgesia,* V.108, No.4, pp.1132-8. ISSN 0003-2999.

Gómez -Arnau, J.I., Yangüela, J., González, A., Andrés, Y., García del Valle, S., Gili, P., Fernández-Guisasola, J., Arias, A. (2003) Anaesthesia-related diplopia after cataract surgery. *British Journal of Anaesthesia,* V.90, No.2, pp.89-92. ISSN 0007-0912.

Gomez, R.S., Andrade, L.O., Costa, J.R. (1997) Brainstem anaesthesia after peribulbar anaesthesia. *Canadian Journal of Anaesthesia,* V.44, No.7, pp.732-4. ISSN 0832-610X.

Hamilton, R.C., Gimbel, H.V., Strutin, L. (1988) Regional anesthesia for 12000 cataract extraction and intraocular lens implantation procedures. *Canadian Journal of Anaesthesia,* V.35, No.6, pp.615-23. ISSN 0832-610X.

Hamilton, R.C. (1996) Local anesthetics and adjuvant drugs. In Smith GB, Hamilton RC, Carr CA. *Ophtalmic anesthesia: a practical hand book.* (2nd ed.) Oxford university. pp.84-103. ISBN 340567570, New York.

Hirschman, D.R., Morby, L.J. (2006) A study of the safety of continued anticoagulation for cataract surgery patients. *Nursing Forum* V.41, No. 1, pp.30-7. ISSN 1538-0688.

Hodgkins, P.R., Teye-Botchway, L., Morrel, A.J., Fetherston, T.J., Perthen, C., Brown. N.E. (1992) Neuroleptanalgesia and extracapsular cataract extraction. *British Journal of Ophtalmology,* V.76, No.3, pp.153-6. ISSN 1468-2079.

Kallio, H., Paloheimo, M., Maunuksela, E.L. (2000) Haemorrhage and risk factors associated with retrobulbar/peribulbar block: a prospective study in 1383 patients. *British Journal of Anaesthesia,* 85: No.5, pp.708-11. ISSN 0007-0912.

Katz, J., Feldman, M.A., Bass, E.B., Lubomski, L.H., Tielsch, J.M., Petty, B.G., Flesher, L.A., Schein, O.D. (2001) Adverse intraoperative medical events and their association with anesthesia management strategies in cataract surgery. *Ophtalmology,* V.108, No.10, pp.1721-6. ISSN 03656691.

Kim, S.J., Flach, A.J., Jampol, L.M. (2010) Nonsteroidal anti-inflammatory drugs in ophthalmology. *Survey of Ophtalmology,* V55, No.2, pp.108-33. ISSN 0039-6257.

Kumar, C.M., Williamson, S., Manickam, B. (2005) A review of sub-Tenon's block: current practice and recent development. *European Journal of Anaesthesiology,* V.22, No.8, pp.567-577. ISSN 02650215.

Lambert, S.R., Lynn, M.J., Reeves, R., Plager, D.A., Buckley, E.G., Wilson, M.E. (2006) Is there a latent period for the surgical treatment of children with dense bilateral congenital cataracts? *Journal of American Association for Pediatric Ophtalmology and Strabismus,* V.10, No.1, pp.30-6. ISSN 1091-8531.

Madan, R., Bharti, N., Shende, D., Khokhar, S.K., Kaul, H.L. (2001) A dose response study of clonidine with local anesthetic mixture for peribulbar block: a comparison of three doses. *Anesthesia & Analgesia,* V.93, No.6, pp.1593-7. ISSN 0003-2999.

Mahfouz, A.K., Kalteri, H.M. (2007) Randomized trial of superficial peribulbar compared with conventional peribulbar anesthesia for cataract extraction. *Clinical Ophtalmology,* V.1, No.1, pp.55-60. ISSN 1177-5467.

McGoldrick, K.E., Gayer, S.I. (2006) Anesthesia and the eye. In *Clinical anesthesia* (5th ed.) Barash PG, Cullen BF, Stoelting RK eds. Lippincott Williams and Wilkins, 995. ISBN-13:970-07817-5745-4, Philadelphia.

Murodch, J.A., Grant SA, Kenny, G.N. (2000) Safety of patient-maintained propofol sedation using a target controlled system in healthy volunteers. *British Journal of Anaesthesia,* V.85, No.2, pp.299-301. ISSN 0007-0912.

Nicoll, J.M.V., Acharya, P.A., Ahlen, K., Beguneid, S., Edge, K.R. (1987) Central nervous system complications after 6000 retrobulbar block. *Anesthesia & Analgesia,* V.66, No.12, pp.1298-1302. ISSN 0003-2999.

O'Brien, P.D., Ho, S.L., Fitzpatrick, P., Power, W. (2007) Risk factors for a postoperative intraocular pressure spike after phacoemulsification. *Canadian Journal of Ophtalmology,* V.42, No.1, pp.51-5. ISSN 0008-4182.

Page, M.A., Fraunfelder, F.W. (2009) Safety, efficacy, and patient acceptability of lidocaine hydrochloride ophthalmic gel as a topical ocular anesthetic for use in ophthalmic procedures. *Clinical Ophtalmology,* V.3, pp.601-9. ISSN 1177-5467.

Ramsay, M.A., Savage, T.M., Simpson, B.R., Goodwin, R. (1974) Controlled sedation with alphaxalone-alphadolone. *British Medical Journal,* V.22, No.2, pp.656-9. ISSN 09598138.

Ramsay, R.C., Knobloch W.H. (1978) Ocular perforation following retrobulbar anesthesia for retinal detachment surgery. *American Journal of Ophtalmology,* V.86, No.1, pp.61-4. ISSN 0002-9394.

Reah G, Bodenham AR, Braitwaite P, Esmond J, Menage MJ. (1998) Peribulbar anesthesia using a mixture of local anesthetic and vecuronium. *Anaesthesia,* V.53, No.6, pp.551-4. ISSN 1365-2044.

Reinhardt, S., Buckhardt, U., Nestler, A., Wiedemann, R. (2002) Use of piritramide for analgesia and sedation during peribulbar nerve block for cataract surgery. *Ophtalmologica,* V.216, No.4, pp.256-60. ISSN 0030 3755.

Rewari, V., Madan, R., Kaul, H.L., Kumar, L. (2002) Remifentanil and propofol sedation for retrobulbar block. *Anaesthesia & Intensive Care,* V.30, No.4, pp.433-7. ISSN 0310-057X.

Ripart, J., Lefrant, J.Y., de La Coussaye, J.E., Prat-Pradal, D., Vivien, B., Eledjam, J.J. (2001) Peribulbar versus retrobulbar anesthesia for ophtalmic surgery: an anatomical comparison of extraconal and intraconal injections. *Anesthesiology,* V.94, No.1, pp.56-62. ISSN 0003-3022.

Ripart, J., Lefrant, J.Y., Vivien, B., Charavel, P., Fabbo-Peray, P., Jassaud, A. (2000) Ophtalmic regional anesthesia: medial canthus episcleral (Sub-Tenon) anesthesia is more efficient than peribulbar anesthesia. *Anesthesiology,* V.92, No.5, pp.1278-85. ISSN 0003-3022.

Ripart, J., Nouvellon, E., Chaumeron, A. (2005) Regional anesthesia for eye surgery. *Regional Anesthesia and Pain Medicine,* V.30, No.1, pp.72-82. ISSN 1098-7339.

Rizzo, L., Marini, M., Rosati, C., Calamai, I., Nesi, M., Salvini, R., Mazzini, C., Campana, F., Brizzi, E. (2005) Peribulbar anesthesia: a percutaneous single injection technique with a small volume of anesthetic. *Anesthesia & Analgesia,* V.100, No.1, pp.94-6. ISSN 0003-2999.

Ryu, J.H., Kim, M., Bahk, J.H., Do, S.H., Cheong, I.Y., Kim, Y.C. (2009) A comparison of retrobulbar block, sub-Tenon block and topical anesthesia during cataract surgery. *European Journal of Ophtalmology,* V.19, No.2, pp.240-6. ISSN 1120-6721.

Schein, O.D., Katz, J., Bass, E.B., Tielsch, J.M., Lubomski, L.H., Feldman, M.A., Petty, B.G., Steinberg, E.P. (2000) The value of routine preoperative medical testing before cataract surgery. *New England Journal of Medicine,* V.342, No.3, pp.168-75. ISSN 0028-4793.

Steeds, C., Mather, S.J. (2001) Fasting regimens for regional ophthalmic anaesthesia. A survey of members of the British Ophtalmic Anaesthesia society. *Anaesthesia,* V.56, No.7, pp.638-42. ISSN 1365-2044.

Stevens, J.D. (1992) A new local anaesthesia technique for cataract extraction by one quadrant sub-Tenon's infiltration. *British Journal of Ophtalmology,* V.76, No.11, pp.670-4. ISSN 1468-2079.

Swan, K.C. (1956) New drugs and techniques for ocular anesthesia. *Transactions of the American Academy of Ophtalmology & Otolaryngology.,* V.60, No.3, pp.368-75. ISSN 0002-7154.

Tan, C.S.H., Kumar, C.M., Fanning G.L., Lai, Y.C., Au Eong, K.G. A survey on the knowledge and attitudes of anaesthesia providers in the United States of America, United Kingdom and Singapore on visual experiences during cataract surgery. *European Journal of Anesthesiology,* 2006; V.23, No.4, pp.276-81. ISSN 02650215.

Vohra, S.B., Good, P.A. (2000) Altered globe dimensions of axial myopia as a risk factors for penetrating oclar injury during peribulbar anesthesia. *British Journal of Anaesthesia,* V.85, No.2, pp.242-5. ISSN 0007-0912.

Weindler, J., Kiefer RT, Rippa A, Wiech K, Ruprecht KW. (2000) Low-dose oral clonidine premedication before intraocular surgery in retrobulbar anesthesia. *European Journal of Ophtalmology,* V.10, No.3, pp.248-56. ISSN 1120-6721.

Weindler, J., Weindler, M., Ruprecht, K.W. (2004) Lokalanästhesie in der ophtalmochirurgie. *Ophtalmologe,* V.101, No.8, pp.847-65. ISSN 1682-3974.

5

Anticoagulant and Antiplatelet Use in Cataract Surgery and Combined with Posterior Vitrectomy

Hiroshi Kobayashi
Department of Ophthalmology, Kanmon Medical Center, Shimonoseki, Japan

1. Introduction

Patients receiving long-term anticoagulant and antiplatelet medications pose a clinical challenge when therapy needs intraocular surgery, including cataract surgery and vitrectomy [1-3]. Maintaining antiplatelet and anticoagulation places them at risk for serious bleeding complications, whereas discontinuing these medications puts them at risk of thromboembolic complications [4-6]. Currently, there is little consensus on the appropriate perioperative treatment of patients on long-term acetylsalicylic acid (aspirin) and warfarin therapy [7-9]. In this study, we compared the incidence of hemorrhagic and non-hemorrhagic complications and visual course of phacoemulsification alone and combined phacoemulisification and vitrectomy between patients who maintained or discontinued anticoagulant and/or antiplatelet medications.

2. Patients and methods

A total of 824 consecutive cases of 532 patients undergoing cataract surgery alone and of 69 consecutive cases of 69 patients undergoing combined cataract and vitreous surgery for the treatment of epiretinal membrane and macular hole who had been administered warfarin and/or aspirin for 6 months or longer between April 2005 and March 2009 were studied (Table 1). Before April 2007, all patients discontinued the drugs prior to the surgery. After

	Anticoagulant and antiplatelet medications	Number of patients (Number of cases)
Phacoemulsification alone group	Discontinuation subgroup	274 (421)
	Maintenance subgroup	258 (403)
Combined phacoemulsification and vitrectomy group	Discontinuation subgroup	33 (33)
	Maintenance subgroup	36 (36)

Table 1. Outline of patients with discontinuation and maintenance of anticoagulant and/or antiplatelet medications

No Financial support has been received by any authors and none of the authors has any proprietary interest in the subject matter presented.

April 2007, all patients maintained the treatment at the time of surgery (Table 1). The discontinuation subgroups consisted of patients who ceased taking warfarin and/or aspirin 1 week before the surgery, with their therapies then restarted 2 days postoperatively. The study protocol and consent forms were approved by the Human Subjects Committee.

2.1 Surgical procedure and postoperative interventions

Cataract surgery

Phacoemulsification and intraocular lens implantation was performed through a superior sclerocorneal incision after scleral cauterization. Sub-Tenon anesthesia with 2% lidocaine (Xylocaine, Asteras, Tokyo, Japan) was employed using Fukasaku's blunt subtenon's cannula (Handaya, Tokyo, Japan). A standard phacoemulsification technique was used. In all cases, a three-piece hydrophobic acrylic intraocular lens (AcrySof™ MA30BM; Alcon, Fort Worth, TX, USA) was implanted. Sodium hyaluronate 1% (Healon, AMO, Santana, CA, USA) was used as viscoelastics.

Vitrectomy for epiretinal membrane and macular hole

A standard three port pars plana vitrectomy was performed in all patients after sub-Tenon anesthesia, phacoemulsification and intraocular lens implantation. We achieved a complete posterior vitreous detachment during pars plana vitrectomy using a vitreous cutter. For patients with epiretinal membrane, the membranes were removed with a slightly bent microvitreoretinal blade or internal limiting membrane forceps. For patients with macular hole, the internal limiting membranes around the macular hole were removed in assistance with triamcinolone acetonide or indocyanine green. Sulfur hexafluoride (20%) was used for gas tamponade. Patients remained in the prone position for 7-10 days postoperatively.

Postoperative management

In both groups, all patients were given topical levofloxacin, dexamethasone and diclofenac three times daily during the first 2 weeks, with the drugs then tapered off over the next 3 months.

Evaluation of outcomes

Before enrollment, patients had an ocular and systemic history taken as well as slit-lamp biomicroscopy, visual acuity, a physical examination, and dilated fundoscopy. Best-corrected visual acuity (BCVA) was measured, with the log of the minimum angle of resolution (LogMAR) then calculated and used for all statistical analyses. Intraocular pressure was measured using Goldmann applanation tonometry while a slit-lamp examination was used to clinically grade the preoperative nuclear sclerosis as per the method of Emery and Little [10]. After pupil dilation, ophthalmoscopic and slit-lamp biomicroscopic examinations were employed to assess retinal, vitreous and choroidal/suprachoroidal hemorrhages. For patients with epiretinal membrane and macular hole, we performed optical coherence tomography (OCT) scanning (OCT scanner 3000 and Cirrus, Humphrey Instruments, San Leandro, California) before and 1, 3, and 6 months after surgery. The fovea was identified as the patient's fixation point or with the fundus monitor in the OCT device. The cross-sectional images were normalized and smoothed using OCT plug-in software. Patients were also assessed intraoperatively and at every postoperative visit for the presence of general complications, which included cerebral events such as transient ischemic attack and cerebral infarction and hemorrhage, and cardiovascular events such as deep vein thrombosis, myocardial ischemia, and myocardial infarction. Hemorrhagic complications were defined as subconjunctival hemorrhage and hyphema, or retinal, vitreous and choroidal/suprachoroidal hemorrhage. Hypotony was defined as an intraocular pressure of less than 4 mmHg after surgery, while the criteria of Teehasaenee and Ritch [11] were used to define shallow anterior chamber. An intraocular pressure spike was defined as an intraocular pressure on the first postoperative day that was greater than or equal to 3 mmHg higher than the level observed preoperatively.

2.2 Statistical analysis

A Student's t-test was used to evaluate the continuous variables, while a paired t-test was used was used to evaluate the difference in intraocular pressures between the follow-up intervals. All t-tests were two-tailed. Categoric variables were evaluated by using the chi-square test, the Fisher exact test, or the Spearman rank correlation, as appropriate. Results were defined as being statistically significant when $P < 0.05$.
For the pairing of groups, baseline values for age, sex, BCVA, and prothrombin time-international normalized ratio (PT-INR) were used for matching. When correlations between paired observations were noted, we used the F-test to examine the variances between the two populations.

3. Results

Baseline

Patient demographics are summarized in Table 2. No significant differences were found between the two subgroups for age, sex, or BCVA in the phacoemulsification alone group and the combined phacoemulsification and vitrectomy group. In patients who were administered warfarin, mean PT-INR was 1.94 ± 0.77 in the maintenance subgroup and 1.87 ± 0.62 in the discontinuation subgroup in the phacoemulsification alone group ($P = 0.3$) and 1.89 ± 0.57 in the maintenance subgroup and 2.23 ± 0.66 in the maintenance subgroup in the combined phacoemulsification and vitrectomy group ($P = 0.0249$).

3.1 Hemorrhagic and non-hemorrhagic complications

Phacoemulsification alone group: As seen in Table 3, there were no systemic complications or any significant intraoperative bleeding noted for the two subgroups. There were 87 eyes (21.6 %) in the maintenance subgroup and 46 eyes (10.9%) in the discontinuation subgroup that exhibited subconjunctival hemorrhage of greater than one quadrant ($P < 0.0001$). On the first postoperative day, microscopic hyphema was seen in 26 eyes (6.5%) in the maintenance subgroup and in 11 eyes (2.6%) in the discontinuation subgroup ($P = 0.0078$), whereas no apparent hyphema was found in the two subgroups. Within 1 week of the surgical procedure, all bleeding had stopped without affecting the visual acuity. There was also no vitreous or choroidal/ suprachoroidal hemorrhage found in either of the two subgroups. There were 5 posterior capsule rupture and 2 vitreous loss in the maintenance subgroup and 7 posterior capsule rupture and 3 vitreous loss in the discontinuation subgroup, respectively (posterior capsule rupture: $P = 0.6$; vitreous loss: $P = 0.7$) (Table 3). No significant differences were noted for the incidence of non-hemorrhagic intraoperative complications between the two subgroups.

Phacoemulsication alone group			
	Maintenance subgroup	Discontinuation subgroup	P
No.of patients (no. of eyes)	258 (403)	274 (421)	-
Age	74.3±7.7 (46 – 88)	73.7±8.4 (48 – 90)	0.4
Gender	135 females, 122 males	147 females, 127 males	0.8
Best-corrected visual acuity	0.313 (20/64.0) (0.01 – 0.8)	0.326 (20/61.3) (0.01 – 0.8)	-
LogMAR ± SD	0.505 ± 0.391	0.486 ± 0.393	0.5
Nuclear sclerosis	2.4 ± 0.8 (1 - 5)	2.3 ± 0.8 (1 - 5)	0.1
Administration			
Warfarin only	51 (83)	61 (96)	0.7
Aspirin only	194 (299)	197 (302)	
Both	13 (21)	16 (23)	
PT-INR	1.89±0.56 (1.17-3.54)	1.95±0.58 (1.20-3.47)	0.4
Duration of warfarin administration	4.2±2.1 (1 -14)	4.5±1.8 (2-12)	0.3

Combined phacoemulsication and vitrectomy group			
	Maintenance group	Discontinuation group	P
No.of patients (No. of eyes)	36 (36)	33 (33)	
Age	63.8±7.1 (51 – 78)	64.6±7.2 (52– 76)	0.6
Gender	23 females, 13 males	20 females, 13 males	0.8
Epiretinal membrane	22	19	0.8
Macular hole	14	14	
Best-corrected visual acuity	0.290 (20/68.9) (0.08-0.5)	0.311 (20/64.1) (0.1-0.6)	-
LogMAR ± SD	0.537 ± 0.216	0.506 ± 0.193	0.5
Nuclear sclerosis	2.2 ± 0.6 (1 - 4)	2.1 ± 0.7 (1 - 3)	0.5
Administration			
Warfarin only	7	8	0.7
Aspirin only	26	22	
Both	3	3	
PT-INR	1.89±0.57 (1.31-3.14)	2.23±0.66 (1.38-3.46)	0.0249
Duration of warfarin administration	4.1±1.7 (2-8)	4.4±1.6 (2-7)	0.5

LogMAR ± SD: Log of the minimum angle of resolution ± Standard Deviation
PT-INR: prothrombin time-international normalized ratio

Table 2. Demographics of Patients

Combined phacoemulsification and vitrectomy group: Hyphema, apparent or microscopic, was seen on the first postoperative day in 15 eyes (41.7%) in the maintenance subgroup and in 3 eyes (45.5%) in the discontinuation subgroup (P = 0.6). Minor postoperative vitreous and retinal hemorrhage was found in 3 eyes (7.7%) and 6 eyes (15.4%) in the maintenance subgroup and in 2 eyes (5.6%) and 8 eyes (22.2%) in the discontinuation subgroup, respectively (vitreous hemorrhage: P = 0.3; retinal hemorrhage: P = 0.3) (Table 3). Within 1 month of the surgical procedure, bleeding was not found without affecting the visual acuity. There was no vitreous or choroidal/suprachoroidal hemorrhage found in either of the two subgroups. No significant difference was found in non-hemorrhagic complications between the two subgroups (Table 3).

Phacoemulsification alone group			
	Maintenance group	Discontinuation group	P
	403 eyes	421 eyes	
Systemic complications			
Cerebral events	0 (0.0%)	0 (0.0%)	-
Cardiovascular events	0 (0.0%)	0 (0.0%)	-
Hemorrhagic complications			
Subconjunctival hemorrhage	87 (21.6%)	46 (10.9%)	< 0.0001
Hyphema (> 1mm)	0 (0.0%)	0 (0.0%)	-
Microscopic hyphema	26 (6.5%)	11 (2.6%)	0.0078
Vitreous hemorrhage	0 (0.0%)	0 (0.0%)	-
Retinal hemorrhage	6 (1.4%)	3 (0.7%)	0.3
Choroidal/suprachoridal hemorrhage	0 (0.0%)	0 (0.0%)	-
Non-hemorrhagic complications			
Intraoperative complications			
Early perforation	7 (1.7%)	9 (1.1%)	0.7
CCC tear	13 (4.0 %)	18 (4.3%)	0.4
Posterior capsule rupture	5 (1.2%)	7 (1.7%)	0.6
Vitreous loss	2 (0.4%)	3 (0.3%)	0.7
Nucleus drop	0 (0.0%)	0 (0.0%)	-
Early postoperative complications			
Hypotony	0 (0.0%)	0 (0.0%)	-
IOP spike	16 (3.9%)	13 (3.1%)	0.5
Corneal edema	8 (2.0%)	10 (2.4%)	0.7
Shallow/flat anterior chamber	0 (0.0%)	0 (0.0%)	-
Distorted pupil	2 (0.0%)	3 (0.0%)	0.7
IOL dislocation	0 (0.0%)	0 (0.0%)	-
Vitreous herniation	0 (0.0%)	0 (0.0%)	-
Retinal detachment	0 (0.0%)	0 (0.0%)	-
Endophthalmitis	0 (0.0%)	0 (0.0%)	-

Combined phacoemulsification and vitrectomy group			
	Maintenance group	Discontinuation group	P
	36 eyes	33 eyes	
Systemic complications			
Cerebral events	0 (0.0%)	0 (0.0%)	
Cardiovascular events	0 (0.0%)	0 (0.0%)	

Hemorrhagic complications			
Hyphema (> 1mm)	1 (2.8%)	0 (0.0%)	0.3
Microscopic hyphema	14 (38.9%)	15 (45.5%)	0.6
Vitreous hemorrhage	3 (7.7%)	2 (5.6%)	0.3
Retinal hemorrhage	6 (15.4%)	8 (22.2%)	0.3
Choroidal/suprachoridal hemorrhage	0 (0.0%)	0 (0.0%)	-
Non-hemorrhagic complications			
Intraoperative complications			
Early perforation	0 (0.0%)	0 (0.0%)	-
CCC tear	2 (5.6%)	1 (3.0%)	0.6
Posterior capsule rupture	0 (0.0%)	0 (0.0%)	-
Vitreous loss	0 (0.0%)	0 (0.0%)	-
Early postoperative complications			
Hypotony	0 (0.0%)	0 (0.0%)	-
IOP spike	4 (11.1%)	2 (6.1%)	0.4
Corneal edema	0 (0.0%)	0 (0.0%)	-
Shallow/flat anterior chamber	0 (0.0%)	0 (0.0%)	-
Distorted pupil	0 (0.0%)	0 (0.0%)	-
IOL dislocation	0 (0.0%)	0 (0.0%)	-
Retinal detachment	1 (2.8%)	0 (0.0%)	0.3
Endophthalmitis	0 (0.0%)	0 (0.0%)	-

Table 3. Incidence of hemorrhagic and non-hemorrhagic complications in the discontinuation and maintenance group

3.2 Visual acuity change

Phacoemulsication alone group: Mean BCVA before and at 1 month postoperative were 0.312 and 0.917 in the maintenance subgroup and 0.326 and 0.925 in the discontinuation subgroup, respectively (Table 4). The mean changes for the LogMAR BCVA during the 1-month postoperative period were -0.467 ± 0.339 in the maintenance subgroup and -0.453 ± 0.342 in the discontinuation subgroup. These differences were not significant between the two subgroups (P = 0.6) (Table 4).

Combined phacoemulsification and vitrectomy group: In patients undergoing surgery for the treatment of epiretinal membrane, mean BCVA before and at 6 months postoperative were 0.337 and 0.757 in the maintenance subgroup and 0.359 and 0.737 in the discontinuation subgroup, respectively (Table 4). The mean changes for the LogMAR BCVA during the 1-month postoperative period were -0.351 ± 0.173 in the maintenance subgroup and -0.312 ± 0.164 in the discontinuation subgroup (P = 0.5) (Table 4). In patients with macular hole, all patients had macular hole closure in the two subgroups. Mean BCVA before and at 6 months postoperative were 0.229 and 0.774 in the maintenance subgroup and 0.257 and 0.796 in the discontinuation subgroup, respectively (Table 4). The mean changes for the LogMAR BCVA during the 6-month postoperative period were -0.528 ± 0.195 in the maintenance subgroup and -0.491 ± 0.216 in the discontinuation subgroup (P = 0.6) (Table 4).

Phacoemulsification alone group			
	Maintenance group	Discontinuation group	
No.of eyes	403	421	
Baseline			
BCVA	0.312 (20/64.0)	0.326 (20/63.3)	-
Mean (LogMAR) ± SD	0.505±0.391	0.486±0.393	0.45
1day			
BCVA	0.849 (20/23.6)	0.853 (20/23.4)	-
Mean (LogMAR) ± SD	0.071±0.187	0.069±0.181	0.9
Change of LogMAR	-0.434±0.325	-0.415±0.328	0.4
1 week			
BCVA	0.899 (20/22.3)	0.903 (20/22.1)	-
Mean (LogMAR) ± SD	0.047±0.163	0.044±0.157	0.8
Change of LogMAR	-0.459±0.333	-0.442±0.340	0.5
1 month			
BCVA	0.917 (20/21.8)	0.925 (20/21.6)	-
Mean (LogMAR) ± SD	0.039±0.155	0.034±0.151	0.6
Change of LogMAR	-0.467±0.339	-0.453±0.342	0.6

Table 4. A Change of Best-corrected Visual Acuity

4. Discussion

In patients who maintained warfarin and/or aspirin treatment, no increase was identified in potentially sight-threatening complications in the phacoemulsification group and the combined phacoemulsification and vitrectomy group compared with those who discontinued the treatment. In patients undergoing phacoemulsification alone, the incidence of subconjunctival hemorrhage and microscopic hyphema in the maintenance subgroup was significantly higher compared with the discontinuation subgroup; all subconjunctival hemorrhage and hyphema in both subgroups were self-limiting and spontaneously resolved within one week.

In patients undergoing combined phacoemulsification and vitrectomy, there was no significant difference in hemorrhagic complications between patients with and without interruption of anticoagulant and/or antiplatelet therapy. In patients undergoing cataract surgery alone, several investigators have demonstrated that the incidence of hemorrhagic complications was approximately 9-10% (range 0 to 36.1%, mean 13.0±13.3%) in anticoagulated patients without discontinuation of warfarin. Postoperative hemorrhagic complications typically consisted of mild hyphemae and subconjunctival hemorrhage, all of which were self-limiting and without further clinical consequences. [12-27]. Several studies have compared postoperative bleeding in anticoagulant-treated patients with that of normally coagulated patients. Even patients with normal coagulation undergoing cataract surgery may have postoperative hemorrhage. Patients without warfarin discontinuation have an approximately 3-fold greater risk for postoperative bleeding than normally anticoagulated patients who have cataract surgery [14,21,23-27].

The variance of the incidence of hemorrhagic complications previously reported may result from inconsistency of their definition and the duration and methods of their observation

[12-27]. Hemorrhagic complication rates may have also been influenced by the anesthetic and surgical techniques used. It is difficult to accurately measure risks of local anesthetic blockade in anticoagulated patients since anesthetic techniques varied as studies done after the late 1990s tended towards use of topical or sub-Tenon anesthesia [21-27], whereas, before then, retrobulbar or peribulbar anesthesia had been commonly used [13,15,20,21] Retrobulbar hemorrhage is more frequent even when anticoagulation is discontinued prior to surgery when compared to normally coagulated patients [27]. Prognosis for visual acuity with retrobulbar hemorrhage is generally good, provided an experienced surgeon is present to rapidly decompress the eye. However, sub-Tenon block and topical techniques appear safer still, and acceptable provided both patients and surgeons are satisfied. In the studies after the mid-1990s phacoemulsification was in common use [16,17,21-24,26,27]. Before then, the extracapsular extraction technique, which needed a larger wound and caused greater tissue injury and bleeding than the phacoemulsification technique, had been employed. [12-15,17,20]. However, hemorrhagic complication rates did not appear to differ based on surgical technique.

Benzimra et al. showed a significant increase in hemorrhagic and non-hemorrhagic complications without discontinuation of continuous antiplatelet medications [27], whereas other studies have demonstrated no increase [28-30]. These complications had no significant effect on visual improvement [27-30].

In this study, patients undergoing vitreous surgery with epiretinal and macular hole in combination with phacoemulsification were studied. Even normally coagulated patients undergoing vitrectomy have a risk of hemorrhagic complications from other diseases, including retinal detachment and proliferative diabetic retinopathy, which were hence excluded from this study. In patients without interruption of anticoagulant and/or antiplatelet medications, there were 14 microscopic hyphema and 6 retinal hemorrhages, whereas 15 microscopic hyphema and 8 retinal hemorrhage were found in patients who discontinued the medications. Most of the retinal hemorrhages occurred during the peeling of the epiretinal and internal limiting membranes, and hyphema developed from a postoperative prone position in patients who underwent macular hole surgery. Several investigators demonstrated the incidence of hemorrhagic complications in vitrectomy was less than 1% [31-35], the vast majority of which was transient vitreous hemorrhage, which was self-limiting and without any significant effect on visual improvement. There was only one potentially serious subretinal hemorrhage, which required retinotomy, in patients on anticoagulation [34]. Therefore, there has been no reported evidence that perioperative continuation of anticoagulant therapy may a deleterious impact on cataract surgery and postoperative visual improvement related to either continuation of anticoagulation or hemorrhagic complications [1-9].

In this study, no systemic complications were noted in patients with and without anticoagulant and antiplatelet therapy in the phacoemulsication group and combined phacoemulsication and vitrectomy group. Many believe that there may be minimal risk of thromboembolism in patients whose anticoagulant therapy is discontinued for surgery [36]. Less than a half of reported hospitals continued antiplatelet or anticoagulant regimen at the time of surgery in Japan [37], although the majority of the Canadian Society of Cataract and Refractive Surgery members reported that they did not stop either warfarin or aspirin for cataract surgery during the perioperative period [38]. Current evidence suggests that warfarin therapy significantly improves prognosis in patients with atrial fibrillation with coexisting cerebrovascular disease, and those with non-tissue prosthetic heart valves [1].

Attempted cessation and recommencement of warfarin therapy may not only reverse anticoagulation for unpredictable periods of time but may also expose patients to a transient yet dangerous hypercoagulable state [39,40]. The discontinuation of warfarin does not prevent thromboembolism. There have been several documented cases of serious embolic complications, including deaths, after discontinuing warfarin therapy. Cosgriff reported that thromboembolisms occurred in14 of 17 patients (71% of cases) of dental extractions whose warfarin therapy was discontinued [41]. In 542 documented cases of discontinuing anticoagulant therapy for dental procedures, five cases (0.9%) had serious embolic complications, including four deaths [42]. Another study showed that discontinuation of anticoagulant therapy did not increase the incidence of thromboemobolitic events, but caused it to become serious and to increase the morbidity once the events occur [1]. However, in patients with cataract surgery, there was one (2.4%) thromboembolic complication in 36 cases of discontinuing anticoagulant treatment [14]. There were none (0%) in 208 patients discontinuing anticoagulant therapy whereas two thromboembolisms (0.4%) were reported in 524 anticoagulated patients and 15 thromboembolisms (0.08%) in 18,215 normally coagulated patients [21].

This study has important limitations. The study design was non-randomized, and the sample size of this study was relatively small and therefore not powered to detect small differences. Small sample size also precluded an assessment of safety. A large-scale randomized study is required to assess the safety of continuous anticoagulant and antiplatelet treatment associated with phacoemulsification alone and in combination with vitrectomy.

In cataract surgery blood vessels likely to cause persistent hemorrhage are unlikely to be encountered [6]. Although there is a theoretical risk of hemorrhagic complications after cataract surgery in patients at therapeutic levels of anticoagulation, the risk may be greatly outweighed by the risk and morbidity of thromboembolism after discontinuation of anticoagulant therapy [2-9]. There are several documented cases of serious thromboembolic complications, including deaths, in patients after discontinuation of anticoagulant therapy [41,42]. Patients receiving anticoagulant therapy who undergo cataract surgery have been reported to have more hemorrhagic complications than patients with normal coagulation. The vast majority of these complications are self-limiting and without significant effect on visual improvement. Ophthalmologists and physicians should collaborate closely in treating their patients who are taking anticoagulants, especially to make sure that the patient's INR is within the therapeutic range before cataract surgery [1-9]. Good surgical and anesthetic techniques and local measure, including cautery, to control bleeding are also important in all patients undergoing intraocular surgery, especially those receiving continuous anticoagulant and antiplatelet medications [3-9,23].

Although the sample size in each group was small, the current study demonstrated that (1) patients undergoing cataract surgery alone who maintained warfarin and/or aspirin experienced a significantly higher incidence of subconjunctival hemorrhage and hyphema compared with those who discontinued them; and (2) there was no significant difference in the incidence of intraoperative and postoperative complications and visual improvement between patients with and without interruption of anticoagulant and antiplatelet medications in patients undergoing cataract surgery alone and in combination with vitrectomy. Future study of a large population is needed to verify these observations. However, this information may be clinically valuable when treating patients with cataract and long-term administration of anticoagulant or antiplatelet medication.

5. References

[1] Hirsh J, Fuster V, Ansell J, Halperin JL. American Heart Association/American College of Cardiology Foundation guide to warfarin therapy. Circulation. 2003;107:1692–1711.

[2] Douketis JD. Perioperative anticoagulation management in patients who are receiving oral anticoagulant therapy: a practical guide for clinicians. Thromb Res. 2002;108:3–13.

[3] Dunn AS, Turpie AG. Perioperative management of patients receiving oral anticoagulants: a systematic review. Arch Intern Med 2003;163:901-8.

[4] Jafri SM. Periprocedural thromboprophylaxis in patients receiving chronic anticoagulation therapy. Am Heart J 2004;147:3-15.

[5] Douketis JD, Berger PB, Dunn AS, et al. The perioperative management of antithrombotic therapy: American College of Chest Physicians Evidence-Based Clinical Practice Guidelines (8th Edition). Chest 2008;133(6 Suppl):299S-339S.

[6] Michael J. Wahl. Dental Surgery in Anticoagulated Patients. Arch Intern Med. 1998;158:1911-1916.

[7] Hodge W, Horsley T, Albiani D, Baryla J, Belliveau M, Burhmann R, et al. The consequences of waiting for cataract surgery: a systematic review. Can Med Assoc J. 2007;176:1285–1290.

[8] Dunn AS, Turpie AGG. Perioperative management of patients receiving oral anticoagulants: a systematic review. Arch Intern Med. 2003;163:901–908.

[9] Jamula E, Anderson J, Douketis JD. Safety of continuing warfarin therapy during cataract surgery: A systematic review and meta-analysis. Thromb Res 2009;124:292-299.

[10] Emery JM, Little HY. Phacoemulsification and aspiration of cataract: Surgical techniques, complications and results. CY Mosby, St Louis, pp45-48, 1979.

[11] Teehasaenee C, Ritch R. The use of PhEA 34c in trabeculectomy. Ophthalmology 1986;93:487-490.

[12] McMahan LB. Anticoagulants and cataract surgery. J Cataract Refract Surg. 1988;14:569–571.

[13] Hall DL, Steen WH, Drummond JW, Byrd WA. Anticoagulants and cataract surgery. Ophthalmic Surg.1988;19:221–222.

[14] Gainey SP, Robertson DM, Fay W, Ilstrup D. Ocular surgery on patients receiving long-term warfarin therapy. Am J Ophthalmol. 1989;108:142–146.

[15] Robinson GA, Nylander A. Warfarin and cataract extraction. Br J Ophthalmol. 1989;73:702–703.

[16] Hall DL. Cataract surgery and anticoagulants. J La State Med Soc. 1996;148(10):431–433.

[17] Saito AK, Saito A, Taniguchi H, Amemiya T. Anticoagulation therapy and ocular surgery. Ophthal Surg Lasers 1998;29:909-15.

[18] Morris A, Elder MJ. Warfarin therapy and cataract surgery. Clin Experiment Ophthalmol. 2000;28:419-22.

[19] Rotenstreich Y, Rubowitz A, Segev F, et al. Effect of warfarin therapy on bleeding during cataract surgery. J Cataract Refract Surg. 2001;27:1344-6.

[20] McCormack P, Simcock PR, Tullo AB. Management of the anticoagulated patient for ophthalmic surgery. Eye. 1993;7:749-50.

[21] Katz J, Feldman MA, Bass EB, et al. Risks and benefits of anticoagulant and antiplatelet medication use before cataract surgery. Ophthalmology. 2003;110:1784–1788.

[22] Wirbelauer C, Weller A, Haberle H, Pham DT. Cataract surgery under topical anesthesia with oral anticoagulants. Klin Monatsbl Augenheilkd. 2004;221:749–752.

[23] Jonas JB, Pakdman B, Sauder G. Cataract surgery under systemic anticoagulant therapy with coumarin. Eur J Ophthalmol. 2006;16:30–32.

[24] Kumar N, Jivan S, Thomas P, McClure H. Sub-Tenon's anesthesia with aspirin, warfarin, and clopidogrel. J Cataract Refract Surg. 2006;32:1022–1025.

[25] Gauba V, Saleh GM, Watson K, Chung A. Sub-tenon anaesthesia: Reduction in subconjunctival haemorrhage with controlled bipolar conjunctival cautery. Eye. 2007;21:1387–1390.

[26] Barequet IS, Sachs D, Priel A, et al. Phacoemulsification of cataract in patients receiving Coumadin therapy: Ocular and hematologic risk assessment. Am J Ophthalmol. 2007;144(5):719–723.

[27] Benzimra JD, Johnston RL, Jaycock P, et al. The Cataract National Dataset electronic multicentre audit of 55 567 operations: antiplatelet and anticoagulant medications. Eye 2008;23:10-16.

[28] Assia EI, Raskin T, Kaiserman I, Rotenstreich Y, Segev F. Effect of aspirin intake on bleeding during cataract surgery. J Cataract Refract Surg.1998;24:1243-6.

[29] Carter K, Miller KM. Phacoemulsification and lens implantation in patients treated with aspirin or warfarin. J Cataract Refract Surg. 1998;24:1361-4.

[30] Kobayashi H. Evaluation of the need to discontinue antiplatelet and anticoagulant medications before cataract surgery. J Cataract Refract Surg. 2010;36:1344-6.

[31] Dayani PN, Grand MG. Maintenance of warfarin anticoagulation for patients undergoing vitreoretinal surgery. Trans Am Ophthalmol Soc. 2006;104:149-60.

[32] Dayani PN, Grand MG. Maintenance of warfarin anticoagulation for patients undergoing vitreoretinal surgery. Arch Ophthalmol. 2006;124:1558-65.

[33] Fu AD, McDonald HR, Williams DF, Cantrill HL, Ryan EH Jr, Johnson RN, Ai E, Jumper JM. Anticoagulation with warfarin in vitreoretinal surgery. Retina. 2007;27:290-5.

[34] Chauvaud D. Anticoagulation and vitreoretinal surgery. Bull Acad Natl Med. 2007;191:879-84.

[35] Mason JO 3rd, Gupta SR, Compton CJ. Comparison of hemorrhagic complications of warfarin and clopidogrel bisulfate in 25-gauge vitrectomy versus a control group. Arch Ophthalmol 2011;118:543-7.

[36] Tinker JH, Tarhan S. Discontinuing anticoagulant therapy in surgical patients with cardiac valve prostheses: observations in 180 operations. JAMA.1978;239:738-739.

[37] Yasaka M, Okada Y, Inoue T, et al. Questionnaire survey to investigate correspondence of medical doctors and dentists in Japan for antithrombotic therapy at surgeries or biopsy. Brain Nerve 2007;59:871-6.

[38] Ong-Tone L, Paluck EC, Hart-Mitchell RD. Perioperative use of warfarin and aspirin in cataract surgery by Canadian Society of Cataract and Refractive Surgery members: survey. Cataract Refract Surg. 2005;31:991-6.

[39] Grip L, Blomback M, Schulman S. Hypercoagulable state and thromboembolism following warfarin withdrawal in post-myocardial infarction patients. Eur Heart J. 1991;12:1225-1233.

[40] Michaels L, Beamish RE. Relapses of thromboembolic disease after discontinued anticoagulant therapy: a comparison of the incidence after abrupt and after gradual termination of treatment. Am J Cardiol. 1967;20:670-673.
[41] Cosgriff SW. Chronic anticoagulant therapy in recurrent embolism of cardiac origin. Ann Intern Med. 1953;38:278-287.
[42] Akbarian M, Austen WG, Yurchak PM, Scannell JG. Thromboembolic complications of prosthetic cardiac valves. Circulation. 1968;37:826-831.

Section 2

Operative Surgery and the History of Cataract Surgery

6

The History of Cataract Surgery

F.J. Ascaso[1] and V. Huerva[2]
[1]*University of Zaragoza,*
[2]*University of Lleida,*
Spain

1. Introduction

Cataracts were undoubtedly very common in antiquity (Aruta et al., 2009; Bernscherer, 2001; Muhkopadhyay & Sharma, 1992; Shugar, 1997). The current word *cataract*, which means both an opacity of the lens and a torrent of water, comes from the Greek word *υπόχυσις* (kataráktēs) meaning the fall of water. The Latins called it *suffusio*, an extravasation and coagulation of humors behind the iris; and the Arabas, *white water* (Ascaso & Cristóbal, 2001). The old Egyptian name for the lens is not yet known and the medical literature does not let us conclude that old Egyptians were able to diagnose cataracts (Ghalioungui, 1973). The only possible reference to cataract is the *ꜥh.t* disease mentioned in the Ebers Papyrus (about 1525 B.C.). Ebbel translated the *ꜥh.t* disease as cataract (Ebbel, 1937). However, other distinguished linguistists interpreted it as a discharge or accumulation of water in the eyes (Hirschberg, 1899; Deines et al., 1958; Andersen, 1997). According to Ebers Papyrus, the old Egyptians tried to treat cases of *ꜥh.t* disease by eye ointments and magic spells. It is hardly believable that such remedies had any effect on the cataract, since the extraction of the lens is the only effective measure.

2. Cataract surgery in ancient cultures: *"Couching"* technique

The oldest documented case of cataract throughout history was reported in a famous and small statue from the 5th dynasty (about 2457-2467 B.C.) contained in the Egyptian Museum in Cairo, Egypt. This statue, discovered in 1860 in Saqqāra, dates from the Old Kingdom and represents a male figure, the priest reader Ka-āper, also called Cheikh el-Beled (Figure 1A).
We found an obvious white pupillary reflex in the left eye (Figure 1B). This finding, in an aged man, probably indicates a mature cataract; moreover, it does not appear in the right eye. We suggested that the author carefully inspected a man with cataract and accurately reproduced the physical sign in wood (Ascaso & Cristóbal, 2001). This fact confirms that old Egyptian knew the disease. By analysis of ancient surgical instruments it is possible to define the history of medical specialties, and acquaint the evolution of specific surgical techniques and operations through the centuries (Aruta et al., 2009). Scientists have often discussed whether cataract was firstly operated in Ancient Egypt (Bernscherer, 2001). This hypothesis seems plausible (Ascaso et al., 2009). Thus, a wall painting in the tomb of the master builder Ipwy at Thebes (about 1200 B.C.) reveals an oculist treating the eye of a craftsman. Because of the length of the instrument, the scene might also be interpreted as a cataract surgery by couching of the lens into the vitreous cavity (Figure 2).

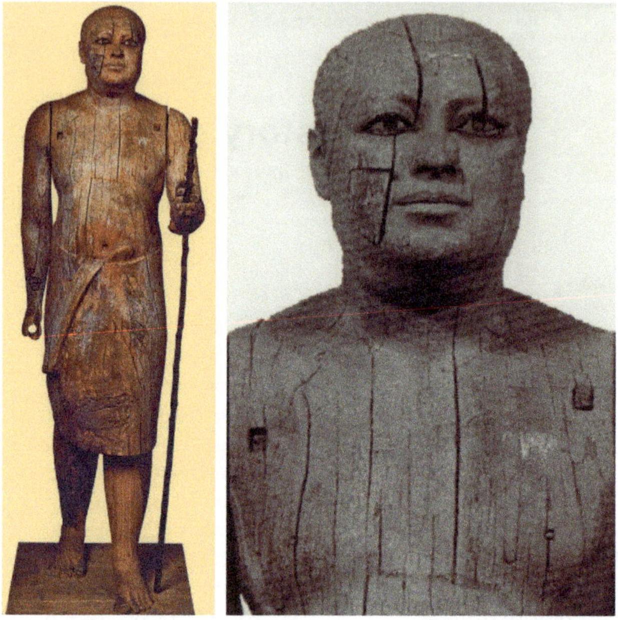

A B

Fig. 1. A: Ka-aper´s statue *(Egyptian Museum, Cairo, Egypt)*. B: Detail of the white pupillary reflex in the left eye indicating a mature cataract *(taken from J Cataract Refract Surg 2001;27(11):1714-5)*

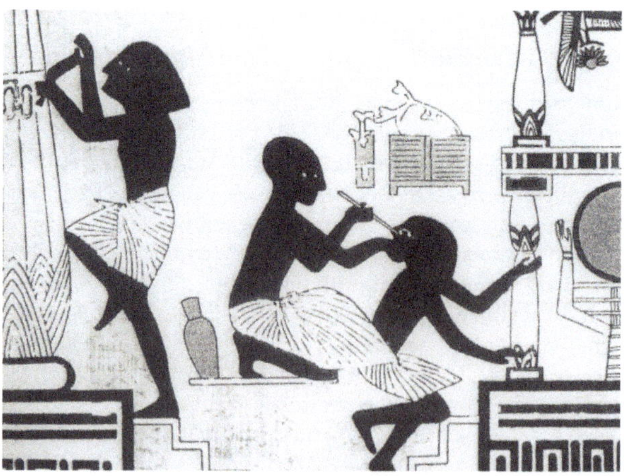

Fig. 2. A wall painting in the tomb of the master builder Ipwy at Thebes (about 1200 B.C.). An oculist treats the eye of a workman. *(Modern copy of the painting at the entrance to the Cornea Bank at Ain Sham´s University Hospital, Cairo, Egypt).*

The temple of Kom Ombo, constructed by Tutmes III (1479-1425 B.C.), shows a relief on the internal facade of the second wall, which depicts a series of surgical instruments carved in stone, including several needles (Figure 3).

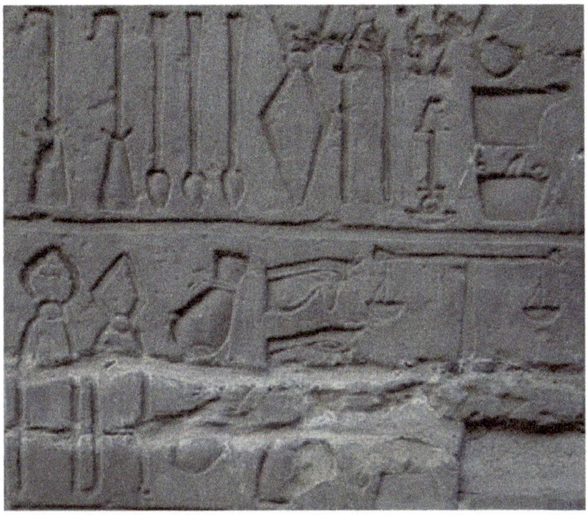

Fig. 3. Detail from the relief on the internal facade of the second wall in the temple of Kom Ombo, Egypt.

National Museums in Liverpool, England, contain a series of ancient cooper needles having neither hooks nor eyes. They were found in 1900 by Flinders Petrie in the tomb of King Khasekhemwy (c. 2700 B.C.), in the Royal Necropolis at Abydos, Upper Egypt (Petrie et al., 1900) (Figure 4).

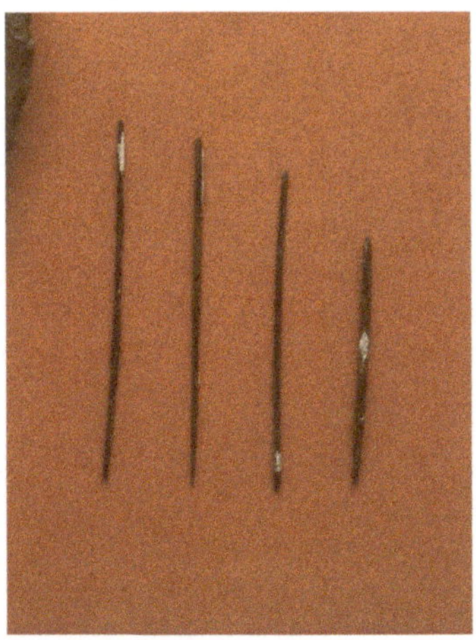

Fig. 4. A series of cooper needles from the tomb of King Khasekhemwy at Abydos, Egypt (c. 2700 B.C.). *(Courtesy by National Museums Liverpool, England).*

In 2001, near the Saqqara pyramid complex (built *c.* 2630 BC), about 19 miles south of Cairo, archaeologists made a fascinating discovery: the oldest-known tomb of a pharaonic surgeon, dating back more than 4000 years. This was the tomb of Skar, the chief physician of one of Egypt's Fifth Dinasty rulers. In the writing on its walls was a hint that surgery had actually been practised in ancient Egypt, the first hard evidence of it being performed as early as this. It contained about 30 bronze surgical tools used by the ancient Egyptian doctor, the oldest ever found, including several needles. The above mentioned findings confirm the high surgical skill level achieved, and the possibility that old Egyptian and Babylonian used, before Indian surgeons, the couching operation for dislodging the cataract away from the pupil. The surgeon used a lancet to push the clouded lens backward into the vitreous body of the eye. The relative simplicity of this technique was probably the major reason why it was the procedure of choice through thousands of years until 1748, when the French doctor Daviel performed the first known cataract extraction (Floyd, 1994).

Cataract surgery by "couching" (lens depression) was, without a doubt, one of the oldest surgical procedures. This technique involved using a sharp instrument to push the cloudy lens to the bottom of the eye. Perhaps this procedure is that which is mentioned in the articles of the Code of Hammurabi (Cotallo & Esteban, 2008; Ascaso et al., 2011). Hammurabi (ca. 1792-1750 BC), the greatest ruler in the first Babylonian dynasty became king of all Mesopotamia, the land what is today known as Iraq. He established the greatness of Babylon, transforming a small Mesopotamian city-state into the world's first metropolis (Horne, 2010). His long reign was for about 40 years, extending his empire northward from the Persian Gulf through the Tigris and Euphrates river valleys and westward to the coast of the Mediterranean Sea. Although he was a successful military leader and administrator, Hammurabi is primarily remembered for his celebrated codification of the laws governing Babylonian life called the Code of Hammurabi (*Codex Hammurabi*) (Bartz & König, 2005). This primitive form of what would be now known as a constitution began and ended with addresses to the gods, and regulated in clear and definite strokes the organization of society. The ancient law code, based on older Sumerian codes, was engraved on a large upright black stone monument which was set in front of one of the major temples, where it could be seen by the public. One nearly complete example of the Code survives today, inscribed on an eight feet high basalt stele in the Akkadian language in the cuneiform script (Hammu, 2010; Graves & Graves, 2010). This noted stone was discovered in 1901 by the Egyptologist Gustav Jéquier, not in Babylon, but in a city of the Persian mountains- in what is now Khūzestān (ancient Elam) in the southwest of Iran, to which some later conqueror must have carried it in triumph in the 12th century BC (Bartz & König, 2005). It is currently on display at the Louvre Museum in Paris, France (Hooker, 1996) (Figure 5).

The Code of Hammurabi contains 282 laws, each usually no more than a sentence or two. Thus, the law number 196 says: *"If a man put out the eye of another man, his eye shall be put out"*. There, we can see where the Hebrews learned their law of "*an eye for an eye*". Medical information included in King Hammurabi´s Code gives a picture of a highly organized society where medical care was regulated. Moreover, it contained a number of sections related to the eye which let to understand the state of ophthalmological knowledge in the Ancient River Cultures (Bieganowski, 2003). So, the code shows the first known sliding fee schedule for services, where the amounts are specified according to how prosperous the patient was. *"The surgeon who has successfully operated on a patrician´s eye with a bronze lancet, shall charge 10 shekels of silver. The fee will be only five shekels and two shekels in the case of a plebeian and owned slave, respectively"*. Five shekels (Jewish silver coin) was equivalent to the yearly rent of a good type of house and represented 150 times the daily wage of a workman (1/30 shekel) (Albert, 1996). However, Hammurabi´s Code discouraged the pursuit of a career in Ophthalmology specifying the penalties for "medical malpractice". They varied with the economic status of the patient: *"If a doctor operates (...) on the eye of a* patrician *who loses his eye in consequence, his hands shall be cut off". In the case of a slave, if the surgeon has caused his death the penalty was to replace him by another, and if he made the slave lose his eye, he shall pay half his value"* (Fishman, 1999). At the dawn of civilization, about 4,000 years ago, the Codex Hammurabi already prescribed the concepts of managed care for the practice of medicine. Tempered by time, its managed care mandates can still be considered the genesis of the current concepts of managed care (Spiegel, 1999).

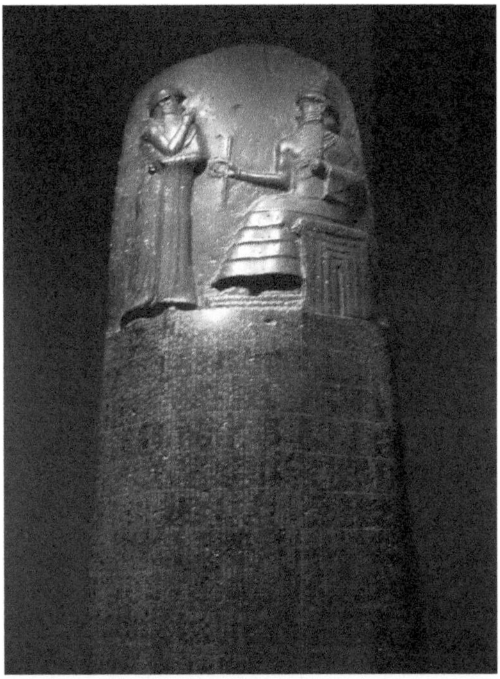

Fig. 5. Detail of the stela inscribed with Hammurabi´s code, showing the king before the Mesopotamian Sun God Shamash; bas-relief from Susa, ancient Elam (Khūzestān, southwest of Iran), 18th century BC *(Courtesy of the Louvre Museum, Paris, France).*

However, there are some doubts about the real meaning of the term "na-kap-tu", which someone translated as "cloud", and other directly as "waterfall." It is even possible that these articles of the Code of Hammurabi made some reference to treatment of corneal pathology instead of cataract (Gorin, 1982).

So, couching for cataract is one of the most ancient surgical procedures; however, Maharshi Sushruta, an ancient Indian surgeon, first described the procedure in "Sushruta Samhita, Uttar Tantra", an Indian medical treatise (800 B.C.) (Duke-Elder, 1969; Chan, 2010) (Figure 6).

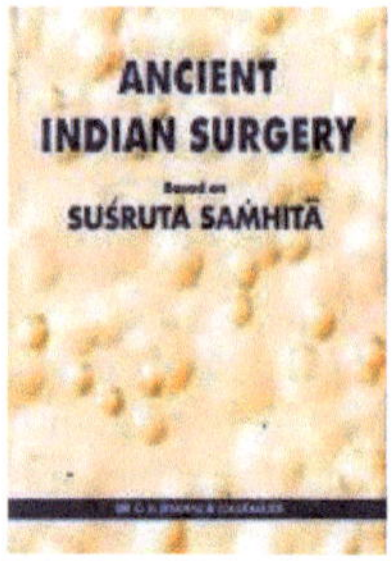

Fig. 6. Sushruta Samhita, Uttar Tantra, an Indian medical treatise (800 B.C.)

This text describes an operation called "couching", in which a curved needle was used to push the lens into the rear of the eye and out of the field of vision. The eye would later be soaked with warm clarified butter and then bandaged. Sushruta claimed success with this method but cautioned that this procedure should only be performed when absolutely necessary. This method may have been brought to the West by Greek travelers from India and the Middle East (Wales, 2010). The removal of cataract by surgery was also introduced into China from India (Lade & Svovboda, 2000). The procedure, also known as *jin pi shu* in Mandarin, was introduced to China via the Silk Road during the late West Han Dynasty (206 B.C.-9 A.C), and it spread throughout China during the Tang Dynasty (618-907 A.C.). As the procedure was combined with the Chinese concept of acupuncture, *jin pi shu* was integrated into Chinese medical practice until the founding of the Republic of China in 1911 (Chan, 2010).

In the Western world, bronze instruments that could have been used for cataract surgery have been found in excavations in Babylonia, Greece, and Egypt. The first references to cataract and its treatment in the West are found in 29 B.C. in *De Medicinae*, the work of the Latin encyclopedist Aulus Cornelius Celsus (Figure 7), which also describes the couching operation (Wales, 2010)

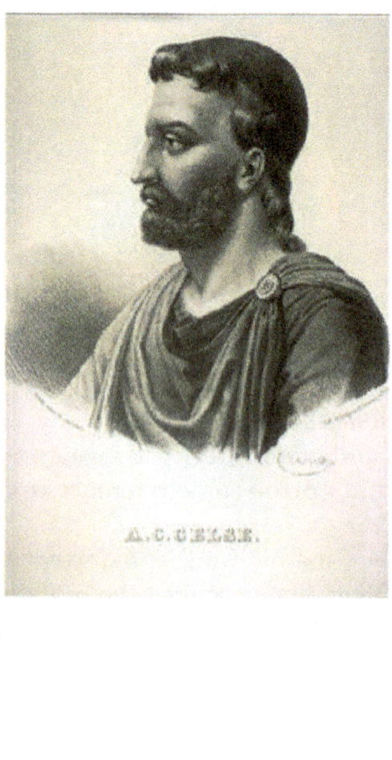

Fig. 7. Aulus Cornelius Celsus

"Couching" technique continued to be used throughout the Middle Ages and is still used in some parts of Africa and in Yemen (Savage-Smith, 2000). However, it was an ineffective and dangerous method of cataract therapy, and often resulted in patients remaining blind or with only partially restored vision.

3. A New revolution: Cataract extraction surgery

Later, *"couching"* technique would be replaced by cataract extraction surgery. The lens could be removed by suction through a hollow instrument. Bronze oral suction instruments that have been unearthed seem to have been used for this method of cataract extraction during the 2nd century A.C. Such a procedure was described by the 10th-century Persian physician Muhammad ibn Zakariya al-Razi, who attributed it to Antyllus, a 2nd-century Greek physician. The procedure "required a large incision in the eye, a hollow needle, and an assistant with an extraordinary lung capacity" (Savage-Smith, 2000). This suction procedure was also described by the Iraqi ophthalmologist Ammar ibn Ali of Mosul, in his *Choice of Eye Diseases*, also written in the 10th century (Savage-Smith, 2000). He presented case histories of its use, claiming to have had success with it on a number of patients. Extracting the lens has the benefit of removing the possibility of the lens migrating back into the field of vision (Finger, 2001). A later variant of the cataract needle in 14th-century Egypt, reported by the oculist Al-Shadhili, used a screw to produce suction. It is not clear, however, how often this method was used as other writers, including Abu al-Qasim al-Zahrawi and Al-Shadhili, showed a lack of experience with this procedure or claimed it was ineffective (Savage-Smith, 2000).

The French ophthalmologist Jacques Daviel (1696–1762) was the first modern European physician to successfully extract cataracts from the eye. He performed the first extracapsular cataract extraction on April 8, 1747. It was the first significant advance in cataract surgery since *couching* was invented. Daviel earned his medical degree from the Medical School of Rouen. He was on the staff of Hospital d'Invalides and became oculist to Louis XV. He died of apoplexy in 1762 while on a trip to Geneva, Switzerland. His technique marked the beginning of the modern era in cataract surgery (Dolezalova, 2005; Obuchowska & Mariak, 2005) (Figure 8).

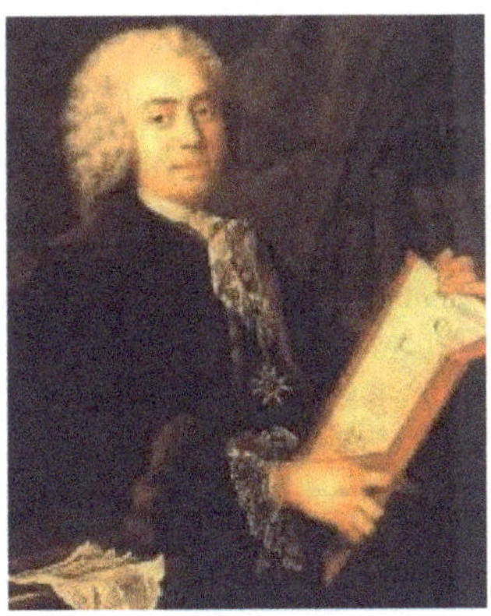

Fig. 8. The French ophthalmologist Jacques Daviel (1696–1762) performed the first extracapsular cataract extraction on April 8, 1747.

The increasing importance of the "extraction" versus traditional "couching" of the lens made both entered in competition. None of the two techniques was free of complications. Thus, in 1750, the famous German composer Johann Sebastian Bach (1685-1750), underwent bilateral cataract surgery by the British surgeon John Taylor (1703-1772), who employed the standard couching. A week later, Bach was reoperated due to cataract recurrence. Nevertheless, the musician was blind and died four months later (Zegers, 2005). Another example is the famous composer George Frideric Händel (1685-1759), who underwent "couching" cataract surgery by the same surgeon and suffered blindness during the last years of his life (Figure 9).

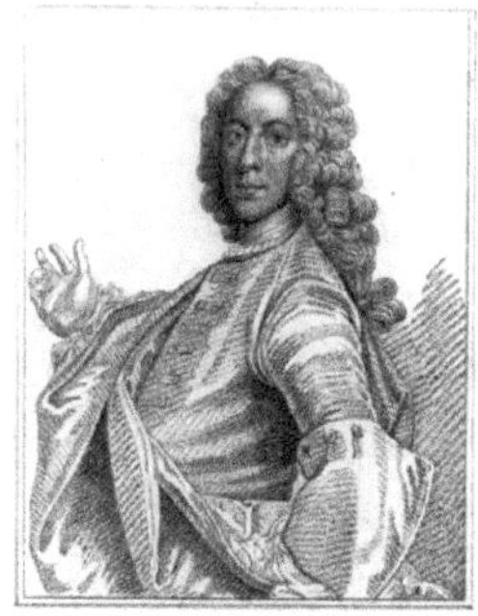

JOANNES TAYLOR, MEDICUS,
In Optica expertissimus.

Fig. 9. John Taylor (1703-1772)

John Taylor was a coucher, or cataract surgeon, who performed removal of cataracts by breaking them up into pieces. His major talent was that of self-promotion, becaming the self-proclaimed personal eye surgeon to King George II, the Pope and number of European royal families. He was as famous for his womanizing as for his surgical skills. Prior to performing each surgical procedure, he would deliver a long, self-promoting speech in an unusual oratorial style. He traveled throughout Europe in a coach painted with images of eyes. His arrival in a town would be publicised several days in advance to draw the largest crowd and he claimed to be able to cure misaligned eyes with his surgical skills. His trick was to make a small incision in the conjunctiva of the eye and cover the other eye. He would then instruct the patient to leave the eye covered for seven days. During this interval he would contrive to leave town and be as far away as possible, when the eye covering was removed. Not even the extraction guaranteed the result. So, in 1775, the poet Goethe witnessed the failure of a bilateral cataract extraction performed in Frankfurt to a distinguished patient, by the famous German surgeon Johann Heinrich Jung-Stilling (1740-1817) (Figure 10).

Albrech von Graefe (1828-1870), who was of tremendous importance in Ophthalmology, died at the early age of 42. By the age of 39 Von Graefe was internationally a unique figure and presided and dominated over the entire 3rd International Congress of Ophthalmology held in Paris in 1867. He read four papers including a classic description of choroid tubercles, but his most important contribution was his exposition of his "modified linear extraction" as a new technique for the operation of cataract. His contributions to Ophthalmology were multiple. His name is eponymously remembered in the von Graefe sign in exophthalmic goitre and the von Graefe extraction knife. Ophthalmology developed through the application of the ophthalmoscope by von Graefe.

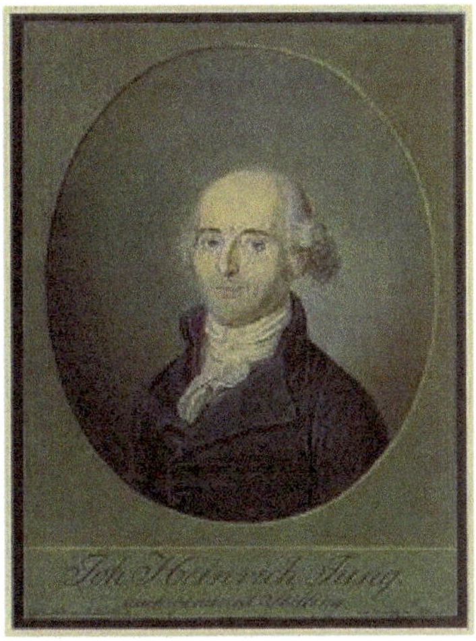

Fig. 10. Johann Heinrich Jung-Stilling (1740-1817)

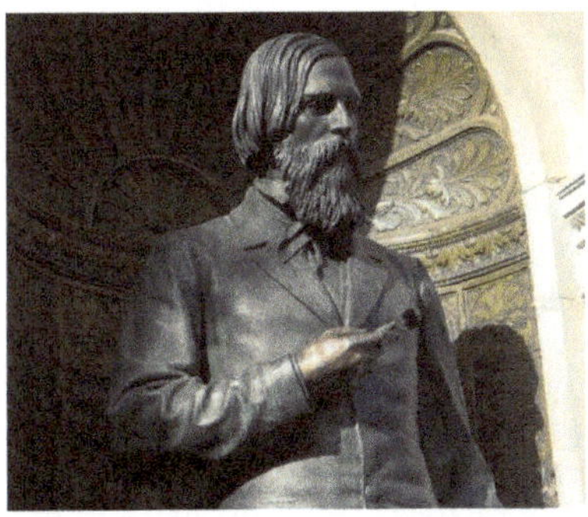

Fig. 11. Monument to the memory of the great German ophthalmologist Albrecht von Graefe, which can be admired on the Charité-Medical University terrain (Berlin)

John Louis Borsch Jr. (1873-1929), was an ophthalmologist from Philadelphia who spent most of his career in France. During his lifetime he was probably best known as the inventor of the first fused bifocal lens, which was marketed very successfully as the Kryptok lens. He may be better known today for performing cataract surgery on Mary Cassatt (1844-1926), the American Impressionist artist, and on James Joyce (1882-1941), the Irish author (Ravin, 2009; Ascaso & Bosch, 2010).

4. The era of Intraocular Lenses (IOLs)

Sir Nicholas Harold Lloyd Ridley (1906, Kibworth Harcourt, Leicestershire - 2001, Salisbury, Wiltshire) was an English ophthalmologist who pioneered artificial intraocular lens transplant surgery for cataract patients. He worked as a surgeon at Moorfield Eye Hospital and St Thomas' Hospital in London, specialising in Ophthalmology (Figure 12).

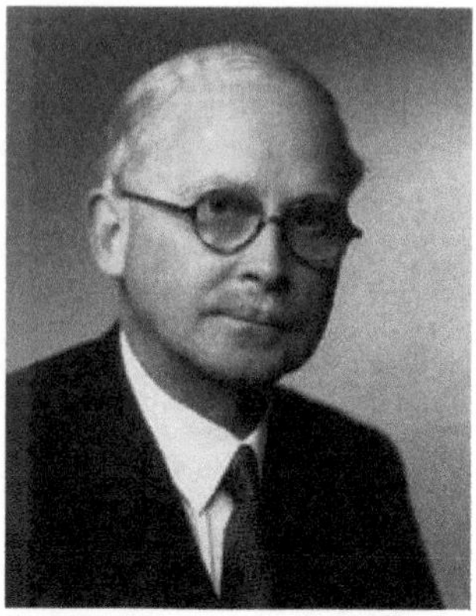

Fig. 12. Harold Ridley, circa 1950, at the time of the first IOL

Dissatisfied with the poor acuity and loss of binocular single vision following unilateral cataract extraction and the poor outcome, particularly in children, with the contact lenses then available, he had early in his career envisaged using an artificial lenticulus. His research was catalysed by the now famous remark of a medical student, that it was a pity that the cataract he had seen extracted could not be replaced by a clear lens. Ridley described his threefold problem. Firstly, he had to find an inert material for what would be an intraocular foreign body. He was inspired in his choice of polymethylmethacrylate (PMMA) which became the gold standard of implant materials. This lack of inflammatory response to glass and plastic intraocular foreign bodies, provided they did not touch the iris, had been observed in the eyes of injured aircrew who survived aerial combats. Ridley thought to use an artificial lens after observing the eye's tolerance of PMMA following eye injuries in Royal Air Force pilots. When the pilots' plastic canopies were struck with bullets, they shattered, leaving small pieces of PMMA in the pilots' eyes. Ridley observed, however, that the pilots' eyes were compatible with them and did not reject the inert PMMA substance. This inspired him to use this material in early intraocular lens (IOL) implantations to correct cases of cataracts (William, 2001). In the 1940s, he introduced the concept of implantation of the intraocular lens which permitted more efficient and comfortable visual rehabilitation possible after cataract surgery. Thus, on 29 November 1949, Harold Ridley successfully implanted the first IOL at St. Thomas' Hospital in London (Figure 13).

The implant was made of an inflexible material called PMMA. It was not until 1950 that he left an artificial lens permanently in place in an eye. The first lens was manufactured by the Rayner company of Brighton & Hove, East Sussex (Spalton, 2009). Despite Ridley's success, the technique did not catch on in the wider ophthalmic community for a number of decades, as many were adverse to the idea of replacing the eye's natural lens with an artificial one. During the years since 1949, however, IOL technology continued to advance. In 1951, Ridley presented his paper *"Intra-Ocular Acrylic Lenses"* at the Oxford Ophthalmological Congress, which was met with significant opposition from Ridley's professional colleagues. Furthermore, Ridley's work was condemned as reckless the following year, at the American Academy meeting in Chicago. In 1952 the first IOL implant was performed in the United States, a Ridley-Rayner lens implanted at the Wills Eye Hospital in Philadelphia. After years of progress, as Ridley and others continued to work to refine the surgery, the first international symposium on intraocular lenses and implants was held in 1966 at the Royal Society of Medicine in London. Through this, the Intraocular Implant Club (IIC) was formed, with Ridley as the first President.

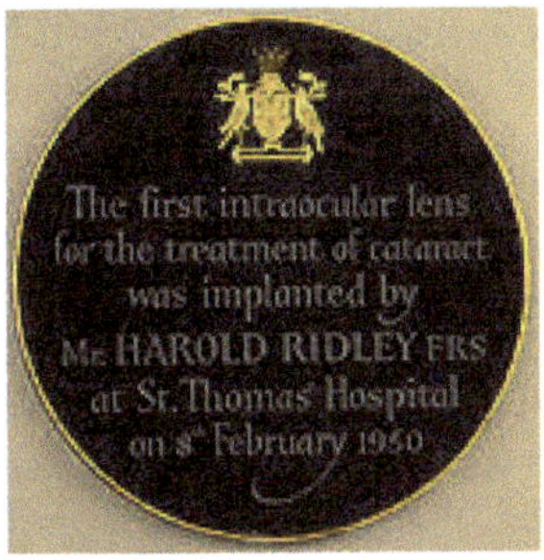
The first intraocular lens
for the treatment of cataract
was implanted by
Mr HAROLD RIDLEY FRS
at St. Thomas' Hospital
on 8th February 1950

Fig. 13. First permanent insertion of intraocular lens, 8 February 1950

Ridley went on to develop comprehensive programmes for cataract surgery with intraocular implants and pioneered this treatment in the face of prolonged strong opposition from the medical community. He worked hard to overcome complications, and had refined the technique by the late 1960s.

Harold Ridley with his pupil Peter Choyce (Figure 14) cofounded the International Intraocular Implant Club in 1966, which was responsible for the gradual acceptance of artificial lens implantation. Peter Choyce developed several models of IOLs, but did not patent the majority of them. The Choyce Mark IX, manufactured by Rayner Intraocular Lenses, became the first US Food and Drug Administration-approved IOL in 1981.

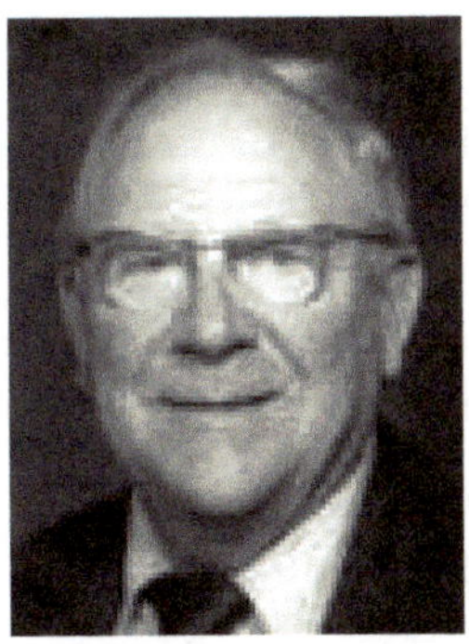

Fig. 14. Peter Choyce

Cataract extraction surgery with IOL implantation is now the commonest type of eye surgery. Ridley retired from NHS hospital service in 1971 and received many awards over the next 29 years. He was a Fellow of the Royal College of Surgeons and a Fellow of the Royal Society. In February 2000, Harold Ridley was knighted by HM Queen Elizabeth II at Buckingham Palace in London. Sir Harold Ridley resided in Wiltshire until his death on 25 May 2001 (Encyclopaedia Britannica, 2010; Apple, 2006).

In so doing he changed the practice of Ophthalmology. Ridley's invention provided not only superior visual rehabilitation to cataract patients for generations to come, but also, without it the IOL has been a major factor in changing the way Ophthalmology is practiced. The fact that lens implantation is by far the commonest and one of the most successful of all eye operations has virtually created a medical-industrial complex. In business terms, the IOL procedure - and its cousin, refractive surgery - have become "products" that can be marketed and sold to a wide base of consumers. In the United States, the economic fallout of these procedures changed ophthalmic practice patterns and accelerated the pace towards managed care (Apple & Sims, 1996).

Now, his discoveries affect virtually all human beings. Over 14 million individuals annually worldwide who have their vision restored with the Ridley-cataract-IOL-operation across the globe. The procedure has came a long way to mean that patients are treated now under a local anesthetic meaning that the visit to the clinic is an out-patient basis and they can return home as soon as the day of the procedure. Visual recovery tends to be very fast, and many patients achieve an excellent level of visual acuity the same day of surgery. Unfortunately, in poor countries around the world, there are still over 25.000.000 unoperated people with cataracts who cannot receive this treatment because of financial/logistical reasons.

Ridley's invention is of much more than historical interest. It is now possible to take plastic implants analogous to his designs and embed high technology micro-devices such as silicone microchips micro-telescopes, mini-cameras and the like, into them. These can then receive light and images from the environment and transmit, visual impulses to a blind person's brain, thus at least partially restoring vision. With such gadgetry it would be possible to treat blindness of all possible conditions and diseases, for example, macular degeneration and retinitis pigmentosa, glaucoma, destruction of the eye by severe eye trauma and many others. This is the concept of the "*eye transplant*" or "*bionic eye*" (see USA Today "Tiny Chip May Restore Vision to Patients", by Kathleen Fackelmann, August 1, 2001) that is now under intense research. Such futuristic devices that can be implanted in the eye are no doubt going to be developed and applied. Therefore, complete eradication of blindness - only a dream until now - will become a reality. Ridley's contribution has been to provide the needed break-through towards successful intraocular prosthesis implantation.

In large part because of his invention, the last half-decade of the 20th century has been termed the Golden Age of Ophthalmology and visual sciences. His discovery has indeed changed the world so that we might better see it with our eyes. It has brought forth a miracle by helping all of us see better by preserving our gift of sight. Even when a miracle might appear to become routine over time, it still remains a miracle (Apple et al., 2002; Kohnen, 2009).

5. The modern phacoemulsification technique

In 1967, Charles D. Kelman (1930, Brooklyn, New York–2004, Boca Raton, Florida), an ophthalmologist pioneer in cataract surgery, introduced phacoemulsification after being inspired by his dentist's ultrasonic probe. This technique uses ultrasonic waves to emulsify the nucleus of the crystalline lens in order to remove the cataracts without a large incision. This new method of surgery decreased the need for an extended hospital stay and made the surgery less painful. Dr. Kelman did his residency (1956-1960) at Wills Eye Hospital in Philadelphia, then worked as an ophthalmologist at the Manhattan Eye, Ear and Throat Hospital in New York. He received the National Medal of Technology from President

George H. W. Bush in 1992, was inducted [in February 2004] into the National Inventors Hall of Fame in Akron, Ohio (Figure 15).

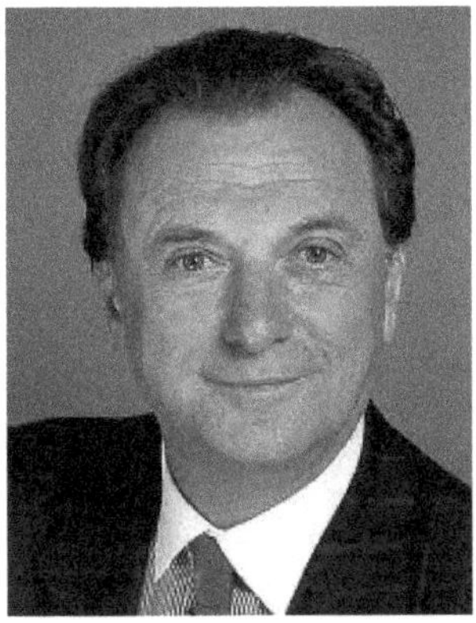

Fig. 15. Charles D. Kelman (1930-2004), best known as the father of phacoemulsification

6. Conclusion

In conclusion, cataract surgery is a technique described since recorded history. Nevertheless, it has greatly evolved only in the latter half of the past century. The development of the intraocular lenses and phacoemulsification as a procedure for cataract extraction could be considered as the two most significant strides that have been made in this surgical field (Ashwin et al., 2009).

Before the introduction of modern ophthalmic surgical technology following World War II, cataract surgery was easier and safer to perform if the cataract was mature and both eyes were involved. The surgeon was constrained from early surgery by the frequency of severe complications, the long recovery period, and the distortions secondary to aphakic glasses. Now it is easier to perform phacoemulsification and implant lenses in the early stages of cataract formation when the nucleus is soft and the posterior lens capsule has not been weakened with age. Also, modern small-incision extracapsular cataract extraction has a low rate of complications and a short convalescent period. It is feasible to extract a clear lens or one with minimal opacifications and have a grateful patient. The surgeon is able to improve the refractive state of the eye by selecting the IOL power (Jampel, 1999).

The techniques and results of cataract surgery have changed dramatically during the past four decades. We have moved from intracapsular cataract extraction as the preferred technique to exclusively extracapsular procedures. Smaller incisions have become the standard, with phacoemulsification now being the method of choice for all surgeons. Along with these advances have come improved IOL materials and designs, especially well suited for use with smaller incisions. Phacoemulsification as a method to remove the cataractous lens was first proposed more than 30 years ago. Advances in techniques and equipments have led to a dramatic increase in the popularity of phacoemulsification with increased safety and efficiency. Viscoelastic agents have been developed synchronously with modern phacoemulsification techniques, playing an integral role in the success of this new technology. Improved surgical techniques for removing the anterior lens capsule have decreased the incidence of both intraoperative and postoperative capsular complications. Nucleus removal, formerly performed primarily in the anterior chamber, is now performed in the posterior chamber, decreasing damage to the corneal endothelium. Improved wound construction allows many wounds to be left unsutured, and smaller wounds allow shorter recovery time and greater intraoperative control and safety. IOLs can have smaller optic sizes and still maintain accurate centration. Foldable IOLs can take advantage of the smaller incision, even further shortening the time to visual recovery. Continual evolution of this technology promises to further improve patient outcomes after cataract surgery (Linebarger et al., 1999).

7. References

Albert DM, Edwards DD. (1996). Ophthalmology before Hippocrates, In: *The History of Ophthalmology*, Albert DM, Edwards DD. Cambridge, Mass., Blackwell Science.

Andersen Ry S. (1997). The eye and its diseases in Ancient Egypt. *Acta Ophthalmol Scand* 1997;75:338-344.

Aplle DJ, Sims J. (1996). Harold Ridley and the Invention of the Intraocular Lens. *Surv Ophthalmol*, 40(4):279-292.

Apple DJ, Werner L, Werner LP. (2002). He changed the world ¾ So that we might better see it. *Arq Bras Oftalmol*, 65(1):137-140.

Apple DJ. (2006). Sir Harold Ridley and His Fight For Sight: He Changed the World So That We May Better See It. SLACK Incorporated. Thorofare.

Aruta A, Marenco M, Marinozzi S. (2009). History of cataract surgery. *Med Secoli*, 21(1):403-428.

Ascaso FJ, Cristóbal JA. (2001). The Oldest Cataract in the Nile Valley. *J Cataract Refract Surg*, 27:1714-1715.

Ascaso FJ, Lizana J, Cristóbal JA. (2009). Cataract surgery in ancient Egypt. *J Cataract Refract Surg*, 35(3):607-608.

Ascaso FJ, Bosch J. (2010). Uveitic secondary glaucoma: influence in James Joyce's (1882-1941) last works. *J Med Biog*, 18(1):57-60.

Ascaso FJ, Singh AD, Dua HS. (2011). Decoding eyes in the Code of Hammurabi. *Br J Ophthalmol*, 2011;95(6):760

Ashwin PT, Shah S, Wolffsohn JS. (2009). Advances in cataract surgery. *Clin Exp Optom*, 92(4):333-42.

Bartz G, König E. (2005). Arts and Architecture. Köln: Könemann. http://www.commonlaw.com/Hammurabi.html (accessed 5 Aug 2010).

Bernscherer G. (2001). Selection from the history of cataract surgery from 2640 B.C. to 1750 A.D. *Orv Hetil*, 142(30):1623-1625.

Bieganowski L. (2003). Ophthalmology in the ancient river cultures. Was cataract surgery performed during the time of King Hammurabi? *Klin Oczna*, 105(3-4):240-4.

Cotallo JL, Esteban M. (2008). La catarata en la historia de la humanidad (de la Prehistoria al siglo XX). In: *Cirugía del cristalino*, Lorente R, Mendicute J, pp. 1-29, Sociedad Española de Oftalmología, Madrid.

Cristóbal JA, Ascaso FJ. (2007). Historia de la Cirugía de la Catarata. In:. *El Libro del Cristalino de las Américas*, Centurión V, Nicoli C, Villar-Kuri J, pp. 25-37. Livraria Santos Editora. Sao Paulo.

Chan CC. (2010). Couching for cataract in China. *Surv Ophthalmol*, 55(4):393-8.

Deines H, Grapow H, Westendorf W. (1958). *Grundriss der Medizin der alten Ägypter*, Berlin, Akademic Verlag, vol IV, I, 43. Ebers 378 (60, 3-6) and 44. Ebers 385 (60, 16-61, 1)

Dolezalova V. (2005). Jacques Daviel, 11 August 1696--30 September 1762. *Cesk Slov Oftalmol*, 61(1):73-5.

Duke-Elder S. (1969). "Sushruta Samhita-Uttar Tantra", chap. 17, verses 57-70. In: *System of Ophthalmology*. Duke-Elder S. Vol. II, pp. 249, Kimpton. London.

Ebbel B. (1937). *The Ebers Papyrus; the Greatest Egyptian Medical Document*, pp. 72-73, Levin & Munksgaard, Copenhagen.

Finger, Stanley (2001). *Origins of Neuroscience: A History of Explorations Into Brain Function*. US: Oxford University Press.

Fishman RS. (1999). The History of Ophthalmology. *Bull Hist Med*, 73:174-175.

Floyd RP. (1994). History of cataract surgery. In: *Principles and practice of Ophthalmology*. Vol. I, Albert DM, Jakobiec FA. pp. 606-608. W.B. Saunders Company. Philadelphia.

Ghalioungui P. (1973). The *House of Life: Per Ankh, Magic and Medical Science in Ancient Egypt*. pp. 130-132, Israël BM, Amsterdam.

Gorin G. (1982). *History of Ophthalmology*. Delaware: Publish or Perish; 16.

Graves D, Graves J. (1995). Archaeological History of the Code of Hammurabi. In: *Electronic Christian Media*, (accessed 3 Jun 2010), Available from: <http://www.abu.nb.ca/ecm/topics/arch2.htm#1>

Hammu HG. (accessed 4 Aug 2010). Available from: <http://www.historyguide.org/ancient/hammurabi.html >

Hirschberg J. (1899). Geschichte der Augenheilkunde im Alterrum, Band I, I. Die Augenheilkunde der alten Ägypter. Vol XII: Pathologie und Terapie. In: *Handbuch der Gesamten Augenheilkunde*. Graefe A, Saemisch T, eds, pp. 17-18, Engelmann Verlag, Leipzig.

Hooker R. (1996). Mesopotamia: The Code of Hammurabi. In: *Washington State University*, (accessed 5 Aug 2010), Avalilable from: <http://www.wsu.edu/~dee/MESO/CODE.HTM>

Horne C.H. The Code of Hammurabi: Introduction The Avalon Project at Yale Law School. (accessed 6 Jul 2010), Available from: <http://avalon.law.yale.edu/subject_menus/medmenu.asp>

Jampel RS. (1999). The effect of technology on the indications for cataract surgery. *Doc Ophthalmol*, 98(1):95-103.

Johns CHW. (1987). Babylonian and Assyrian Laws, Contracts and Letters.1904. In: *The Library of Ancient Inscriptions, from a facsimile produced by The Legal Classics Library*, Division of Gryphon Editions, New York.

Kohnen T. (2009). How far we have come: from Ridley's first intraocular lens to modern IOL technology. *J Cataract Refract Surg*, 35(12):2039.

Lade A, Svoboda R. (2000). Chinese Medicine and Ayurveda. Motilal Banarsidass. McGrath D. Couching' for cataracts remains a persistent problem in Yemen. EuroTimes, September 2005, p. 11. http://www.escrs.org/Publications/Eurotimes/05September/pdf/couching.pdf

Linebarger EJ, Hardten DR, Shah GK, Lindstrom RL. (1999). Phacoemulsification and modern cataract surgery. *Surv Ophthalmol*, 44(2):123-47.

Mukhopadhyay B, Sharma KR. (1992). History of cataract surgery. *Bull Indian Inst Hist Med Hyderabad*, 22(2):105-10.

Obuchowska I, Mariak Z. (2005). Jacques Daviel-the inventor of the extracapsular cataract extraction surgery. *Klin Oczna,* 107(7-9):567-71

Pandey SK, Apple DJ. (2005). Professor Peter Choyce: an early pioneer of intraocular lenses and corneal/refractive surgery. *Clin Experiment Ophthalmol,* 33(3):288-93.

Petrie WMF, Griffith FL. (1900). Sold at the Offices of the Egypt Exploration Fund. The Royal Tombs of the First Dynasty. London.

Ravin JG. (2009). The multifaceted career of Louis Borsch. *Arch Ophthalmol,* 127(11):1534-7.

Savage-Smith E (2000). The Practice of Surgery in Islamic Lands: Myth and Reality. *Soc Hist Med,* 13 (2): 307-321.

Shugar JK. (1997). History of cataract surgery. *Ophthalmology,* 104(2):173-174.

Sir Harold Lloyd Ridley. (2010). In: *Encyclopædia Britannica Online,* (Retrieved November 20, 2010), Available from: <http://www.britannica.com/EBchecked/topic/761211/Sir-Nicholas-Harold-Lloyd-Ridley>

Spalton DJ. (2009). Diamond jubilee of the first intraocular lens implantation? *J Cataract Refract Surg,* 35(12):2040-1.

Spiegel AD, Springer CR. (1997). Babylonian medicine, managed care and Codex Hammurabi, circa 1700 BC. *J Community Health,* 22(1):69-89.

Wales J. Cataract surgery. (accessed 4 Nov 2010), Available from: < http://en.wikipedia.org/wiki/Cataract_surgery>

Williams HP. (2001).. Sir Harold Ridley´s vision. *Br J Ophthalmol,* 85:1022-1023.

Zegers RH. (2005). The eyes of Johann Sebastian Bach. *Ned Tijdschr Geneeskd,* 149(52):2927-2932.

7

Major Advances in Cataract Surgery

Farhan Husain Zaidi
Consultant Ophthalmic Surgeon, Maidstone and Tunbridge Wells NHS Trust, Kent,
Honorary Fellow, Moorfields Eye Hospital, London,
UK

1. Introduction

Cataract is the leading cause of blindness worldwide and likely has been since at least ancient times [1]. Consequently cataract surgery is recorded to have attracted the interest of surgeons for thousands of years [2,3]. During this period physicians and scientists have tried to improve the results of cataract surgery [1]. Cataract surgery is the most frequently performed operation in the world. In this chapter the principal concepts and pathways in thinking which have driven the development of the operation forward as well as some of the causes for resistance to change are discussed.

2. The Platonic theory of vision - The operations and observations of Susruta, Celsus and Galen

The first record of cataract being surgically treated is from 600 B.C. by Susruta of India [1]. It is quite possible that cataract surgery was performed by other surgeons before him including outside India but no reliable record from them has been found. Susruta used couching wherein the cataract is surgically dislocated away from the visual axis by a surgical instrument inserted into the eye [4]. Modernday cataract surgery has moved considerably beyond couching but it is worth noting in this context that couching is still performed by 'quack' doctors and also some traditional 'healers' for example in many underdeveloped parts of Africa, in the Yemen, and in rural China. Modern couching uses a long needle-like device inserted just behind the limbus - thereby crudely clearing the visual axis for light transmission by displacing the cataract into the anterior chamber or vitreous cavity [5]. The result is fairly unpredictable and the rate of blindness is high including many years after surgery. Retained lens matter is known to elicit a potentially very marked inflammatory reaction within the eye risking intractable glaucoma while vitreous loss risks both the latter complication as well as a significantly increased risk of retinal detachment and maculopathy. Siddig and Ali studied outcomes of this 'modern' form of couching done by rural 'healers' in the Darfur region of Sudan and found that 22% of patients develop endophthalmitis, and 38% develop longterm optic nerve atrophy from glaucoma [5]. Overall in the longterm they found that 60% of patients eventually had no perception of light in the operated eye after undergoing couching. It is likely that these outcomes would have been even worse in ancient times when there was no recourse to modern antibiotics for endophthalmitis or treatments for glaucoma. Yet couching remained the norm as far as surgical management of cataract went for many centuries.

With the conquest of northern India by Alexander the Great his physician brought knowledge of couching to Alexandria in Egypt [1]. It is possible the technique was in use even before this time in Egypt. Celsus in 25 A.D. provided the earliest extant description of the couching operation [1]. However the first recorded major advance in the practice of cataract surgery was not in finding a technique to supercede couching but in assessing the visual potential of an eye being considered for cataract surgery [1]. In this context Galen's records are worth scrutiny [1,2]. Galen (died 199 A.D.) was born and trained in medicine in Pergamon in Asia Minor (in modernday Turkey). After completing additional clinical work in the main medical cities of his time, Galen moved practice to Rome where he records couching cataracts [2]. Galen noticed that before cataract surgery a visible inequality of static pupil size was of limited prognostic value as the pupil can be of normal size with even severe cataract or many other disease processes in the eye or the opposite fellow eye [1,2]. He also noted what is now called the "consensual" light reflex and he also made an association between it and visual potential in the fellow eye. He observed that if a diseased eye is occluded there will be less dilation of the fellow eye than otherwise expected, and sometimes there is none. He also noted that if positive this test may be associated with a poor visual prognosis for cataract surgery in the affected eye [2,6]. However Galen's proposed mechanism to explain this correct observation was flawed. The Platonic schematic inherited from Ancient Greece by the Romans exerted a retarding influence in this context since it proposed a "pneuma" emerging from the eye which was responsible for sight. According to Plato, whose views dominated much of Ancient Greece and Rome, light was not thought of as the stimulus for vision, but rather sight was falsely regarded as a consequence of the emission of the 'visual spirit' from the brain, optic nerve and finally the eye, passing through its pupil to the outside world [2]. On the basis of the Platonic schematic Galen therefore mistakenly proposed that the 'pneuma' was responsible for pushing the pupil aside which thereby caused the pupil's movement in the light [2]. This faulty Platonic model of vision would act as a conceptual barrier to advances in the field of vision science and ophthalmology including cataract surgery for hundreds of years to come.

3. A different perspective to visual perception by the Imams Jafar ibn Mohammad and Mohammad ibn Ali – The Platonic schematic of vision discarded

Galen's "prognostic pupillary signs" were translated and transcribed into Arabic thereby preserving them during the European Dark Ages [2]. It was in the Middle East that the Platonic schematic of visual perception would eventually be discarded leading to important advances in optics and successful clinical outcomes in ophthalmology [1,2]. These observations were original and not a rehashing of older Greek, Persian or Coptic knowledge nor was it knowledge that was, as some have rather fancifully advanced, secretly saved from being burned in the library of Alexandria [1,2,7].

The key advance made during this period of history was the fundamental observation wherein light was recognised as the stimulus for vision, a belief recorded to have first been made by the Imam Jafar ibn Mohammad (702-765 A.D.) who taught at the academy started by his father the Imam Mohammad ibn Ali in the Arabian city of Medina [1,7,8,9]. The Imam Jafar ibn Mohammad stated that for every sensory phenomenon, including sight, there was an organ (in the case of vision the eye) to perceive it, and in the case of vision the stimulus was light, and it was this which gave rise to the visual phenomena including colour vision [1,7,8]. The Imam Jafar ibn Mohammad is also recorded to have stated the concept that rays of light are emitted, reflected or transmitted by objects, and also that it is the entry of these rays of light into the eye that causes vision (as opposed to the Greco-Roman pneuma, which postulated the reverse) - he thereby undid the age-old Platonic schematic for vision which had retarded advance in vision science and ophthalmology [1,7,8]. Using a clear logical argument he correctly stated for the first recorded time what eventually became a scientific truism:

"The rays of light from different objects come to our eyes and enable us to see them. The rays of light from our eyes do not go out and fall on other objects, otherwise we could have seen them in the darkness also. We see only those objects which are luminous. If they are not luminous themselves, they must reflect the light falling upon them by some luminous object." [1,7,8]

The profundity of the above statements in the face of the Platonic schematic of vision which had dominated the scientific and medical world cannot be overestimated. The first recorded mathematical concepts in geometric optics were also proposed by the Imam Jafar ibn Mohammad on the basis of which he proved that light scatter can be explained by regarding light as rays and this scatter is the cause of unclear vision for distant objects [1,7,8]. In these contexts he stated:

"If we make a device through which all the rays of light coming from the camels grazing at a distance of 3000 Zirah [One Zirah = 40 inches] entered our eyes we would see them grazing at a distance of only 60 Zirah and all other objects would look 50 times nearer to us." [1,7,8]

He also stated that since minification of objects occurs as little light is geometrically entering the eye (a small angle object) that the opposite, magnification, would occur when more light enters the eye and the angle increases - and hence distant objects could be magnified if the rays of light from the object could be concentrated to increase the angle by suitable employment of a technical instrument [1,7,8]. This is the first description of a theory for magnifying instruments, both simple lenses as well as microscopes and telescopes, and also for key functions of the crystalline lens including accommodation. These new beliefs about optics and vision carried far and wide owing to the immense number of students of the Imam Jafar ibn Mohammad – which included eminent scientists like Jabir bin Hayan (also known in the West as 'Geber', a man universally regarded as the scientific 'father' of chemistry) [1,9]. The Imam Jafar ibn Mohammad also stated that light and time were related, that light had a motion, and, additionally, that this motion was very rapid. Light was in his opinion capable of moving objects if concentrated, an important principle that while technically unfeasible in ancient times is an important principle associated with the mechanism of lasers in the modern world [1,7,8].

4. Applications of the new model for vision to optics, clinical diagnosis and cataract surgery in the Middle East

In the 9th and 10th centuries physicians in the Middle East applied Galen's prognostic pupillary signs to decide which cataracts carried a good visual prognosis [1,2,10,11]. The influence of the new teachings on vision and optics by the Imam Jafar ibn Mohammad is once again hard to overestimate since he taught innumerable major scholars in the eighth century. Applying his teachings on vision both Ammar ibn Ali and Ibn Sina (also known as

Avicenna) are recorded to have likewise discarded Plato's theory which had been incorrectly used by Galen in their correct explanation of the pupil's movement which correctly stated that it was a light stimulus which entered the pupil from outside which drove the pupil's movement and not a visual 'pneuma' being emitted from within the eye [2,12]. Both men noted additionally the existence of a direct pupil response to light for the first time in the literature, in distinction to Galen who had noted only the consensual response [2].

The erudite German ophthalmologist and medical historian Julius Hirschberg, speaking in 1905 at the American Medical Association in California, after dedicating 5 years to the study of the field noted how great his initial surprise was at the rapid advance in the field of ophthalmology in the Middle East during the period which would have been just after the Imam Jafar ibn Mohammad proposed his correct explanation for how vision arises [13]. Hirschberg does not seem to have been familiar with the details of the works of the latter since in 1905 few works by the Imam Jafar ibn Mohammad had been translated into English or German. Consequently Hirschberg was unable to fully explain how ophthalmologists of this period in the Middle East based their clinical practice on a rejection of the older Platonic schematic of vision inherited from the Greco-Roman world, since they otherwise frequently used such sources like Galen's Ten Treatises of the Eye by Ammar ibn Ali in *Choice of Eye Diseases*. In the absence of Ancient Greek or Roman sources (which all upheld the erroneous Platonic schematic of visual perception) the origin of the new theory for vision could only have come from within this part of the world and the Imam Jafar ibn Mohammad since the latter was widely influential, had innumerable eminent students including students of science who spread across the Islamic world, and since his recorded statements exist to this day showing his thinking was logical and went unchallenged [1,7,8].

Following on from the theoretical advances of the Imam Jafar ibn Mohammad the first recorded advance in the technique of cataract surgery since couching occurred. In *Choice of Eye Diseases* written in Egypt by the Iraqi Ammar ibn Ali, who invented the hollow needle and syringe for clinical use (hence his invention of the hypodermic syringe), he describes adapting one of his hollow needles for the purpose of cataract extraction:

"Then I constructed the hollow needle, but I did not operate with it on anybody at all, before I came to Tiberias. There came a man for an operation who told me: Do as you like with me, only I cannot lie on my back. Then I operated on him with the hollow needle and extracted the cataract; and he saw immediately and did not need to lie, but slept as he liked. Only I bandaged his eye for seven days. With this needle nobody preceded me. I have done many operations with it in Egypt." [14]

Was this operation of cataract aspiration as described by Ammar ibn Ali an intracapsular cataract extraction (ICCE) wherein the posterior capsule is removed with the cataract or an extracapsular cataract extraction (ECCE) wherein the posterior capsule is left intact hence reducing significantly the risk of vitreous loss and its attendant complications? Given that the mechanism of aspiration seems to have been fairly crude by modern standards it is unlikely that the posterior capsule survived, but this is not known with certainty. It is also likely that this technique would have been used for softer cataracts for obvious reasons. What is known with certainty is that it represents the first recorded description of *extraction* of a cataract, the first major advance in ophthalmic surgery since couching.

This major technical advance in cataract surgery took place after a very prolonged period of stagnation in surgical advance in the field. It took place shortly after the Platonic schematic for vision had been discarded - and combined with the long history of couching that preceded it – it would seem unlikely to have been a coincidence. The likely reason for this is as follows. Galen, who is often referred to by Middle Eastern physicians including Ammar ibn Ali in his *Choice of Eye Diseases*, had wrongly viewed the Platonic pneuma as pushing the pupil aside as it exited the eye - hence it was proposed to account for the pupillary movement [1,2]. This theory, albeit deeply flawed, had fitted well conceptually with the couching operation - it made thematic sense that the lens likewise could be pushed out of the way, this time by a surgical instrument, in the same way the pneuma was held responsible for pushing the pupil out of the way causing it to dilate or constrict. The abandonment of this Platonic schematic for vision beginning with the Imam Jafar ibn Mohammad (8th century) was hence likely to have been a factor giving rise to the birth of new conceptual approaches to cataract surgery resulting in the aspiration of the lens as an alternative to couching, aided by the coincidental technical invention of the hypodermic syringe which was adapted for this purpose. Whether Ammar ibn Ali's cataract aspiration operation was truly the first of its kind or an inadvertent revision of a much older technique hence becomes irrelevant in this context. The Persian physician Mohammad ibn Zakariya al-Razi also described such an aspiration technique for cataract and there is a suggestion by him it may have been performed even earlier by Antyllus, a 2nd-century Greek physician though unlike Ammar ibn Ali and Mohammad ibn Zakariya al-Razi there is no original record of the operation from Antyllus himself should he have undertaken the procedure [15]. In the Middle East a knife to create a wound and oral suction were in use to assist the aspiration procedure - like sucking on a straw [15].

Building on the teachings of the Imam Jafar ibn Mohammad on geometrical optics in approximately 984 Ibn Sahl wrote a treatise entitled 'On Burning Mirrors and Lenses' laying out his understanding of how curved mirrors and lenses bent and focussed light, and on which basis Ibn Sahl has been credited with the first recorded description of what was much later called Snell's law of refraction [16]. Ibn Sahl also used this law to work out the shapes of lenses that focus light with no geometric aberrations, known as anaclastic lenses, an important fundamental advance in what would one day become an applied science of clinical optics including intraocular lens design [16]. Rashed has shown that Ibn Sahl's treatise was used in part by Abu Ali al-Hasan ibn al-Hasan ibn al-Haitham of Basra in Iraq (often called Ibn al-Haitham, also known in the West as Al Hazen) (965-1039 A.D.) in his Book of Optics which brought together much of the work up to that time, including dispersion of white light into its constituent colours [16,17]. Al-Haitham also described the geometry of the reflection of light and built the first pinhole camera showing an intra-ocular image of the outside world formed by inversion of the image passing through the cornea and lens in the pupil plane [1,9].

5. Advances in cataract extraction in Europe

The technique of cataract extraction by aspiration, though practised in the Middle East alongside couching, seems to have been performed only by a small number of surgeons such as the pioneering Ammar ibn Ali. The rate of such progress in science, medicine and surgery within the Middle East seems to have started to wither away after the 10th century and there is little evidence that the practice of cataract surgery reverted to anything more than couching once again.

It was in Europe in 1748 where cataract surgery was next extensively developed by the French ophthalmologist Jacques Daviel who used an extracapsular technique made public in 1753 [18]. Daviel incised the inferior cornea at the limbus with a myrtiform or triangular knife and enlarged the incision on both sides with a thin, blunt pointed, double-edged knife as far as was possible till the cornea became too unsupported to cleanly incise after which he completed the incision superiorly within the cornea to above the pupil with curved scissors. The anterior capsule of the lens was incised with a sharp-edged needle and with a spatula the cataractous lens loosened which he then delivered. The corneal flap was replaced without sutures and then covered with a compress to protect against disturbing the wound so as to allow it to eventually heal sufficiently so as to seal the eye. In effect this is a similar technique to modern extracapsular surgery except for significant advances in instrumentation, suturing and capsulorhexis technique.

By the late nineteenth century the ECCE operation had progressed little more save for the adoption by many European surgeons of the von Graefe knife to make the corneal section - an instrument invented by the celebrated German surgeon after whom it is named. Even as late as the end of the twentieth century some surgeons in England were still using this technique in a highly developed form employing a 'no-touch' technique (that is no contact between hands and the eye). Some surgeons took this to unusual lengths and did not even glove.

6. Intraocular lens implantation

A very major advance in cataract surgery was implantation of a lens within the eye to replace the crystalline lens removed during cataract extraction - and called 'the intraocular lens' (IOL). The theoretical benefit of this had been acknowledged ever since the first studies of the function of the lens in the Middle East from the 8th to the 10th centuries A.D. Yet it was not performed successfully till the mid-twentieth century. It has been suggested by Fechner and Fechner that Tadini, an Italian-born ophthalmologist living in the second half of the eighteenth century, is likely to have been the first European to have conceived of the possibility of intraocular correction of aphakia [19]. Running contrary to popular belief amongst many ophthalmologists a detailed literature review also suggests that the first IOL was not implanted by the English surgeon Harold Ridley in London but, as researched by Fechner and Fechner, as follows [19]. They note that Casanova recorded that Tadini possessed a box of artificial glass lenses for intraocular use - they suggest that the latter passed Tadini's idea onto Casaamata, an ophthalmic surgeon in Dresden, Germany and who is the first surgeon recorded to have implanted an intraocular lens (IOL) to correct aphakia in 1795 [19]. However being made of glass the IOL sank in the eye owing to its weight and the idea for IOL implantation did not seem to catch on till it was revisited in the twentieth century in London [19]. As a result, even into the present day patients exist who underwent bilateral cataract extractions in the age before IOL implantation was near-universal and who wear highly plus spectacle-mounted lenses which cause considerable image magnification (aphakic spectacles) including 'jack in the box' aberrations. Other problems are associated with aphakia in addition to poor visual acuity. Unless corrected by a lens there is a loss of binocular single vision following unilateral cataract extraction, and in children the outcome was even poorer not only because of amblyopia but because of the poor quality of contact lenses which were available till the fairly recent past.

The problem of post cataract extraction aphakia would be revisited by a London medical student who would change the history of ophthalmology forever - incidentally it does not seem the unknown medical student himself ever became an ophthalmologist himself. The medical student remarked in the presence of Harold Ridley, an ophthalmic surgeon in London, how theoretically the outcome of cataract surgery could be improved considerably if the lens that Ridley had extracted during a cataract operation could be replaced. Ridley seized upon this idea with practical determination. He found an inert material for an artificial lens in the form of polymethylmethacrylate (PMMA). It had already been observed by ophthalmologists that glass and plastic intraocular foreign bodies in injured aircrew during World War II did not elicit a significant inflammatory response provided the iris was not touched, so the choice of PMMA seemed a good one. In 1949 Ridley implanted the first such IOL in London and set about trying to popularise the practice. He met for many years with severe resistance from many other surgeons, some of which seems to have been likely due to an element of professional rivalry [20]. Ridley's attempts to popularise IOLs were not helped by the fact that the early surgeons performing the procedure forgot that the refractive index of PMMA was different in air and in water (and hence inside the eye) - leading to a massive miscalculation of the postoperative refraction. This however opened the door to the applied science of biometry, which would eventually spawn a large number of mathematical equations to accurately compute the target IOL power within the eye, a field which has had many contributors from both sides of the Cold War which was going on at the time including the Russian surgeon Fyodorov, and which continues to advance with equations such as the SRK-T, Hoffer Q and Holladay 2 which are currently the most widely used formulae to calculate the IOL power. Ridley and another British surgeon Peter Choyce co-founded the International Intraocular Implant Club in 1966, an organisation which was in large part responsible for the gradual acceptance of artificial lens implantation [20]. Nevertheless for these and related reasons IOL implantation took a long time to became standard spreading slowly and haphazardly to different parts of the world. Subsequent design modifications have considerably improved the lens design.

Above all the vogue for newer methods of cataract extraction would drive the development of newer IOLs. A drawback of the PMMA lenses is that they were rigid and could not be folded. Initially this did not seem to matter as the early IOLs were anterior chamber (AC) IOLs such as iris clip-on lenses. However clinical experience in their use would prove to surgeons that AC IOLs had many problems, many of which have not even yet been fully resolved, including corneal decompensation from corneal endothelial loss, uveitis and hyphaema. By the 1990s with the beginning of the widespread popularity of phacoemulsification newer IOLs made of acrylic and silicone would become popular since they could be folded to take advantage of the much smaller wound offered by phacoemulsification, and being flexible they could also more readily be placed within the capsular bag or even ciliary sulcus should the latter lack support rather than in the anterior chamber. Once the technique of phacoemulsification eventually became routine these lenses also thereby came into routine use. IOLs made of PMMA did not cause much posterior capsule opacity (PCO) when placed in the capsular bag as the rigid lens had a sharp edge and was also more adherent to the posterior capsule preventing migration of cells responsible for PCO. The newer IOL materials of silicone and acrylic induced more PCO, which temporarily slowed down their acceptance by some units, though fortunately this was countered in the 1980s by the increasing use of pulsed Neodymium:Ytrrium, Aluminium, Garnet (Nd:YAG) laser used in the Q-switched mode for posterior capsulotomy

- obviating the need for an invasive procedure such as posterior capsulectomy to deal with the PCO.
Since the 1990s injectable foldable IOLs have become more and more popular. These are deployed within the eye from within a cartridge inserted into the eye instead of manually using forceps. They however require familiarity with the exact specific mechanism of insertion including loading the IOL to be used safely and the ease, safety and reliability varies a great deal between different manufacturers.

7. Advances in cataract extraction – ECCE and ICCE

There was little advance in the actual technique of cataract extraction for a long period of time - the extracapsular technique popularised by Daviel in the late eighteenth century remained – except that the von Graefe knife came to be used by many European surgeons for making the corneal section. Instead of a spatula as used by Daviel in the twentieth century 'needling' was frequently the method employed to remove the cataract, which involved making a corneal incision and scraping the cataract out with (ideally) an intact posterior capsule, a technique used in children till the late twentieth century.
In the twentieth century advances in surgical cryotherapy permitted an application to cataract surgery with what came to be called 'intracapsular cataract extraction' (ICCE). In 1962 Dr Charles Kelman devised a modern version of the cryoprobe, a freezing instrument for the extraction of cataracts within their capsules (and also later applied by him for sealing retinal breaks). In ICCE, after making an incision into the eye similar to the large incision used in traditional extracapsular surgery, a cryoprobe is inserted into the eye which because of the extremely cold temperature it 'freezes' anything it comes into contact with – in this case it is made to stick to the anterior capsule and the entire lens with its anterior and posterior capsules are extracted 'en bloc'. A modification was administration of intracameral zonulolysins to facilitate this process by dissolving the zonules, and also liquid nitrogen could be applied to the anterior capsule to enhance the stickiness of the adhesion. Vitreous loss was common and de Wecker's scissors evolved to excise vitreous – a technique now almost replaced by anterior vitrectomy. Owing to vitreous loss being fairly common the risk of retinal detachment was much higher than more modern techniques of cataract extraction, and the corneal incision was also much larger. ICCE is still extremely rarely used to extract a hypermobile lens by some surgeons, though a posterior pars plana approach to remove the cataract using phacoemulsification may be preferred by many faced with this situation. Since there is no capsular bag left after ICCE the only option for IOL implantation is an anterior chamber design.
Both traditional ECCE and ICCE were used by different surgeons in different institutions till the 1980s. Advances in the ability to perform posterior chamber IOL implantation, and the gradual introduction of operating microscopes during the 1970s offering better intraocular visibility and ability to safely place multiple corneal sutures, led to modifications in key steps of the old ECCE operation. The modernday ECCE operation consequently comprises extraction of the crystalline lens using a can-opener capsulorhexis and controlled irrigation to dislocate the lens into the anterior chamber with the modern irrigating vectis instrument from where the lens is delivered and after anticipated IOL implantation 'in the bag' closure of the corneal section using several 10-0 sutures. This operation is still recommended in cases where phacoemulsification is not safe such as some cases of loss of the anterior capsular edge during capsulorhexis, or if phacoemulsification is impractical such as in some

eye camps in developing countries. An advance in the field of ECCE has been 'small incision' ECCE using a scleral tunnel to perform the operation. This avoids the need for sutures and permits increased recuperation time and higher volume surgery since it does not require suturing of the section.

It is also worth noting that rehabilitation from older forms of cataract surgery (whether ECCE or ICCE) which pre-date the widespread use of the operating microscope (a 1970s development) was very prolonged as corneal suturing could not be safely performed in anything but a most rudimentary fashion without the magnification and stereopsis afforded by the operating microscope. Furthermore corneal suturing materials were crude - 10-0 sutures were not available- and at best a single silk suture could be temporarily placed to seal a corneal wound by the 1960s. In the 1950s and before even this was not possible. Patients would consequently have to lie with their heads sand-bagged flat on their backs for weeks in hospital while the incision into the eye healed sufficiently for them to be allowed to move. Indeed this was a familiar sight to those who visited eye wards in the 1950s in many countries from the United Kingdom to India.

8. Dr Charles Kelman and the age of phacoemulsification

The revolutionary introduction by Dr Charles Kelman of New York of the phacoemulsification technique ('phaco') in 1967 had at least three main implications. First it would eventually permit surgeons to reduce the morbidity from cataract surgery considerably as it allowed access to the cataract using a much smaller incision than ECCE or ICCE. In the early years of the procedure this meant that recovery would be much faster as patients would not have to lie sandbagged for weeks. However even with modern ophthalmic surgical suturing techniques phaco offers great advantages in terms of reducing the risk of endophthalmitis and refractive problems associated with larger wounds. Second the development of phaco spurred on interest in foldable IOLs as discussed above. Third it permitted very high volume cataract surgery to be performed as a day case - indeed it thereby had major ramifications for the expansion of day case surgery in the overall field of surgery.

The principal clinical advantage of phaco is consequent to the small wound size afforded by the ultrasound-emitting tip of a handpiece used by the surgeon to cut the cataract inside the eye - this is the core feature of the technique. The cut fragments of the crystalline lens are removed from the eye by holes for vacuum and aspiration which are built into the phaco handpiece. These parameters can all be adjusted by the surgeon. Modern phaco machines employ a titanium or steel tip inserted via a main incision typically less than 3.0 mm and emitting ultrasonic frequency of 40,000 Hz thereby emulsifying the lens material. A second instrument inserted via a much smaller side port augments the surgeon's ability to manually crack or chop the nucleus into smaller fragments alongside use of ultrasound to emulsify the lens. In a throwback to the distant past aspiration is still used in virtually all modern cataract surgery. After all 'hard' parts of the cataract have been removed a dual irrigation-aspiration (I-A) instrument or a bimanual I-A system is used to aspirate the remaining peripheral cortical material. In very soft cataracts the entire procedure can be done using aspiration obviating the need for ultrasound altogether.

The phaco handpiece can be inserted into the eye through a much smaller incision than for ECCE or ICCE. Typical modern wounds for phaco are 2 to 3 mm wide (and can in the latest microincisions be less than 2 mm in width) The small incision size used in phacoemulsification permits the option of "sutureless" wound closure in contrast to ECCE which utilises a larger wound (10-12mm) requiring stitching; further, although sutureless ECCE via a scleral tunnel may be used the incision is still larger than for phaco.

The early phaco operations were complicated by very significant corneal endothelial loss creating resistance to the use of the technique since visual outcomes from ECCE were, despite the prolonged period of recuperation, nevertheless good in the longterm. Kelman himself noted that there was a period when after pioneering 'phaco' he was banned from operating altogether at the hospital in New York where he had done the first operation. Kelman persisted in improving his technique. With persistence in improving his technique Kelman was able to obviate complications of early phaco operations such as significant corneal endothelial damage. By the mid-1990s the operation he pioneered in 1967 had come to be the most widely used method for cataract extraction in the developed world. In addition to showing the sometimes very long period required for acceptance of a fundamentally good surgical technique (such as IOL implantation) the prolonged time course for the acceptance of phaco also underlines the very long learning curve to the operation. This is owing to the number of complex steps being performed, some simultaneously, in a very limited physical space within the anterior chamber - a learning curve which is probably longer than that of any other operation in the book of surgery and which took intraocular surgery into a new level of technical skill. Simply put no other operation takes many hundreds of independent procedures to become confident at it, and the operation is sometimes wrongly dismissed as minor or easy to perform based upon misleading impressions arising from the often high turnover in expert hands and the implications for revenue generation and payment.

9. Phaco-refractive surgery

Recuperation has been much faster with phaco than with ECCE surgery - astigmatism and other wound-related complications like pain and infection are all reduced. But it has also allowed refractive modification of the cornea in a more predictable manner. Once the risk of corneal decompensation was reduced phaco was found to leave a less damaged corneal surface than the large wound of ECCE of ICCE surgery, a surface that was much closer to the ideal optical sphere of textbooks on physiological optics. This of course meant surgeons could manipulate the cornea more predictably - the era of phaco-refractive surgery burgeoned in the 1990s.

A wide variety of methods were devised to deal with corneal astigmatism at the same time as phaco. This began with modifying wound construction - 'on-axis' corneal incisions flattened the steep meridian; temporal corneal sections could reduce the astigmatic effect of an incision compared with other incisions; phaco wound incisions further from the visual axis were noted to have less effect on astigmatism just as with other corneal sections. Later coupled limbal relaxing incisions were popularised by some surgeons, which can now be planned using biometry inputted into a computer algorithm, though the refractive effect diminishes with time. Finally toric IOL design provided the definitive solution to astigmatism allowing surgeons to make safe triplanar wounds to reduce the risk of endophthalmitis and simultaneously reduce postoperative astigmatism.

Alongside modifications to the cornea, the other ocular refracting surface of the lens was also subject to further manipulation in terms of IOL design in addition to toric IOLs. Monofocal IOLs were supplemented with a variety of new generic IOL designs which could compensate in theory for the loss of accommodation with cataract extraction - accommodative (i.e. pseudo-accommodative) and multifocal IOLs. These designs of IOLs could be combined within a toric IOL design to also address the issue of astigmatism. However apart from toric design the other generic modifications to IOL design remain somewhat controversial, with at present only multifocals gaining reasonable popularity, though with a risk of glare and reduction in contrast sensitivity. For those myopes wishing to avoid spectacles for reading the option of monovision is still favoured by many surgeons, leaving one eye myopic enough to read with (typically about -1.5D to -1.75D) and the other emmetropic for distance and intermediate vision.

'Intracor' refractive laser treatment has very recently offered the option of reducing presbyopia without cataract extraction and IOL implantation by modifying the corneal thickness centrally, but its only niche should it become more widely used would be as a neo-adjunctive therapy for presbyopia prior to eventual cataract surgery with IOL implantation as the patient ages and develops significant lenticular opacity. Corneal refractive surgery with LASIK (Laser-Assisted in Situ Keratomileusis), LASEK (Laser Epithelial Keratomileusis) and PRK (photorefractive keratectomy) can help patients with high order aberrations following cataract surgery in whom the aberrations can be identified using wavefront technology.

10. Fluidics and adjuncts to phacoemulsification

The most recent innovations have sought to extent Kelman's principal success in using phaco to use bimanual instrumentation separating the phaco tip (cum aspirator) from irrigation and to make the wound smaller and smaller - sub-2mm wounds are now feasible and have given rise to smaller bimanual instruments and readily insertable IOLs.

Alongside these major advances other developments have included modifications to the original phaco machine fluidics. The older peristaltic pumps notoriously suffered the risk of occlusion (suction) breaks during the procedure. Venturi pumps overcame this problem. Further hybrid-like pumps using elements from both basic designs have been developed. The field has come full circle in fact in the past decade with many pumps employing a superior peristaltic design with more rigid tubing to prevent the infamous occlusion breaks which risked tearing the posterior capsule in earlier designs. By far the biggest advantage of all these advances has been the maintenance of a much more stable anterior chamber than with earlier machines dating to the 1990s.

More evolved phaco tip design has come to be used over the past couple of decades with the general abandonment of the old-fashioned Kelman tip and also the successful development of phaco tips that can vibrate not only in continuous mode but in burst and pulse modes. The latter modes enable more efficient removal of lens fragments and reduce the risk of corneal burns from the high frequency ultrasound tip of the phaco handpiece, a complication which has consequently significantly reduced in frequency. Adjunctive techniques include the development of capsule tension rings, dyes to optimise visibility, ophthalmic viscosurgical devices, sharp disposable knives and advances in microbiology especially the use of pre-operative povidone iodine and antibiotics administered intracamerally or subconjunctivally which significantly reduce the risk of endophthalmitis. These are just a selection of the more significant advances in cataract surgery which have accompanied the phaco revolution over the past 3 decades. Awareness and understanding of the effects of phacoemulsification on the retina have given rise to peri-operative drugs such as intracameral or subconjunctival or peribulbar steroids and topical non-steroidal anti-inflammatory agents (NSAIDs) to reduce the risk of macular oedema in select patients. Yellow-tinted IOLs have been employed to reduce the potentially hazardous effect of blue light on the macula, an area of research that has become topical once again more recently owing to the discovery of blue light sensitive inner retinal photoreceptors involved in circadian rhythms, the pupil light reflex and perception of light [21].

Finally phacoemulsification has permitted the field of ophthalmic anaesthesia to change massively during the past 30 years. The eye is the most sensitive structure in the body and is associated with a number of specialised techniques of anaesthesia to permit surgery on the organ. Early phacoemulsification operations were all done under general anaesthesia where this was feasible, and carried the risks of a general anaesthetic. Regional anaesthetic blocks could also be employed. Retrobulbar injections with their higher risks of potentially very serious local and systemic complications such as globe perforation and cardiorespiratory depression have moreoless fallen out of use in favour of the less risky peribulbar injections. In many countries during the 21st century newer soft-needle techniques such as sub-Tenon's local anaesthesia displaced other needle-based techniques as the standard technique to administer regional anaesthesia in cataract surgery (and this has been extended from cataract surgery to many other intraocular operations). Owing to the small corneal wound size used in phacoemulsification the possibility of topical anaesthesia has been found to be feasible, ideally supplemented with intracameral anaesthesia, and is a viable option for anaesthesia in selected patients.

11. Laser cataract surgery

Most base modifications to the fundamental phacoemulsification ultrasound technique have come and gone or simply not caught on. Aqualase is essentially defunct after a brief flurry of interest - it employed a water jet in place of ultrasound. Torsional ultrasound is a newer development which is still being used in some phaco machines – it reduces the amount of phaco power expended during most operations. While the latter can work well for dense cataracts and the former for softer cataracts phaco has been able to cope well with all densities of cataract leading to its great versatility as the preferred technique for cataract extraction in most situations.

The only significant promise of a major advance beyond phacoemulsification is at present femtosecond laser which cuts the cataract using a laser after a corneal section and anterior capsulorhexis have been made (the latter can also be made by the laser). This leaves only extraction of the cataract to the surgeon after which the soft lens matter may be aspirated, IOL inserted under a viscoelastic which is aspirated and the wound closed. The longer term outcomes of this technique are in the process of evaluation [22]. Femtosecond cataract surgery may come to occupy a niche within the overall field of cataract surgery, even though the procedure is at present slow to perform on a high volume basis generally requiring two operating theatres – one for the laser and one for the surgery.

12. Conclusion - The future

Whether femtosecond laser cataract surgery replaces or gains a niche alongside phacoemulsification and extracapsular cataract extraction is unknown. However it is interesting to note that the full femtosecond technique, which is the most recent technique in cataract surgery, requires utilisation of all the theoretical and practical advances described at the start of this chapter which were made in the 8th to 10th centuries. These are the rejection of the Platonic schematic for vision, understanding of the function of the crystalline lens, the theory of lasers including their ability to disrupt matter, and the extraction of cataract by aspiration. It is always risky predicting the future, but it is a fair guess that the major advances in cataract surgery in the future, should they occur, will likely proceed along similar conceptual pathways.

13. Acknowledgements

The author is grateful to doctors from older generations for sharing their experiences and knowledge of the past of clinical ophthalmology in the UK, US and India - in particular Mr Adrian Macfarlane (Consultant Ophthalmic Surgeon, Maidstone Hospital, Kent), Mr Paul Hunter (Consultant Ophthalmic Surgeon, Kings College Hospital, London; former President of the Royal College of Ophthalmologists), Professor Alistair Fielder (Emeritus Professor of Ophthalmology, City University, London), Mr Gregory Munton (retired Consultant Ophthalmic Surgeon, Maidstone Hospital, Kent), Dr Zafar Husain Zaidi (deceased, late Consultant Paediatrician, London and Essex), Mr John Ormerod (deceased, late Consultant Ophthalmic Surgeon, Kent) and Dr Charles Kelman (deceased, late Ophthalmic Surgeon, New York, US).

14. References

[1] Zaidi FH. Novel photoreceptor cells, pupillometry and electrodiagnosis in orbital, vitreo-retinal and refractive disorders. PhD thesis. University of London, Imperial College London; 2008.

[2] Thompson HS. The vitality of the pupil: a history of the clinical use of the pupil as an indicator of visual potential. Journal of Neuro-ophthalmology 2003;23:213-224.

[3] Fishman GA. When your eyes have a wet nose: the evolution of the use of guide dogs and establishing the seeing eye. Survey of Ophthalmology 2003;48:452-458

[4] Rucker CW. Cataract: a historical perspective. Investigative Ophthalmology 1965;4:377-383.

[5] Siddig MA, Ali NAM. Complications of couching and visual outcome after IOL implantation. Sudanese Journal of Ophthalmology 2009;1:33-36

[6] Galen C. On the Usefulness of the Parts. Ithaca, New York: Cornell University Press, 1968. Book 10, II/72, p 476. Translated by May MT. Originally written in the second century.

[7] Mirza KA and the Research Committee of the University of Strasbourg. Imam Jafar Ibn Muhammad As-Sadiq A.S.: The Great Muslim Scientist and Philosopher. Ontario: Willowdale, 1997. 2nd edition.

[8] Al Majlisi MB. Bihar al Anwar. London, 1994. Translation. Vol. 111, pp 57-151. Originally published in the 1600s.

[9] Sarton G. Introduction to the History of Science. Baltimore: Williams and Wilkins, 1927. Vol. 1.

[10] Hunain ibn Is'haq. The Book of the Ten Treatises of the Eye Ascribed to Hunain Ibn Is'haq (809-877 AD). Oculist in Cairo. Government Press, 1928. Translated by Max Meyerhof. Originally written in the ninth century.

[11] Ali Ibn Isa. Memorandum Book of a Tenth-Century Ophthalmologist. Chicago: Northwestern University, 1936. Translated by Wood CA. Originally published in the tenth century.

[12] Hirschberg J. The History of Ophthalmology. Wayenborgh Verlag, 1985. Vol. 2. The Middle Ages, p 145, note no 427 on Ammar. Translated by Blodi FC and Bonn JP.

[13] Koelbing HM. Julius Hirschberg (1843-1925), ophthalmologist and medical historian. Klinische Monatsblätter für Augenheilkunde 1976;168: 103-8

[14] Finger S. Origins of Neuroscience: A History of Explorations Into Brain Function. Oxford: Oxford University Press, 1994, p70.

[15] Savage-Smith E. The Practice of Surgery in Islamic Lands: Myth and Reality. Social History of Medicine 2000;13:307-321.

[16] Rashed R. Géométrie et dioptrique au Xe siècle: Ibn Sahl, al-Quhi et Ibn al-Haytham. Paris: Les Belles Lettres, 1993.

[17] Al Deek M. Ibn Al-Haitham: Master of Optics, Mathematics, Physics and Medicine. Al Shindagah, 2004, November-December.

[18] Floyd RP. History of cataract surgery. In: Albert DM, Jakobiec FA (ed). Principles and Practice of Ophthalmology. Philadelphia: W.B. Saunders Company, 1994. Vol. 1 pp 606-608.

[19] Fechner PU, Fechner MU. Tadini, the man who invented the artificial lens. Journal of the American Intra-ocular Implant Society 1979;5:22-3.

[20] Pandey SK, Apple DJ. Professor Peter Choyce: an early pioneer of intraocular lenses and corneal/refractive surgery. Clinical and Experimental Ophthalmology 2005;33:288-93.

[21] Zaidi FH, Hull JT, Peirson SN, Wulff K, Aeschbach D, Gooley JJ, Brainard GC, Gregory-Evans K, Rizzo JF 3rd, Czeisler CA, Foster RG, Moseley MJ, Lockley SW. Short-wavelength light sensitivity of circadian, pupillary, and visual awareness in humans lacking an outer retina. Current Biology 2007;17:2122-8.

[22] Bali SJ, Hodge C, Lawless M, Roberts TV, Sutton G. Early experience with the femtosecond laser for cataract surgery. Ophthalmology 2012;119:891-9.

8

Dual OVD (Ophthalmic Viscosurgical Devices) Sealing Technique

Takao Tanaka[1,*], Maiko Hirose[1], Shigemitu Ishii[1], Satoshi Fujita[1] and Keisuke Kimura[2]

[1]*Hachioji Medical Center, Tokyo Medical University Hospital, Hachioji Tokyo*

[2]*Department of Ophthalmology, Tokyo Medical University, Tokyo, Japan*

1. Introduction

The soft shell technique (Arshinoff SA) is an excellent technique for protecting the corneal endothelium, particularly when performing microincision cataract surgery (MICS) (Tsuneoka H, et al.; Osher RH; and Agarwal A, et al.). We have observed that this technique is often associated with an increase in intraocular pressure (IOP) after surgery (Figure 1). Here we conducted a preliminary retrospective study to evaluate increases in IOP after surgery using the soft shell technique with different incision sizes. The incidence of an IOP of at least 22 mmHg at 1 day after surgery is increased when a narrow incision size is made during surgery. Therefore, the IOP spike may depend on the incision size.

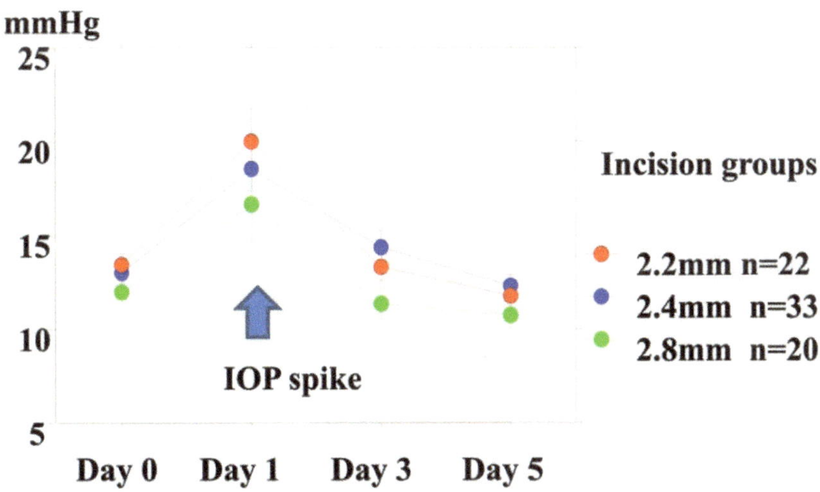

Fig. 1. IOP Values after Surgery Using the Soft Shell Technique

* Corresponding Author

This was a preliminary retrospective study (n=75 cases). For cataract surgery, the soft shell technique is excellent for protecting the corneal endothelium. In our experience, however, the use of this technique during minimal incision cataract surgery (MICS) is often associated with an increase in postoperative intraocular pressure, especially 1 day after surgery in cases in which a 2.2-mm clear corneal incision was made.

Based on this impression, we designed a dual Ophthalmic Viscosurgical Device (OVD) sealing technique, anticipating that use of this sealing technique in combination with MICS would attenuate the IOP elevation and better protect the cornea as by contributing to maintain the appropriate anterior chamber depth during surgery.

The technique involves filling the anterior chamber with a low-molecular-weight ophthalmic viscosurgical device (LMW-OVD), using sodium hyaluronate (SH; Opegan®, Santen) for corneal protection (Nagahara M & Shimizu K). In addition, another OVD with a different surface tension, preferably one containing SH and chondroitin sulfate (SH/CS; Viscoat®, Alcon) is used to seal the wound to prevent marked leakage of the LMW-OVD from the anterior chamber. The purpose of this study was to evaluate the effect of this dual OVD sealing technique, combined with MICS, on the postoperative IOP and corneal protection.

2. Methods

Technique: After the initial paracentesis, a cannula was inserted into the anterior chamber and the LMW-OVD was injected. After filling 70% of the anterior chamber, the secondary SH/CH-OVD was injected around the wound. Injection of the LMW-OVD was resumed, penetrating the SH/CS-OVD mass and sealing the wound (Figure 2).

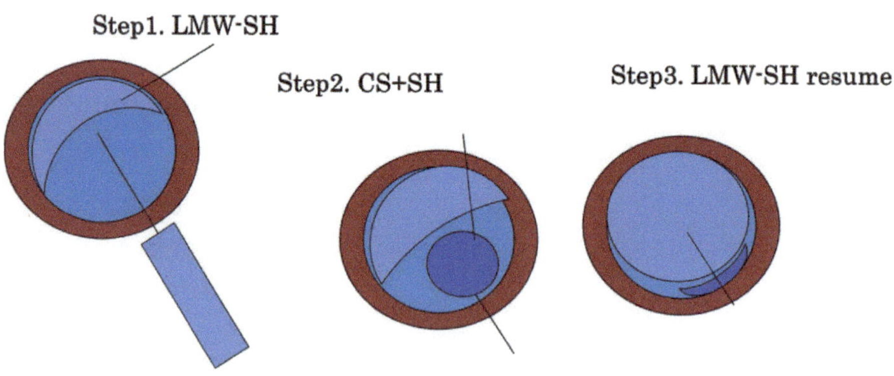

Fig. 2. The dual-OVD sealing technique
The anterior chamber is filled with LMW-OVD. The inside wound is sealed using a secondary OVD SH/CS-OVD with a different surface tension.

3. Clinical evaluation

The retrospective study involved a total of 165 eyes that underwent MICS by the same surgeon (T.T.). Subjects that underwent MICS with a 2.2-mm clear corneal incision and micro co-axial phaco were classified into five groups as follows: Group 1 (n=29), the soft shell technique (SH/CS-OVD and HMW-OVD, Healon ®, AMO); Group 2 (n= 29): a high molecular weight OVD (HMW-OVD1: Healon ®) was used; Group 3 (n=33) HMW-OVD2 (Opegan Hi ®, Santen); Group 4 (n=40): dual-OVD sealing technique (DOS) using a LMW-OVD and SH/CS-OVD; and Group 5 (n=34): LMW-OVD alone. Intraocular pressure and percent corneal endothelial cell loss were measured before surgery, and at 1, 3, and 5 days after surgery.

4. Results

At day 1 after surgery, IOP was increased in all cases (Figures 3 and 4) and did not significantly differ between groups. After day 1, however, IOP was significantly higher in Group 1, in which the soft shell technique was used, compared to Groups 2-5.

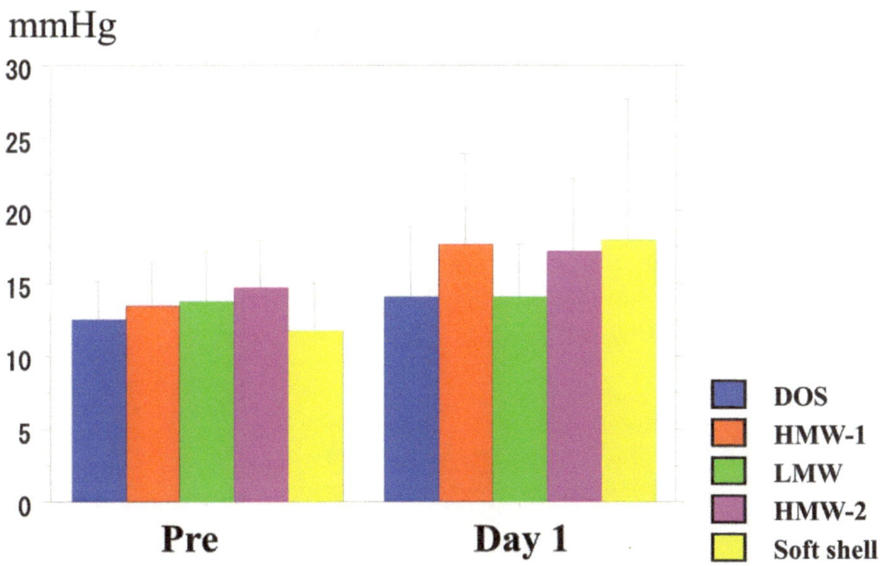

Fig. 3. Intraocular pressure

These findings suggest that the soft shell technique tends to induce an increase in the IOP compared with the non-soft shell techniques. The OVD used did not significantly affect corneal endothelial loss rate; mean cell area and the coefficient of variation did not differ significantly between groups (Figures 5,6, and 7).

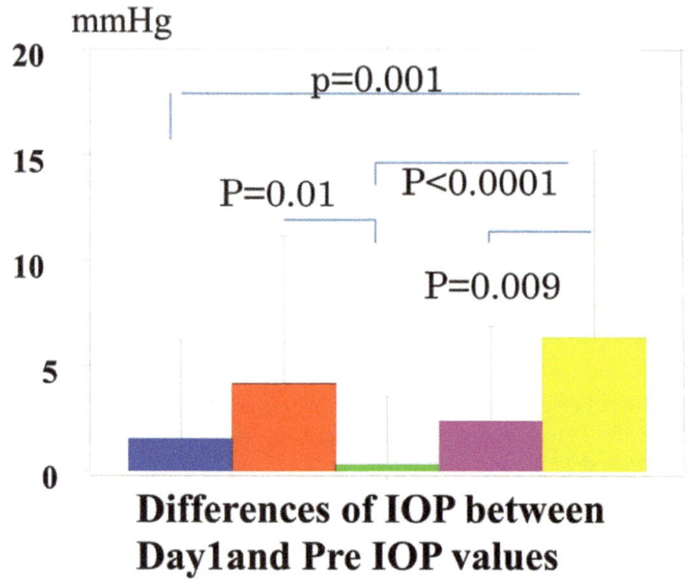

Fig. 4. Differences in the IOP elevation values

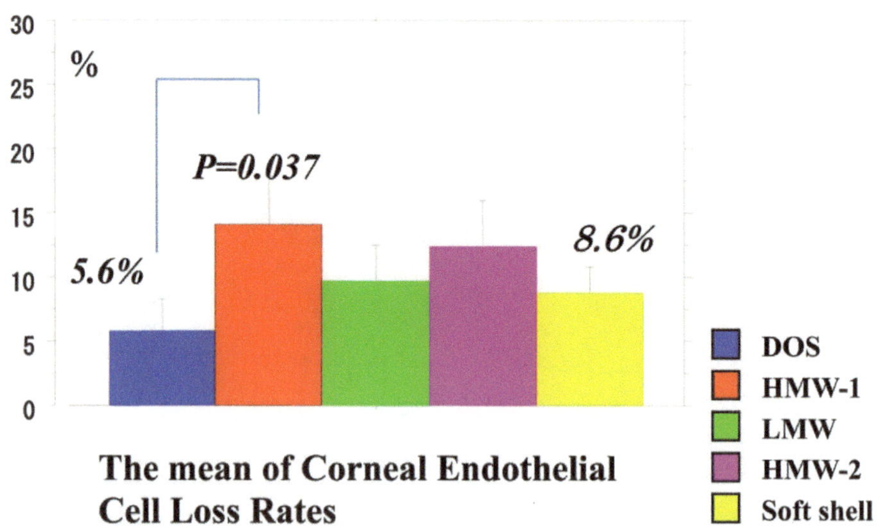

Fig. 5. Mean corneal endothelial cell loss rate

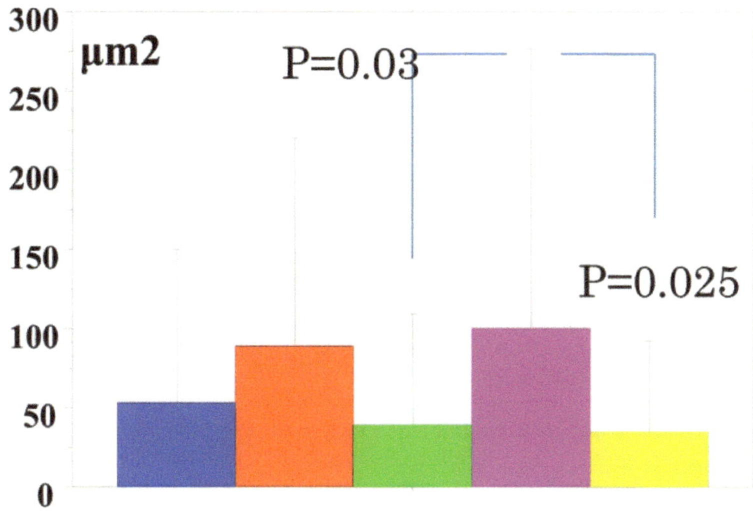

Fig. 6. Difference in mean cell area between before and after surgery

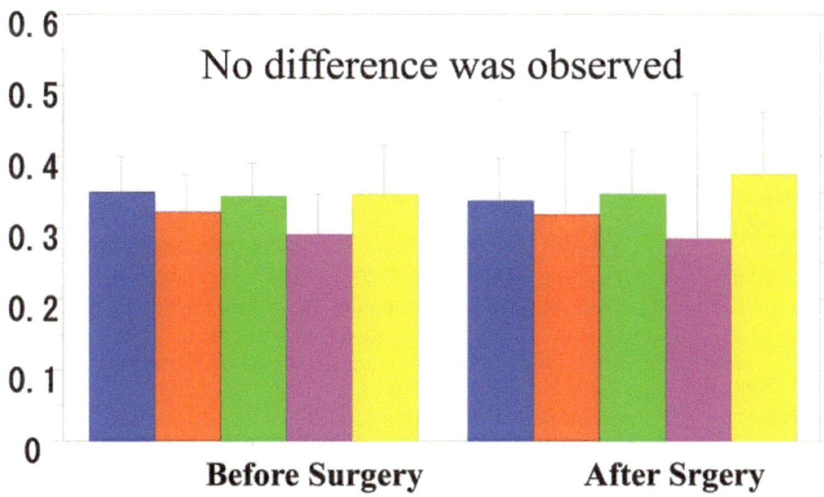

Fig. 7. Coefficient of variation

5. Discussion

Sodium hyaluronate demonstrates remarkable viscoadaptability and prolonged retention at the lower flow rate is associated with a high residual volume (Tanaka T, et al.). Leakage of the LMW-OVD is prevented when using the dual OVD sealing technique because the injection of a secondary OVD with a different surface tension facilitates maintenance of the anterior chamber depth.

Although the soft shell technique (Arshinoff SA) is useful for protecting the cornea, it is sometimes associated with an increased postoperative IOP when MICS is performed with a small incision. Thus, the IOP elevation may be due to residual OVD. Longer wash periods are therefore required to wash out the residual OVD or, when performing MICS, the irrigation volume must be very low. In such cases, the use of a LMW-OVD is expected to prevent the IOP elevation.

In our dual sealing procedure, a lower volume of the OVD is used than in the soft shell technique, allowing for the use of a LMW-OVD instead of a high molecular of OVD as the main filling in the anterior chamber. The SH/CS-OVD may prevent leakage and help to maintain an adequate anterior chamber depth. Thus, the dual OVD sealing technique appears to be more appropriate for small incision surgery.

The advantages of the dual sealing technique include: 1. Corneal protection by the LMW-OVD and 2. Low residual OVD, which helps prevent the elevation in IOP.

6. Financial disclosure

Takao Tanaka received partial support in the form of grants from Santen Pharmaceutical Company, Ltd., Osaka, Japan.

7. References

Agarwal A, Agarwal A, Agarwal S, Narang P, Narang S. Phaconit: phacoemulsification through a 0.9 mm corneal incision. J Cataract Refract Surg 2001; 27:1548–1552

Arshinoff SA. Soft Shell technique, Dispersive-cohesive viscoelastic soft shell technique J Cataract Refract Surg 1999; 25:167-173

Nagahara M, Shimizu K. Protecting the corneal endothelium with viscoelastic material during phacoemulsification. Rinsho Ganka (Written in Japanese) 1994; 48:900-901

Osher RH. Micro coaxial phacoemulsification. Part 2: clinical study. J Cataract Refract Surg 2007; 33:408–412

Tsuneoka H, Shiba T, Takahashi Y. Ultrasonic phacoemulsification using a 1.4 mm incision: clinical results. J Cataract Refract Surg 2002; 28:81–86

Tanaka T, Kimura K, Usui M. Adhesive retention of sodium hyaluronate ophthalmic viscosurgical devices in an acrylic tube model and in porcine-eye corneal endothelium with different irrigation rates. J Cataract Refract Surg 2009 ; 35: 2008-2013

9

Management of Intraocular Floppy Iris Syndrome (IFIS) in Cataract Surgery

Allan Storr-Paulsen
Department of Ophthalmology, Cataract Outpatient Surgery Unit, Frederiksberg University Hospital, Frederiksberg, Denmark

1. Introduction

Intraoperative floppy iris syndrome (IFIS) was first described in 2005 (Chang & Campbell 2005; Parssinen 2005). The fullblown syndrome comprises a triad of: 1) billowing of the iris stroma in response to normal irrigation currents, 2) the floppy iris tends to prolapse through the phaco and the side port incisions, and 3) a progressive pupillary constriction during the surgical procedure. Although IFIS may be multifactorial in etiology, systemic treatment with α-1_a adrenergic receptor (AR) antagonists, and tamsulosin in particular, seems to play a pivotal role. The clinical presentation varies widely, from a mild form with a fluttering iris only, to the more severe case with the complete triad (Chang et al. 2007). The condition potentially increases the risk of intraoperative complications, such as iris trauma, zonular dehiscence, posterior capsule rupture, vitreous loss, as well as postoperative complications, including increased intraocular pressure and cystoid macular oedema. The prevalence of IFIS in cataract surgery varies among different countries, from 0.5 % to 2.0 % (Chang & Campbell 2005; Cheung et al. 2006; Chadha et al. 2008). The incidence of IFIS during cataract surgery in patients on tamsulosin medication varies from 43 - 100%. In contrast, the incidence of IFIS in patients taking one of the other α-1a AR antagonists, e.g. alfuzosin, is 10-15% (Blouin et al. 2007).

2. Etiology

Adrenergic α-1 receptors are frequently found in smooth muscles of the human prostate / bladder neck, and in the iris dilator muscle of the eye, predominantly the subtypes α-1_a and the α-1_d. Stimulation of the iris dilator muscle and the smooth muscles in the prostate and the bladder neck is mediated by the adrenergic α-1_a and α-1_d receptors.

Lower urinary tract symptoms (LUTS) suggestive of benign prostatic hyperplasia (BPH) is a common condition among elderly male patients and the prevalence of BPH and cataract is similar, increasing with age. Benign prostatic hyperplasia implies both a static and a dynamic component. The static component is characterized by an increased prostatic mass, and the dynamic component by an increased α-1 AR mediated tone in the smooth muscles of the bladder neck and in the prostate. Inhibition of the α-1_a ARs relaxes the muscular tone, which decreases the pressure within the lower urinary tract improving urinary outflow, and at the same time produces relaxation of the iris dilator muscle causing a floppy iris and miosis. Thus, systemic treatment with α-1 AR inhibitors (alfuzosin, doxazosin, tamsulosin and terazosin) has been a successful therapy of LUTS including benign prostatic hyperplasia, but the same treatment may cause some degree of IFIS during cataract surgery. Due to a better cardio-vascular profile tamsulosin and alfuzosin seems to be better tolerated than doxazosin and terazosin (Djavan et al. 2004). However, tamsulosin also has a very high affinity for the α-1a and α-1d ARs in the smooth muscular tissue of the iris. On the other hand, alfuzosin acts clinically in a more uro-selective manner, which may explain, why alfuzosin causes IFIS less frequent than tamsulosin, decreasing the odd ratio for IFIS to 1:32 compared to patients exposed to tamsulosin (Blouin et al. 2007).

3. Management of IFIS

3.1 Preoperative precautions

3.1.1 Medical history

The risk of unexpectedly encountering IFIS during surgery in cataract patients should be minimized through a thorough questioning of the previous and the current medical history. Of particular interest is a history of symptoms from the lower urinary tract and the prostate. This also applies to women, as α-1a AR inhibitors may be prescribed for LUTS and arterial hypertension in females. IFIS may develop in patients treated with tamsulosin for only a few months. It might seems rational to stop the treatment with α-1 AR antagonists preoperatively, but there is little or no clinical effects on the severity of IFIS by stopping the treatment with tamsulosin, although the preoperative pupil diameter may be larger (Chang et al. 2007; Nguyen et al. 2007). The authors´ institution does not recommend the patients stop treatment with α-1 AR inhibitors prior to surgery.

3.1.2 Preoperative dilatation

A preoperative maximum pupillary dilatation is mandatory. The author recommends an anticholinergic agent to relax the sphincter of the pupil (cyclopentolate 1%) combined with an α-1 AR agonist (phenylephrine 2.5 - 10%) to enhance the dilatation and increase the tone of the iris dilator stroma administrated twice at 15-20 minutes interval before surgery. The author adds a non-steroid anti-inflammatory drug (diclofenac 0.1% / ketorolac 0.5%) to provide a more stable dilatation throughout the surgery. A poorly dilated pupil preoperatively may predict eyes likely to manifest IFIS during operation. At the authors´ institution, a preoperative pupil diameter ≤ 6 mm in IFIS patients indicates the need for iris retractors, pupil expansion rings or intracameral phenylephrine.

Atropine 1% applied topically prior to cataract surgery in patients on tamsulosin has been recommended to obtain a maximum preoperative dilatation (Bendel & Phillips 2006; Masket & Belani 2007). In the case series by Bendel & Philips, atropine 1% was prescribed twice daily for 10 days. Thirteen out of 16 patients (81%) on tamsulosin did not require other modification of their cataract surgery. Masket & Belani used a presurgical administration of topical atropine 1% three times daily for two days in addition to routine preoperative mydriatics. During the operative procedure, 0.3 to 0.5 mL intracameral epinephrine diluted 1:2500 with BSS was placed under the iris. They reported 19 eyes out of 20 to have an excellent pupil dilatation without signs of IFIS.

Atropine, a potent anti-cholinergic agent, relaxes the sphincter of the pupil, but care should be taken due to the risk of intensified LUTS and acute urinary retention, especially if tamsulosin is stopped preoperatively. Treatment with atropine 1% also represent a risk in the elderly group of cataract patients because of atropine's well-know cardiac and cerebral side-effects.

3.2 Operative strategies

3.2.1 Epinephrine in irrigation solution

Epinephrine, a combined α- and β- AR agonist, should be added to the irrigation solution. The author recommends 1 mL epinephrine 1 mg/mL (preservative- and sulphite free) in 1000 mL balanced salt solution (1: 1 000 000) with a pH within the range of 6.5 - 8.5. Irrigation and aspiration flow rates should be reduced to prevent iris fluttering.

3.2.2 Intracameral injection of epinephrine

Myers & Shugar reported good effect of an intracameral mydriatic and anesthetic mixture, the "epi-Shugar" solution, comprised of epinephrine 0.025% and lidocaine 0.75% in BSS Plus. The technique showed excellent results in a paired prospective single masked study (Myers & Shugar 2009). The epi-Shugar solution consists of a 1 : 4000 epinephrine mixture with a pH of 6.9. There was no report of corneal endothelial cell damage (Shugar 2006). Masket & Belani injected 0.3 - 0.5 mL epinephrine diluted with BSS (1 : 2500) intracameral and placed under the iris with excellent results (Masket & Belani 2007). Takmaz & Can suggested a mixture of 0.1 mL non-preserved epinephrine (0.5 mg / mL) diluted with 2 mL BSS (1 : 4000 solution) (Takmaz & Can 2007). They reported no change in the incidence of IFIS, but the mixture seemed effective in order to prevent miosis.

However, intracameral injection in these concentrations may cause local damage, since severe changes has been described in corneal endothelial cell morphology after intracameral use of 0.5 mL epinephrine in a 1:10.000 solution (Edelhauser et al. 1982; Pong et al. 2008).

3.2.3 Intracameral injection of phenylephrine

Intracameral injection of phenylephrine, an α-1 AR agonist, has been recommended to reverse intraoperative iris fluttering and pupil constriction (Manvikar & Allen 2006; Gurbaxani & Packard 2007). In both studies diluted phenylephrine 2.5% was used (Minims®, buffered with bisulphite and edetate). Manvikar & Allen used a solution with 0.25 mL unpreserved phenylephrine 2.5% (Minims) diluted with 2 mL BSS. This corresponds to a 1:360 dilution with a pH of 6.4. The authors argued in a study comprising 32 eyes that the solution had a good effect in order to prevent IFIS. Gurbaxani & Packard reported on the use of intracameral phenylephrine 2.5% mixed with 1 mL BSS in a study with seven patients on tamsulosin. All patients had significant reduction in the signs of IFIS, and a sustained pupillary dilation in all cases. No clinical signs of corneal edema were reported, but unfortunately the density of endothelial cell was not evaluated.

In an early report by Edelhauser et al., a cytotoxic effect on the endothelium of phenylephrine at a concentration of 2.5% was described in cases where the epithelium was removed (Edelhauser et al. 1979). In a recent report on corneal endothelial cell changes in cataract patients on tamsulosin we found no association between the intracameral use of 0.25 mL phenylephrine 2.5% (Minims®) in 2 mL BBS and postoperative endothelial cell loss (Storr-Paulsen et al. 2013).

3.2.4 Capsular staining

Capsular staining with trypan blue 0.06% (Vision Blue, DORC, The Netherlands) is an excellent technique to visualize an obscured leading edge of the capsulorrhexis at the beginning of the operation due to a small pupil or a mature cataract. Trypan blue is also very effective to visualize the border of the rhexis, if iris retractors are required later in the procedure due to progressive miosis. Trypan blue is safe and effective as an adjunct for capsule visualization (de Waard et al. 2002; Jacobs et al. 2006)

3.2.5 Use of ophthalmic viscosurgical devices (OVDs)

Injection of Healon5 was one of four different surgical strategies used to manage IFIS in a multicenter study. A total of 98 of 103 cases were completed with Healon5 alone and the remaining five cases required additional use of iris retractors / iris expansion rings (Chang et al. 2007). In a survey of surgeons' experiences with IFIS in the UK, 27% of the responding surgeons answered that they used Healon5, and 85% found it effective (Nguyen et al. 2007). In 1999, Arshinoff described a technique, where a lower viscosity dispersive OVD was used together with a higher viscosity cohesive OVD (Arshinoff 1999). This "soft-shell" technique is performed with the dispersive injected into the anterior chamber until the chamber is 75-80% full. The cohesive is then injected on the surface of the anterior capsule, pushing the dispersive OVD upward and outward until the pupil stops dilating. The technique was later modified to improve surgery, especially in IFIS patients (Arshinoff 2006).

3.2.6 Use of iris retractors

The use of flexible iris retractors to enlarge the pupil was originally described in the early 1990s (de Juan E Jr & Hickingbotham 1991; Nichamin 1993) and later modified to create a diamond shape, which is very suitable in IFIS surgery (Oetting & Omphroy 2002). In the UK survey of surgeons´ preferences in cases of IFIS, 61% of the responders chose iris retractors, and 72% of that group found them effective (Nguyen et al. 2007). In the American multicenter study, iris retractors were only used in 31% of the cases. The difference may be explained by the fact that the British survey questioned all UK eye surgeons about their experiences; whereas the American study only asked 15 selected and highly experienced surgeons (Chang et al. 2007). Pupil stretching and sphincterotomies are usually of no effect because of the elasticity of the pupil margin, and may on the contrary worsen the constriction of the pupil (Chang & Campbell 2005).

3.2.7 Use of pupil expansion rings

Pupil expansion rings have been used to enlarge the pupil and to maintain the size throughout the surgery. Expansion rings were only used by 3% of the surgeons in the UK survey (Nguyen et al. 2007), and expansion rings were the least used of four alternatives (4% of cases) in the American multicenter study (Chang et al. 2007). The expansion rings were found to cause less trauma to the iris, but was the most time- and cost consuming method, when compared to the use of iris retractors (Akman et al. 2004).

4. Conclusion

To reduce possible complications in cataract patients taking α-1 AR antagonists (especially tamsulosin), the surgeon should:

1. highlight the patient´s medical history, particularly for symptoms of LUTS and benign prostate hyperplasia. A thorough questioning regarding current and previous therapy is strongly recommended. Remember that α-1 AR antagonists are also prescribed for LUTS and arterial hypertension in women.

2. use a preoperative dilation including cyclopentolate, phenylephrine, and a NSAID. Atropine may be used, but cautions should be taken in elderly patients because of the risk of cardiac side effects and acute urinary retention.
3. use capsular staining in order to facilitate visualization of the rhexis edge.
4. use a viscoadaptive or the soft-shell technique in all cases of IFIS.
5. keep phenylephrine ready for intracameral injection in case of a progressive pupil constriction during surgery.
6. consider the use of iris retractors or iris expansion rings if preoperative dilation is ≤ 6 mm.

5. References

Akman A, Yilmaz G, Oto S, Akova YA. (2004): Comparison of various pupil dilatation methods for phacoemulsification in eyes with a small pupil secondary to pseudoexfoliation. Ophthalmology 111: 1693-1698.

Arshinoff SA. (1999): Dispersive-cohesive viscoelastic soft shell technique. J Cataract Refract Surg 25: 167-173.

Arshinoff SA. (2006): Modified SST-USST for tamsulosin-associated intraoperative [corrected] floppy-iris syndrome. J Cataract Refract Surg 32: 559-561.

Bendel RE, Phillips MB. (2006): Preoperative use of atropine to prevent intraoperative floppy-iris syndrome in patients taking tamsulosin. J Cataract Refract Surg 32: 1603-1605.

Blouin MC, Blouin J, Perreault S, Lapointe A, Dragomir A. (2007): Intraoperative floppy-iris syndrome associated with alpha1-adrenoreceptors: comparison of tamsulosin and alfuzosin. J Cataract Refract Surg 33: 1227-1234.

Chadha V, Borooah S, Tey A, Styles C, Singh J (2007): Floppy iris behaviour during cataract surgery: associations and variations. Br J Ophthalmol 91: 40-42

Chang DF, Campbell JR. (2005): Intraoperative floppy iris syndrome associated with tamsulosin. J Cataract Refract Surg 31: 664-673.

Chang DF, Osher RH, Wang L, Koch DD. (2007): Prospective multicenter evaluation of cataract surgery in patients taking tamsulosin (Flomax). Ophthalmology 114: 957-964.

Cheung CM, Awan MA, Sandramouli S. (2006): Prevalence and clinical findings of tamsulosin-associated intraoperative floppy-iris syndrome. J Cataract Retract Surg 32: 1336-1339

de Juan E Jr, Hickingbotham D. (1991): Flexible iris retractor. Am J Ophthalmol 111: 776-777.

de Waard PW, Budo CJ, Melles GR. (2002): Trypan blue capsular staining to "find" the leading edge of a "lost" capsulorhexis. Am J Ophthalmol 134: 271-272.

Djavan B, Chapple C, Milani S, Marberger M. (2004): State of the art on the efficacy and tolerability of alpha1-adrenoceptor antagonists in patients with lower urinary tract symptoms suggestive of benign prostatic hyperplasia. Urology 64: 1081-1088.

Edelhauser HF, Hine JE, Pederson H, Van Horn DL, Schultz RO. (1979): The effect of phenylephrine on the cornea. Arch Ophthalmol 97: 937-947.

Edelhauser HF, Hyndiuk RA, Zeeb A, Schultz RO. (1982): Corneal edema and the intraocular use of epinephrine. Am J Ophthalmol 93: 327-333.

Gurbaxani A, Packard R. (2007): Intracameral phenylephrine to prevent floppy iris syndrome during cataract surgery in patients on tamsulosin. Eye 21: 331-332.

Jacobs DS, Cox TA, Wagoner MD, Ariyasu RG, Karp CL. (2006): Capsule staining as an adjunct to cataract surgery: a report from the American Academy of Ophthalmology. Ophthalmology 113: 707-713.

Manvikar S, Allen D. (2006): Cataract surgery management in patients taking tamsulosin staged approach. J Cataract Refract Surg 32: 1611-1614.

Masket S, Belani S. (2007): Combined preoperative topical atropine sulfate 1% and intracameral nonpreserved epinephrine hydrochloride 1:4000 [corrected] for management of intraoperative floppy-iris syndrome. J Cataract Refract Surg 33: 580-582.

Myers WG, Shugar JK. (2009): Optimizing the intracameral dilation regimen for cataract surgery: prospective randomized comparison of 2 solutions. J Cataract Refract Surg 35: 273-276.

Nguyen DQ, Sebastian RT, Kyle G. (2007): Surgeon's experiences of the intraoperative floppy iris syndrome in the United Kingdom. Eye 21: 443-444.

Nichamin LD. (1993): Enlarging the pupil for cataract extraction using flexible nylon iris retractors. J Cataract Refract Surg 19: 793-796.

Oetting TA, Omphroy LC. (2002): Modified technique using flexible iris retractors in clear corneal cataract surgery. J Cataract Refract Surg 28: 596-598.

Parssinen O. (2005): The use of tamsulosin and iris hypotony during cataract surgery. Acta Ophthalmol Scand 83: 624-626.

Pong JC, Tang WW, Lai JS. (2008): Toxic endothelial cell destruction syndrome after intraocular lens repositioning with intracameral epinephrine. J Cataract Refract Surg 34: 1990-1991.

Shugar JK. (2006): Use of epinephrine for IFIS prophylaxis. J Cataract Refract Surg 32: 1074-1075.

Storr-Paulsen A, Skovlund J, Norregaard JC, Thulesen J. (2013): Corneal endothelial cell changes after cataract surgery in patients on systemic sympathetic alpha-1a medication (tamsulosin). Acta Ophthalmol Scand 91: In press

Takmaz T, Can I. (2007): Clinical features, complications, and incidence of intraoperative floppy iris syndrome in patients taking tamsulosin. Eur J Ophthalmol 17: 909-913.

10

In-Vitro Thermal Study of Different Tips in Various Operating Modes of the Sina Phacoemulsification System

Radin Tahvildari[1,2], Hanieh Fattahi[1,3] and Ahmad Amjadi[1]
[1]Sharif University of Technology,
[2]University of Ottawa,
[3]Max Planck Institute of Quantum Optics,
[1]Iran
[2]Canada
[3]Germany

1. Introduction

Ultrasonic surgery units operating in the frequency range 20-60 kHz for tissue fragmentation and removal have been available for over 20 years. Such devices are widely used in phacoemulsification (phaco), in the recanalization of coronary arteries and related procedures and in a range of soft tissue procedures, in particular neurosurgery. Cataract consists of opacification of the crystalline lens, causing a decrease in vision. To restore transparency and vision to the eye it is necessary to proceed surgically, removing the lens and restoring the eye's refractive power by inserting an artificial lens. A foldable intraocular lens implant (IOL) is placed into the remaining lens capsule. Phacoemulsification refers to modern cataract surgery in which the eye's internal lens is emulsified with an ultrasonic hand piece, and aspirated from the eye. Three components constitute the heart of all phaco systems: irrigation, aspiration and ultrasound. This surgical procedure requires eye-hand-foot coordination. The ultrasound generating mechanism of the phaco hand piece causes the tip attached to it to vibrate rapidly back and forth. Sharpness of the tip is directly proportional to the tip angle and its selection is dependent on aspirated fluids being replaced with irrigation of balanced salt solution, thus maintaining the anterior chamber, as well as cooling the hand piece.

Phacoemulsification is the preferred technique because of the lower incidence of wound-related complications and quicker healing times than with other surgery methods. So the patient's recovery time is usually faster.

One of the primary challenges is managing the heat generated be the tip at the incision site. With an increase in the use of phacoemulsifiation concern about the potential for thermal wound injuries during surgery has increased, such as burns on the cornea and the sclera. These are due mainly to a rise in heat in the area around the phaco tip. In some cases burns can result in fusion of the cornea or the sclera, wound gape, and damage to the corneal endothelium.

It is important to note that the aim of this chapter is to compare and analyze in vitro the changes of temperature around the different tips for three operating modes of the Sina Phacoemulsification System which is one of the products of an Iranian medical engineering company (Aali-Payam Corporation).
This chapter is based on study in which two different types of thermocouples, digital and thin wires, have been used as instruments for measuring and monitoring the temperature changes around different tips for three operating modes of the system (Constant, Linear and Pulse). The proposed in-vitro approach has been investigated in detail.
Phacoemulsifier tips come in a number of variations; the three common ones are named for the angle of the cutting area. These are the 15 degree, the 30 degree and the 45 degree tips. Some surgeons like to vary the tip depending on the density of the cataract: using a 45 degree tip for a hard cataract and a 30 degree tip for softer cataracts - as these latter are the most popular all of the measurements and comparisons have been done for these two tips.
On the other hand bubbles which form at the tip during surgery by phacoemulsification damage the corneal endothelium. The principal source of them is the degassing of the irrigation solution by ultrasonic agitation.
In part 5 of the chapter, it will be shown that the quantity of bubbles is modulated by the partial pressure of air in the irrigation solution and the intensity of the ultrasonic energy.

2. How a phacoemulsification system works

When the natural lens of eye becomes cloudy, usually because of the aging process, it blocks light rays from passing through or diffuses the light in such a way that vision becomes fuzzy or hazy. This cloudy lens is called a cataract. The object of cataract surgery is to remove this hazy lens and to replace it with a plastic prescription lens that is permanently implanted in the eye.
At present, the most widely used surgical technique is phacoemulsification, developed by Charles Kelman (Kelman, 1967), in which ultrasonic emissions are utilized to fragment the crystalline lens inside the eye, the fragments then being drawn out through a very small incision - about 2.8-3 mm - at the zone where the cornea meets the sclera. This technique has several advantages such as faster surgical times, smaller incisions which make healing times quicker and increased surgeon control (Packer et a1., 2005; Corvi et a1., 2006).
Three components constitute the heart of all phaco systems which are irrigation, aspiration and ultrasound (Yow et al., 1997). According to the position of operator's foot on the pedal of system, four positions are defined (Maloney et al., 1988)
Position 0: Foot is off the pedal, no action.
Position 1: Initial depression of foot pedal. Fluid flows from the bottle, no aspiration or emulsification.
Position 2: Pedal pushed to the detent. Aspiration now accompanies irrigation.
Position 3: Pedal pressed to the next detent. With phaco hand piece, emulsification now is added to irrigation and aspiration.
Three operating modes were analyzed;

- **Linear mode,** in this mode the power of ultrasound waves are increased gradually from zero to the preset power of the system and it directly depends on how far down the pedal is pushed
- **Constant mode,** in this mode the power of ultrasound emissions are equal to the preset power of system immediately in the stages in which waves were used

- **Pulse mode,** in this mode the ultrasonic stream is not continuous but pulsed (Aali-Payam Corporation, 2006)

The ultrasonic hand piece (**Figure 1**) incorporates a transducer for converting high frequency, alternating current in to mechanical vibrations. By piezoelectric crystals electrical energy converts to mechanical energy and causes the hollow cylindrical tip attached to oscillate at a frequency around 40 KHz to break up (emulsify) the cataract into tiny pieces (Bond et a1., 2003; Packer et a1., 2005).

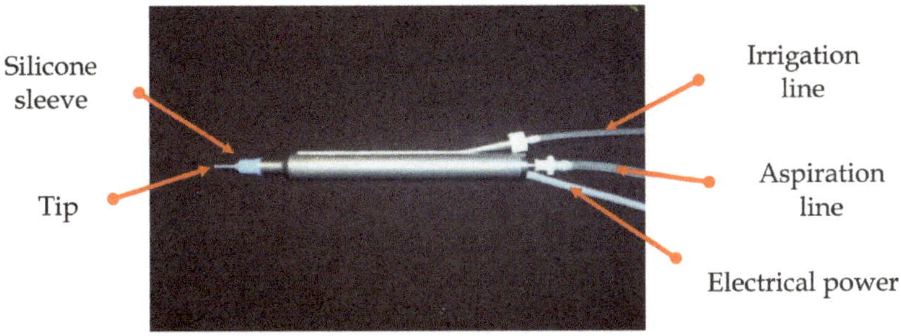

Fig. 1. Phacoemusification hand piece

The emulsified material is simultaneously suctioned from the eye by the tip. A special titanium alloy is the material of choice for such applications because of a favorable strength-to-weight ratio as well as biocompatibility and resistance to fragmentation. Phacoemulsifier tips come in a number of variations; the three common ones are named for the angle of the cutting area. They are the 0 degree, the 15 degree, the 30 degree and the 45 degree. The 45 degree tip has the longest bevel and therefore the sharpest tip, so it cuts most easily. Because of the large bevel of the aspiration port it occludes less easily. The 30 degree tip has a smaller bevel. Therefore the port is smaller and occludes more easily so it is more efficient for the aspiration. Some surgeons like to vary the tip depending on the density of the cataract: using a 45 degree tip for a hard cataract and a 30 degree tip for softer cataracts and they are the most popular so measurements and comparisons have been made for these two tips. The front (anterior) section of the lens capsule is removed along with the fragments of the natural lens. The back (posterior) portion of the capsule is left in place to hold and maintain the correct position for the implanted intraocular lenses.

2.1 Discussion

With an increase in the use of phacoemulsification concern about potential for thermal wound injuries during surgery has increased (Ernest et a1., 2001). Phacoemulsification requires more attention to detail than any other ophthalmic surgical procedure. The success of each step of the procedure is critically dependent upon how well each previous step was performed. Errors early in the procedure will almost inevitably result in subsequent problems. The small incision is what gives phaco most its advantages but, as with all steps in phacoemulsification, it must be fashioned very exactly (Osher et a1., 2006). The location, the size, the depth and configuration of the incision are all critical factors in determining the final outcome in phaco. In some cases burns can result in fusion of the cornea or the sclera, damage to the corneal endothelium, wound gape and delayed wound healing.

It is important to note that the aim of this study is to compare and analyze the changes of temperature around the different tips for three operating modes of the Sina Phacoemulsification System (**Figure 2**) which is one of the products of an Iranian medical engineering company (Ernest et a1., 2001; Tahvildari et a1., 2008).

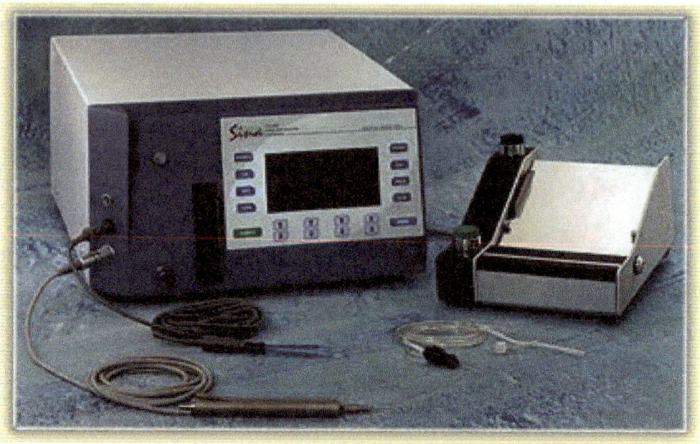

Fig. 2. Sina Phacoemulsification System (Aali-Payam Co.)

3. Test instruments and methodology

In this study, for the purpose of monitoring in vitro the changes of temperature values are based on the utilization of two different types of thermocouples;

a. Digital Thermocouple
b. Thin wires Thermocouple

In all of the experiments the phaco tip is in the chamber with dimension of 10 cm × 18 cm × 23 cm and is full of serum solution (Sodium Chloride 0.9%). The size of chamber is big enough for it to act as a thermal bath. The power of the system was on its pre-set value of 50% and the intensity of waves for this power are about 155 W/cm^2 (Tahvildari et a1., 2008, 2007).

3.1 Digital thermocouple

The digital thermocouple has a probe and can measure temperatures near the phaco tip with sensitivity of 0.01 °C. In measurement with a digital thermocouple, each experimental test is repeated 5 times for every mode and the averages of temperature change in a period of 60 seconds are plotted.

3.2 Thin wires thermocouple

The thin wires thermocouple is made of two different metal wires with sealing wax on them for prevention of RF (radio frequency) waves (Jones & Chin, 1991) In our experiments thin wires themocouple had been made of Nickel-Nickel, Chrome (Ni-NiCr). With four thin wires thermocouple temperatures are measured in four different areas (**Figure 3**) near the tip indirectly by the changes of voltage with sensitivity of 1 μV and simultaneously are drawn by an X-Y recorder.

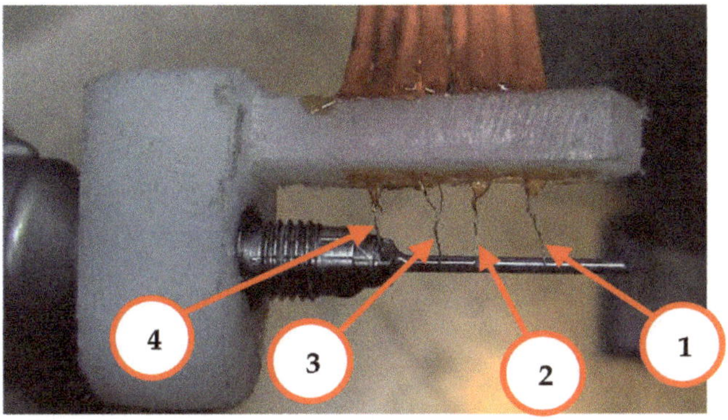

Fig. 3. Four different thin wires thermocouples monitor the temperature changes of the tip

On the next stage temperature changes are measured by the thin wires thermocouple for the same tip in a period of 60 seconds with the same initial conditions.
Because voltage changes are in the order of μV, then the numbers of peaks in a specific period of time are greater so in these graphs four points are important for us in comparison: the starting point, maximum, minimum and ending.

4. Analysis of results

In this study, for the purpose of monitoring in vitro the temperature values around two tips with the angle of 30 and 45 degree, first the measurements were performed using the digital thermocouple for different operating modes of the phaco system. In the next stage the same measurements were performed but with the thin wires thermocouple.

4.1 30 Degree tip – Digital thermocouple

Shown in **Figure 4** and **Table 1** are the temperature values monitored by digital thermocouple when the system is operating in linear and constant modes for the 30 Degree tip. In linear mode maximum temperature increase is 0.5 °C but in constant mode it is 0.47 °C.

	Average of Starting	Average of Maximums	Average of Minimums	Average of Endings
LINEAR MODE	21.62	22.12	21.87	22.1
CONSTANT MODE	21.65	22.12	21.87	22.12

Table 1. Temperature Values for Linear and Constant modes measured by Digital Thermocouple

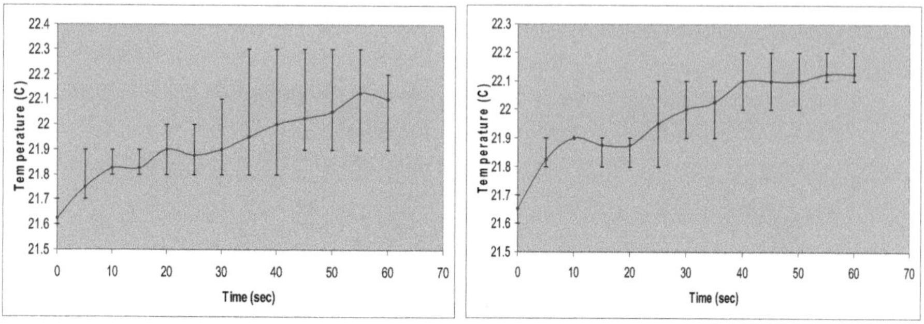

Fig. 4. Linear Mode - Temperature values versus Time [top]; Constant Mode - Temperature values versus Time [bottom]

Shown in **Figure 5** and **Table 2**, in pulse mode, when the system is set to emit 10 pulses per second (pps), maximum temperature increase for linear - pulse mode around the tip is 0.2 °C but for constant - pulse mode this value is 0.23 °C.

	Average of Starting	**Average of Maximums**	**Average of Minimums**	**Average of Endings**
LINEAR PULSE MODE	22.05	22.25	22.1	22.27
CONSTANT PULSE MODE	21.62	21.85	21.72	21.82

Table 2. Temperature Values for Linear - Pulse and Constant - Pulse modes measured by Digital Thermocouple

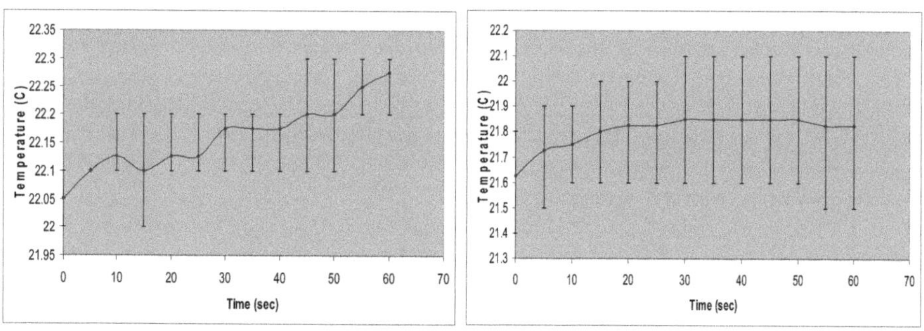

Fig. 5. Linear-Pulse Mode (10 pps) - Temperature values versus Time [top]; Constant-Pulse Mode (10 pps) - Temperature values versus Time [bottom]

4.2 30 Degree tip – Thin wires thermocouples

In **Table 3**, the temperature values reached in linear and constant modes around the tip which are measured by thin wires thermocouples in four different areas around the 30 Degree tip is shown.

		Starting	Maximum	Minimum	Ending
LINEAR MODE	THERMO NO.1	-10	38	8	22
	THERMO NO.2	-3	12	-1	-2
	THERMO NO.3	-10	102	35	80
	THERMO NO.4	-4	65	41	50
CONSTANT MODE	THERMO NO.1	-2	54	12	31
	THERMO NO.2	-2	17	1	2
	THERMO NO.3	3	100	59	89
	THERMO NO.4	1	84	21	67

Table 3. Temperature Values for Linear and Constant modes measured by thin wire thermocouples

Figure 6 are the temperature changes that are plotted according to the voltage changes of each thermocouple versus time in linear mode.
The maximum temperature increase in this mode for thermocouples No.1 is 48, No.2 is 15, No.3 is 112 and No.4 is 69 μV.

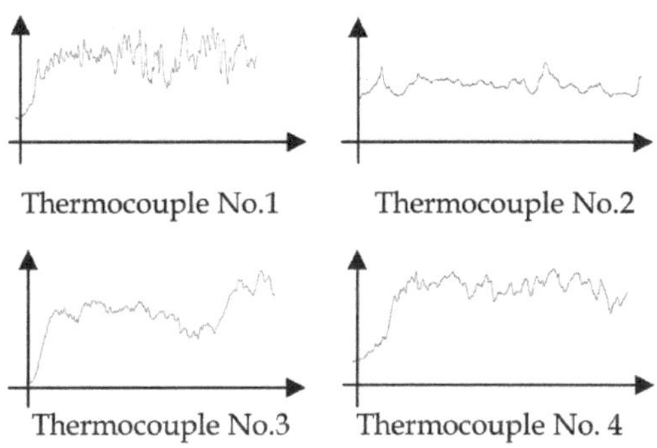

Fig. 6. Linear Mode - Voltage changes (μV) versus Time (sec.) for each thermocouple

Figure 7 are the temperature changes that are plotted according to the voltage changes of each thermocouple versus time in constant mode.
The maximum increase in this mode for thermocouples No.1 is 56, No.2 is 19, No.3 is 97 and No.4 is 83 μV.

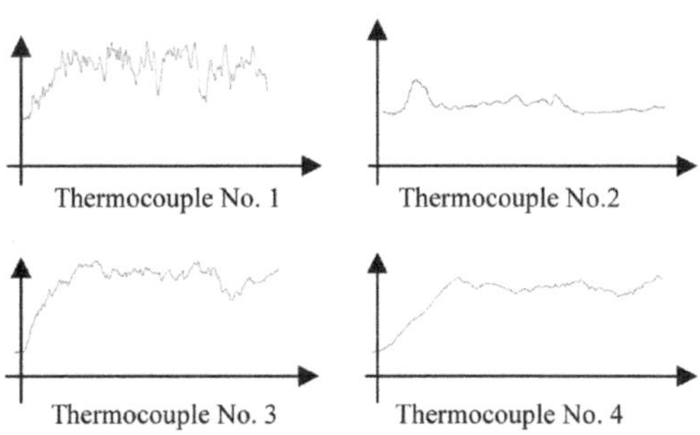

Fig. 7. Constant Mode - Voltage changes (μV) versus Time (sec.) for each thermocouple

In **Table 4**, the temperature values reached in linear - pulse and constant - pulse modes around the tip which are measured by thin wires thermocouples in four different areas around the tip is shown.

		Starting	Maximum	Minimum	Ending
LINEAR PULSE MODE	THERMO NO.1	2	31	18	27
	THERMO NO.2	-8	8	1	2
	THERMO NO.3	-3	57	38	37
	THERMO NO.4	-5	61	53	52
CONSTANT PULSE MODE	THERMO NO.1	-11	21	8	10
	THERMO NO.2	-2	17	9	11
	THERMO NO.3	12	63	48	57
	THERMO NO.4	6	90	78	9

Table 4. Temperature Values for Linear - Pulse and Constant - Pulse modes measured by thin wire thermocouples

Figure 8 are the temperature changes that are plotted according to the voltage changes of each thermocouple versus time in linear - pulse mode when the system is set to emit 10 pulses per second (10 pps). The maximum increase in this mode for thermocouples No.1 is 29, No.2 is 16, No.3 is 60 and No.4 is 66 μV.

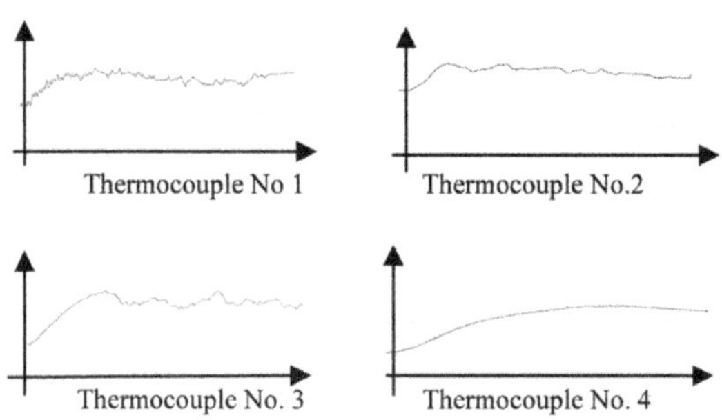

Fig. 8. Linear - Pulse Mode (10 pps) - Voltage changes (μV) versus Time (sec.) for each thermocouple

Figure 9 are the temperature changes that are plotted according to the voltage changes of each thermocouple versus time in constant - pulse mode when again the system is set to emit 10 pulses per second (10 pps). The maximum increase in this mode for thermocouples No.1 is 32, No.2 is 19, No.3 is 51 and No.4 is 84 μV.

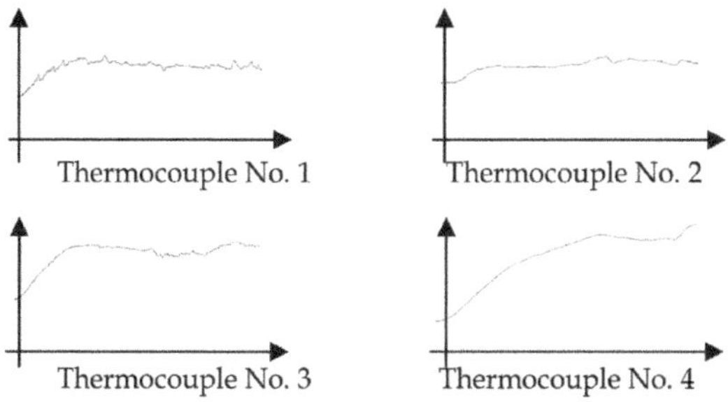

Fig. 9. Constant - Pulse Mode (10 pps) - Voltage changes (μV) versus Time (sec.) for each thermocouple

4.3 45 Degree tip – Digital thermocouple

Shown in **Figure 10** and **Table 5** are the temperature value monitored by digital thermocouple during the system is operating in linear and constant modes for the 45 Degree tip. In linear mode maximum increase is 0.72 °C but in constant mode it is 0.67 °C.

	Average of Starting	Average of Maximums	Average of Minimums	Average of Endings
LINEAR MODE	20.35	21.07	20.92	20.97
CONSTANT MODE	20.35	21.02	20.85	21.12

Table 5. Temperature Values for Linear and Constant modes measured by Digital Thermocouple

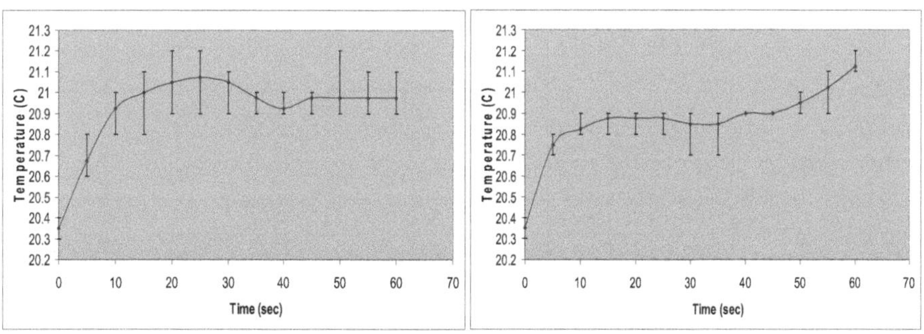

Fig. 10. Linear Mode - Temperature values versus Time [top]; Constant Mode - Temperature values versus Time [bottom]

Shown in **Figure 11** and **Table 6**, in pulse mode, when the system is set to emit 10 pulses per second (10 pps), maximum increase for linear - pulse mode around the tip is 0.17 °C but for constant - pulse mode this value is 0.13 °C.

	Average of Starting	Average of Maximums	Average of Minimums	Average of Endings
LINEAR PULSE MODE	21.40	21.57	22.55	21.62
CONSTANT PULSE MODE	20.57	20.70	20.65	20.72

Table 6. Temperature Values for Linear - Pulse and Constant - Pulse modes measured by Digital Thermocouple

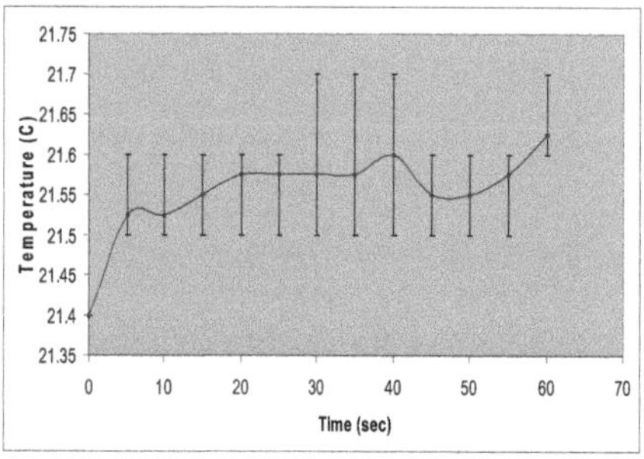

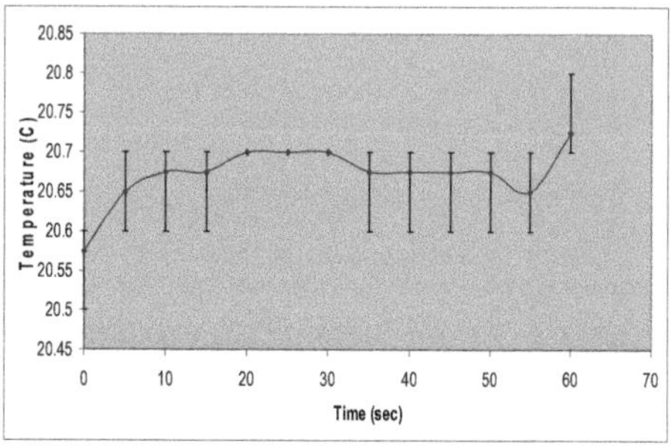

Fig. 11. Linear -Pulse Mode (10 pps) - Temperature values versus Time [top]; Constant - Pulse Mode (10pps) - Temperature values versus Time [bottom]

4.4 45 Degree tip – Thin wires thermocouples

In **Table 7**, the temperature values reached in linear and constant modes around the tip which are measured by thin wires thermocouples in four different areas around the tip is shown.

		Starting	Maximum	Minimum	Ending
LINEAR MODE	THERMO NO.1	0	40	-2	9
	THERMO NO.2	-9	23	7	18
	THERMO NO.3	-7	40	0	8
	THERMO NO.4	-7	6	0	2
CONSTANT MODE	THERMO NO.1	-5	4	-10	2
	THERMO NO.2	-8	11	-2	2
	THERMO NO.3	-14	50	10	15
	THERMO NO.4	-5	62	32	56

Table 7. Temperature Values for Linear and Constant modes measured by thin wire thermocouples

Figure 12 are the temperature changes that are plotted according to the voltage changes of each thermocouple versus time in linear mode.

The maximum increase in this mode for thermocouples No.1 is 40, No.2 is 32, No.3 is 47 and No.4 is 13 μV.

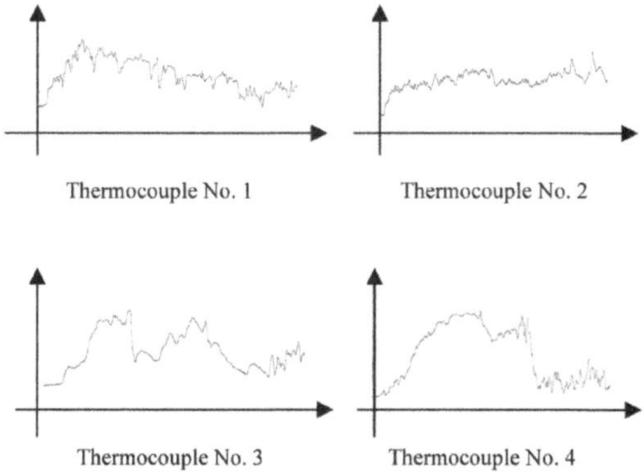

Fig. 12. Linear Mode - Voltage changes (μV) versus Time (sec.) for each thermocouple

Figure 13 are the temperature changes that are plotted according to the voltage changes of each thermocouple versus time in constant mode. The maximum increase in this mode for thermocouples No.1 is 9, No.2 is 19, No.3 is 64 and No.4 is 67 μV.

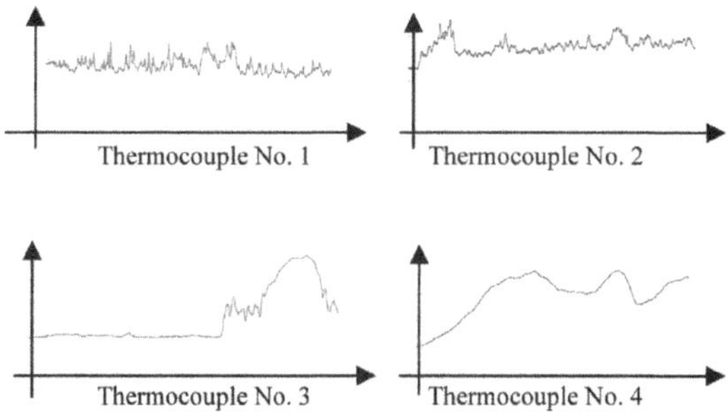

Fig. 13. Constant Mode - Voltage changes (μV) versus Time (sec.) for each thermocouple

In **Table 8**, the temperature values reached in linear - pulse and constant - pulse modes around the tip which are measured by thin wires thermocouples in four different areas around the tip is shown.

		Starting	Maximum	Minimum	Ending
Linear Pulse mode	Thermo No.1	0	12	-4	6
	Thermo No.2	0	26	16	23
	Thermo No.3	-2	12	-1	0
	Thermo No.4	4	58	33	54
Constant Pulse mode	Thermo No.1	-12	4	-8	2
	Thermo No.2	6	30	8	21
	Thermo No.3	-5	18	-7	-3
	Thermo No.4	9	40	16	33

Table 8. Temperature Values for Linear - Pulse and Constant - Pulse modes measured by thin wire thermocouples

Figure 14 are the temperature changes that are plotted according to the voltage changes of each thermocouple versus time in linear - pulse mode when the system is set to emit 10 pulses per second (10 pps). The maximum increase in this mode for thermocouples No.1 is 12, No.2 is 26, No.3 is 14 and No.4 is 54 μV.

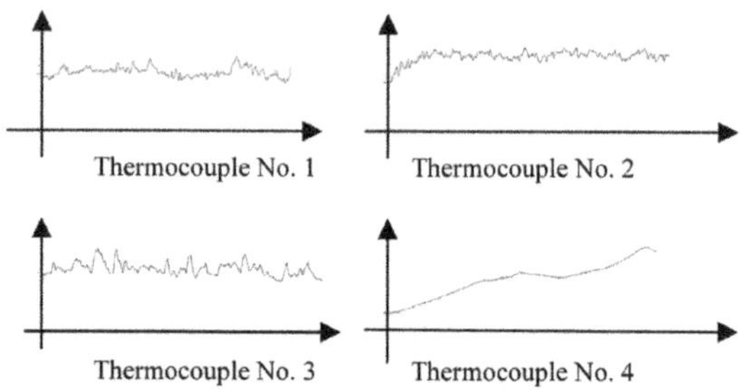

Fig. 14. Linear - Pulse Mode (10 pps) - Voltage changes (μV) versus Time (sec.) for each thermocouple

Figure 15 are the temperature changes that are plotted according to the voltage changes of each thermocouple versus time in constant - pulse mode when the system is set to emit 10 pulses per second (10 pps).
The maximum increase in this mode for thermocouples No.1 is 16, No.2 is 24, No.3 is 23 and No.4 is 31 μV.

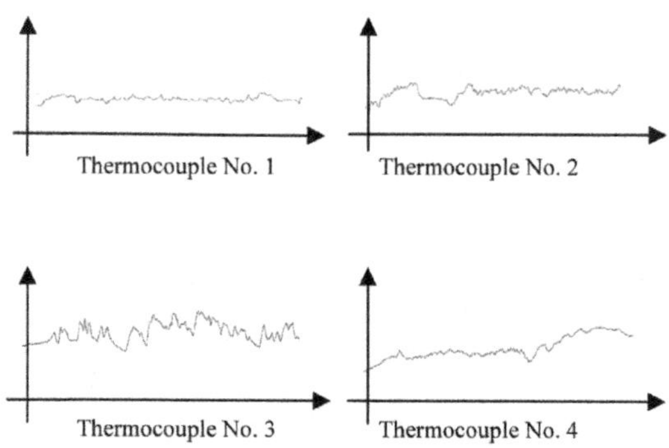

Fig. 15. Constant - Pulse Mode (10 pps) - Voltage changes (μV) versus Time (sec.) for each thermocouple

5. Air bubble effects on temperature changes

Bubbles generated during phacoemulsification damage the corneal endothelium. The principal source of the bubbles is the degassing of the irrigation solution by ultrasonic agitation. The quantity of bubbles is modulated by the partial pressure of air in the irrigation solution and the intensity of the ultrasonic energy. Bubbles reaching the endothelium can destroy cells (Kim et a1., 2002).

In this study all experiments were done in 60 seconds for the 45 degree tip using three solutions with different partial pressures of gas: ordinary, low-gassed and high-gassed. The phaco system was operating in constant mode with 50% power.
In **Table 9**, the temperature changes around the tip which are measured by digital thermocouple for three solutions is shown.

	Average of Starting	**Average of Maximums**	**Average of Minimums**	**Average of Endings**
ORDINARY	21.9	22.6	22.4	22.7
LOW-GASSED	21.9	22.9	22.6	22.9
HIGH- GASSED	22.1	22.8	23.3	23.3

Table 9. Temperature changes for different solutions measured by digital thermocouples shown in **Figure 16** the temperature value monitored by digital thermocouple during the system is operating in constant modes and the 45 Degree tip for three different solutions.

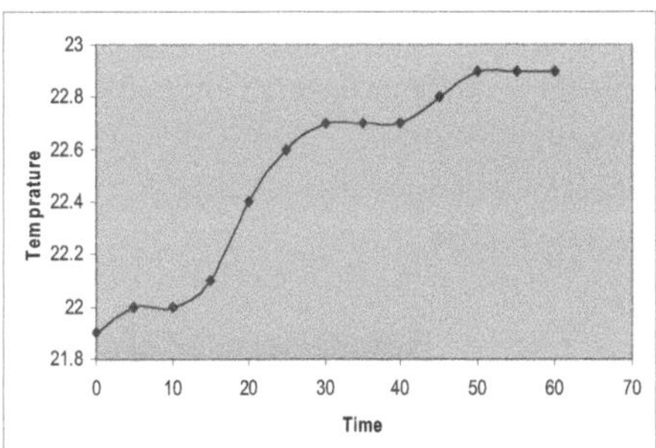

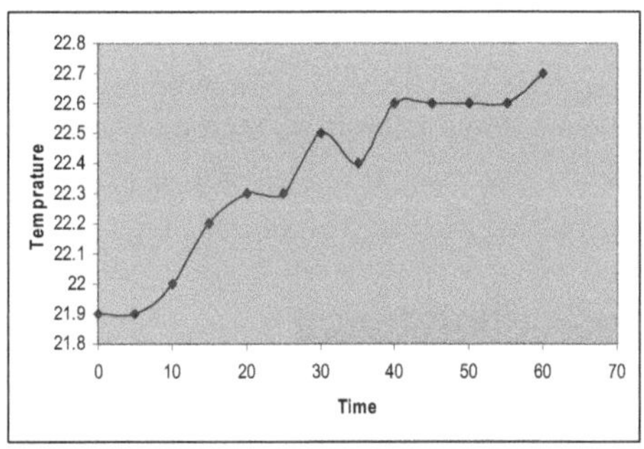

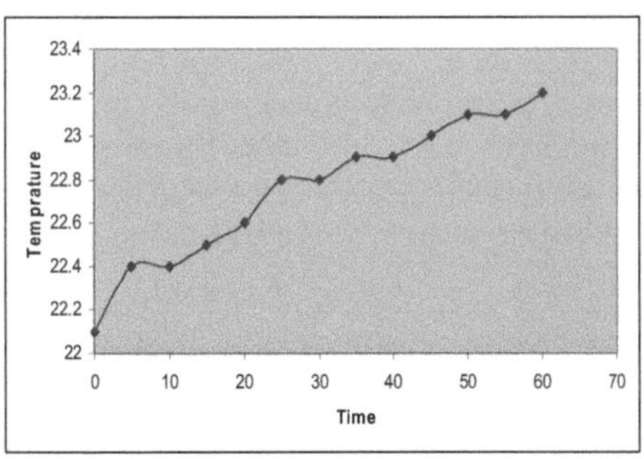

Fig. 16. Constant Mode - Temperature values versus Time for ordinary solution [top]; low-gassed solution [middle]; high-gassed solution [bottom]

According to these plots the changes of temperature for ordinary solution is is 0.7 °C, for low-gassed solution is 1.0 °C and for the high-gassed one is 1.2 °C.

In **Table 10**, the temperature changes around the tip where it is inserted to the eye exactly under the endothelium measured by digital thermocouple number 1 for three solutions is shown.

	Average of Starting	Average of Maximums	Average of Minimums	Average of Endings
Ordinary	68	75	71	73
Low-gassed	76	100	79	79
High- gassed	76	113	69	84

Table 10. Temperature changes for different solutions measured by thin wire thermocouple (Number 1)

Figure 17 are the temperature changes that are plotted according to the voltage changes of each thermocouple versus time in constant mode when the system is set to its 50% power.

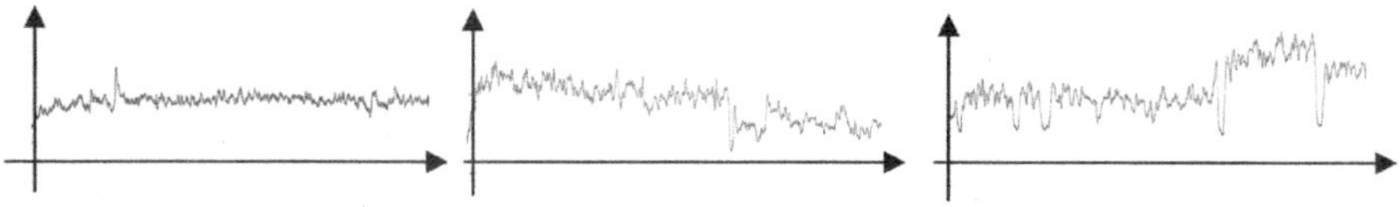

Fig. 17. Constant Mode – Temperature values versus Time for ordinary solution [left]; low-gassed solution [middle]; high-gassed solution [right] messured by thin wire thermocouples

According to these results the changes of temperature for ordinary solution is 7, for low-gassed solution is 23 and for the high-gassed solution is 27μV.

6. Conclusion

In this study thermocouples have been used as an instrument for measuring the temperature changes of different phaco tips for the purpose of monitoring and comparing three operating modes of a phacoemulsification system.

All in vitro measurements were done with the same initial conditions. In evaluating the maximum temperatures reached in each operating mode, it has been found that for both tips temperature changes in pulse mode (linear - pulse and constant - pulse) have fewer and lower peaks. The main reason for this is that the short periods of time between each pulsed wave allow the tip to cool between two successive emissions. Moreover, in these modes, the system produces a lower thermal increase with respect to the linear and constant modes.

It is strongly recommend that in cataract surgery employing the Sina phaco system only linear - pulse and constant - pulse modes should be used, so to reduce any possible surgical complications caused by the excessive release of heat.

Accordingly keeping the levels of partially dissolved gas in the irrigation solution low is a strategy for avoiding bubble formation and corneal endothelial damage.

Although all the experiments were performed in vitro, and increases in tip temperature during surgical operations is even higher than in these data, the results suggest the modern procedure of phacoemulsification can be performed at a safe temperature through an informed manipulation of surgeon-controlled parameters.

7. Acknowledgment

This research based on a collaboration research between Applied Physics Center at Sharif University of Technology and an Iranian medical engineering company (Aali-Payam Corporation).

I would like to thank Dr. M. Hashemi, Department of Ophthalmology at Iran University of Medical Sciences, for his guidance, helpful comments and support throughout this research. Special thanks to all the members of Aali-Payam Co. for giving us the opportunity to do this research on the Sina phacoemulsification system which is one of their products. I also thank the anonymous reviewers for providing insightful comments.

At the end, I owe an immense debt of gratitude to my beloved parents (The late Louise Tahvildary and the late Amanollah Tahvildari) for all of their support.

8. References

Aali-payam Corporation (2006), Instruction manual of phaco system; Sina model., pp. 23-24

Bond, L.J., Flake, M.D. and Tucker, B.J., (2003) Physics of phacoemulsification. Conference: World Conference on Ultrasound, Paris (FR)

Corvi, A., Innocenti, B., Mencucci, R., (2006) Thermography used for analysis and comparison of different cataract surgery procedures based on phacoemulsification. *Physiological Measurements*,Vol. 27, pp. 371-384

Ernest, P., Rhem, M., McDermott, M. and Lavery, K., (2001) Phacoemulsification conditions resulting in thermal wound injury," *Journal of Cataract & Refractive Surgery*, Vol. 27, pp. 1829-1839

Jones, L.D. and Chin, A.F. (1991) Electronic instruments and measurements, Prentice-Hall, New Jersey, 300-303.

Jones, L.D., and Chin, A.F., (1991) Electronic Instruments and Measurements Prentice-Hall, 300-303

Kelman, C.D., (1967) Phaco-emulsification and aspiration. A new technique of cataract removal. A preliminary report. *American journal of ophthalmology*, Vol. 64, pp. 23-35

Kim, E., Cristol, S., Kang, S. J. and Edelhauser, H., (2002) Endothelial protection: Avoiding air bubble formation at the phacoemulsification tip," *Journal of Cataract & Refractive Surgery*, Vol. 28, pp. 531-537

Maloney, William, F., Grindle, L. and Fallbrook, (1988) Textbook of phacoemulsification, CA: Lasenda Publishers

Osher, R.H., Injev, V.P., (2006) Thermal study of bare tips with various system parameters and incision. *Journal of Cataract & Refractive Surgery*,Vol. 32, pp. 867-872

Packer, M., Fishkind, W.J., Howard Fine, I. and Hoffman, R.S., (2005) The physics of phaco: A review. *Journal of Cataract & Refractive Surgery*,Vol. 31, pp. 424 - 431

Tahvildari, R., Fattahi, H. and Amjadi, A., (July 2010) Thermal analysis of different tips for various operating modes of phacoemulsification system. *Journal of Biomedical Science and Engineering (JBiSE)*, Vol. 3, No. 7, pp. 727 - 734

Tahvildari, R., Fattahi, H. and Amjadi, A., (May 2008) An in-vitro Measurement of Temperature Changes in Phacoemulsification System during Different modes.

Proceedings of the 2nd International Conference on Bioinformatics and Biomedical Engineering, Shanghai, China, pp. 1569-1574

Yow, L., Basti, S., (1997) Physical and mechanical principles of phacoemulsification and their cilinical relevance. *Indian Journal of Ophthalmology*, 45, 241-249

11

Hydrodynamic Analysis and Irrigation Device Design for the Coaxial and Bimanual Phacoemulsification Techniques in Cataract Surgery

Yury Spirochkin
Engineering Centre of Nuclear Equipment Strength (ENES)
Russia

1. Introduction

The phacoemulsification method, being in use in cataract surgery, includes mechanical disintegration of the lens of the human eye by special tools introduced into the anterior chamber of the eye through small incisions. The generated fragments of the lens are removed together with the intraocular fluid by aspiration. An artificial lens of transparent plastic is then inserted into the eye to replace the eliminated lens.

To avoid collapse of the anterior chamber because of the rarefaction (collapse may cause irreversible tissue injury), irrigation is carried out simultaneously with aspiration using a replacing fluid. Several phacoemulsification techniques are elaborated. Key ways in which they differ one from another are in the method of lens disruption and in the organization of aspiration-irrigation flow. Each technique requires adequate surgical tips to the instrument.

The basic technique now widely used is a combination of eye lens disintegration, aspiration and irrigation functions in one tip made of two coaxial tubules. The inner tubule is periodically subjected to longitudinal oscillations with an ultrasonic frequency in order to crush the lens fragments situated near the tubule end. The emulsion formed by these fragments and the fluid filling the anterior chamber are eliminated trough this tubule. The irrigation fluid is brought into the chamber through the annular channel between the inner and external tubules (Fig. 1).

Bimanual phacoemulsification is an alternative technique based on the use of two separated tips: one for aspiration and the other for irrigation. They are introduced into the anterior chamber through two incisions separated by a distinct distance and positioned angularly (Fig. 2). As a result, the fluid flow pattern across the surgical field changes substantially in comparison with the basic (coaxial) technique.

The decision to perform coaxial phacoemulsification is by many ophthalmic surgeons influenced by the greater experience with this technique and the desire of surgeons to avoid additional incisions. It was however observed in a series of operations that the bimanual technique is accompanied by a decrease of adverse hydrodynamic effect on eye tissues and of irrigation fluid consumption (Trubilin et al., 2005). A reduction of operation time was also observed. It was supposed that these favorable tendencies (which directly effect the quality of ophthalmic surgical care) are caused by the differences mentioned above in the intraocular hydrodynamics.

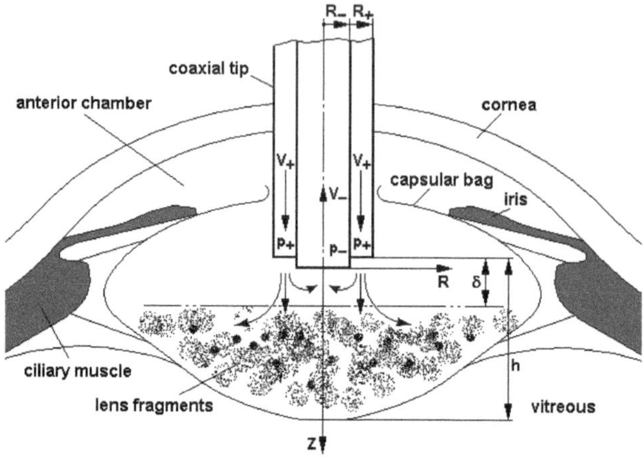

Fig. 1. Flow in the coaxial phacoemulsification technique

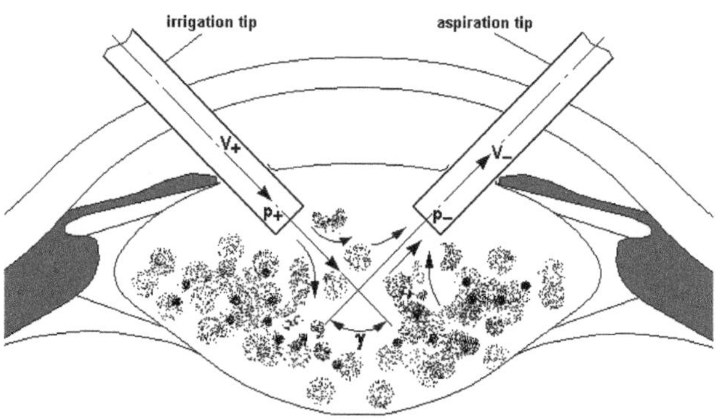

Fig. 2. Flow in the bimanual phacoemulsification technique

The possibilities of experimental validation of this assumption on natural eye specimens are limited because of high preparation costs, difficulties in physical data recording within small volumes, etc. Under these circumstances, mathematical modeling is the most accessible method for study of intraocular fluid flow.

Generally, both the empirical approach to the choice of ophthalmic surgical tools, which is widespread now, and the subjectivism in the clinical appraisal of their advantages or disadvantages lead to difficulties in design and development of tools which could ensure minimal tissue damage and maximal efficiency of the corresponding operation technique. Therefore, analysis of a new surgical method or a technique and the tools that will be used therein by means of an adequate mathematical model is quite an urgent problem. Its solution is demanded by ophthalmic surgeons as well as by designers of surgical tools.

In order to prove the advantages of the bimanual phacoemulsification technique the following steps are necessary:

- building an adequate mathematical model in the form of equations describing the fluid movements in the capsule bag volume during the operation
- clarifying on the basis of solution of these equations the main capabilities of this technique concerning the decrease of the injury from surgery, irrigation fluid consumption and operation time (relative to the coaxial technique)
- determining a set of quantitative parameters that characterize the operation technique and values of these parameters which could ensure its maximal efficiency.

The following parameters are taken as the efficiency criteria: reduction of tissue trauma caused by hydrodynamic forces, lowering of irrigation fluid consumption and decrease of the operation time. The tissue trauma can be associated with, amongst other causes:

- high fluid pressure including the dynamic sinusoidal and pulsation components
- inadvertent entry of the posterior lens capsule into the aspiration tubule
- collapse of the capsule chamber resulting from high difference between the internal and external pressure.

Hense, the required mathematical model should allow determination of the hydrodynamic pressure in zones of the anterior eye (as a trauma index) and the irrigation fluid consumption (as an economic index) as well as evaluation of the operation time.

In this Chapter, a simplified analytical model and analysis of hydrodynamic processes during phacoemulsification are presented; on the basis of the analysis, advantages of the bimanual technique are revealed and the favourable effect of this technique on operation time is evaluated. Subsequently, a review of applications of the sophisticated numerical analysis method - the finite element method (FEM) - applied to ocular biomechanics is given; use of this method for simulation of cataract surgery techniques could make analytical results more exact. As a practical embodiment of the ideas of the hydrodynamic analysis, designs of irrigation devices intended for the bimanual phacoemulsification technique are considered.

2. Simplified mathematical model of hydrodynamic processes

Mathematical modeling of the intraocular fluid flow is based on the mass, impulse and energy conservation laws. Assuming some simplifications, these laws allow series of relations to be obtained between the required values of pressure and irrigation fluid consumption, and the known geometric, physical and mechanical parameters. The fluid is assumed as incompressible viscose medium under stationary flow conditions. This assumption is valid even when oscillations of irrigation fluid rate exist over a wide frequency range. Indeed, the frequency value f, over which the non-stationary wave-propagation processes must be taken into account, can be evaluated by the formula

$$f \approx \frac{c}{L} \tag{1}$$

where c is the acoustic speed in the irrigation fluid, and L denotes the characteristic dimension of the flow domain.

As to the eye, L is about 10 mm, while c is about 1000 m/s. Therefore, the threshold value of f is not less than 10^5 Hz, and the slow dynamic processes in consideration can be regarded as stationary ones.

When building an adequate mathematical model, it is important to determine whether the fluid flow is turbulent or laminar one. The boundary between both flow types is determined by the Reynolds criterion

$$\mathrm{Re} = \frac{\rho L V}{\nu} \tag{2}$$

where ρ is the density of the fluid; for the irrigation fluid $\rho = 1000$ kg/m^3, for the emulsion $\rho = 998$ kg/m^3 (Malygin, 2002); V is the flow velocity of the irrigation fluid and of the emulsion; it ranges from 0.2 to 0.6 m/s; the mean value is 0.4 m/s (Malygin, 2002); ν denotes the dynamic viscosity coefficient; for the aqueous $\nu = 0.014$ Pa·s (Malygin, 2002).
In the case of the irrigation fluid outflow, the characteristic dimension L is the tubule diameter, up to 3 mm. Based on these values, Re is not more than 90, this is far from the critical value $Re_C = 2300$ typical for tube flows. Therefore, the irrigation fluid flow is laminar one. For the emulsion flow, L can be taken equal to capsular bag diameter (10 mm), so the Reynolds criterion can reach 300. However even in this case, it is substantially lower than the critical value quoted just now, or typical for free flow ($Re_C = 10^5$). The introduction of viscoelastic substances essentially increases the emulsion viscosity (Malygin, 2002), and this leads to corresponding decrease of the Reynolds criterion. Similar evaluation is also valid for the aspiration flow. Consequently, there is no reason to speak about the presence of flow instability, i.e. the appearance of turbulence in the irrigation and aspiration flows, and also in the emulsion within the operation field.
The laminar character of the flows under consideration makes their mathematical modeling easier. Usually, the equations in partial derivatives, e.g. the Navier-Stocks equations, are used for modeling in hydrodynamics (Landau and Livshits, 1988). They are solved by numerical methods taking into account given boundary conditions. As a result, the required parameters of the fluid flow in different points of the investigated domain are found: pressure, velocity, etc. However, solution of these equations for domains with intricate shapes, such as the anterior chamber of the eye is a difficult problem, especially when taking into account the configurations of the irrigation and aspiration flows, the biphasic character of the emulsion, the spatial diffusion of the lens fragments, the presence of an acoustic (ultrasonic) action, the movements of the surgical instruments, the flexibility of the eye tissues, etc.
Moreover, many physical parameters of the eye taken as input data for mathematical modeling have a significant scattering from one individual to another, and can not be exactly measured in each case with certainty. Additional uncertainties are caused by elasticity (flexibility) parameters of the ocular tissue or position of the aspiration-irrigation tip, which is manipulated by the surgeon's hand. Therefore the model needs to be simplified to obtain approximate solutions with acceptable precision and reasonable computing expenses for the calculations. But every simplification must be carefully grounded – in particular by means of special experiments. Otherwise the calculation errors may become unacceptable high.
Taking these factors into account it may not seem worthwhile creating complicated numerical approximations of the fluid movements. On the contrary, it is reasonable to use simple and evident physical relations resulting from the fundamental conservation laws. A basis for this approach lies correct choice of the surface on which flow parameters are checked, i.e. *the checking surface* (Abramovich, 1969). If a quantitative correlation between pressure and velocity

(correspondingly, the flow rate) can be established for various zones of this surface, without going into details concerning the flow in the internal domains, this correlation gives the required solution for each of the analyzed cases. Correspondingly, a comparison of the cases in dependence on the mentioned parameters is possible.

The simplified model described below is intended for comparative analysis of the two techniques of the phacoemulsification method under consideration. It takes into account the most substantial factors in which their differences may arise. In this case, the factors simultaneously inherent to both methods present no interest and are not subjected to the analysis. In particular, this model does not simulate the lens disintegration process, movement/shifting of surgical tools during the operation, finite dimensions of the lens particles, their motions, emulsion inhomogeneity, etc. Therefore it may be called the 1st approach model.

Let us first turn to the more established and in some ways more basic operation technique, i.e. the coaxial technique. The checking surface is chosen as the outlet cross section of the irrigation and aspiration tubules of the tip, which are considered being situated on one plane. The irrigation fluid is introduced into the anterior eye through the external annular part of this surface with the cross section area S_+ with the velocity V_+. The aspiration of the emulsion is carried out through the internal part with the cross section area S_- with the velocity V_-. According to the law of continuity, the irrigation volume flow must be equal to the aspirating one, i.e.

$$S_+V_+ = S_-V_- \tag{3}$$

from which is obtained an expression for the aspiration velocity:

$$V_- = \alpha V_+,\ \alpha = \frac{S_+}{S_-} = \left(\frac{R_+}{R_-}\right)^2 - 1 \tag{4}$$

where R_+ and R_- are the internal radii of the irrigation and aspiration tubules, correspondingly.

As follows from the Bernulli equation (which presents one of the forms of the law of conservation of energy), the pressure at the entry into the aspiration tubule comes to

$$p_- = p_+ - \frac{\rho V_+^2}{2}\left(\alpha^2 - 1\right) \tag{5}$$

while at the internal surface of the lens posterior capsule, against the edge of the irrigation-aspiration tip, where the irrigation flow completely loses the velocity (on the wall), the pressure value is

$$p_c = p_+ + \frac{\rho V_+^2}{2} \tag{6}$$

The parameter p_+ denotes the static pressure at the irrigation tubule outlet. For the coaxial tip of the above described design, R_+ is about 2 - 3 times greater than R_-. It follows that a may range from 3 up to 8. The pressure at the entry into the aspiration tubule p_-, as it seen from formula (4), is significantly lower than the pressure p_+ (about a half if a = 8), while the pressure p_c exceeds the latter by the velocity head $\rho V_+^2/2$. The approximate pattern for pressure distribution within the fluid volume between the edge of the coaxial irrigation-aspiration tip and the posterior lens capsule (the latter is an additional part of the checking surface) is shown in Fig. 3.

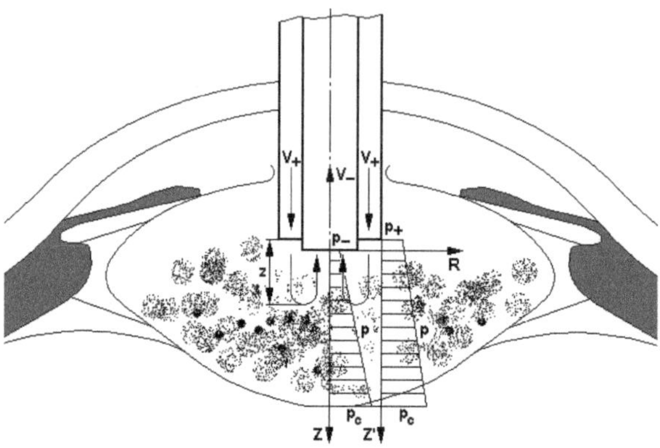

Fig. 3. Pressure distribution (p) and displacement of fluid particles (z) in the coaxial technique

The irrigation flow passes across this volume filled with the lens fragments, mixes with them (forming an emulsion), changes its movement direction into the opposite one and then is sucked into the aspiration tubule. The impulse value change is proportional to the vector difference between the aspiration and irrigation flow velocities and has in this case a maximal value. It produces a load on the internal surface of the capsular bag and can be estimated by the value p_c. With the actual pressure distribution a part of the irrigation fluid, moving near the aspiration tubule, has no time to mix with the lens fragments and does not dilute the emulsion, but is at once moved away by the aspiration flow. It does not have any useful effect and is merely pure losses. These shall now be estimated.
The displacement of the irrigation fluid particles along the Z axis (see Fig. 3) up to the stopping, i.e. up to the change of velocity sign, depends on their initial velocity V_+ and on the pressure gradient $\partial p/\partial z$

$$z = \frac{\rho V_+^2}{2} \frac{1}{\partial p / \partial z} \tag{7}$$

On the basis of the obtained pressure distribution (Fig. 3) the $\partial p/\partial z$ value at various points of the area in view can be evaluated, and so the z value can be found. In particular, at $R = R_-$

$$\frac{\partial p}{\partial z} \approx \frac{p_c - p_-}{h} = \frac{\rho V_+^2}{2h} \alpha^2 \tag{8}$$

where from follows $z = \dfrac{h}{\alpha^2}$,

and if $R = R_+$

$$\frac{\partial p}{\partial z} \approx \frac{p_c - p_+}{h} = \frac{\rho V_+^2}{2h} \quad (9)$$

then $z = h$

Here, h denotes the distance between the tip edge and the posterior lens capsule (see Fig. 1). Thus, the particles of irrigation fluid, which are moving near the internal surface of the irrigation tubule (at $R \approx R_+$), pass the entire distance to the posterior lens capsule ($z = h$). That means they run through the entire emulsion volume, dilute it and are sucked together with the lens fragments. The particles of irrigation fluid, which run directly near the aspiration tubule (at $R \approx R_-$), are sharply decelerated and may pass only a much shorter path ($z=h/a^2$) due to the great pressure drop near the edge. If the lens fragments are situated at a greater distance from the tip edge than h/a^2, they do not mix with these particles and exit into the aspiration tubule instead of the emulsion.

Assuming a linear pressure distribution along the radial coordinate, the following approximation for the displacement z of the particles is obtained, depending on the distance from the tubule axis R

$$z(R) = h\left[\frac{1}{\alpha^2} + (1 - \frac{1}{\alpha^2})\frac{R - R_-}{R_+ - R_-}\right] \quad (10)$$

Based on this approximate correlation, shown in Fig. 4, and starting from the distance between the tip edge and the conventional boundary of the lens fragments position δ (see Fig. 1) it is possible to determine the radial coordinate $R(\delta)$ that corresponds to the dividing of the irrigation flux in two parts Q_p and Q_n

$$R(\delta) = R_- + \frac{\frac{\delta}{h} - \frac{1}{\alpha^2}}{1 - \frac{1}{\alpha^2}}(R_+ - R_-) \quad (11)$$

The particles, which meet the condition $R > R(\delta)$, form the flux part

$$Q_p = V_+\pi[R_+^2 - R(\delta)^2] \quad (12)$$

which dilutes the emulsion. Therefore it exerts a useful action. The particles with the coordinates $R \leq R(\delta)$ do not reach the emulsion boundary. They form the flux part

$$Q_n = V_+\pi[R(\delta)^2 - R_-^2] \quad (13)$$

which presents pure losses.

As follows from equations (11) - (13), the less the distance between the edge of the irrigation-aspiration tip and the conventional boundary of where the zone with the lens fragments δ is, the nearer the radial coordinate $R(\delta)$ to the radius value R_- is, and the less the losses Q_n are. Correspondingly, the further the tip edge from the above mentioned boundary lies, the greater the losses are. In particular, for a tip with the parameters $R_- \approx 0.5$ mm and $R_+ \approx 1.5$ mm, when the edge is situated at 2 mm from the internal surface of capsular bag and at 1 mm from the indicated boundary, about 40% of the infused fluid is useless taken away through the aspiration tubule. When $\delta = h/a^2$ the losses become almost zero. However this distance is difficult to control and it is impossible to avoid losses completely. The calculation shows that losses of the irrigation fluid are a fundamental disadvantage of the coaxial technique, which lowers its efficiency.

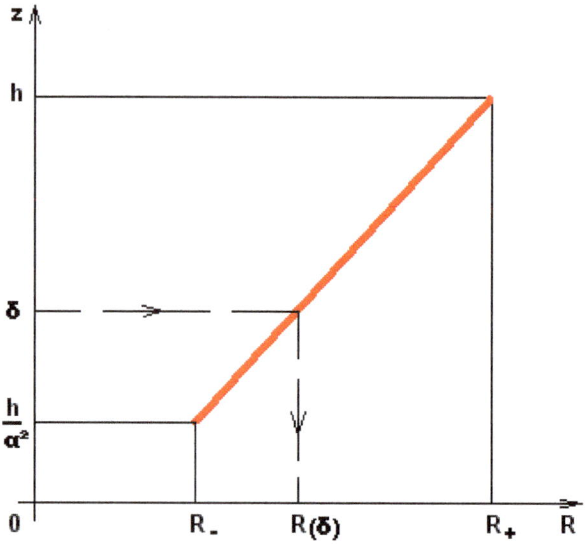

Fig. 4. Displacement of fluid particles, z, in dependence on distance from the tubule axis, R

Let us examine the bimanual technique which uses separated irrigation and aspiration tubules. As done formerly, the control surface will be considered to consist of the tubules' end section areas and of the internal surface of capsular bag (the posterior lens capsule).

If the tubules are positioned parallel (Fig. 5) there is no practical difference in the hydrodynamic situation as compared to the coaxial method.

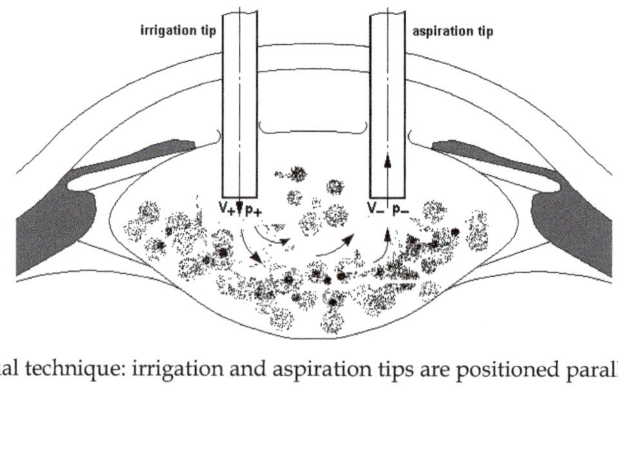

Fig. 5. Bimanual technique: irrigation and aspiration tips are positioned parallel

The irrigation flow changes the direction into the opposite one, the momentum increment is maximal, and the pressure on the internal surface of capsular bag comes to $p_c = p_+ + \rho V_+^2/2$ as in the precedent example. If the tubules are situated at some angle one to another, the momentum increment decreases proportional to cos (γ/2), where γ denotes the angle between the tubules' axes (see Fig. 2), and the pressure correspondingly decreases. The flatter the tubules are situated one to another, the less is the pressure on the wall. It reaches a minimum value when γ = 180°, i.e. the tubules are situated on one axis. Thus the bimanual technique allows control of the pressure by positional relationship of the tubules.
As to the irrigation fluid consumption, the irrigation and aspiration tubules may be placed at different sites of the volume occupied by the lens fragments. In this case it is possible to direct the flux Q across this volume that insures maximal dilution of the emulsion and its aspiration, practically without losses i.e.

$$Q_p = Q = V_+ \pi R_+^2 ,\ Q_n = 0 \tag{14}$$

Thus far the quasi-static component of the fluid pressure has been analyzed. Pulsation of the hydrodynamic pressure under the conditions of laminar flow may be caused by oscillations of fluid consumption only. As for the pulsation due to transient processes, these do not exceed several percents of the flowing fluid velocity head (Aviation acoustics, 1986). In reality, the pulsation component does not appreciable change the velocity of the irrigation-aspiration flow and the whole modeled situation. Taking this into account would therefore not exert a substantial influence on the results that have been obtained.
The modeling that has been described shows that the bimanual technique is more efficient than the coaxial one in reducing both the traumatic factor (pressure on the eye tissues) and the irrigation fluid consumption.

3. Evaluation of operation time

The time necessary to clean the operative field from the lens fragments in many respects depends on the cleaning method and on the degree of homogeneity of the emulsion formed after the irrigation fluid infusion. Several typical cases of the development of this process may be analyzed.
Case 1. The irrigation and aspiration flows are laminar and cover the entire anterior chamber of the eye. In this case, the emulsion is smoothly eliminated from the operative field and the time of full cleaning t can be determined by the formula

$$t = \frac{\theta}{Q} \tag{15}$$

where θ denotes the volume of the anterior chamber.
Case 2. The emulsion is maintained in a homogeneous state during the entire aspiration process. The necessary degree of homogeneity can be achieved by continuous mixing the fluid. In this case, the concentration of the lens fragments decreases with time governed by exponential law with the exponent proportional to t.
Case 3. Laminar flow of the irrigation and aspiration fluids occurs only in a part of the operative field while in the remaining domain stagnation zones are observed. In these zones, the fluid circulates in a circle. In this domain the elimination of the emulsion occurs

only from the above mentioned area, where the irrigation-aspiration flow (laminar flow with running off) is organized.
Of course, none of the cases mentioned is realized in a pure form, but nevertheless they ensure a qualitative comparison between the cleaning time values for the anterior chamber when using the coaxial and the bimanual phacoemulsification techniques. Case 3 gives the best fit for characterization of the coaxial technique. Here, laminar flow with running off occupies a relatively small part of the operative field. According to the estimation above, under these conditions only somewhat more than a half of the infused irrigation fluid volume is effectively used. To clean the stagnation zones the aspiration tip must be shifted. This necessitates the skill of the surgeon and takes an amount of time also.
The bimanual technique is instead characterized rather by Case 1. Laminar flow with running off occupies the major part of the anterior chamber of the eye and correspondingly of the cloud of lens fragments so that shifting of the tip is not necessary.
When using both the coaxial and the bimanual techniques, any shift of the tip (casual or intentional) leads to mixing of the emulsion. The process then tends to follow the characteristics of Case 2 that results in increasing the cleaning time.
Thus, it may be affirmed that in all cases the cleaning time depends to a great extent on the surgeon's skill. However, the bimanual technique does not need a large tip shift and is potentially less traumatic. Besides, the theoretic cleaning time (as follows from the calculations above), which is determined by the loss of the irrigation fluid, is lower by some ten percent.

4. Review of finite element analyses

More precise mathematical modeling of hydrodynamic processes during surgical operation is able to increase the efficiency of the bimanual technique both in lowering pressure further and in obtaining a faster cleaning of the operating field from lens fragments. For modeling, the sophisticated numerical approximations based on FEM are applicable.
A short summary review of finite element simulations applied to several problems of eye biomechanics is presented below; it gives information on how investigations develop and which issues arise. The summary does not pretend to be a comprehensive review of the topic and only touches on some key achievements.
One of the first applications of FEM to modeling of the human eye seems to have been carried out by Pinsky and Datye (Pinsky & Datye, 1991). A finite element model was built to examine effects of radial keratotomy. It assumed horizontal and vertical corneal symmetry and linear elastic material for mechanical behavior of eye tissues.
Bryant and his colleagues have used finite element analysis to investigate the susceptibility of the human cornea with fully healed radial keratotomy incisions (Bryant et al., 1994). The material was assumed to be homogeneous, isotropic, and nonlinearly elastic, with the elastic modulus defined as the derivative of the average stress-strain curve of control strips cut from fresh human donor corneas subjected to tensile testing and failure. Differences between analysis and experimental data have been observed, accounted for by variation in stiffness between the uncut stroma and the wound collagen, and the effect of stress concentration at the wound.
Researchers from the Department of Ophthalmology, Yokohama City University School of Medicine, have applied FEM to determine mechanical behaviour of human eye when loading by impacts of foreign bodies causing intraocular injuries (Uchio at al., 1999). Solid

modeling was based on information obtained from cadaver eyes. Blunt-shaped missile impacts onto the surface of the cornea or sclera at velocities 30 to 60 m/s have been simulated; simulations have been carried out using a supercomputer.

In sequential investigations, finite element modeling technique of the eye has been developed; the main developments were the following: improved approximation of complex geometry (Belezza et al., 2000), (Sigal et al., 2004), anisotropic fiber-matrix material properties (Amini and Barocas, 2009), and nonlinear anisotropic, inhomogeneous, collagen fiber-reinforced structure of eye tissues (Girard et al., 2009). For modeling and calculations, ANSYS software is widely used now. All the investigations noted above focused on improved approximations of eye tissues without adequite modeling of intraocular fluid.

In the Department of Biomechanical Engineering in University of Minnesota Supercomputing Institute, a coupled-flow finite element model of the iris and the aqueous humor has been developed (Elastohydrodynamics of the Anterior Eye, 2002). This model accounts for the passive deformation of the solid iris in response to flow of aqueous humor fluid. The problem is fully coupled because the location of the iris depends on the flow pressure, but the fluid flow pattern depends on the location of the iris (Fig. 6). This relative simple model is already large enough to require considerable computational resources because of the fluid-solid coupling, and the rapidity of ocular events (the lens accommodates from far-viewing to near-viewing in a few tenths of a second).

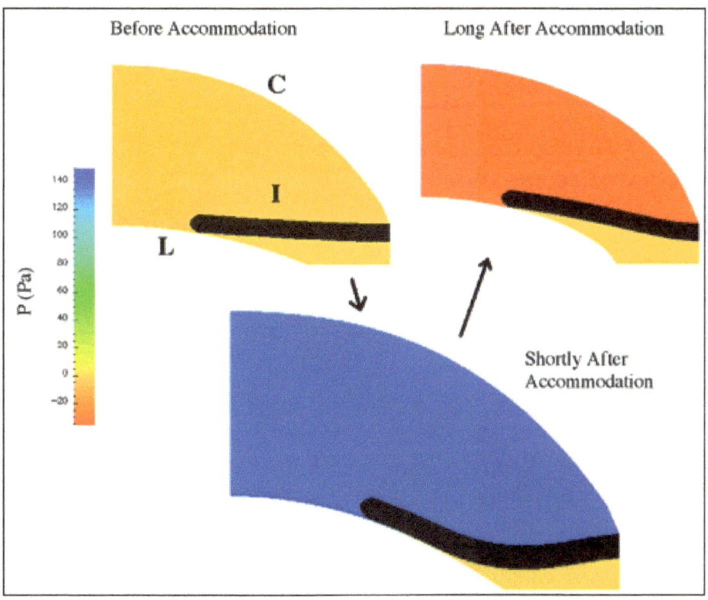

Fig. 6. Iris deformation in response to lens motion (Elastohydrodynamics of the Anterior Eye, 2002)

This coupled-flow finite element model does not cover cataract surgery. An approximation relating to cataract surgery was developed in order to predict changes in the corneal curvature after surgery based on investigations into the material properties of the cornea

(Crouch et al., 2005). A linear elastic material model was used for the entire eye. To examine the effect of surgical incisions, a cut in the initial eye mesh was made representing the incision made in an extra-capsular cataract extraction procedure. The authors note that extensive future work is needed to produce and validate a biomechanical model that could be used to help predict surgical outcomes. This work may expand on the current work in the following ways:

- apply an oriented fiber tissue model
- augment the finite element model with a time-dependent simulation of the healing response
- experiments with individualized eye models.

With participation of the author of this Chapter, a group of researchers at the Helmholtz Moscow Research Institute of Eye Diseases have started with investigation of accommodation processes using FEM (Poloz et al., 2008).

Scientists and engineers of University of Minnesota now run patient-specific computational fluid dynamics (CFD) and finite element simulations to support medical device innovation and validation (Medical Device Invention and Evaluation through Simulation, Visualization, and Interactive Design, 2010). Simulation could reduce the time it takes to reach bench tests and animal trials, make these trials more effective, and, in time, overtake these methods as the primary evaluative approach in device design. A group of researchers have begun to work on design environment composed of coupled components for running simulations, visualization and comparing massive numbers of results, and interacting directly with the parameter space to explore new device designs. The approach is very promising, but for the moment, the latter innovations do not cover cataract surgery and ophthalmology.

5. Irrigation device design based on hydrodynamic analysis

Based on mathematical modeling, surgical tool design can be carried out in a rational and validated manner. For example, it is known that sudden expansion of a channel is accompanied by significant hydraulic resistance i.e. decrease of the total flow pressure (Abramovich, 1969). The pressure drop in expanding stream of the irrigation fluid (in absence of a wall) may be evaluated as follows:

$$\Delta p = \frac{\rho V_+^2}{2}(1 - \frac{S_+}{S}) \tag{16}$$

where S is the surface area formed by the expanding stream (the sum of end surface areas of separate fluid jets). Consequently, the greater S is, the smaller the hydrodynamic effect of the fluid on eye tissue is exerted.

The stream, which outflows from the tubule with normal (perpendicular to the axis) outlet cross section into a great volume cavity, has a shape nearing to a cone. If series of holes are made in the tubule wall and their number and arrangement are correctly chosen, an almost spherically expanding stream can be obtained, and consequently the maximal area S. In this case, it is possible to approach almost the minimal pressure value on the wall determined by the formula (16).

The idea has been embodied in a device for irrigation (Pletnev et al., 2005) intended for the bimanual phacoemulsification technique. The device contains the hollow tube 1 with the hooked end 2 as shown in Fig. 7. A part of cylindrical surface 2 has at least two rows of irrigation holes 3. Each three of these holes are situated at the corners of equilateral triangles and form equilateral triangles with the neighbouring holes. The closed end surface 4 of the hooked end is furnished with at least one irrigation hole. The total area of all holes lies within the range 20% to 25% of the area of the cylindrical surface of the hooked end.

The device is designed so that the fluid outflows from irrigation holes in the form of fluid jets oriented normally to the cylindrical surface. In all holes, approximately the same flow rate and hydraulic drop are realized. The fluid jets interflowing form a closed frontal surface akin to spherical one, where hydrodynamic pressure is at the minimum.

An advanced device for irrigation which functions in a similar way is shown in Fig. 8 (Spirochkin et al., 2008). This device contains the hollow tube 1 with the closed end surface furnished with irrigation holes 2. The end surface is designed in the form of an ellipsoid of revolution 3 extended along the tube axis. This form of the end surface is chosen to ensure nearly spherical front surface of the outflowing irrigation fluid and approximate equidistance to the crystalline lens inner surface inside which this end enters. The holes 2 are situated at equal spatial angles 4 measured relative to the ellipsoid center. The total area of the irrigation holes lies within the range 40% to 50% of the ellipsoid surface area.

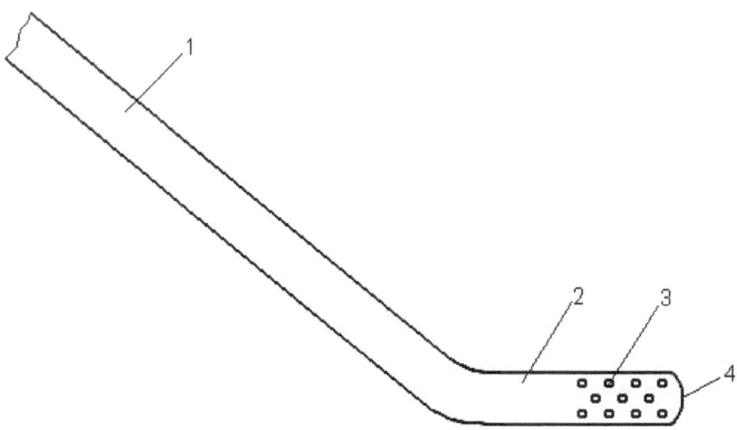

Fig. 7. Device for irrigation (Pletnev et al., 2005). See text for details.

The irrigation fluid outflowing through the holes 2 forms a closed frontal ellipsoid surface and effects with nearly minimum hydrodynamic pressure on the internal surfaces of eye tissues. Hence use of these inventions theoretically reduces trauma to eye tissues.

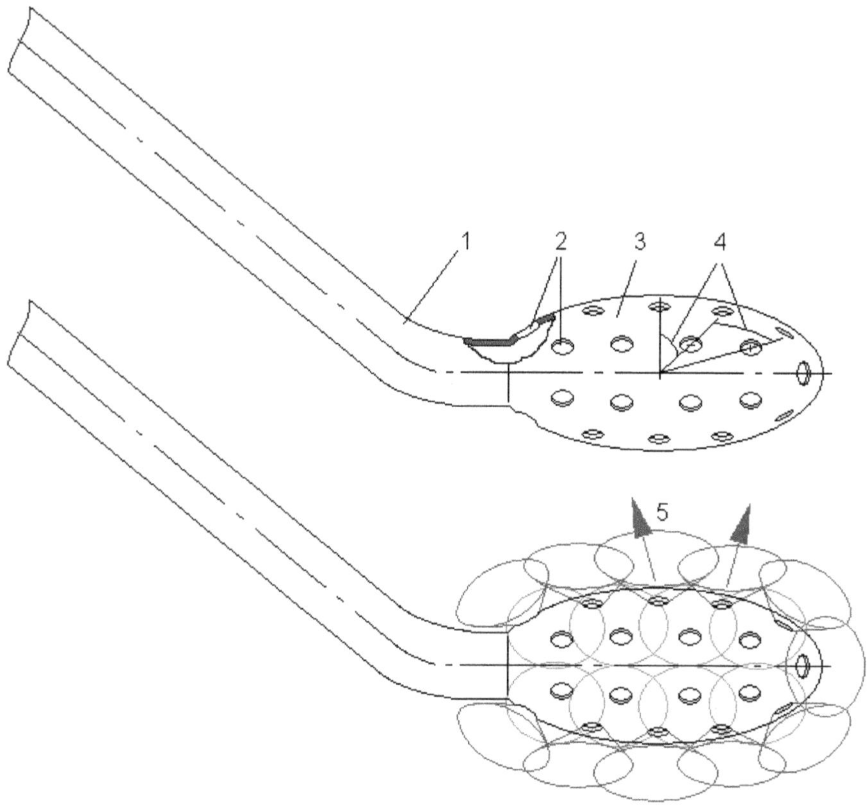

Fig. 8. Advanced device for irrigation (Spirochkin et al., 2008). See text for details.

6. Conclusion

The analytical approach, which has been presented, provides a rational basis for evaluation of new surgical methods in ophthalmology and for design of surgical tools. Simplified mathematical modeling of hydrodynamic processes during surgical operations is similar to the technique of structure dimensioning, or sizing, commonly used in engineering practice, e.g. in nuclear engineering (with which the author is especially familiar). Surgical procedures or structural parameters of surgical tools obtained at the stage of dimensioning can be checked and corrected at the next stage of engineering: coupled structure-fluid analysis using the finite element method. However techniques of finite element analysis for support of cataract surgery need to be developed.

7. Acknowledgment

The problem has been introduced to the author by Dr. Zimina (Moscow). Her assistance during its formulation and solution is invaluable. The author is thankful to Mr. Pletnev, the head of experimental test laboratory in the Energia Corp. (Korolyov near Moscow), for enormous intellectual contribution to this work.

8. References

Abramovich, G.N (1969). Applied Gasdynamics (3rd Edition). - Moscow: Science (in Russian)

Amini, R. and Barocas, V.H. (2009). Anterior Chamber Angle Opening during Corneoscleral Indentation: The Mechanism of Whole Eye Globe Deformation and the Importance of the Limbus. *Investigative Ophthalmology & Visual Science*. Vol. 50, No. 11, pp. 5288-5294

Aviation acoustics (1986). Ed. by A.G. Munin. In 2 parts. Part 2. - Moscow: Machine-building (in Russian)

Belezza, A.J.; Hart, R.T.; Burgoyne, C.F. (2000). The Optic Nerve Head as a Biomechanical Structure: Initial Finite Element Modeling. *Investigative Ophthalmology & Visual Science*. Vol. 41, No. 10, pp. 2991-3000

Bryant, M.R.; Szerenyi, K., Schmotzer, H.; McDonnel, P.J. (1994). Corneal Tensile Strength in Fully Healed Radial Keratotomy Wounds. *Investigative Ophthalmology & Visual Science*. Vol. 35, No. 7, pp. 3022-3031

Crouch, J.R.; Merriam, J.C.; Crouch, E.R. (2005). Finite Element Model of Cornea Deformation. *Medical Image Computing and Computer-Assisted Intervention - MICCAI 2005. Lecture Notes in Computer Science*. Vol. 3750/2005, pp. 591-598, Available from: http://www.springerlink.com/content/3vc2ua4tjqdf2vw9

Elastohydrodynamics of the Anterior Eye (2002). *Supercomputing Institute Research Bulletin. Summer 2002*. University of Minnesota. Vol. 18, No. 2, Available from: http://static.msi.umn.edu/research_bulletin/Vol.18-No.2

Girard, M.J.A.; Suh, J.-K.F; Bottlang, M.; Burgoyne, C.F.; Downs, J.C. (2009). Scleral Biomechanics in the Aging Monkey Eye. *Investigative Ophthalmology & Visual Science*. Vol. 50, No. 11, pp. 5226-5237

Landau, L.D. and Livshits, E.M. (1988). Hydrodynamics. - Moscow: Science (in Russian)

Malyugin, B.E. (2002). Medical and Technological System for Surgical Rehabilitation of Patients with Cataract on the Base of Ultrasonic Phacoemulsification and Intraoculare Lens Implantation.Dissertation. - Moscow: Fedorov's Center of Eye Microsurgery (in Russian)

Medical Device Invention and Evaluation Through Simulation, Visualization, and Interactive Design (2010). *Supercomputing Institute Research Bulletin. Fall 2010*. University of Minnesota. Vol. 26, No. 3, Available from: http://static.msi.umn.edu/research_bulletin/2010-26-3.pdf

Pinsky, P. and Datye, D. (1991). A Microstructurally Based Finite Element Model of the Incised Human Cornea. *Journal of Biomechanics*, Vol. 24, pp. 907-992

Pletnev, I.V.; Spirochkin, Yu.K.; Zimina, T.Yu., Trubilin, V.N. (2005). Device for Irrigation. Patent of Russian Federation for useful model, No. 51869 (in Russian)

Poloz, M.V.; Iomdina, E.N., Spirochkin, Yu.K. (2008). Numerical Modeling for Optical and Mechanical Proccesses of Accomodation, Available from: http://www.helmholtzeyeinstitute.ru/photo/406.doc

Sigal, I.A.; Flanagan, J.G.; Tertinegg, I.; Ethier, C.R. (2004). Finite Element Modeling of Optic Nerve Head Biomechanics. *Investigative Ophthalmology & Visual Science*. Vol. 45, No. 12, pp. 4378-4387

Spirochkin, Yu.K.; Takhchidi, Kh.P., Karavaev, A.A. (2008). Device for Irrigation. Patent of Russian Federation for invention, No. 2331395 (in Russian)

Trubilin, V.N; Zimina T.Y., Spirochkin, Yu.K. (2005). Comparative Analysis of Hydrodynamic Streams during the Coaxial and the Bimanual Phacoemulsification. *Refractive Surgery and Ophthalmology*, Vol. 5 (No.1), pp. 19-25 (in Russian)

Uchio, E.; Ohno, S.; Kudoh, J.; Aoki, K.; Kisielewicz, L. (1999). Simulation Model of an Eyeball Based on Finite Element Analysis on a Supercomputer. *British Journal of Ophthalmology*, Vol. 83, pp. 1106-1111

12

Intracameral Mydriatics in Cataract Surgery

Anders Behndig, Björn Lundberg and Gunnie Bäckström
Department of Clinical Sciences, Ophthalmology, Umeå University, Umeå, Sweden

1. Introduction

The routines for cataract surgery have undergone a remarkable development over the past two to three decades (Lundstrom, Stenevi et al. 2002). Surgical techniques have improved constantly, and now require less extensive anesthesia (Behndig and Linden 1998), decreased need for hospitalization (Oshika, Amano et al. 2001; Yi, Flanagan et al. 2001) and fewer postoperative controls (Edwards, Rehman et al. 1997). Still, it is remarkable that some perioperative routines have undergone very little change, despite the general improvement. One of those more or less unchanged routines have been the routine for preoperative pupil dilatation.

In a phacoemulsification cataract procedure, a large proportion of the work is done within the eye, and sufficient mydriasis is a prerequisite to allow for visualization of the capsulorhexis and the lens. Conversely, poor mydriasis during cataract surgery increases the risk of intraoperative complications such as posterior capsule rupture (Artzen, Lundstrom et al. 2009), A small pupil can make instrument maneuvering within the eye more difficult, make the capsulorhexis hydrodissection and phacoemulsification more difficult to perform of the lens nucleus can lead to an increased risk of iris damage, and increases the risk also for other complications, including sphincter tear, bleeding and dropped nucleus. Iris damage due to a small pupil can result in an irregular and atonic pupil with photophobia and other types of discomfort.

Traditionally, topical administration of a combination of anticholinergic (passive) mydriatic agents such as cyclopentolate 1%, tropicamide 1%, homatropine 5% or scopolamine 0.25% and sympathomimetic (active) mydriatic agents such as phenylephrine 2.5% to 10% has been the preferred way to achieve mydriasis. Often, topical nonsteroidal antiinflammatory drops such as indomethacin 1%, flurbiprofen 0.03%, or suprofen 1% are also added, to enhance and prolong the mydriatic effect. The administration of the eye drops is typically started 45 minutes to 1 hour before the surgical procedure. It is clear that this regimen has some disadvantages. First, it is well known that the slow penetration of mydriatic substances through the cornea renders a slow pupil enlargement (Lovasik 1986; Chien and Schoenwald 1990) with a maximum mydriatic effect at 30 minutes for cyclopentolate (Haaga, Kaila et al. 1998) and as much as 75 minutes for phenylephrine. (Matsumoto, Tsuru et al. 1982) In practice, this means that the waiting time for the pupil to dilate often is several-fold longer than the surgical procedure itself. Second, limited bioavailability of topically administered substances means a significant systemic absorption (Doane, Jensen et al. 1978; Kaila, Huupponen et al. 1989; Haaga, Kaila et al. 1998) which in turn may increase the risk for cardiovascular side-effects, (Fraunfelder and Scafidi 1978; Fraunfelder and Meyer 1985) especially in high-risk groups such as persons with hypertension, (Hakim, Orton et al. 1990) or cardiovascular diseases, (Meyer and Fraunfelder 1980) and in children. (Ogut, Bozkurt et al. 1996; Elibol, Alcelik et al. 1997), Third, even if a good mydriasis is achieved initially, the mydriatic effect often tends to diminish during the operation, and especially when the procedure takes longer than expected. Different solutions have been suggested to prolong the mydriatic effect from topical mydriatics such as preoperative treatment with diclofenac (Antcliff and Trew 1997), viscous 10% phenylephrine, (Duffin, Pettit et al. 1983) or intraoperative intracameral epinephrine. (Duffin, Pettit et al. 1983; Liou and Yang 1998). In 2003, we first introduced the concept of intracamerally injected mydriatics, in which mydriatic substances were mixed with the intracameral lidocaine given at the start of the phacoemulsification cataract procedure. As we will see below, a local anesthetic will also have an additive, passive mydriatic effect when injected intracamerally (Cionni, Barros et al. 2003). We early found that when using a regimen involving intracameral mydriatics, some of the disadvantages with topical mydriatics are avoided, since the method means no preoperative waiting time and also reduced doses of the mydriatic substances - and thereby likely lowers the risk for systemic side-effects (Lundberg and Behndig 2003) (Morgado, Barros et al. 2010). In our own current setting, a preservative-free mixture of phenylephrine 1.5% and lidocaine 1% is used, but other solutions have been proposed and used clinically, mainly preservative-free epinephrine 0.025% with lidocaine 0.75%, or lidocaine 1% only. Other substances have been tried experimentally and proven efficient, such as epinine 0.3% - 3.0% and isoprenaline 0.3%. An interesting consequence of the concept of intracameral mydriatics in intraocular surgery is also that is provides us with a possibility to use other mydriatic substances than the traditional anticholinergics and α_1-adrenergics (Cionni, Barros et al. 2003; Lundberg and Behndig 2009; Myers and Shugar 2009), since the doses of potentially cardiotoxic drugs can be reduced, and we no longer have to consider limitations in bioavailability because of the corneal barrier. Cyclopentolate, whether given topically or intracamerally, has been demonstrated not to contribute to increased mydriasis when using intracameral mydriatics (Lundberg and Behndig 2008), and neither has epinephrine added to the intraoperative infusion (Lundberg and Behndig 2007). Cyclopentolate and similar substances are therefore often abandoned in intracameral mydriatics regimens today, and accordingly, intraoperative epinephrine infusion is more seldom used today by surgeons using intracameral mydriatics. With intracameral mydriatics, the mydriasis generally reaches 95% its final value within 20-30 seconds. Intracameral mydriatics render slightly smaller pupils than topical mydriatics at a maximum dosage, but with intracameral mydriatics, the pupils do not contract intraoperatively, as with topical mydriatics. As insufficient adrenergic stimulation of the pupil dilator appears to be a major factor causing intraoperative pupil contraction during phacoemulsification cataract surgery (Antcliff and Trew 1997; Liou and Yang 1998; Backstrom and Behndig 2006), intracameral mydriatics containing an adrenergic substance is effective in re-dilating the pupil (Backstrom and Behndig 2006; Mori, Miyai et al. 2010), and are also used to prevent intraoperative floppy iris syndrome (IFIS) (Gurbaxani and Packard 2007; Takmaz and Can 2007; Cantrell, Bream-Rouwenhorst et al. 2008). With intracameral mydriatics, the patients perceive less initial glare from the operation microscope light, as the pupil is small at the beginning of the procedure. The intracameral mydriatics concept has been extensively studied from a safety perspective by us and others, and is found to be safe with no increase in corneal endothelial cell loss (Lundberg and Behndig 2003) (including at long-term follow-up), inflammatory reaction, postoperative corneal swelling (Lundberg and Behndig 2003) or macular edema (Johansson, Lundberg et al. 2007). Furthermore, in routine surgery, the surgical performance does not differ from when a standard topical mydriatic regimen is used (Behndig and Eriksson 2004). Intracameral mydriatics comprise a rapid, effective and safe alternative to topical mydriatics in phacoemulsification surgery. It has a potential to simplify the preoperative routines, and for certain high-risk groups, it may reduce the risk for cardiovascular side effects.

2. Intracameral mydriatics

2.1 Published studies

Several studies have been published suggesting different routines for the use of intracameral mydriatics, and evaluating the various regimens. This chapter aims to give a brief overview of the published studies.

2.1.1 Initial studies: Cyclopentolate/phenylephrine/lidocaine

In 2003 our group published a prospective, randomized, double-masked study (Lundberg and Behndig 2003) in which the patients were randomly assigned either of two treatments: traditional topical mydriatics with 3 drops each of cyclopentolate 1% and phenylephrine 10% with 15 minutes interval plus 150µl of preservative-free xylocaine 1% intracamerally at the beginning of the procedure, or intracameral mydriatics with placebo eye drops and 150 µl of a preservative-free mixture of cyclopentolate .1%, phenylephrine 1.5% and lidocaine 1% intracamerally. In this study, the intracameral injection was given by the other surgeon, and thus, neither the operating surgeon nor the patients were aware of which of the two treatments was given, allowing for the double-masked design. The pupil sizes were recorded during surgery using video recordings, and also at one day and one month postoperatively, using the Orbscan II®, (Marsich and Bullimore 2000) (Bausch & Lomb Surgical, Inc., San Dimas, CA). In addition, corneal endothelial morphometry, ETDRS visual acuity (Camparini, Cassinari et al. 2001) intraocular pressure (IOP) and intraoperative blood pressure and pulse were measured.
After injection of intracameral mydriatics, the pupils reached 95±3% of their maximum size after 20 seconds (Figure 1). In the intracameral mydriatics group, the pupil size after viscoelastic injection was 6.7±1.0 mm, which was about 1 mm smaller than with topical mydriatics, but when using intracameral mydriatics the pupils continued to enlarge throughout the procedure as opposed to when topical mydriatics were used. The corneal endothelial morphometry did not differ between intracameral and topical mydriatics. A significant pulse deceleration was seen with topical, but not with intracameral mydriatics. This likely resulted from the fact that the total dose of phenylephrine with intracameral mydriatics in this setting was only 23% of that with topical mydriatics. The results of this study were confirmed in a small pilot series of 10 patients published by Soong *et al* in 2006 (Soong, Soultanidis et al. 2006), where it was also concluded that the intracameral technique is a safe, rapid, and effective alternative to conventional topical mydriasis in phacoemulsification cataract surgery, and that it can reduce the duration of stay within the outpatient surgical units. The latter is not least important considering the high turnover of modern cataract surgery. The authors had also, at the time of publication, continued with another 280 uneventful routine cases using the same technique.

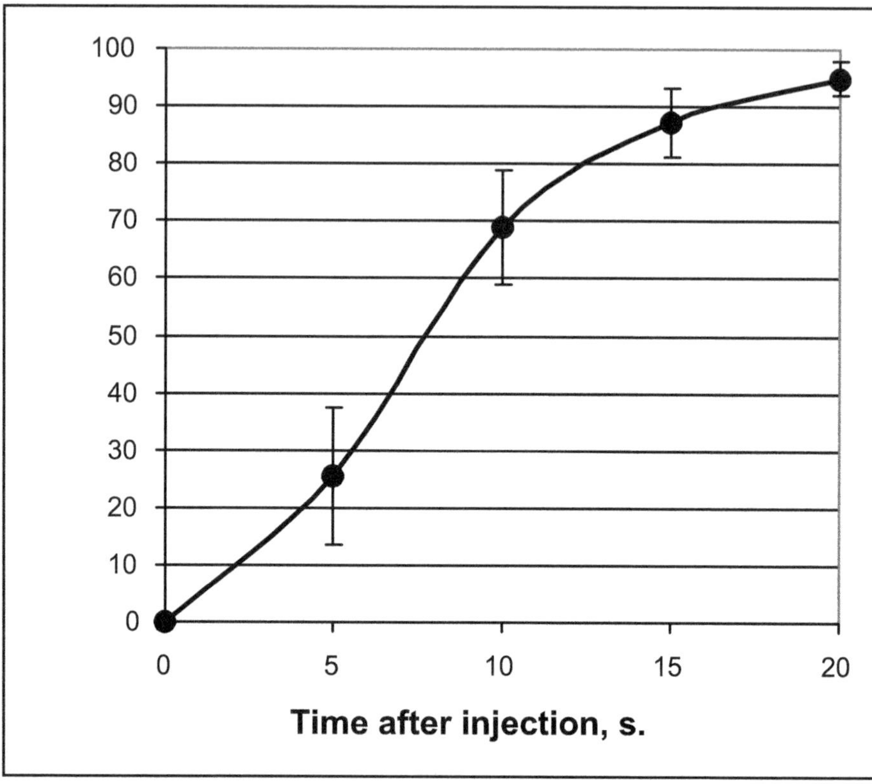

Fig. 1. Pupil size after injection of intracameral mydriatics. Pupils reached 95±3% of their maximum size after 20 seconds.

2.1.2 Initial studies: Lidocaine

At the same time as the above mentioned study (in fact in the same number of Journal of Cataract and Refractive Surgery) Robert J Cionni *et al* published an article describing the use of 300 to 500µl of Xylocaine-MPF 1% injected intracamerally as the sole mydriatic agent (Cionni, Barros et al. 2003). Epinephrine 0.3 cc of 1:1000 was also added to the infusion. The authors state that "Mydriasis begins immediately, enabling the surgeon to proceed within 90 seconds." In this study, the first 12 patients had adequate mydriasis, with a mean pupil size before dilation of 2.4 mm (range 1.5 to 3.1 mm) and after intracameral Xylocaine-MPF 1%, 6.5 mm (range 5.2 to 7.2 mm).

2.1.3 Further studies on lidocaine

The results from Cionni's study were confirmed in 2007 by Nikeghbali *et al* (Nikeghbali, Falavarjani et al. 2007) in a prospective comparative case series including 57 patients randomized to receive either topical mydriatics (30 eyes) or intracameral lidocaine (27 eyes) to dilate the pupil. The topical mydriatics given consisted of 3 drops of cyclopentolate 1%

and phenylephrine 5% given 5 minutes apart starting 60 minutes before surgery. The intracameral group received 0.2-0.3 ml of preservative-free lidocaine 1% intracamerally. Noteably, in this study, no epinephrine was added to the irrigating solution. The mean pupil dilation was 4.52±0.08mm in the intracameral group and 4.06±0.09 mm in the topical group, and no difference in the overall subjective surgical performance was noted. Similar results were also published the following year in the Indian Journal of Ophthalmology by the same group; in a case series of 31 consecutive cases the pupils dilated from 2.63±0.33 mm to 7.03±0.61 90 seconds after injection of 0.2 to 0.3 ml of preservative-free lidocaine 1%, and no negative effects on the surgical performance were noted (Nikeghbali, Falavarjani et al. 2008). Jayadev and Nayak also published a short report on this regimen in 2007 (Jayadev and Nayak 2007).

Noticeably, both the studies by Nikeghbali (Nikeghbali, Falavarjani et al. 2007; Nikeghbali, Falavarjani et al. 2008) and Jayadev (Jayadev and Nayak 2007) demonstrate significantly larger pupils after intracameral lidocaine without preoperative topical mydriatics, than we have seen in our investigations (Lundberg and Behndig 2008). This difference in effect from intracameral lidocaine may be due to population differences, differences in lidocaine dosage, or the fact that the pupil size was measured 90 seconds after the intracameral lidocaine injection in the studies in question. Generally, the onset of mydriasis from a passive dilator such as lidocaine, administered intracamerally will be a bit slower than from the combination of an active and a passive dilator.

2.1.4 Surgical performance

In 2004, a series of 198 consecutive cases operated with intracameral mydriatics was compared to the previous 198 cases operated with traditional topical mydriatics (Behndig and Eriksson 2004). Several pre- intra- and postoperative parameters were registered, the subjective surgical performance was graded after each procedure, and the change in pulse and oxygen saturation induced by the ICM injection was registered. Despite the smaller pupils at the initiation of the procedures, no increase in operation time or complication rates was seen with with intracameral mydriatics, compared to when standard topical mydriatics were used. Furthermore, the subjective surgical performance was ranked as equally good for both groups. The studies from Nikeghbali *et al* (Nikeghbali, Falavarjani et al. 2008) confirmed the results of a surgical performance similar to when using topical mydriatics.

2.1.5 Handling intraoperative pupil constriction

In 2006, a prospective, randomized, placebo-controlled, double-masked study study involving 80 patients was published, aiming to determine whether intracameral mydriatics can redilate pupils that contract during phacoemulsification cataract surgery (Backstrom and Behndig 2006). Patients were randomized to receive or not receive an addition of 0.6 μg/ml of epinephrine to the irrigation solution, and further randomized to have an injection of our original intracameral mydriatics mixture or placebo after the phacoemulsification and cortex cleaning. The pupil sizes were registered at different time points during surgery and the day after surgery. There was a greater degree of pupil contraction in the absence of epinephrine in the irrigation solution compared to in the presence of epinephrine. In cases where no epinephrine was added to the irrigation solution, the intracameral mydriatics solution given significantly redilated the pupils at 30 seconds ($p<0.001$ compared with placebo) as well as at 2 mins ($p = 0.015$ compared with placebo). These findings are also well in accordance with the later findings of Mori *et al*, demonstrating a satisfactory pupil ditatation with an intracameral solution containing phenylephrine and tropicamide in cases with insufficient pupil dilatation from topical mydriatics (Mori, Miyai et al. 2010). The findings of the 2006 study also confirms earlier reports that insufficient adrenergic stimulation of the pupil dilator is a major factor causing intraoperative pupil contraction during phacoemulsification cataract surgery (Antcliff and Trew 1997; Liou and Yang 1998). Likely, this factor also contributes to the absence of pupil contraction seen when using a large bolus dose of an adrenergic substance at the beginning of a surgical procedure (as with intracameral mydriatics), as opposed to when topical mydriatics are employed (Lundberg and Behndig 2003; Lundberg and Behndig 2007).

2.1.6 Omitting epinephrine infusion

It has long been known that addition of epinephrine to the irrigating solution prevents intraoperative pupil constriction in phacoemulsification surgery with topical mydriatics (Antcliff and Trew 1997; Liou and Yang 1998; Backstrom and Behndig 2006). To investigate whether this holds true also with intracameral mydriatics, we performed a study in 2007 to evaluate the possibility of removing epinephrine from the irrigating solution in phacoemulsification surgery when using intracameral mydriatics (Lundberg and Behndig 2007). In this prospective, randomized, double-masked study involving a total of 140 cataract patients, the first part of the study included 90 patients divided into two groups. Patients in both groups were given 150 µl of the intracameral mydriatic solution at the beginning of the procedure. In the first group, 0.6 µg/ml epinephrine was added to the irrigating solution; no epinephrine was added to the irrigation solution used in the second group. The second part of the study involved 50 patients, all of whom were given topical mydriatics and then similarly divided into two groups and treated as in the first part of the study. As noted in our initial studies (Lundberg and Behndig 2003), the pupil sizes generally increased during the procedures with intracameral mydriatics. Interestingly, this increase was significantly greater without epinephrine (13 +/- 19% versus 4 +/- 14%; $p = 0.02$). In the topical mydriatics setting, pupil sizes decreased intraoperatively in both groups; significantly more without epinephrine (- 5 +/- 4% versus - 12 +/- 7%; $p < 0.001$). We concluded that an irrigating solution without epinephrine can safely be used with intracameral mydriatics. The increase in pupil size during the procedure was even shown to be greater without epinephrine. As epinephrine is unstable in a solution with physiological pH, time-consuming repeated blending procedures are needed, which can be avoided if intracameral mydriatics are used. The study also confirms earlier findings that epinephrine is beneficial when using topical mydriatics (Antcliff and Trew 1997; Liou and Yang 1998; Backstrom and Behndig 2006).

2.1.7 Omitting cyclopentolate

Since we suspected that the onset of mydriasis from intracameral cyclopentolate was too slow for the substance to be meaningful as an intracameral mydriatic, and that the passive dilating effect of lidocaine would be quite sufficient together with an adrenergic substance such as phenylephrine, we decided to assess the separate mydriatic effects of intracameral cyclopentolate hydrochloride, lidocaine hydrochloride and phenylephrine hydrochloride in another prospective randomized double-masked study published in 2008 (Lundberg and Behndig 2008). The study involved a total of 56 cataract patients: in 16 patients, lidocaine 1%, phenylephrine 1.5%, and cyclopentolate 0.1% were injected sequentially one after the other.

Phenylephrine and cyclopentolate were randomized to switch in order, creating 2 study groups with 8 patients in each. In part two of the study, an additional 40 patients were randomized to receive either all three substances intracamerally (lidocaine 1%, phenylephrine 1.5%, and cyclopentolate 0.1%) or intracameral lidocaine 1% and phenylephrine 1.5% only.
Lidocaine alone gave a significant pupil dilation to 4.9±0.6 mm. When cyclopentolate was injected next, the pupil size increased further by 1.3±0.6 mm. When phenylephrine was added, the pupil increased an additional 0.7±0.4 mm. In the second group, in which phenylephrine was given directly after lidocaine, the pupil size increased by 2.1±0.5 mm. When cyclopentolate was added as the third substance, no significant change in the pupil size could be seen (Figure 2). Accordingly, no statistically significant differences in pupil size were observed between the 20+20 patients who were given intracameral mydriatics with or without cyclopentolate. Noteably, though, the day after surgery, the pupils were significantly larger in the cyclopentolate group (4.7±1.1mm) than in the group without cyclopentolate 2.9±0.8 mm. We concluded that cyclopentolate administrated intracamerally has no immediate additive mydriatic effect to intracameral lidocaine plus phenylephrine, or to put it more precisely, intracameral cyclopentolate dilates the pupil after surgery, but not during surgery. After this study, cyclopentolate was omitted from our clinical routine preparation.

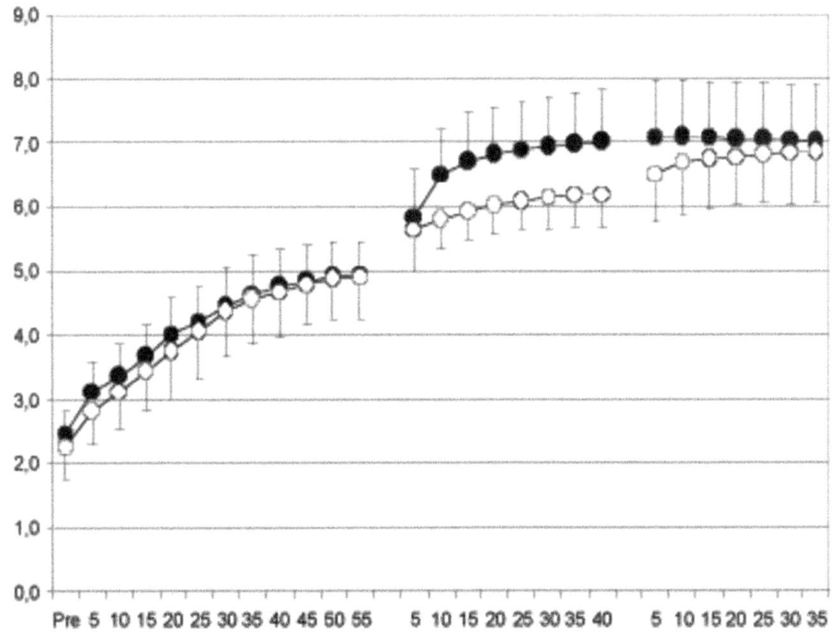

Fig. 2. The figure shows the pupil sizes (in mm, Y-axis) at different time points (in seconds, X-axis) after stepwise intracameral injections of lidocaine 1% (given first in both gruops, left part of the diagram), phenylephrine 1.5% and cyclopentolate 0.1%, 150 mL each. The order of the latter 2 injections was randomized (black circles: phenylephrine first; n=7; white circles: cyclopentolate first; n=8). Note that the addition of phenylephrine has a pronounced mydriatic effect, as opposed to cyclopentolate. Cyclopentolate given after phenylephrine has no detectable additive mydriatic effect.

A later study showed that when 2 drops of topical phenylephrine 10% combined with 150µl of intracameral lidocaine 1% is given at the beginning of a phacoemulsification procedure, no additive mydriatic effect can be seen from administrating preoperative topical cyclopentolate (Lundberg and Behndig 2009). The study was designed as a prospective, double-masked, randomized trial including 20 patients with age-related cataract. Initially, the pupil sizes were significantly smaller in the group where no topical cyclopentolate had been given - 4.8±1.2 mm compared to 6.5±1.4 mm, but the lidocaine injection increased the pupil sizes significantly in the absence of cyclopentolate, so that the pupil sizes were equalized throughout the surgical procedure for the both treatments. These findings show that the passive diating effect from intracameral lidocaine is sufficient, without topical passoive diating agents, and that preoperative topical cyclopentolate can be omitted when intracameral lidocaine is used.

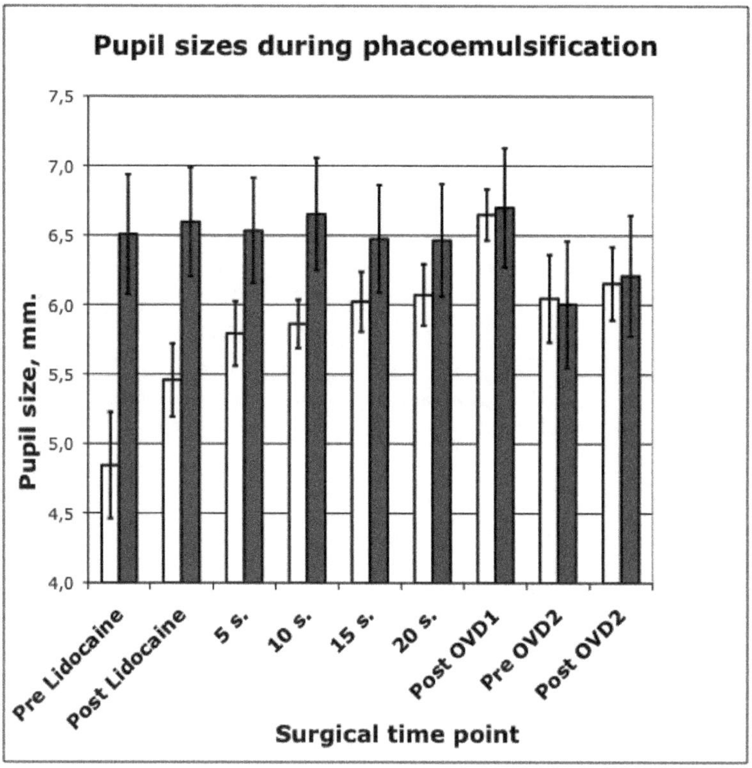

Fig. 3. The figure demonstrates the pupil sizes (in mm, Y-axis) at different time points during the phacoemulsification process (X-axis) before and after the intracameral injection of 150µl lidocaine 1% Both treatment groups were given 2 drops of topical phenylephrine 10%; group 2 (grey bars) were also given 2 drops of topical cyclopentoloate 1%. Note that intracameral lidocaine has a pronounced mydriatic effect, noticeable when preoperative cyclopentolate is not given, and that both groups have practically identical pupil sizes throughout the procedure from after the injection of the ophthalmic viscosurgical device (OVD) and on.

2.1.8 Epinephrine/lidocaine

In their paper "Optimizing the intracameral dilation regimen for cataract surgery: prospective randomized comparison of 2 solutions" from 2009, William G Myers and Joel K Shugar compared the efficacy of a solution of epinephrine 0.025% and lidocaine 0.75% in fortified balanced salt solution ("epi-Shugarcaine") and the original solution from our group (cyclopentolate 0.1%, phenylephrine 1.5%, and lidocaine 1%). The study was designed as a pair-eye single-masked prospective study involving 84 eyes of 42 patients. Topical tropicamide was given to both treatment groups. The pupils were statistically significantly larger with epi-Shugarcaine; 0.528 mm larger 1 minute after instillation and 0.34 mm larger at the end of the procedure (Myers and Shugar 2009). Since epinephrine is a much more unspecific adrenergic stimulator than the specific α_1-receptor phenylephrine, the findings of this important study indirectly indicate that adrenergic receptors other than the α_1-receptor stimulated by phenylephrine may be involved in the mydriatic response from intracamerally administered mydriatics. Subsequent studies have lent further support to this theory, as we will see below.

2.1.9 Tropicamide/phenylephrine

In a study from 2010, Mori *et al* investigated the efficacy and safety of intracameral injection of a commercially available eye drop containing 0.5% tropicamide and 0.5% phenylephrine hydrochloride (Mori, Miyai et al. 2010), demonstrating no increased damage to cultured human corneal endothelial cells, and a good mydriatic effect in cases with poor mydriasis after preoperative topical mydriatics.

2.1.10 Cardiovascular safety

Cardiovascular effects from topical mydriatic substances have been reported by many authors thoughout the years (Fraunfelder and Scafidi 1978; Meyer and Fraunfelder 1980; Fraunfelder and Meyer 1985; Hempel, Senn et al. 1999; Motta, Coblentz et al. 2009). A rapid absorption of anticholinergic and/or adrenergic substances via the nasal mucosa can render surprisingly high systemic levels of the substance. In our first two studies, we could se no signs of negative cardiovascular effects from intracameral myriatics (Lundberg and Behndig 2003; Behndig and Eriksson 2004), which is well in accordance with the facts that the doses of the adrenergic and anticholinergic substances are lower when the substance is administered intracamerally, and that there is likely to be a smaller proportion of the drug that enters the lacrimal drainage system with intracameral administration. Morgado *et al* confirmed in a study from 2010 involving 90 patients that topical mydriatics is more efficient from an initial mydriatic point of view, but intracameral mydriatics are safer from a cardiovascular point of view (Morgado, Barros et al. 2010). Taken together, the reports on cardiovascular safety combined with the widespread clinical routine use of intracameral mydriatics are reassuring - the risk of systemic side effects is not likely to be higher with the intracameral route of administration.

2.1.11 Macular safety

Many investigators have reported an association between the use of epinephrine and macular edema in glaucoma patients (Kolker and Becker 1968; Thomas, Gragoudas et al. 1978; Classe 1980; Mehelas, Kollarits et al. 1982), particularly in aphakia, but also in pseudophakia, a condition known as epinephrine maculopathy (Miyake, Shirasawa et al.

1989). It has been hypothesized that epinephrine maculopathy is induced by a mechanism involving prostaglandins or other eicosanoids and not directly by epinephrine (Miyake, Shirasawa et al. 1989). Whatever the exact mechanisms behind epinephrine maculopathy may be, it is particularly important to rule out negative effects on the macula from the rather large doses on adrenergics given in intracameral mydriatics. Therefore, in 2007, an investigation aiming to quantify the macular edema induced by intracameral phenylephrine and lidocaine in phacoemulsification surgery was undertaken (Johansson, Lundberg et al. 2007). Optical coherence tomography (OCT) has been used in several studies to assess the macular thickness after cataract surgery (Sourdille and Santiago 1999; Biro, Balla et al. 2006; Ching, Wong et al. 2006), including randomized trials to evaluate intraoperative treatments (Ball and Barrett 2006). With this highly sensitive instrument, minute postoperative macular thickness increases can be detected in a high proportion of cataract patients, also after uneventful surgery (Sourdille and Santiago 1999; Biro, Balla et al. 2006). Such changes, although subtle, can have a clinical relevance, being associated with decreased contrast sensitivity (Ball and Barrett 2006) or visual acuity (Sourdille and Santiago 1999). In a randomized study of 22 patients, 11 patients were given 150 µl of a mixture of phenylephrine 1.5% and lidocaine 1% intracamerally for mydriasis and anesthesia. The control group (n = 11) was given conventional topical mydriatics and intracameral lidocaine. No differences in macular edema between the 2 treatments could be noted on optical coherence tomography. The degree of foveal thickness increase found in the study, with a thickness increase exceeding 15µm in about 20% of the cases, is in the same range as previously reports from other reports with topical mydriatics (Sourdille and Santiago 1999; Ball and Barrett 2006).

Similar results have later been reported also for intracameral epinephrine from Bozkurt *et al.* In a consecutive, randiomized case series of a total of 158 uneventful cataract procedures half of the eyes were given 0.2 ml of 0.02% epinephrine as an intracameral injection. No difference was seen in central macular thickness with optical coherence tomography at any time point up to 6 months after surgery. In both treatment groups, the increase in macular thickness from preoperatively to 1, 3, and 6 months postoperatively was significant. In this rather large series, clinically significant macular edema was noted in 3 eyes in the epinephrine group and 3 eyes in the control group. The authors concluded that intracameral injection of 0.2 ml of 0.02% epinephrine did not increase the risk for macular edema after uneventful phacoemulsification.

2.1.12 Long term follow-up

The results from 40 of the cases from the original 2003 study on intracameral mydriatics were evaluated after 6 years, to assess if any long term complications such as posterior capsule opacification would be more frequent in patients operated with intracameral mydriatics. In the study, the visual acuity was measured using the ETDRS-fast protocol (Klein, Klein et al. 1983; Camparini, Cassinari et al. 2001), and the intraocular pressure, the grade of inflammation inflammation, the corneal thickness and the corneal endothelial cell loss were evaluated. The degree of posterior capsule opacification was assessed from standardized photographs using a digital camera. The grading of the posterior capsule opacifiaction (fraction and severity) was done with the POCOman program (Accessed from James Boyce, PhD (Bender, Spalton et al. 2004; Ronbeck, Zetterstrom et al. 2009)). The same masked observer performed the measurements twice for every image and the mean of the 2 measurements was calculated.

At 6 years, no statistically significant differences could be observed in visual acuity, intraoucular pressure and pupil size. The corneal thickness and endothelial cell loss did not differ significantly between the two treatment groups. At the 6 year follow up the total endothelial cell loss was 16.5 ± 14.6% in the TM group vs. 15.0 ± 15.4 % in the intracameral mydriatics group (P=0.73). Furthermore, the endothelial cell morphology showed no statistical differences between the cases where intracameral mydriatics had been used and the control cases with traditional topical dilatation at surgery. The median posterior capsule opacification fraction was 9 % in the TM group vs. 7.5 % in the intracameral mydriatics group (P=0.8). Similarly, the median severity grade of the posterior capsule opacification was 0.12 vs. 0.10 (P=0.7). Two patients in each group had YAG laser capsulotomy (P=1.0). A hydrophobic acrylic intraocular lens (MA60BM, Alcon Laboratories, Fort Worth, TX) was implanted in all cases in this study. The posterior capsule opacification scorings are in accordance with the results of other studies using the POCOman program, hydrophobic acrylic intraocular lenses and similar or shorter time for follow up (Kang, Choi et al. 2009; Ronbeck, Zetterstrom et al. 2009). Also, the rate of YAG capsulotomy in the present study was similar to reported rates from previous studies done with a comparable follow up times and acrylic hydrophobic lenses (Boureau, Lafuma et al. 2009; Boureau, Lafuma et al. 2009; Ronbeck, Zetterstrom et al. 2009).

Studies concerning corneal endothelial cell loss predominantly have follow up times of a year or less and there is a wide range in reported corneal endothelial cell loss after cataract surgery (Werblin 1993; Dick, Kohnen et al. 1996; Mathys, Cohen et al. 2007). However, it is stated that there is a progressive corneal endothelial cell loss after cataract surgery that exceeds the physiological cell loss (Lesiewska-Junk, Kaluzny et al. 2002). In the present study, the 6 year corneal endothelial cell loss appears to be comparable with other studies with longer follow up times] (Werblin 1993; Dick, Kohnen et al. 1996) (Lesiewska-Junk, Kaluzny et al. 2002).

In summary, the study showed that the concept of using intracameral mydriatics in phacoemulsification cataract surgery is safe, also in a long perspective.

2.1.13 Epinine

Other candidate substances for intracamral use have also been evaluated. In 2009, we performed a study of intracamerally injected N-methyl-3,4-dihydroxyphenylamine (epinine) to phenylephrine in a porcine eye model involving 112 eyes from newly slaughtered pigs (Lundberg and Behndig 2009). Epinine is an adrenergic substanse that also shows dopaminergic properties (Pyman 1909) (Barger and Dale 1910). Epinine is known to stimulate all six known receptors in cardiovascular tissues: α_1, α_2, β_1, β_2, DA_1 and DA_2 (Itoh 1991), and can be regarded as one of the most unspecific adrenergic/dopaminergic stimulators in this respect. In the study, after contracting the pupils with acetylcholine, 0.15 mL epinine or phenylephrine 0.3%, 1.5%, or 3.0% was given as an intracameral injection. Interestingly, epinine was significantly more potent than phenylephrine at equal concentrations. Similar results have also been demonstrated for related topical substances: ibopamine, an ester of epinine, is hydrolyzed to epinine during its passage through the cornea and exerts its pharmacological effects within the eye as epinine (Soldati, Gianesello et al. 1993). Topical ibopamine is routinely used as a mydriatic in some countries due to its interesting pharmacological profile: 2% ibopamine is a more potent mydriatic than 10% phenylephrine (Marchini, Babighian et al. 2003), and the mydriatic effect is reversed within 4 hours (Gelmi, Palazzuolo et al. 1989), making ibopamine the most short-acting and most effective topical mydriatic agent studied this far. Given these circumstances, we think epinine cold be a promising candidate substance for intracameral injection to achieve mydriasis in cataract surgery.

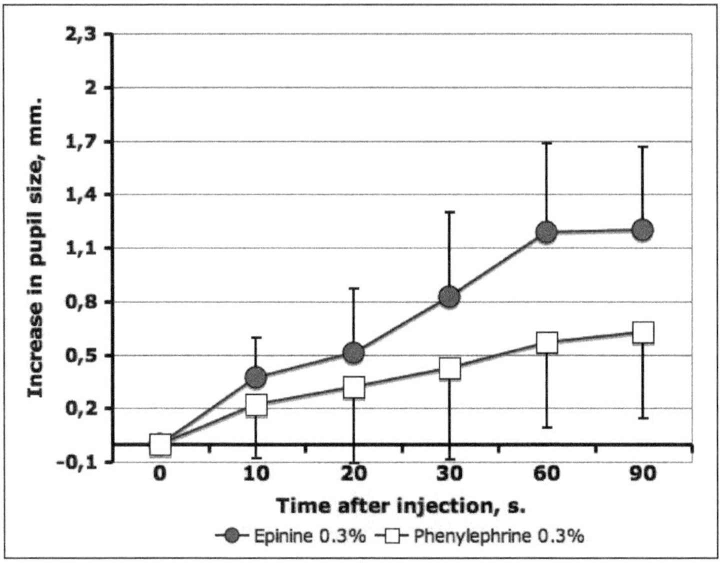

A

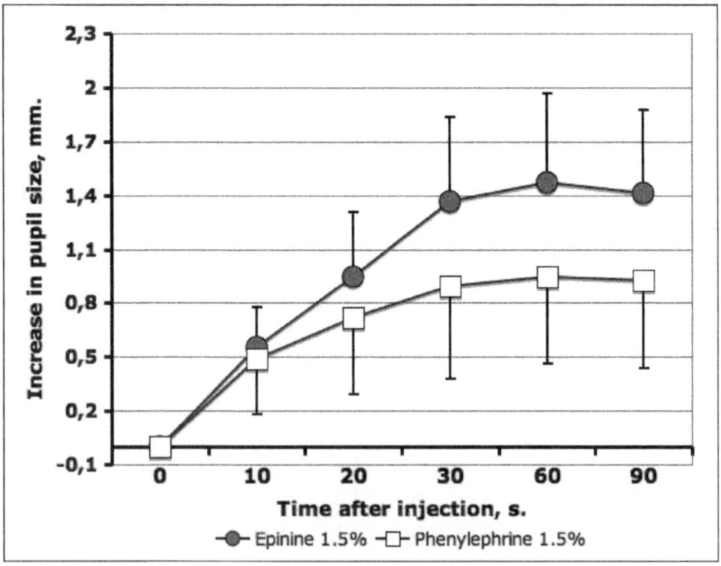

B

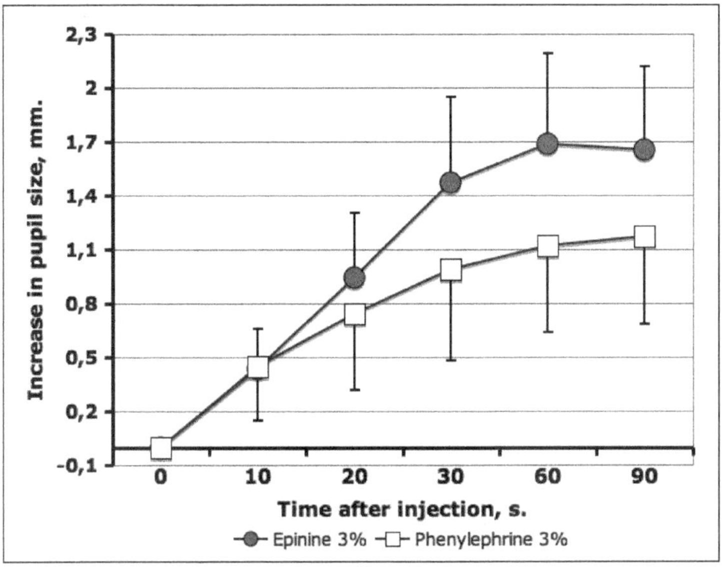

C

Fig. 4. The figure shows the increase in pupil size in porcine eyes after an intracameral injection of 150µl epinine hydrochloride (grey circles) or phenylephrine hydrochloride (white squares): 0.3% (4A) 1.5% (4B) and 3% (4C). Epinine has a more pronounced mydriatic effect at all concentrations.

2.1.14 Isoprenaline

In 2011, we compared the mydriatic effect of intracamerally injected isoprenaline (a β-receptor stimulator) plus phenylephrine to phenylephrine alone and to epinephrine in a porcine eye model with 89 intact porcine eyes; 0.3% isoprenaline and 0.15 ml 3.0% phenylephrine were injected sequentially in the mentioned or the reverse order. The control groups were treated with 0.025% epinephrine intracamerally or placebo. Phenylephrine injected after isoprenaline had a larger mydriatic effect than epinephrine, but without isoprenaline pretreatment, the mydriatic effect of phenylephrine was significantly smaller than that of epinephrine. Isoprenaline also showed a small mydriatic effect of its own. The β-receptor stimulator isoprenaline enhances the mydriatic effect of intracameral phenylephrine, indicating a role for the β-receptor in the mydriatic response. Mydriasis mediated by β-receptors may explain why non-specific adrenergic stimulators such as epinine and epinephrine can have larger mydriatic effects than the specific α_1-receptor stimulator phenylephrine (Janbaz, Lundberg et al. 2011).

2.2 Adrenergic receptors

Phenylephrine, commonly used as an intracameral mydriatic, is characterized as a specific α_1-receptor agonist. In rats and rabbits, it has been shown that the alpha(1A)-adrenoceptor is the chief mediator of the adrenergic mydriatic effects of the iris dilator muscle (Yu and Koss 2002; Yu and Koss 2003), but the mydriatic effect from an adrenergic substance may still be a bit more complex; as an example, stimulation of iris β□-receptors can cause a relaxation of the pupil sphincter (Toda, Okamura et al. 1999). The study of Myers and Shugar indicates that epinephrine may be a more potent mydriatic agent than phenylephrine when injected intracamerally (Myers and Shugar 2009), and indeed, epinephrine has a larger affinity for the β-receptor than phenylephrine (Mishima 1982). Accordingly, we have shown in a porcine eye model that the β-receptor stimulator isoprenaline fortifies mydriasis from intracameral phenylephrine (Janbaz, Lundberg et al. 2011), which further suggests a role for the β-receptor in the mydriatic response. Mydriasis mediated by β-receptors may explain why non-specific adrenergic stimulators such as epinephrine can have larger mydriatic effects than the specific α_1-receptor stimulator phenylephrine.

Epinine has a broad spectrum of adrenergic and dopaminergic effects (Itoh 1991), and the fact that epinine stimulates all adrenergic receptors, including the β_1-receptor (Itoh 1991) may contribute to a mydriatic effect superior to that of phenylephrine.

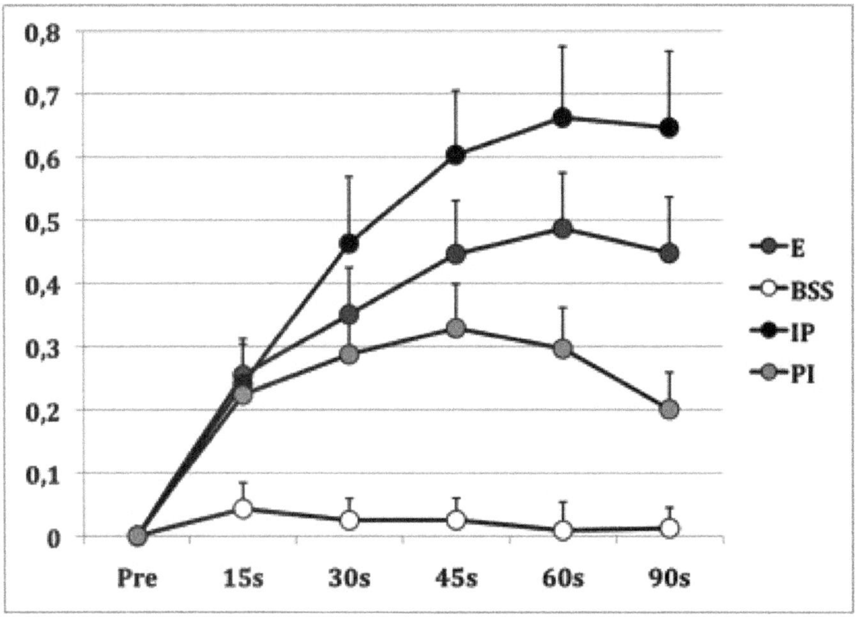

Fig. 5. The increase in pupil size in porcine eyes after an intracameral injection of 0.15 ml 0.025% epinephrine (E; n=20), Balanced Salt Solution (BSS; n=26), 0.3% isoprenaline followed by 3.0% phenylephrine (IP; n=21) or the latter two in the reversed order (PI; n=22), means and standard errors of the mean. The mydriatic effect of phenylephrine is significantly enhanced after pretreatment with isoprenaline ($p<0.05$ from 30-60 s), making it even larger than that of epinephrine ($p<0.05$ at 30 s; $p<0.01$ at 45-90 s).

(It is worth noting that due to logistic reasons, we were unable to receive the porcine eyes within 24 hours in this study, as opposed to in the epinine material (see 2.1.8) Therefore, the mydriatic responses in this study were generally smaller, but still fully measurable and possible to quantify and compare between the groups.)

2.3 Using intracameral mydriatics in intraoperative floppy iris syndrome (IFIS)

Intraoperative floppy iris syndrome (IFIS) is a condition often associated with systemic medication with α_1 adrenergic receptor antagonists for benign prostatic hyperplasia. The substances most often discussed are tamsulosin, terazosin, doxazosin and alfuzosin. Of these, tamsulosin predominates in the literature. IFIS was first described and defined in 2005 as a clinically observed triad: fluttering and billowing of the iris stroma, tendency for iris prolapse, and pupil constriction. As any cataract surgeon will realize, such conditions will make the surgical procedure more difficult and increase the risk for complications. The presumed mechanism by which tamsulosin causes IFIS is by blocking α_1 receptors in the iris dilator muscle, and thereby preventing mydriasis during cataract surgery. Certain measures can be taken to reduce the risk of surgical complications in patients with IFIS, including iris hooks, preoperative topical atropine (Masket and Belani 2007), and - perhaps most interesting in this context - intracameral phenylephrine or epinephrine (Gurbaxani and Packard 2007; Masket and Belani 2007). Manvikar *et al* first described the use of intracameral phenylephrine to enhance mydriasis in patients with IFIS (Manvikar and Allen 2006). In their series of 32 cases on tamsulosin medication, the degree of IFIS varied among cases: 53% eyes had good mydriasis preoperatively from topical mydriatics but of these 43% showed intraoperative pupil constriction. Thirty- eight percent had semi-dilated pupils, and 9% had poor preoperative dilation. Intracameral phenylephrine, when needed, was efficient in dilating the insufficiently dilated pupils. It is well known that pupil sizes get generally smaller with age. It has been demonstrated, however, that there is no difference in α_1-adrenoceptor sensitivity in the elderly and the young, and thus, age related miosis is not attributable to an alteration in the iris α_1-receptors with age (Buckley, Curtin et al. 1987). Takmaz and Can published a large material in 2007, where the incidence of IFIS was determined to be 1.6% in the whole material of 858 eyes, and in no less than 14 of the 18 eyes of patients using tamsulosin (77.8%). Intracameral epinephrine was effective in preventing intraoperative miosis in the IFIS cases (Takmaz and Can 2007). A similar frequency of IFIS - just above 1% - has been reported also by other groups (Oshika, Ohashi et al. 2007; Keklikci, Isen et al. 2009). Gurbaxani and Packard showed in 2007 in a series of seven cases who were on systemic tamsulosin for benign prostatic hyperplasia that intracameral phenylephrine gave a significant reduction in iris mobility and fluttering, as well as a sustained mydriasis, in accordance with most other reports on intracameral mydriatics (Lundberg and Behndig 2003; Behndig and Eriksson 2004; Lundberg and Behndig 2007; Myers and Shugar 2009). In a retrospective material by Chen *et al* (Chen, Kelly et al. 2010), the incidence of IFIS among patients operated by resident physiciancs was 29.6% among patients taking tamsulosin, and more common among patients with a preoperative dilated pupil diameter of less than 6.5 mm. The authors concluded from their findings that the use of intracameral lidocaine-epinephrine did not reduce the incidence of IFIS.

To conclude, most authors agree that although intracameral adrenergics may not affect the incidence of IFIS *per se*, the enlargement of the pupils obtained in these difficult cases is still of benefit for the surgical handling and outcome. The published data support the intuitive impression that adrenergic substances at high doses should be beneficial in cases where the iris has an insufficient muscle tone, as in IFIS.

2.4 Pharmacokinetics of intracameral mydriatics

Generally, diffusion through the cornea is considered to be the main penetration route for topically applied drugs (Mishima 1981; Grass and Robinson 1988), and the corneal epithelium is considered to be the main barrier (Sieg and Robinson 1976; Mishima 1981; Grass and Robinson 1988). Topically applied drugs generally penetrate the cornea slowly, with aqueous peak times ranging from 0.7 hours to 2.2 hours for various substances (Mishima 1981; Grass and Robinson 1988). For topically applied mydriatics the slow penetration through the cornea means a slow mydriatic onset (Lovasik 1986; Chien and Schoenwald 1990). For example, the peak mydriatic effect for cyclopentolate is at 30 minutes (Haaga, Kaila et al. 1998) and for phenylephrine 75 minutes (Matsumoto, Tsuru et al. 1982). In addition the bioavailability is limited for topically administered substances, which means a significant proportion of the drug will be absorbed systemically (Doane, Jensen et al. 1978; Kaila, Huupponen et al. 1989; Haaga, Kaila et al. 1998). Injecting a substance directly intracamerally will increase its bioavailability substantially, and accordingly decrease the systemic absorption. The onset of the effect will generally be very rapid after intracameral injection. Below, the research fields of intracameral pharmacokinetics will be briefly exemplified by lidocaine and phenylephrine.

2.4.1 Lidocaine

In a study from 1998, we determined the intracameral concentrations of lidocine after topical administration or intracameral injection (Behndig and Linden 1998). After 3 drops of topical lidocaine, the aqueous humour lidocaine concentration was 1.4±0.5 µg/ml and with 6 drops, 4.3±1.5µg/ml. With an intracameral injection, a concentration of 341.8 +/- 152.6 µg/ml was reached. We concluded that measurable amounts of lidocaine entered the anterior chamber in topical anesthesia, and that more entered when more drops were given. It is likely that concentrations in this range could anesthetize the iris, but they are far lower than the concentrations after an intracameral injection. This is probably the reason why the mydriatic effect from topical anesthetics is very minute - although it is indeed detectable and quantifyable with sensitive methods (Behndig 2007). Thus, topically administered lidocaine is found in low, but likely pharmacologically effective levels in the aqueous humor (Behndig and Linden 1998), and it has a measurable direct mydriatic and cycloplegic effect, at least in eyes with pale (blue) irides and less pigment binding of the substance (Behndig 2007). Since anesthetic agents lack adrenergic or anticholinergic properties, these mydriatic and cycloplegic effects can be ascribed a paralytic effect on the iris, analogous to the marked pupil dilation seen after intracameral lidocaine (Cionni, Barros et al. 2003).

In the beforementioned study, the lidocaine measured concentrations after an intracameral injection were about 10 times lower than what could be expected from simple dilution of the aqueous humor, meaning that just below 10 % of the injected lidocaine was found in the aqueous after 2 minutes. The rapid increase in anterior chamber volume and pressure upon injecting a volume of 100 µl might lead to diffusion of aqueous (and lidocaine) into the posterior chamber. An unknown proportion of the drug may also bind to iris pigment, as has been shown to occur for the related substance cocaine, and also for other drugs.

2.4.2 Phenylephrine

A dose-response study for intracameral phenylephrine from 2010 (Behndig and Lundberg 2010) showed that phenylephrine when injected intracamerally in human subjects has a rather moderate mydriatic effect at low concentrations and that the effect is very similar in concentrations ranging from 0.015-0.5%. Higher concentrations, however, (1.5 or 3.0%) give significantly larger pupils. Noticeably, a similar lack of dose-response relationship has been noted by several investigators for topical phenylephrine when comparing 2.5% to 10% (Weiss, Weiss et al. 1995; Tanner and Casswell 1996; Motta, Coblentz et al. 2009). Applying experimental bioavailability data (Mishima 1981) and assuming an aqueous humor volume of 160 μl (Jonsson, Markstrom et al. 2006) and a dose of three 37μl drops (Behndig and Linden 1998), three drops of 2.5 -10% would give intracameral doses of 0.14 and 0.57 mg phenylephrine, respectively, which is in the same range as the four lower concentrations in the dose-response study (0.02 mg - 0.73 mg). One point five and 3.0% would thus give 3.9 and 7.7 times higher intracameral phenylephrine doses, respectively, than a standard "maximum dilatation" regimen involving 3 drops of phenylephrine 10%. The effects of such high doses of phenylephrine have never been studied in humans, since the maximum recommendable topical dose is limited by potential systemic side effects (Hakim, Orton et al. 1990; Ogut, Bozkurt et al. 1996; Elibol, Alcelik et al. 1997; Lundberg and Behndig 2003), but it appears that increasing the dose of phenylephrine further would increase also the mydriatic effect beyond what can be reached with the standard topical "maximum dilatation". It may also be of interest to note that a lack of dose-response relationship similar to that of intracameral phenylephrine has been noted also for intracameral epinephrine in dilutions ranging from 0.00025% to 0.004% (Liou and Chen 2001).

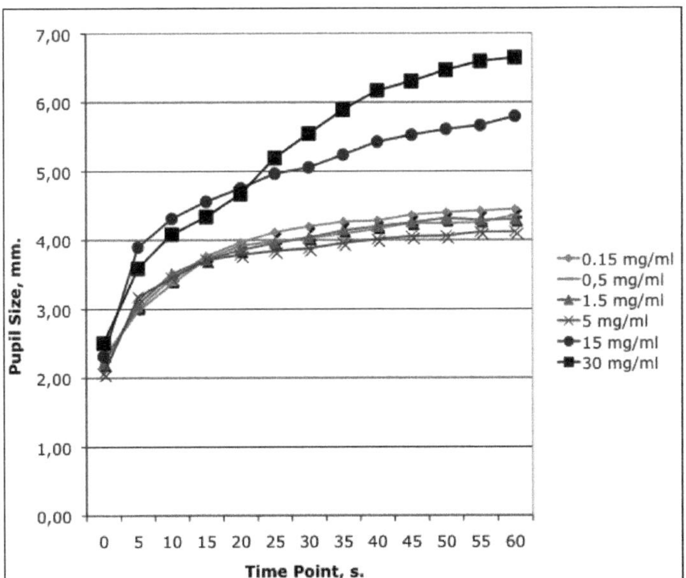

Fig. 6. The increase in pupil size after different concentrations of intracameral phenylephrine in cataract patients. Note that the mydriatic effect, including the time course, is very similar in concentrations ranging from 0.015-0.5% (0.15-5.0 mg/ml). At higher concentrations, 1.5 or 3.0%, a larger mydriatic effect is seen.

The rather weak effect of phenylephrine at low doses is a bit puzzling given that the α_1-receptors of the iris dilator are considered to be the most important mediators of the adrenergic mydriatic response (Yu and Koss 2002; Yu and Koss 2003). The binding of phenylephrine to the α_1-receptor is rather weak - less than 1/5 of that for epinephrine (Besse and Furchgott 1976). This may in part - but not fully - explain why comparably high doses of phenylephrine are required to achieve mydriasis. Although phenylephrine has a high specificity for the α_1-receptor, it may not be 100% specific (Mishima 1982), and at very high concentrations such as when using intracameral mydriatics, stimulation of other receptors, for example the β-receptor, could also be speculated to contribute to the mydriatic effect.

2.5 Preparation of intracameral mydriatics

It was early noted that sodium bisulfite-containing solutions of epinephrine damaged the corneal endothelium (Hull, Chemotti et al. 1975). Solutions containing sodium bisulfite are therefore usually not recommended for intracameral use, although some authors claim they may be safe from an endothelial perspective if sufficiently diluted (Hull, Chemotti et al. 1975; Hull 1979). Epinephrine *per se* is not toxic to the corneal endothelium (Liou, Chiu et al. 2002), but bisulfite-free preparations of epinephrine may not always be easy to purchase in different countries (Myers and Edelhauser 2011). Another putative disadvantage of several adrenergic substances, including epinephrine, is their instability at a neutral pH, which often means they may need to be prepared freshly on a daily basis in clinical routine use. A commercially available eye drop containing 0.5% tropicamide and 0.5% phenylephrine hydrochloride, with addition of benzalkonium chloride, epsilon-amino capronic acid, boric acid, chlorbutanol and pH-adjusting reagents has recently been described as safe for intracameral use by a Japanese group (Mori, Miyai et al. 2010). Else, it is not advisable to try preparations for topical use intracamerally (Hull 1979), and *ex tempore* preparations are usually required for intracameral mydriatics, as we still lack commercially available preparations (Lundberg and Behndig 2003; Myers and Shugar 2009). Soong *et al*, in their publication from 2006 (Soong, Soultanidis et al. 2006), advocated the use of an intracameral cocktail prepared aseptically in the operating room from minims of cyclopentolate hydrochloride 1% phenylephrine hydrochloride 10% and 0.5 mL preservative-free lignocaine hydrochloride 2%. The substances were diluted to final concentrations of 0.1% cyclopentolate, 1.5% phenylephrine and 1.0% lignocaine.

In the studies from our group, as well as in our clinical routine, the sterile solutions of intracameral mydriatics are prepared by the Product and Laboratory Department of the Swedish Pharmacy (Apoteksbolaget AB) from sterile salts of the mydriatic and anesthetic substances. In our current routine this means phenylephrine hydrochloride 15 mg and lidocaine hydrochloride 10 mg, with addition of Sodium edetase 1 mg, boric acid 3,85 mg (for isotony) and *aqua injectabile* ad 1 ml. The sterile solution is supplied in 10 ml airtight glass containers with rubber membranes to allow for use in multiple patients during the same day of surgery. Unopened containers can be used for up to 3 months.

3. Conclusion

In the development of today's highly efficient routines for cataract surgery, the concept of intracameral mydriatics definitely has a place. From our calculations, the time a patient spends in an operating clinic during a visit for a routine cataract operation with traditional topical mydriatics for pupil dilatation consists of 82% waiting for the pupil to dilate and 18% being operated. Based on the available data, we can safely conclude that intracameral mydriatics comprise a safe and efficient alternative to traditional topical mydriatics, with time saving and simplifying potentials.

4. References

Antcliff, R. J. and D. R. Trew (1997). "The maintenance of per-operative mydriasis in phacoemulsification with topical diclofenac sodium." *Eye* 11((Pt 3)): 389-391.

Artzen, D., M. Lundstrom, et al. (2009). "Capsule complication during cataract surgery: Case-control study of preoperative and intraoperative risk factors: Swedish Capsule Rupture Study Group report 2." *J Cataract Refract Surg* 35(10): 1688-1693.

Backstrom, G. and A. Behndig (2006). "Redilatation with intracameral mydriatics in phacoemulsification surgery." *Acta Ophthalmol Scand* 84(1): 100-104.

Ball, J. L. and G. D. Barrett (2006). "Prospective randomized controlled trial of the effect of intracameral vancomycin and gentamicin on macular retinal thickness and visual function following cataract surgery." *J Cataract Refract Surg* 32(5): 789-794.

Barger and Dale (1910). *J. Physiol.* 41: 19.

Behndig, A. (2007). "Effects on pupil size and accommodation from topical lidocaine hydrochloride and tetracaine hydrochloride." *J Ocul Pharmacol Ther* 23(6): 591-598.

Behndig, A. and A. Eriksson (2004). "Evaluation of surgical performance with intracameral mydriatics in phacoemulsification surgery." *Acta Ophthalmol Scand* 82(2): 144-147.

Behndig, A. and C. Linden (1998). "Aqueous humor lidocaine concentrations in topical and intracameral anesthesia." *J Cataract Refract Surg* 24(12): 1598-1601.

Behndig, A. and B. Lundberg (2010). "Mydriatic response to different concentrations of intracameral phenylephrine in humans." *J Cataract Refract Surg* 36(10): 1682-1686.

Bender, L., D. J. Spalton, et al. (2004). "POCOman: new system for quantifying posterior capsule opacification." *J Cataract Refract Surg* 30(10): 2058-2063.

Besse, J. C. and R. F. Furchgott (1976). "Dissociation constants and relative efficacies of agonists acting on alpha adrenergic receptors in rabbit aorta." *J Pharmacol Exp Ther* 197(1): 66-78.

Biro, Z., Z. Balla, et al. (2006). "Change of foveal and perifoveal thickness measured by OCT after phacoemulsification and IOL implantation." *Eye*.

Boureau, C., A. Lafuma, et al. (2009). "Incidence of Nd:YAG laser capsulotomies after cataract surgery: comparison of 3 square-edged lenses of different composition." *Can J Ophthalmol* 44(2): 165-170.

Boureau, C., A. Lafuma, et al. (2009). "Cost of cataract surgery after implantation of three intraocular lenses." *Clin Ophthalmol* 3: 277-285.

Buckley, C., D. M. Curtin, et al. (1987). "Ageing and alpha 1 adrenoceptors in the iris." *Eye* 1((Pt 2)): 211-216.

Camparini, M., P. Cassinari, et al. (2001). "ETDRS-fast: implementing psychophysical adaptive methods to standardized visual acuity measurement with ETDRS charts." *Invest Ophthalmol Vis Sci* 42(6): 1226-1231.

Cantrell, M. A., H. R. Bream-Rouwenhorst, et al. (2008). "Intraoperative floppy iris syndrome associated with alpha1-adrenergic receptor antagonists." *Ann Pharmacother* 42(4): 558-563.

Chen, A. A., J. P. Kelly, et al. (2010). "Pharmacologic prophylaxis and risk factors for intraoperative floppy-iris syndrome in phacoemulsification performed by resident physicians." *J Cataract Refract Surg* 36(6): 898-905.

Chien, D. S. and R. D. Schoenwald (1990). "Ocular pharmacokinetics and pharmacodynamics of phenylephrine and phenylephrine oxazolidine in rabbit eyes." *Pharm Res* 7(5): 476-483.

Ching, H. Y., A. C. Wong, et al. (2006). "Cystoid macular oedema and changes in retinal thickness after phacoemulsification with optical coherence tomography." *Eye* 20(3): 297-303.

Cionni, R. J., M. G. Barros, et al. (2003). "Cataract surgery without preoperative eyedrops." *J Cataract Refract Surg* 29(12): 2281-2283.

Classe, J. G. (1980). "Epinephrine maculopathy." *J Am Optom Assoc* 51(12): 1091-1093.

Dick, H. B., T. Kohnen, et al. (1996). "Long-term endothelial cell loss following phacoemulsification through a temporal clear corneal incision." *J Cataract Refract Surg* 22(1): 63-71.

Doane, M. G., A. D. Jensen, et al. (1978). "Penetration routes of topically applied eye medications." *Am J Ophthalmol* 85(3): 383-386.

Duffin, R. M., T. H. Pettit, et al. (1983). "2.5% v 10% phenylephrine in maintaining mydriasis during cataract surgery." *Arch Ophthalmol* 101(12): 1903-1906.

Edwards, M., S. Rehman, et al. (1997). "Discharging routine phacoemulsification patients at one week." *Eye* 11((Pt 6)): 850-853.

Elibol, O., T. Alcelik, et al. (1997). "The influence of drop size of cyclopentolate, phenylephrine and tropicamide on pupil dilatation and systemic side effects in infants." *Acta Ophthalmol Scand* 75(2): 178-180.

Fraunfelder, F. T. and S. M. Meyer (1985). "Possible cardiovascular effects secondary to topical ophthalmic 2.5% phenylephrine." *Am J Ophthalmol* 99(3): 362-363.

Fraunfelder, F. T. and A. F. Scafidi (1978). "Possible adverse effects from topical ocular 10% phenylephrine." *Am J Ophthalmol* 85(4): 447-453.

Gelmi, C., A. Palazzuolo, et al. (1989). "Pupillographic evaluation of the mydriatic effect of ibopamine solution." *Int J Clin Pharmacol Ther Toxicol* 27(7): 346-351.

Grass, G. M. and J. R. Robinson (1988). "Mechanisms of corneal drug penetration. I: In vivo and in vitro kinetics." *J Pharm Sci* 77(1): 3-14.

Gurbaxani, A. and R. Packard (2007). "Intracameral phenylephrine to prevent floppy iris syndrome during cataract surgery in patients on tamsulosin." *Eye (Lond)* 21(3): 331-332.

Haaga, M., T. Kaila, et al. (1998). "Systemic and ocular absorption and antagonist activity of topically applied cyclopentolate in man." *Pharmacol Toxicol* 82(1): 19-22.

Hakim, O. J., R. B. Orton, et al. (1990). "Topical 2.5% and 5% phenylephrine: comparison of effects on heart rate and blood pressure." *Can J Ophthalmol* 25(7): 336-339.

Hempel, S., P. Senn, et al. (1999). "[Perioperative circulatory side effects of topical 5% phenylephrine for mydriasis]." *Klin Monatsbl Augenheilkd* 215(5): 298-304.

Hull, D. S. (1979). "Effects of epinephrine, benzalkonium chloride, and intraocular miotics on corneal endothelium." *South Med J* 72(11): 1380-1381.

Hull, D. S., M. T. Chemotti, et al. (1975). "Effect of epinephrine on the corneal edothelium." *Am J Ophthalmol* 79(2): 245-250.

Itoh, H. (1991). "Clinical pharmacology of ibopamine." *Am J Med* 90(5B): 36S-42S.

Janbaz, C. C., B. Lundberg, et al. (2011). "Stimulation of adrenergic beta-receptors enhances mydriasis in a porcine eye model." *Acta Ophthalmol.*

Jayadev, C. and B. K. Nayak (2007). "Pupil dilation with intracameral lidocaine during phacoemulsification." *J Cataract Refract Surg* 33(9): 1503; author reply 1503.

Johansson, M., B. Lundberg, et al. (2007). "Optical coherence tomography evaluation of macular edema after phacoemulsification surgery with intracameral mydriatics." *J Cataract Refract Surg* 33(8): 1436-1441.

Jonsson, M., K. Markstrom, et al. (2006). "Slit-scan tomography evaluation of the anterior chamber and corneal configurations at different ages." *Acta Ophthalmol Scand* 84(1): 116-120.

Kaila, T., R. Huupponen, et al. (1989). "Systemic absorption of ophthalmic cyclopentolate." *Am J Ophthalmol* 107(5): 562-564.

Kang, S., J. A. Choi, et al. (2009). "Comparison of posterior capsular opacification in heparin-surface-modified hydrophilic acrylic and hydrophobic acrylic intraocular lenses." *Jpn J Ophthalmol* 53(3): 204-208.

Keklikci, U., K. Isen, et al. (2009). "Incidence, clinical findings and management of intraoperative floppy iris syndrome associated with tamsulosin." *Acta Ophthalmol* 87(3): 306-309.

Klein, R., B. E. Klein, et al. (1983). "Inter-observer variation in refraction and visual acuity measurement using a standardized protocol." *Ophthalmology* 90(11): 1357-1359.

Kolker, A. E. and B. Becker (1968). "Epinephrine maculopathy." *Arch Ophthalmol* 79(5): 552-562.

Lesiewska-Junk, H., J. Kaluzny, et al. (2002). "Long-term evaluation of endothelial cell loss after phacoemulsification." *Eur J Ophthalmol* 12(1): 30-33.

Liou, S. W. and C. C. Chen (2001). "Maintenance of mydriasis with one bolus of epinephrine injection during phacoemulsification." *J Ocul Pharmacol Ther* 17(3): 249-253.

Liou, S. W., C. J. Chiu, et al. (2002). "Effects of intraocular epinephrine on the corneal endothelium of rabbits." *J Ocul Pharmacol Ther* 18(5): 469-473.

Liou, S. W. and C. Y. Yang (1998). "The effect of intracameral adrenaline infusion on pupil size, pulse rate, and blood pressure during phacoemulsification." *J Ocul Pharmacol Ther* 14(4): 357-361.

Lovasik, J. V. (1986). "Pharmacokinetics of topically applied cyclopentolate HCl and tropicamide." *Am J Optom Physiol Opt* 63(10): 787-803.

Lundberg, B. and A. Behndig (2003). "Intracameral mydriatics in phacoemulsification cataract surgery." *J Cataract Refract Surg* 29(12): 2366-2371.

Lundberg, B. and A. Behndig (2007). "Intracameral mydriatics in phacoemulsification surgery obviate the need for epinephrine irrigation." *Acta Ophthalmol Scand.*

Lundberg, B. and A. Behndig (2008). "Separate and additive mydriatic effects of lidocaine hydrochloride, phenylephrine, and cyclopentolate after intracameral injection." *J Cataract Refract Surg* 34(2): 280-283.

Lundberg, B. and A. Behndig (2009). "The mydriatic effect of intracameral epinine hydrochloride." *Invest Ophthalmol Vis Sci* 50(11): 5336-5338.

Lundberg, B. and A. Behndig (2009). "Preoperative topical cyclopentolate can be omitted when using intracameral lidocaine in phacoemulsification surgery." *Acta Ophthalmol* 87(3): 297-299.

Lundstrom, M., U. Stenevi, et al. (2002). "The Swedish National Cataract Register: A 9-year review." *Acta Ophthalmol Scand* 80(3): 248-257.

Manvikar, S. and D. Allen (2006). "Cataract surgery management in patients taking tamsulosin staged approach." *J Cataract Refract Surg* 32(10): 1611-1614.

Marchini, G., S. Babighian, et al. (2003). "Comparative study of the effects of 2% ibopamine, 10% phenylephrine, and 1% tropicamide on the anterior segment." *Invest Ophthalmol Vis Sci* 44(1): 281-289.

Marsich, M. W. and M. A. Bullimore (2000). "The repeatability of corneal thickness measures." *Cornea* 19(6): 792-795.

Masket, S. and S. Belani (2007). "Combined preoperative topical atropine sulfate 1% and intracameral nonpreserved epinephrine hydrochloride 1:4000 [corrected] for management of intraoperative floppy-iris syndrome." *J Cataract Refract Surg* 33(4): 580-582.

Mathys, K. C., K. L. Cohen, et al. (2007). "Determining factors for corneal endothelial cell loss by using bimanual microincision phacoemulsification and power modulation." *Cornea* 26(9): 1049-1055.

Matsumoto, S., T. Tsuru, et al. (1982). "Pharmacokinetics of topical phenylephrine hydrochloride in the normal human eye." *Jpn J Ophthalmol* 26(3): 338-344.

Mehelas, T. J., C. R. Kollarits, et al. (1982). "Cystoid macular edema presumably induced by dipivefrin hydrochloride (Propine)." *Am J Ophthalmol* 94(5): 682.

Meyer, S. M. and F. T. Fraunfelder (1980). "3. Phenylephrine hydrochloride." *Ophthalmology* 87(11): 1177-1180.

Mishima, S. (1981). "Clinical pharmacokinetics of the eye. Proctor lecture." *Invest Ophthalmol Vis Sci* 21(4): 504-541.

Mishima, S. (1982). "Ocular effects of beta-adrenergic agents. XII Jules Stein Lecture. ." *Surv Ophthalmol* 27: 187-208.

Miyake, K., E. Shirasawa, et al. (1989). "Hypotheses on the role of prostaglandins in the pathogenesis of epinephrine maculopathy and aphakic cystoid macular edema." *Prog Clin Biol Res* 312: 265-276.

Morgado, G., P. Barros, et al. (2010). "Comparative study of mydriasis in cataract surgery: topical versus Mydriasert versus intracameral mydriasis in cataract surgery." *Eur J Ophthalmol* 20(6): 989-993.

Mori, Y., T. Miyai, et al. (2010). "Intraoperative mydriasis by intracameral injection of mydriatic eyedrops: in vivo efficacy and in vitro safety studies." *Clin Experiment Ophthalmol.*

Motta, M. M., J. Coblentz, et al. (2009). "Mydriatic and cardiovascular effects of phenylephrine 2.5% versus phenylephrine 10%, both associated with tropicamide 1%." *Ophthalmic Res* 42(2): 87-89.

Myers, W. G. and H. F. Edelhauser (2011). "Shortage of bisulfite-free preservative-free epinephrine for intracameral use." *J Cataract Refract Surg* 37(3): 611.

Myers, W. G. and J. K. Shugar (2009). "Optimizing the intracameral dilation regimen for cataract surgery: prospective randomized comparison of 2 solutions." *J Cataract Refract Surg* 35(2): 273-276.

Nikeghbali, A., K. G. Falavarjani, et al. (2008). "Pupil dilation with intracameral lidocaine during phacoemulsification: Benefits for the patient and surgeon." *Indian J Ophthalmol* 56(1): 63-64.

Nikeghbali, A., K. G. Falavarjani, et al. (2007). "Pupil dilation with intracameral lidocaine during phacoemulsification." *J Cataract Refract Surg* 33(1): 101-103.

Ogut, M. S., N. Bozkurt, et al. (1996). "Effects and side effects of mydriatic eyedrops in neonates." *Eur J Ophthalmol* 6(2): 192-196.

Oshika, T., S. Amano, et al. (2001). "Current trends in cataract and refractive surgery in Japan: 1999 survey." *Jpn J Ophthalmol* 45(4): 383-387.

Oshika, T., Y. Ohashi, et al. (2007). "Incidence of intraoperative floppy iris syndrome in patients on either systemic or topical alpha(1)-adrenoceptor antagonist." *Am J Ophthalmol* 143(1): 150-151.

Pyman (1909). *J. Chem. Soc.* 95(1266): 1610.

Ronbeck, M., C. Zetterstrom, et al. (2009). "Comparison of posterior capsule opacification development with 3 intraocular lens types: five-year prospective study." *J Cataract Refract Surg* 35(11): 1935-1940.

Sieg, J. W. and J. R. Robinson (1976). "Mechanistic studies on transcorneal permeation of pilocarpine." *J Pharm Sci* 65(12): 1816-1822.

Soldati, L., V. Gianesello, et al. (1993). "Ocular pharmacokinetics and pharmacodynamics in rabbits of ibopamine, a new mydriatic agent." *Exp Eye Res* 56(2): 247-254.

Soong, T., M. Soultanidis, et al. (2006). "Safety of intracameral mydriasis in phacoemulsification cataract surgery." *J Cataract Refract Surg* 32(3): 375-376.

Sourdille, P. and P. Y. Santiago (1999). "Optical coherence tomography of macular thickness after cataract surgery." *J Cataract Refract Surg* 25(2): 256-261.

Takmaz, T. and I. Can (2007). "Clinical features, complications, and incidence of intraoperative floppy iris syndrome in patients taking tamsulosin." *Eur J Ophthalmol* 17(6): 909-913.

Tanner, V. and A. G. Casswell (1996). "A comparative study of the efficacy of 2.5% phenylephrine and 10% phenylephrine in pre-operative mydriasis for routine cataract surgery." *Eye* 10((Pt 1)): 95-98.

Thomas, J. V., E. S. Gragoudas, et al. (1978). "Correlation of epinephrine use and macular edema in aphakic glaucomatous eyes." *Arch Ophthalmol* 96(4): 625-628.

Toda, M., T. Okamura, et al. (1999). "Mechanisms underlying the neurogenic relaxation of isolated porcine sphincter pupillae." *Exp Eye Res* 68(4): 505-512.

Weiss, J. S., J. N. Weiss, et al. (1995). "The effects of phenylephrine 2.5% versus phenylephrine 10% on pupillary dilation in patients with diabetes." *Retina* 15(2): 130-133.

Werblin, T. P. (1993). "Long-term endothelial cell loss following phacoemulsification: model for evaluating endothelial damage after intraocular surgery." *Refract Corneal Surg* 9(1): 29-35.

Yi, Q., S. J. Flanagan, et al. (2001). "Trends in health service delivery for cataract surgery at a large Australian ophthalmic hospital." *Clin Experiment Ophthalmol* 29(5): 291-295.

Yu, Y. and M. C. Koss (2002). "alpha(1A)-adrenoceptors mediate sympathetically evoked pupillary dilation in rats." *J Pharmacol Exp Ther* 300(2): 521-525.

Yu, Y. and M. C. Koss (2003). "Studies of alpha-adrenoceptor antagonists on sympathetic mydriasis in rabbits." *J Ocul Pharmacol Ther* 19(3): 255-263.

13

Trans-Scleral Controlled-Release of Drugs for Cataract Surgery

Anselmo G. De Oliveira[1], José A. Cardillo[2,3], Fernando Paganelli[2,3], Acácio A. S. Lima-Filho[2] and Arnóbio A. Da Silva-Júnior[4]
[1]*State of Sao Paulo University-UNESP, School of Pharmaceutical Sciences, Department of Pharmaceutics, Araraquara, SP,*
[2]*Federal University of Sao Paulo-UNIFESP, Department of Ophthalmology, São Paulo, SP,*
[3]*Eye Hospital of Araraquara, Rua Padre Duarte, Araraquara, SP,*
[4]*Federal University of Rio Grande do Norte-UFRN, Health Sciences Centre, Natal, RN, Brazil*

1. Introduction

In the modern cataract surgery era, postsurgical inflammation is minimal, and a more comprehensive medical management strategy to treat such inflammation is still to be determined. Historically, corticosteroids have been the drugs of choice for the prevention or of postoperative ocular inflammation and are commonly used for several weeks. Surodex, an intraocular sustained release pellet of dexametasone has proven to be effective in eliminating the necessity for postoperative topical therapy, at the cost of potential movement and displacement side effects (Tan et al., 1999; Chang et al., 1999; Tan et al., 2001). In addition, there is no sufficient literature evidence to support its routine clinical acceptance. The sustained anti-inflammatory effects associated with the use of triamcinolone in the ophthalmic setting have prompted the authors to consider its therapeutic use for controlling post cataract surgery inflammation. A sub–Tenon's capsule depot corticosteroid injection may satisfy all the requirements for an ideal anti-inflammatory strategy and may have distinct advantages for reducing complications related to patient noncompliance with eye drop administration.

Our published study comparing a single intraoperative sub-Tenon's capsule injection of triamcinolone with conventional prednisolone eye drops substantiates a novel and more comprehensive anti-inflammatory strategy for cataract surgery (Paganelli et al., 2004). Consistent with other investigations (West, Behrens & McDonnell, 2005; Negi, Browning & Vernon, 2006) our results indicated that one 25-mg sub-Tenon's capsule triamcinolone acetonide injection resulted in a therapeutic response and ocular tolerance comparable to 1% prednisolone acetate drops in controlling the signs and symptoms of ocular inflammation after cataract surgery. On the first post-operative day, all patients in both groups had anterior chamber cell and flare scores that gradually decreased over time. The parallel decreases in both groups suggested that triamcinolone is at least as effective as conventional prednisolone eye drops in reducing post-operative inflammation. As a result, a sub-Tenon's capsule injection of depot corticosteroid, an already accepted method for the treatment of various inflammatory ocular diseases, could be useful in the surgical arena. It provides a new way to eliminate patient self-medicating, avoiding problems with compliance and instruction. Furthermore, when this demonstration of the anti-inflammatory effects is coupled with its ability to treat cystoids macular edema and diabetic macular edema aggravated by cataract, (Yoshikawa et al, 1995; Thach et al., 1997; Walton, Wick & Greewald, 1999; Cardillo et al., 2005; Kim et al., 2008) a clear role for triamcinolone as a simple and more rational management strategy for post-cataract surgical inflammation begins to emerge.

One posterior sub-Tenon's capsule triamcinolone injection also had ocular tolerance equivalent to prednisolone eye drops through 4 weeks of follow-up. There were no significant differences between the two treatment groups in the number of adverse events, changes in visual acuity (VA), or lack of response. The potential complications of sub-Tenon's capsule injection of corticosteroids include inadvertent injection into the choroidal or retinal circulation, (McClean, 1975; Ellis, 1978; Morgan et al., 1988) globe perforation, (Giles, 1974; Schlaegel & Wilson, 1974; Schechter, 1985) and occlusion of the central retinal artery (Ellis, 1978), blepharoptosis, proptosis, orbital fat atrophy, delayed hypersensitivity reactions, strabismus, conjunctival hemorrhage, chemosis, and infection also have been reported (Ellis, 1974; Nozik, 1976; O'Connors, 1976; Mathias et al., 1978). Although both studies are not adequately powered to detect rare complications, these complications were not observed.

An increase in intraocular pressure (IOP) after topical or systemic administration of corticosteroids is of particular concern (Herschler, 1976). Patients who receive sub-Tenon's capsule injections of corticosteroids may not respond to maximal anti-glaucomatous therapy and, therefore, may require surgical excision of the depot because of a persistently elevated IOP (Akduman et al., 1996). As increased IOP may be a function of the interaction between the disease itself and the use of topical or systemic corticosteroids - the role of posterior sub-Tenon's capsule corticosteroids in ocular hypertension is not always clear. Therefore these concerns may not apply to patients who underwent surgery whose status in responding to corticosteroids is unknown. Following a posterior 40-mg triamcinolone sub-Tenon's capsule injection, an incidence of increased IOP that was lower than expected was surprisingly observed (Paganelli et al., 2004). In our most recently study, only one eye (triamcinolone group) had an IOP that exceeded 25 mmHg, and the IOP returned to a normal level with topical antihypertensive drops (Paganelli et al., 2009). However, beyond our 28-day follow-up period, delayed onset of increased IOP must be considered. The depot formulation was placed forward under sub-Tenon's capsule and, if an intractable IOP increase occurred, the remainder of the depot could have been easily removed.

Other authors have also confirmed our theory and similar results have been published applying a similar technique targeting operations in cataract and retina surgery (Negi, Browning & Vernon, 2006). Although we cannot draw definitive conclusions based on these initial findings, the results suggest further investigation is needed. A large phase III multicenter trial is being considered to evaluate this potential treatment. Investigation of the latest-generation fluoroquinolone formulation combined with non-steroidal anti-inflammatory drugs is currently underway in our laboratory and will be the next level of improvement for this suggested system.

This suggested anti-inflammatory approach provides the ophthalmologist with an alternative tool to costly controlled drug delivery and eliminates the need for patient self-medication, which avoids problems with compliance and instruction. Such an approach could be especially important in the third world, where topical medications may not be available after intraocular surgery.

2. Anti-infection prophylaxis for cataract surgery

The achievement of high antibiotic concentrations within infected tissue is important for a number of reasons. First of all, in order for the therapy to be effective, the necessary bactericidal concentrations to eradicate the pathogen must be achieved and maintained. The bactericidal activity of fluoroquinolone is largely concentration-dependent, which explains why peak concentration values and the 24-hour area under curve (AUC) are important determinants of individual drug activity (potency). Higher drug exposure and total dosages, as indicated by higher AUCs, may be associated with more effective eradication of the infecting organism (Paccola, Jorge & Barbosa, 2007). Second, the emergence of bacterial resistance to fluoroquinolone also appears to be concentration-dependent (Bui, Dang & Hwang, 1995; MacDonald, 2006). At fluoroquinolone concentrations above the minimum inhibitory concentration (MIC), the frequency of bacterial mutation increases exponentially as the concentration decreases. This means that the employment of fluoroquinolone that can result in tissue concentrations only modestly above the MIC could result in the development of antibiotic resistance to that specific fluoroquinolone (Bui, Dang & Hwang, 1995). Thus, the ability of a drug to produce high drug concentrations within infected tissues may facilitate enhanced antibacterial activity with a reduced likelihood of emergence of resistance. For a future and revolutionizing therapy, this required target could only be achieved by the development of an eye-specific antimicrobial agent or by an appropriate drug delivery approach engineered to enhance drug penetration (Velpandian, 2009).

3. Conventional antimicrobial strategy and its limitations

The route for local ophthalmic drug delivery remains the topical application of solutions at the surface of the eye as drops. Drug delivery to intraocular tissues by this approach, however, is limited by: (A) the significant barrier to solute flux provided by the corneal epithelium; and (B) the precorneal drug loss that occurs by way of the tear fluid turnover. Although a relatively small fraction of the dose applied topically reaches the intraocular tissues, the topical formulations can deliver therapeutic concentrations in tissues of the anterior segment, mainly because the administration of a high dose of the drug is necessary. It has been estimated that typically less than 5% of a topically applied drug actually permeates the cornea and eventually reaches intraocular tissues. The major portion of the instilled dose is absorbed systemically by way of the conjunctiva, through the highly vascular conjunctival stroma and through the lid margin vessels. Additionally, systemic absorption also occurs when the solution enters the nasolacrimal duct and is absorbed by the nasal and nasopharyngeal mucosa (Lang, 1996; Geroski & Edelhauser, 2001).

Conventional ocular pharmacokinetic views have downplayed the possibility of any highly effective transfer of a drug from an eye drop to the aqueous and vitreous humor.

Widely accepted for conjunctival and corneal infection, new antibiotic drops are often exploited for prophylactic use without rationalizing the penetration characteristics in the drug development stage. Interesting, in the currently clinical scenario, in contradiction with the physiological processes involved in guarding the eye against xenobiotics, the newer fluoroquinolone have been marketed partly on the basis of their excellent ocular penetration after topical administration - but at the cost of extremely artificial supportive methods used in their development (Kim et al., 2005; Sollomon, Donnenfeld & Perry, 2005). A careful literature and methods review of the relevant studies will point to an unacceptable high antibiotic loading dose and single point measurement (usually at a short- and higher peak concentration-time point) which is used to demonstrate the potential of the newer-generation fluoroquinolones to overcome these barriers to drug delivery. Tested in a practical clinical setting, where a single drop is instilled ever four to six hours and poor patient compliance to the treatment is a common issue, even later generation antibiotics may face obstacles in reaching high and even more importantly sustained therapeutic levels. In support of our theory against topical antibiotic delivery in cataract surgery, our laboratory has elaborated a more simplistic and realistic investigation method to experimentally address the role of topical prophylaxis in the surgical scenario.

An aqueous humor bioactivity comparison of several fluorquiniolones following a single topical drop delivery was carried out in our laboratory with the single purpose of evaluating quantitatively over time the bioactivity of ciprofloxacin 0.3%, levofloxacin 1.5%. gatifloxacin 0.3% and moxifloxacin 0.5% in the aqueous humor of rabbit eyes. For supportive methods, a total of 64 New Zealand rabbit eyes were topically treated with a commercially available formulation of ciprofloxacin 0.3%, levofloxacin 1.5%, gatifloxacin 0.3% and moxifloxacin 0.5% eye drops. Following an initial loading dose consistent with a single antibiotic drop the aqueous humor was sampled at 30 minutes, 1, 2 and 4 hours post-treatment. Biological activity was indirectly determined from the size of the zone of inhibition (ZOI) of filter paper disc soaked in 25μl of aqueous humor drawn from treated eyes and placed on an agar plate surface-cultured with Staphylococcus Epidermidis. To our amazement, but theoretically expected, although not significant, 0.5% moxifloxacin eye drops showed an initial (30 minutes and 1 hour post-treatment) trend towards superior aqueous bioactivity compared to all other tested formulations (Figure 1). At and following the second hour, the aqueous humor drawn from all treated eyes failed to demonstrate any bacterial inhibitory potential for the four tested formulations, since no zone of inhibition could be observed. The main conclusion of this method of antibiotic-bioactivity exploration is that sole reliance on the minimum inhibitory concentration and artificial pharmacokinetics studies as guides to antibacterial efficacy may be misleading and even newer-generation fluorquiniolones failed to demonstrate a significant aqueous bioactivity using a dosing regimen that simulated prophylactic use after cataract surgery (Paganelli et al., 2010).

Despite surrogate studies showing that topical antibiotics decrease bacteria on the ocular surface and anterior chamber, and that some topical antibiotics can penetrate the cornea and the anterior chamber (Callegan et al., 2003; Price, Quillin & Price Jr, 2005; Sollomon, Donnenfeld & Perry, 2005), there has not been a prospective randomized study showing that topical antibiotics prevent endophthalmitis. Bioavailability has been touted in the literature, but its relationship to endophthalmitis in the human is unknown. In one rabbit study, several drops of moxifloxacin administered preoperatively prevented endophthalmitis from developing (Kowalski et al., 2004). This was the first study to suggest that topical antibiotics alone can prevent endophthalmitis. Once an organism reaches the vitreous, however, topical application of antibiotics is probably not efficacious (Costello et al., 2006). Furthermore, in vitro susceptibility data and animal studies cannot be translated uniformly into a solid and reliable assessment of in vivo efficacy because of additional factors such as anatomic location and pharmacodynamics.

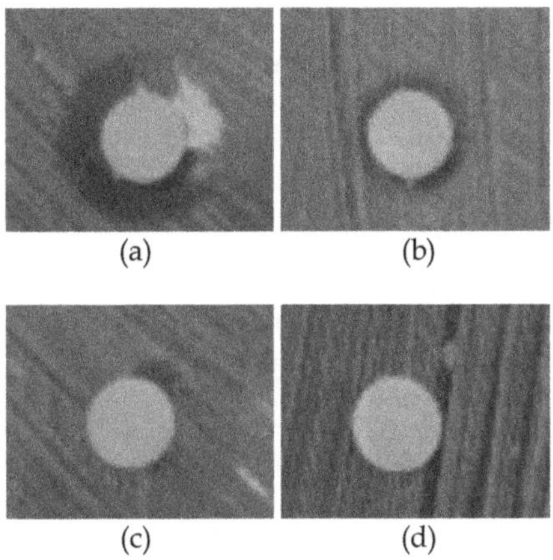

Fig. 1. Aqueous humor bioactivity following the delivery of a single topical drop of moxifloxacin 0.5% evaluated quantitatively over time: (a) 30 minutes, (b) 1 hour, (c) 2 hours and (d) 4 hours post drop-instillation (Paganelli et al., 2010).

4. Technological strategy of micro and nanoparticles for ocular trans-scleral drug delivery

Research and development in the area of pharmaceutical biotechnology has introduced an increasing number of therapeutic possibilities for medical treatment of many diseases, especially ocular diseases. The field of drug-controlled release represents a frontier area in medical science, involves a broad multidisciplinary approach, and has contributed decisively to improving human health. The systems offer clear advantages compared with conventional drug dosage forms, such as increasing the drug efficiency, reduced toxicity, increased patient compliance, improved safety and patient comfort (Zeimer & Goldberg 2001).

Sustained drug delivery devices offer an excellent alternative to solve many problems associated with patient use of postoperative drops in cataract surgery. These devices are made either from biostable (non-biodegradable, non-erodible), or from biodegradable (erodible) polymers. The erodible devices have an inherent advantage over the non-erodible systems in that as they degrade they gradually disappear from the site of implantation. The particles consist of drugs entrapped within a polymer, and are frequently classified by size into microparticles (> 1 μm) and nanoparticles (< 1 μm). According to physical structure, the microparticles are classified as microspheres and microcapsules. Microcapsules have a drug core surrounded by a polymeric film, while in the microspheres the drug is dispersed through the polymeric matrix. The aim in the development of microspheres and microcapsules has been to develop long-acting injectable drug depot formulations with specific drug targeting and delivery optimization (Herrero-Vanrell & Refojo 2001). These systems have been under evaluation for ophthalmic drug delivery purposes for the past 20 years. Among the biodegradable polymers that have been investigated to make microparticles for drug delivery are gelatin, albumin, polyorthoesters, polyanhydrides, and polyesters, particularly polymers of polylactide acid (PLA), polyglicolic acid (PGA), and poly (lactide-co-glycolide) acid (PLGA). These polyesters have been most frequently used to make microspheres for subconjunctival and intravitreous drug delivery. Among the polymeric particles potentially useful for ocular drug delivery, the microspheres have been most commonly used, mainly due to the delivery possibility through conventional small-gauge syringes (Herrero-Vanrell & Refojo, 2001).

In our studies, the spray drying technique was used to produce biocompatible microspheres that were uniform in shape and size, sterilized by gamma radiation, and suitable for ocular administration. The great advantage of this methodology is that it produces dried microspheres of small size and free of solvent residues and other compounds needed in the emulsification methods. The mean particle sizes and encapsulation efficiencies were 1.03 (± 0.30) μm and 97.86% (±0.96%), respectively. These systems have proved to be suitable for subconjunctival and intraocular injection displaying pharmacokinetic profiles with high and prolonged drug concentration in aqueous and vitreous humors (Silva-Jr et al., 2008; Silva-Jr et al., 2009). Figure 2 shows the the images of the scanning electron microscopy of ciprofloxacin-loaded PLGA microspheres utilized in most of our studies.

Subconjunctival ocular drug delivery represents another attempt to elevate intraocular drug concentrations and minimize the frequency of dosing (Hosoya, Lee & Kim, 2005).

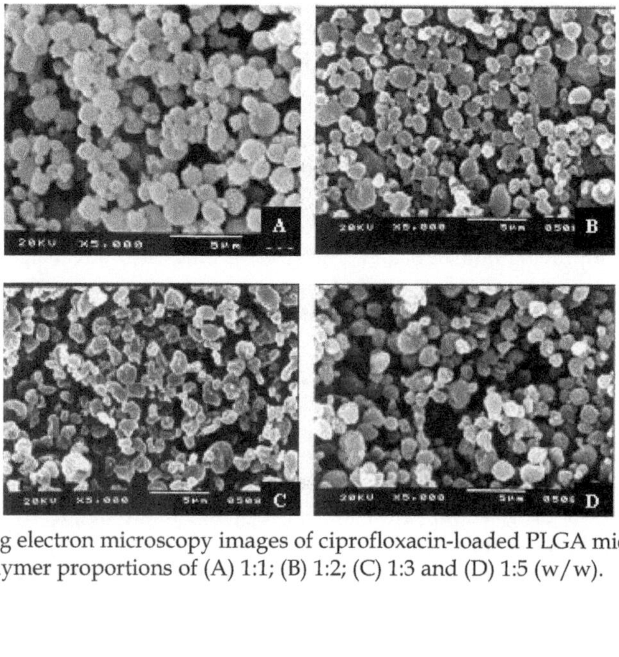

Fig. 2. Scanning electron microscopy images of ciprofloxacin-loaded PLGA microspheres with drug/polymer proportions of (A) 1:1; (B) 1:2; (C) 1:3 and (D) 1:5 (w/w).

Compared with direct intraocular injection, this approach is less risky to the patient and less invasive. Since sclera is much more permeable than conjunctiva, the formidable permeability barrier consisted of both cornea and conjunctiva can be avoided altogether in such approaches (Olsen et al., 1995; Hosoya, Lee & Kim, 2005). The advantage of subconjunctival implants as opposed to conjunctival injection of solution is the achievement of higher drug concentrations and sustained release of the drug in both aqueous and vitreous humor and even retinal areas (Gilbert et al., 2003). Dl-polylactide (PLA) nano- and microparticles containing budesonide (which inhibits the expression of vascular endothelial growth factor (VEGF) for the treatment of angiogenesis in the retina) are reported to afford sustained release of budesonide in vitro. Subconjunctival injection of PLA microparticles (3.6 μm) led to a much higher budesonide concentration in retina and vitreous humor over 14 days, compared with the solution form of dosing and PLA nanoparticle (345 nm) administration (Kompella, Bandi & Yalasomayajula, 2003). It was previously published that the collagen matrix and fibrin sealant provided a better controlled release of cisplatin and carboplatin, respectively, than the conventional drug solution, attaining higher drug concentrations after subconjunctival administration using rabbits in several ocular tissues including retina (Simpson et al., 2002; Gilbert et al., 2003). Trans-scleral delivery is a minimally invasive method that achieves targeted delivery of higher therapeutic levels of anti-infection and anti-inflammatory drugs to the anterior and posterior segments of the eye. This drug delivery modality exhibits linear kinetics of absorption and elimination, with potential to deliver a constant drug concentration. By bridging the potential of later generation antibiotics, trans-scleral delivery of biodegradable microparticles sits at the crossroads of patient comfort, treatment compliance, and enhanced safety.

5. Subconjunctival delivery of antibiotic in controlled-release microspheres

Lack of commercial viability in conjunction with an absence of clarity or consensus about the mechanisms of ocular drug penetration and accurate drug delivery has translated into attenuated enthusiasm among pharmaceutical companies and researchers. This hinders the exploration of novel therapeutic approaches for the eye with appropriate newer molecules and better engineered drug delivery technologies. To the best of our knowledge our recently published investigations open up a new era offering the potential of no need for postoperative drops in cataract surgery (Paganelli et al., 2004; Paganelli et al., 2009; Cardillo et al., 2010). These studies gave new information and substantiated a novel and optimized antibiotic prophylaxis strategy using slow delivery technology. Superior vitreous penetration and immediately higher concentrations of antibiotic in the aqueous humor, when compared with the common practice of dosing eye drops 6-times-daily, both support and add rationale to the use of a slow-release trans-scleral drug delivery system in preventing endophthalmitis after cataract surgery. In addition, when this pharmacologic achievement is coupled with its ability to free the patient from the difficulties posed by topical administration, a clear role for this system as a simple and more comprehensive weapon for fighting postoperative infections begins to emerge.

By exploring superior sclera permeability and to avoid the rate-limiting barriers of the cornea and conjunctiva, subconjunctival routes may offer a promising alternative for enhanced drug delivery and tissue-targeting compared with topical routes (Clements &

Tailor, 1987; Behrens-Baumann & Martell, 1988; Barza, 1989; Starr & Lally, 1995; Prausnitz & Noonan, 1998). Confirming our premise, the controlled-release microsphere delivered therapeutic concentrations of antibiotic greater than the minimum inhibitory concentration for most common ocular pathogens up to 10 days after injection. The dosing regimen tested in this experimental investigation fits into a realistic clinical scenario and may provide a surrogate to assess achievable postoperative concentrations. Similar to previous studies (Gilbert et al., 2003; Kompella & Bandi, 2003; Kosoya, Lee & Kim, 2005) the parallel and higher aqueous and vitreous levels of ciprofloxacin-loaded microspheres, as opposed to the same concentration of ciprofloxacin in its free form after a single subconjunctival injection and to topical ciprofloxacin delivery, are considered a highly desirable pharmacological achievement. Furthermore, given the inherent advantages of intraoperative sustained-release antibiotics, particularly patient compliance and convenience, the studied system may achieve a breakthrough in the development of more successful treatment modalities, suggesting a possible new way to progress anti-infection prophylaxis in parallel with antibiotic drug development.

In an experimental rabbit model of endophthalmitis prophylaxis, we have demonstrated that prophylaxis with a biodegradable controlled-release system trans-scleral delivered through a single subconjunctival injection can reach sustained therapeutic levels in the anterior chamber that predictably reduced bacterial recovery and signs of clinical endophthalmitis (comparable to conventional topical drops). Extrapolating these findings to clinical settings, where typically patients are noncompliant with treatment, we could postulate and expect a superior performance for microspheres system over conventional postoperative drops. The frequency of application is important for attaining adequate antibacterial concentrations, and poor compliance also prevents the drops from reaching efficacious levels. Compliance with topical therapy was studied using an electronic device in ambulatory patients who underwent cataract surgery; all patients were noncompliant regarding total dose, time intervals, and premature discontinuation of therapy (Hermann, Ustundag & Diestelhorst, 2005).

Since adverse events are an important concern with any new dosage form, it is also important to ensure that the system chosen for prophylaxis following cataract surgery is safe and well-tolerated, eliminating any potential toxic effects. The biocompatibility of periocular microspheres of biodegradable polymers has been extensively investigated. In vivo there were no drug or procedure-related adverse events and no inflammatory cells or fibrous tissue response at the site of injection was observed. Clinically, in addition to its minimally invasive and pharmaceutically acceptable nature, no drug or procedure-related adverse events occurred (Paganelli et al., 2009; Cardillo et al., 2010).

Pharmacokinetic profiles of aqueous and vitreous humor in rabbit eyes using 0.2 mg/0.1mL of ciprofloxacin microspheres or 2 mg/0.1mL of free ciprofloxacin were compared to a single drop of 0.3% ciprofloxacin six times a day. In 45 rabbits, Staphylococcus aureus was injected into the anterior chamber and 15 were randomly chosen to receive 1 drop of 0.3% ciprofloxacin every 4 hours during 24 hours, 15 received drops of basic salt solution (BSS), and 15 received ciprofloxacin microspheres. After 24 hours endophthalmitis score were recorded, aqueous and vitreous humors were cultured and histology was performed. The subconjunctival administration of non-encapsulate ciprofloxacin exhibited a rapid absorption and permeation between aqueous and vitreous humors, with sharp decay within 6 hours of application (Fig. 3).

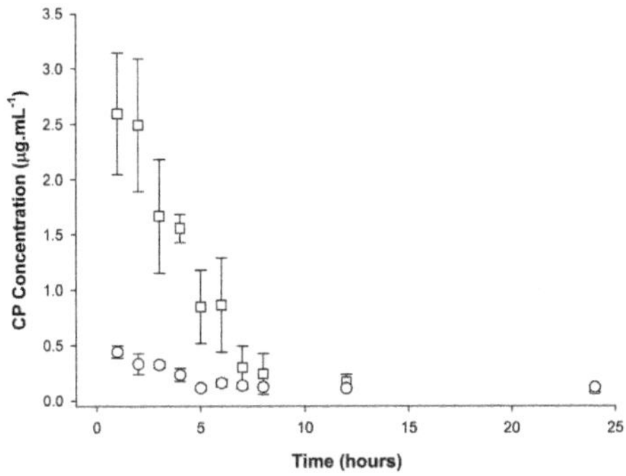

Fig. 3. Comparative pharmacokinetic profiles between the aqueous and vitreous humors after subconjunctival injection of the non-encapsulated ciprofloxacin (2mg/0.1ml). Key: (□) aqueous humor, (O) vitreous humor.

Compared to ciprofloxacin solution injection and ciprofloxacin eye drops, drug levels in the microspheres group showed an immediate and sustained trend towards increased aqueous and vitreous penetration (Fig. 4). A distinct pharmacokinetic trend was observed when the microsphere group was compared with the topical administration group. In the 8 hour-period studied for this group in the design, an immediate higher intraocular antibiotic level was found in the microsphere group, except for the fifth hour that demonstrated comparable measurements. At this time point, one hour prior to sampling, an extra drop of ciprofloxacin was instilled, following the pre-established schedule of one loading drop every 4 hours (Fig. 4).

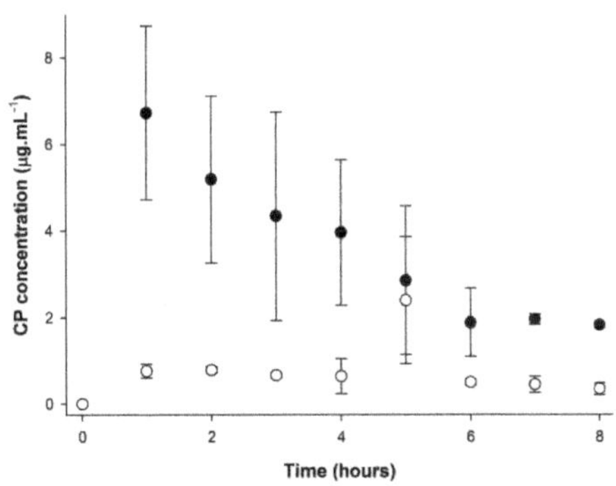

Fig. 4. Comparative pharmacokinetic of ciprofloxacin in the aqueous humor after the single subconjunctival injection of CP (ciprofloxacin)-loaded PLGA microparticles (2mg/0.1ml) (●) and topical CP eye drops 0.3% (O).

Comparing the aqueous concentration following a single subconjunctival injection of the ciprofloxacin-loaded microspheres to the regular ciprofloxacin formulation, a statistically significant difference in favor of the microspheres group was noticed immediately following drug administration and sustained throughout the entire study period. The system allowed sustained aqueous humor concentration of ciprofloxacin in the therapeutic range for most common ocular pathogens (2µg/mL) for up to 8 days (Fig. 5).

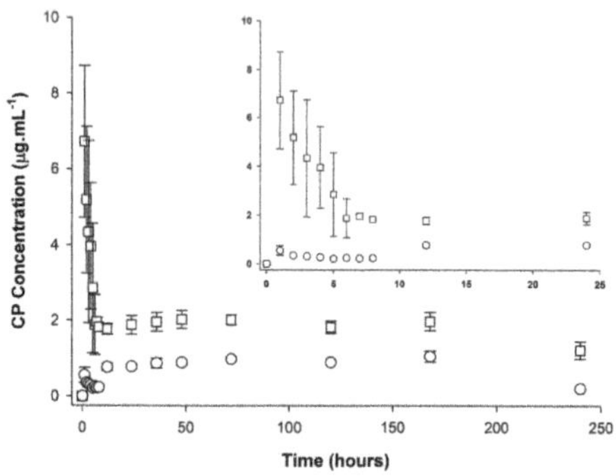

Fig. 5. Comparative pharmacokinetic of ciprofloxacin in the aqueous and vitreous humors subconjunctival administration of 2mg/0.1ml of CP-loaded microparticles. Key: (□) aqueous humor, (O) vitreous humor.

In contrast to the ciprofloxacin microspheres and solution groups, no measurable levels of ciprofloxacin could be detected in the vitreous cavity following topical administration. Assessing the vitreous concentration, a statistical significant difference in favor of the microspheres group was immediately noticed following drug administration and sustained throughout the entire study period.

6. Conclusions

Our scientific observations suggest that a trans-scleral antibiotic delivery system is both effective and may help to eliminate patient noncompliance. By freeing the patient from the hassles and expenses of topical therapy post cataract surgery, a new anti-inflammatory and anti-infection paradigm in modern cataract surgery has been introduced, meriting further consideration. In parallel to antibiotic development, exploiting the routes for trans-scleral delivery or circumventing the cornea-conjunctival barriers will be the key to an ultimate anti-infection strategy in the modern cataract surgery era. While the challenges are formidable, the experimentally and clinically tested systems hold promise for new paradigms in dosing anterior segment drugs. However, no study will provide the final answer regarding optimum antibiotic prophylaxis in this continually developing field. Advances in antimicrobial therapy and modes of delivery make this a dynamic area and highlight the need for continued investigation and periodic guideline reviews to keep pace with new developments to optimize patient care.

7. References

Akduman, L., Kolker, A.E., Black, D.L., Del Priore, L.V. & Kaplan, H.J. (1996)Treatment of persistent glaucoma secondary to periocular corticosteroids. Am. J. Ophthalmol. 122:275-277.

Barza, M. Antibacterial agents in the treatment of ocular infections. (1989) Infect Dis. Clin. North Am. 3:533-551.

Behrens-Baumann W. & Martell, J. (1988) Ciprofloxacin concentration in the rabbit aqueous humor and vitreous following intravenous and subconjunctival administration. Infection 16:54-57.

Bui, D.P., Dang, S.B. & Hwang, D.G. (1995) Effect of ciprofloxacin concentration on mutation resistance rates in S. aureus. Invest. Ophthalmol. Vis. Sci. 36: abstract 4876.

Callegan, M.C., Ramirez, R., Kane, S.T., Cochran, D.C. & Jensen, H. (2003) Antibacterial activity of the fourth-generation fluoroquinolones gatifloxacin and moxifloxacin against ocular pathogens. Adv. Ther. 20:246-252.

Cardillo, J.A., Melo-Jr, L.A.S., Costa R.A., Skaf, M., Belfort, R., Souza-Filho, A.A., Farah, M.E. & Kupperman, B.D. (2005) Comparison of intravitreal versus posterior sub-Tenon's capsule injection of triamcinolone acetonide for diffuse diabetic macular edema. Ophthalmology 112:1557-1563.

Cardillo, J.A., Paganelli, F., Melo-Jr, L.A., Lucena, D., Silva-Jr, A.A., Oliveira, A.G., Pizzolito, A.C., Lavisnk, D., Skaf, M., Hofling-Lima, A.L., Nguyen, Q.D., Keppermann, B.D., Herrero-Vanrell & Belfort, R. (2010) Subconjunctival delivery of antibiotics in a controlled-release system: a novel anti-infection prophylaxis approach for cataract surgery. Arch. Ophthalmol. 128:81-87.

Chang, D.F., Garcia, I.H., Hunkeler, J.D. & Minas, T. (1999) Phase II results of an intraocular steroid delivery system for cataract surgery. Ophthalmology 106:1172-1177.

Clements, DB & Tailor, V.A. (1987) study of aqueous and serum levels of ceftazidine following subconjunctival administration. Br. J. Ophthalmol. 71:433-435.

Costello, P., Bakri, S.J., Beer, P.M., Singh, R.J., Falk, N.S., Peters, G.B. & Melendez, J.A. (2006) Vitreous penetration of topical moxifloxacin and gatifloxacin in humans. Retina 26:191-195.

Ellis P.P. (1978) Occlusion of the central retina artery after retrobulbar corticosteroid injection. Am. J. Ophthalmol. 85:352-356.

Ellis, P.P. (1974) Retrobulbar injections. Surv. Ophthalmol. 18:425-430.

Geroski, D.H. & Edelhauser, H.F. (2001) Trans-scleral drug delivery for posterior segment disease. Adv. Drug Deliv. Rev. 52:37-48.

Gilbert, J.A., Simpson, A.E., Rudnick, D.H., Aaberg-J, T.M. & Edelhauser, H.F. (2003) Trans-scleral permeability and intraocular concentrations of cisplatin from a collagen matrix. J. Control. Rel. 89:409-417.

Giles, C.L. (1974) Bulbar perforation during periocular injection of corticosteroids. Am. J. Ophthalmol. 77:438-441.

Hermann, M.M., Ustundag, C. & Diestelhorst, M. (2005) compliance with topical therapy after cataract surgery using a new microprocessor-controlled eye drop monitor. Invest Ophthalmol. Vis. Sci., 46: E-Abstract 3832.

Herrero-Vanrell, R. & Refojo, M.F. (2001) Biodegradable microspheres for vitreo retinal drug delivery. Adv. Drug Deliv. Rev. 52:5-16.

Herschler, J. (1976) Increased intraocular pressure induced by repository corticosteroids. Am J. Ophthalmol. 82:90-93.

Hosoya, K., Lee, V.H. & Kim, K. (2005) Roles of the conjunctiva in ocular drug delivery: a review of conjunctival transport mechanisms and their regulation. Eur. J. Pharm. Biopharm. 60:227-240.

Kim, D.H., Stark, W.J., O'Brien, T.P. & Dick J.D. (2005) Aqueous penetration and biological activity of moxifloxacin 0.5% ophthalmic solution and gatifloxacin 0.3% solution in cataract surgery patients. Ophthalmol. 112(11):1992-1996.

Kim, S.Y., Yang, J., Lee, Y.C. & Park, Y.H. (2008) Effect of a single intraoperative sub-Tenon injection of triamcinolone acetonide on the progression of diabetic retinopathy and visual outcomes after cataract surgery. J. Cataract Refract. Surg. 34(5):823-6.

Kompella, U.B., Bandi, N. & Ayalasomayajula, S.P. (2003) Subconjunctival nano- and microparticles sustain retinal delivery of budesomide, a corticosteroid capable of inhibiting VEGF expression. Invest. Ophthalmol. Vis. Sci. 44:1192-1201.

Kowalski, R.P., Romanowski, E.G., Mah, F.S., Yates, K.A. & Gordon, Y.J. (2004) Topical prophylaxis with moxifloxacin prevents endophthalmitis in a rabbit model. Am. J. Ophthalmol. 138:33-37.

Lang, L.C. (1996) Ocular drug delivery from conventional ocular formulations. Adv. Drug Deliv. Rev. 16:39-45.

Mathias, C.G.T., Maibach, H.I., Ostler, H.B., Conant, M.A. & Nelson, W. (1978) Delayed hypersensitivity to retrobulbar injections of methylprednisolone acetate. Am. J. Ophthalmol. 86:816-819.

McDonald, M.B. (2006) Research review and update:IQUIX (levofloxacin 1.5%). Int. Ophthalmol. Clin. 46:47-60.

McLean, E,B. (1975) Inadvertent injection of corticosteroid into the choroidal vasculature. Am. J. Ophthalmol. 80:835-837.

Morgan, C.M., Schatz, H., Vine, A.K., Cantrill, H.L., Davidorf,F.H., Gitter,K.A. & Rudich, R. (1988) Ocular complications associated with retrobulbar injections. Ophthalmol. 1988;95:660-5.

Negi, A.K., Browning, A.C. & Vernon, S.A. (2006) Single perioperative triamcinolone injection versus standard post-operative steroid drops after uneventful phacoemulsification surgery: randomized controlled trial. J. Cataract Refract. Surg. 32:468-474.

Nozik, R.A. (1976) Orbital rim fat atrophy after repository periocular corticosteroid injection. Am. J. Ophthalmol. 82:928-9230.

O'Connor. G.R. (1976) Periocular corticosteroid injections: uses and abuses. Eye Ear Nose Throat. Mon. 55:83-8.

Olsen ,T.W., Edelhauser, H.F., Lim, J.I. & Geroski, D.H. (1995) Human scleral permeability. Effects of age, cryotherapy, trans-scleral diode laser, and surgical thinning. Invest. Opthalmol. Vis. Sci. 36:1893-1903.

Paccola, L., Jorge, R. & Barbosa, J.C. (2007) Anti-inflammatory efficacy of a single posterior subtenon injection of triamcinolone acetonide versus prednisolone acetate 1% eyedrops after pars plana vitrectomy. Acta Ophthalmol. Scand. 85:603-608.

Paganelli, F., Cardillo, J.A., Melo-Jr, L.A., Lucena, D.R., Silva-Jr, A.A., Oliveira, A.G., Hofling-Lima, A., Hguyen, Q.D., Kuppermann, B., Belfort, R., Costa, R., Lavinsk, D., Skaf, M. & Lima-Filho, A.A.S. (2009) A single intraoperative sub-tenon's capsule injection of triamcinolone and ciprofloxacin in a controlled-release system for cataract surgery. Invest. Ophthalmol. Vis. Sci. 50:3041-3047.

Paganelli, F., Cardillo, J.A., Melo-Jr, L.A.S., Oliveira, A.G., Skaf, M. & Costa, R.A. (2004) A single intraoperative sub-Tenon's capsule triamcinolone acetonide injection for the treatment of post-cataract surgery inflammation. Ophthalmol. 111:2102-2108.

Paganelli, F., Cardillo, J.A., Dare, A.J.A., Melo-Jr, L.A.S., Lucena, D.R., Silva-Jr, A.A., Oliveira, A.G., Pizzolito, A.C., Lavinsky, D., Skaf, M., Souza-Filho, A.A., Höfling-Lima, A.L., Nguyen, Q.D., Kuppermann, B.D., Herero-Vankell, R. & Belfort, R. (2010) Controlled trans-scleral drug delivery formulations to the eye: establishing new concepts and paradigms in ocular anti-inflammatory therapeutics and antibacterial prophylaxis. Exp. Opin. Drug Deliv. 7(8): 955-965.

Prausnitz, M.R. & Noonan, J.S. (1998) Permeability of cornea, sclera, and conjunctiva: a literature analysis for drug delivery to the eye. J. Pharm. Sci. 87:1479-1488.

Price, M.O., Quillin, C. & Price-Jr, F.W. (2005) Effect of gatifloxacin ophthalmic solution 0.3% on human corneal endothelial cell density and aqueous humor gatifloxacin concentration. Curr. Eye Res. 30:563-567.

Schechter, R.J. (1985) Management of inadvertent intraocular injections. Ann. Ophthalmol. 17:771-775.

Schlaegel, T.F. & Wilson, F.M. (1974) Accidental intraocular injection of depot corticosteroids. Trans. Am. Acad. Ophthalmol. Otolaryngol. 78:847-55.

Silva-Jr, A., Scarpa, M.V., Pestana, K.C., Mercuri, L.P., Matos, J.R. & Oliveira, A.G. (2008) Thermal analysis of biodegradable microparticles containing ciprofloxacin hydrochloride obtained by spray drying technique. Thermochimica Acta 467: 91-98.

Silva-Jr, A.A., Matos, J.R., Formariz, T.P., Rossanezi, G., Scarpa, M.V., Egito, E.S.T. & Oliveira, A.G. (2009) Thermal behavior and stability of biodegradable spray-dried microparticles containing triamcinolone. Int. J. Pharm. 368: 45–55.

Simpson, A.E., Gilbert, .JA., Rudnick, D.H., Geroski, T.M., Aeberg, T.M. & Edelhauser, H.F. (2002) Trans-scleral diffusion of carboplatin: an in vitro and in vivo study. Ophthalmol. 120:1069-74.

Solomon, R., Donnenfeld, E.D., Perry, H.D., Snyder, R.W., Nedrud, C. & Bloom, A. (2005) Penetration of topically applied gatifloxacin 0.3%, moxifloxacin 0.5%, and ciprofloxacin 0.3% into the aqueous humor. Ophthalmol. 112:466-469.

Starr, M.B. & Lally, J.M. (1995) Antimicrobial prophylaxis for ophthalmic surgery. Surv. Ophthalmol. 39:485-501.

Tan, D.T., Chee, S.P., Lim, L., Theng, J. & Van Ede, M. (2001) Randomized clinical trial of Surodex steroid drug delivery system for cataract surgery: anterior versus posterior placement of two Surodex in the eye. Ophthalmol. 108:2172-81.

Tan, D.T., Chee, S.P., Lim, L. & Lim, A.S. (1999) Randomized clinical trial of a new dexamethasone delivery system (Surodex) for treatment of post-cataract surgery inflammation. Ophthalmol. 106:223-31.

Thach, A.B., Dugel, P.U., Flindall, R.J., Sipperley, J.O. & Sneed, S.R. (1997) A comparison of retrobulbar versus sub-Tenon's corticosteroid therapy for cystoid macular edema refractory to topical medications. Ophthalmol. 104:2003-2008.

Velpandian, T. (2009) Intraocular penetration of antimicrobial agents in ophthalmic infections and drug delivery strategies. Expert Opin. Drug Deliv. 3:255-70.

Walton, R.C., Vick, V.L. & Greenwald, M.A. (1999) Sub-tenon's corticosteroid for the treatment of macular edema in bone marrow transplant retinopathy. Retina 19:171-173.

West, E.S., Behrens, A., McDonnell, P.J., Behrens, A., Tielsch J.M., Schein, O.D. (2005) The incidence of endophthalmitis after cataract surgery among the U.S. Medicare population increased between 1994 and 2001. Ophthalmol. 112:1388-1394.

Yoshikawa, K., Kotake, S., Ichiishi, A., Sasamoto, Y., Kosaka, S. & Matsuda, H. (1995) Posterior sub-Tenon injections of repository corticosteroids in uveitis patients with cystoid macular edema. Jpn. J. Ophthalmol. 39:71-76.

Zeimer, R. & Goldberg, M.F. (2001) Novel ophthalmic therapeutic modalities based on noninvasive light-targeted drug delivery to the posterior pole of the eye. Adv. Drug Deliv. Rev. 52:49-61.

14

Chromovitrectomy in Vitreous Loss During Cataract Surgery

Taiji Sakamoto[1] and Toshio Hisatomi[2]
*[1]Department of Ophthalmology,
Kagoshima University Graduate School of Medical and Dental Sciences, Kagoshima,
[2]Department of Ophthalmology,
Kyushu University Graduate School of Medicine, Fukuoka,
Japan*

1. Introduction

Cataract surgery is the commonest surgical operation performed throughout the world, but surgery has always involved some risk. For example, vitreous loss (vitreous breaching the posterior capsule) associated with capsular rupture is a complication that significantly affects postoperative visual acuity. Direct and immediate effects of vitreous loss involve deviation of the pupil (corectopia), inflammation of the anterior chamber, corneal damage, and intraocular pressure elevation; indirect and late effects are cystoid macular edema, vitreous inflammation, and retinal detachment [1-6].

Various factors have been reported to associated with this complication [1]. There is no doubt that the skill of the surgeon is a major factor, and other predisposing factors include white cataract, small pupil, pseudoexfoliation, and a history of previous intraocular surgery. When lost vitreous is treated improperly, it can cause secondary complications, resulting in poor final visual acuity. To prevent these secondary harmful results, good knowledge, experience, and skill are required from surgeons. Specifically, complete removal of the vitreous from the anterior chamber is essential for a favourable postoperative outcome after posterior capsule rupture. However, the surgical procedure for removing the vitreous is difficult because the structure appears transparent under an operating microscope. The vitreous body in the anterior chamber is sometimes difficult even for an experienced surgeon to identify because the cornea is often damaged incidentally in cases involving vitreous prolapse, which are by definition complex cases.

To facilitate this procedure, several approaches have been applied to improve visualisation of lost vitreous. A vital dye has generally been used to stain the lens capsule in standard cataract surgery. This technique is adopted to visualize lost vitreous. Another approach is to stain the components of the vitreous body directly. Recently, triamcinolone acetonide (TA) has been used as an adjunct to visualize the vitreous body during pars plana vitrectomy (PPV) [7]. This technique was originally developed to visualize the vitreous body on the retinal surface. Moreover, it was found to be very helpful for elucidating the pathophysiology of the vitreous body in various retinal diseases [8-10]. Therefore, it has been a natural step to adopt this technique to stain the vitreous in an attempt to facilitate its removal in cases of a ruptured capsule during cataract surgery. The following section presents the concepts behind this methods as well as technical details.

2. History of visualization of the vitreous body

Modern closed vitreous surgery owes much to the work of Machemer [11]. After initial success vitrectomy continued to be developed and has now been established as a standard treatment for vitreoretinal diseases. With advances in instrumentation and understanding of vitreoretinal pathophysiology the indications for vitrectomy have been expanded to include a variety of diseases such as simple rhegmatogenous retinal detachment, macular hole, and macular oedema [8]. In the early days of its use vitrectomy was performed for diseases in which the vitreous body was visible due to vitreous hemorrhage, proliferative diabetic retinopathy, and asteroid hyalosis. At present though indications for vitrectomy include eyes with optically clear vitreous such as in macular hole surgery, and removing transparent hyaloid and/or internal limiting membrane (ILM) has become a standard procedure. Despite advances in surgical instrumentation and techniques, the vitrectomy procedure continues to demand both skill and experience. Removing the vitreous is a particularly challenging procedure, partly due to its transparency. Various approaches have been taken to assist in visualisation of the vitreous during vitrectomy. Recently, intraoperative triamcinolone acetonide has been used in many countries worldwide [7,8].

In the earliest years of retinal surgery, it was recognized that vital dyes could be helpful for facilitating surgery. In such cases, the structure of the vitreous was not the main target, so dyes such as Indian ink, methylene blue and fluorescein were used primarily to visualise retinal breaks. This vital staining was not so commonly used in surgery at that time; however, recently it has been revived as chromovitrectomy. Visualizing ILM is being studied extensively and chromovitrectomy is now one of the most important elements of vitreous surgery.

In terms of the macroscopic structure of the vitreous, important work has been done using cadaveric eyes and living eyes with biomicroscopy or optical coherence tomography (OCT) examinations; the results have contributed extensively to our understanding of the pathology of vitreoretinal diseases [12-14]. Unfortunately, observational techniques cannot be applied during surgery, thus valuable information cannot be fully used during surgery in individual cases, especially during surgical manoeuvres, though of note intraoperative OCT is starting to be used by some surgeons. Abrams et al noticed in the early days of vitrectomy that staining of the vitreous with fluorescein dye improved the ease of vitrectomy by facilitating clear visualization of the vitreous, although this method was used only in animals and for surgical training [15]. Some 20 years later, it was proven in a report which showed that preoperative fluorescein angiography or orally administered sodium fluorescein stained a transparent vitreous, making it visible as light green [16,17]. However, thin posterior hyaloids could not be visualized well by this method, which is indispensable in modern surgery on the retinal surface such as for macular hole or pre-retinal membrane. On the other hand, intravitreous application of autologous blood was used for a similar purpose [18]. It was reported that intravitreous autologous blood could identify the posterior vitreous cortex and facilitate surgical manoeuvres with reduced complications. However, blood is not transparent so it is not necessarily helpful to remove ILM. Furthermore, unclotted erythrocytes may become lysed in the irrigation fluid and swirl the liberated haemoglobin in the vitreous cavity, obscuring the fundus view with a dusty appearance. This characteristic prevents autologous blood from being commonly used in vitrectomy.

3. Visualization of vitreous during cataract surgery

Although vitreous loss is a significant complication of cataract surgery, the outcome can be almost as good as if it had not happened when managed properly - though there nevertheless remains an increased risk of retinal break and retinal detachment. Needless to say, the first and most important step is early recognition that vitreous loss has taken place. The second step is to evaluate the loss of vitreous properly with or without using an anterior vitrector. For that purpose, at present there are the several approaches as described below.

3.1 Trypan blue

Trypan blue has been reported to be effective for staining tissue during anterior and posterior segment surgery without significant toxicity to corneal endothelial cells with short exposure times [19]. In a preliminary study, the dye was injected into the anterior chamber under an air bubble, which prevents dilution of the trypan blue and avoids direct contact between the undiluted dye and the endothelium. Subsequently, the dye was removed with a vitreous cutter as vitrectomy proceeded. On the first postoperative day no residual staining was visualized on inspection with a slit lamp and ophthalmoscope, and no side effects related to intraoperative use of the dye were observed in any patient. This technique was applied to visualize prolapsed vitreous in cataract surgery [20]. Trypan blue does not stain vitreous body directly, but rather allows visualization of the vitreous body by staining the surrounding tissues such as iris and lens capsule. So far there have been no reports on the apparent toxicity of trypan blue in intracameral use [21].

3.2 Triamcinolone acetonide and other related materials

In Japan triamcinolone acetonide (TA) is now the most commonly used agent for pars plana vitrectomy (PPV) for visualization of a transparent vitreous body. A national survey in Japan showed that 75% of PPV comprised TA-assisted PPV in 2005 [22]. When intravitreous TA was first used for PPV, there were strong concerns about its potential adverse effects such as glaucoma, endophthalmitis, or direct toxicity related to preservatives [8]. However, the incidence of these potential adverse events were not significant, probably as most of the TA crystals were removed at the end of surgery [8]. This safety issue was partly supported by the fact that intravitreous injection of TA (without removal) did not cause serious or profound adverse events [23].

Unlike other vital dyes, white granules of TA adhere to the surface of the vitreous, which clearly shows the margin of the vitreous [24,25] This is also the case with intracameral use of TA. Even a small amount of TA can be of great help in visualizing even traces of vitreous in the anterior chamber with a surgical microscope (Figure 1). Theoretically, TA crystals should be removed as much as possible at the end of surgery, because steroid granules left in the anterior chamber might induce secondary glaucoma or infection. But, it might not be necessary because an intracameral depot to release dexamethasone is left safely in the anterior chamber after cataract surgery [26]. In addition, it is impossible in practice to remove all the granules from the anterior chamber.

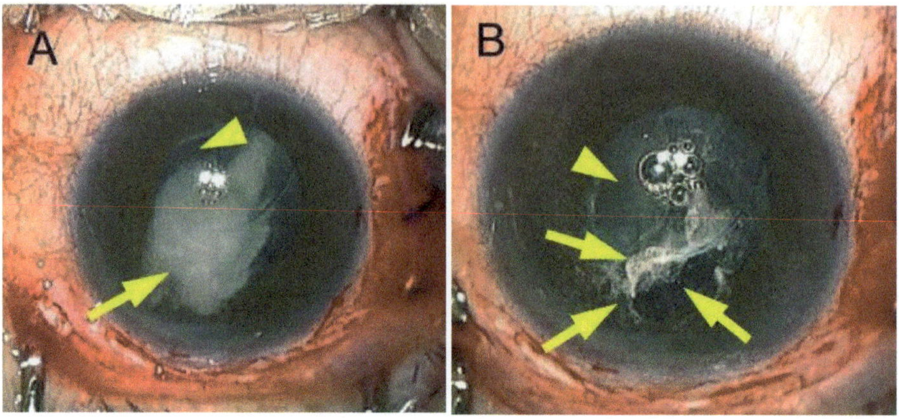

The posterior capsule is ruptured and the vitreous body is moved into the anterior chamber; triamcinolone is sprayed at the location where the vitreous body is likely to have been placed, using a syringe with a dull-edged needle. The vitreous body immediately appears as a white-coloured gel. The vitreous body with TA crystals (arrows) were then easily removed with a vitreous cutter. Arrowhead indicates optic of intraocular lens (A and B). Reprinted from: Yamakiri K et al. (2004), with permission from Elsevier [25].

Fig. 1. Intraoperative photograph of triamcinolone-assisted vitrectomy (cataract surgery after rupture of lens capsule).

A novel approach related to use of TA will be described. Kaji et al reported a new technique for visualising the vitreous in the anterior chamber using 11-deoxycortisol (11-DC) [27]. Its suspension can be prepared without the antiseptic and emulsifying agents contained in commercially available TA. A precursor of cortisol in the cascade of steroid metabolism, 11-DC, is naturally detectable in blood and urine. This material is free from glucocorticoid and mineralocorticoid actions. In addition, the conversion system of 11-DC into cortisol is not present in ocular tissues. Thus, 11-DC injected into the anterior chamber does not induce steroid-related complications such as ocular hypertension. As for the molecular structure, 11-DC contains hydroxyl groups, thus it has some hydrophilic characteristics. Therefore, 11-DC left in the anterior chamber is easily cleared and excreted through the urine. In their study, there were white particles on the surface of the iris or in the vitreous body on the day following surgery, but all the particles had completely disappeared within 2 days after surgery [27]. This hydrophilic characteristic of 11-DC is highly advantageous over hydrophobic cholesterol as a tool to visualize the vitreous body.

There are however concerns about use of 11-DC. Under some circumstances, the steroid activity of TA is advantageous to reduce post-operative inflammation, which 11-DC does not have. The particle size of 11-DC is larger than that of TA. Above all, 11-DC is not commercially available in most of countries at present. Although the use of TA in cataract surgery was off-label, there is a product of TA for general medical use (e.g. Kenalog made by Bristol-Myers Squibb) and products which are licensed specifically for intraocular conditions have also been licensed (e.g. Trivaris made by Allergan). Consequently, TA can be used more easily and in theory more safely than 11-DC. This is a major obstacle to more widespread use of 11-DC.

In an experimental study, Yamashita et al demonstrated that polylactic acid could be applied for this purpose [28]. Polylactic acid is a biodegradable substance without any biological effects. In 2004, the U.S. Food and Drug Administration approved a poly-L-lactic acid (PLLA)-based injectable medical device for restoring and/or correcting signs of facial fat loss in people with human immunodeficiency virus. As a result, the properties of PLLA microparticles have attracted considerable interest in the medical community. PLLA granules are originally white and adhere to the gel-like structure of the vitreous body so easily that they assist in visualizing the transparent vitreous as do TA granules but with no harmful consequences in rabbits and nonhuman primates. In future this agent might be a good alternative in cases where TA is proven to be intolerably harmful such as ocular steroid-responders at risk of glaucoma.

4. Possible adverse events

Although chromovitrectomy is very helpful for facilitating the removal of vitreous in the anterior chamber, to our knowledge there has been no large-scale comparative study. The incidence of vitreous loss in cataract surgery is low and this complication is not predictable [29], therefore it is not possible to conclusively describe any role for chromovitrectomy in preventing adverse events. However, possible adverse events can be described from the results of animal studies, small studies, or chromovitrectomy for vitreoretinal diseases.

4.1 Trypan blue and other vital dyes

At present indocyanine green, trypan blue, and brilliant blue G are commonly used for capsular staining in cataract surgery. Of these, trypan blue has been deemed safe for clinical use [30]. However, non-infectious endophthalmitis has been reported after intracameral use of trypan blue in cataract surgery [31]. In an in vitro study, trypan blue has been shown to be toxic to human corneal endothelial cells at high concentrations or with long exposure [32]. In an animal study conducted by the authors, intracameral injection of each dye resulted in corneal damage to a certain extent and trypan blue was most toxic (Figure 2) [33]. The results of in vitro or animal studies may not necessarily reflect clinical conditions correctly; however, this information should be noted when using trypan blue. Therefore, trypan blue should be removed as much as possible at the end of surgery. The use of trypan blue in cataract surgery does not increase intraocular pressure, nor cause infectious endophthalmitis, or retinal detachment [34].

Most importantly, it should be remembered that these dyes are used in potentially inflamed and/or damaged tissues. The safety issue should be considered more seriously than usual and great caution is warranted.

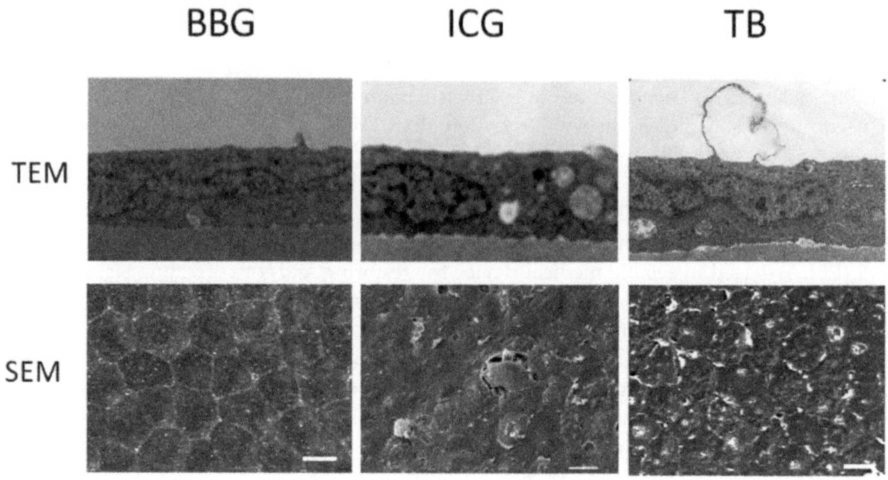

Brown Norway rats received intracameral injection into each eye and the eyes were examined with electron microscopy after 2 months. In the brilliant blue G (BBG) groups, the ultrastructure of the corneal cells and collagen cellular matrix were well preserved (10 mg/mL). The indocyanine green (ICG) group showed mitochondrial swelling at the 5-mg/mL concentration. The trypan blue (TB) group showed cyst formation in the endothelial cell layer due to separation of the cells and degeneration of the corneal endothelium in a sporadic manner (original magnification x6600). The BBG-exposed corneas demonstrated a normal hexagonal endothelial cell sheet with intact borders and no endothelial swelling. The ICG group showed cellular swelling and some degenerated cells in the corneal endothelial cells. C, In the TB group, endothelial cell shrinkage was recognized in a sporadic manner. Cell shrinkage led to endothelial cell loss in the central area of the cornea (original magnification x1000). The detailed method was described by Hisatomi et al [33].

Fig. 2. Ultrastructure of rat corneal cells studied using transmission electron microscopy and scanning electron microscopy.

4.2 Triamcinolone and related materials

Corticosteroids are known to have several adverse effects on an eye, thus this issue was of particular concern from the beginning. However, most of the results have been obtained from the intravitreous use of TA. These should be interpreted carefully.

Corticosteroids are strong inducers of intraocular pressure (IOP) rise. Recent studies have revealed that intravitreous TA without vitrectomy causes a significant rise of IOP in more than 50% of eyes [23]. In comparison, the incidence of IOP rise was not high after TA-assisted vitrectomy, probably due to the fact that TA crystals were almost totally removed at the end of surgery. The largest-scale controlled trial showed that 23 out of 391 eyes (5.9%)

had a significant IOP rise in TA-assisted vitrectomy; while 13 out of 383 eyes (3.4%) did so in conventional vitrectomy, a difference which did not reach statistical significance [35]. Most of these rises in intraocular pressure could be managed with topical treatment, but some of them required filtration surgery [8,35]. It should be noted that patients who had a history of glaucoma were not included in these studies. Because a history of glaucoma is a risk factor for an intraocular hypertensive response to corticosteroid, care must be taken when using TA in patients with such a history.

Corticosteroid has an immune-suppressive effect and endopthalmitis has a poor visual prognosis, thus postoperative infection has been the foremost concern in the intraoperative use of TA. The incidence of acute endophthalmitis was reported to be 7/26,819 cases (0.026%) in the Japan national survey [22]. Therefore, it is not as high as that of simple intravitreous TA injection (0.87%) described by Moshfeghi et al and is similar to the incidence of 20 gauge vitrectomy without TA (0.018 to 0.05%) [36].

The toxicity of TA suspension has been reported in an experimental study. Direct exposure to preserved TA in rabbits damaged the corneal endothelial cells probably due to the preservative benzyl alcohol [37,38]. To avoid potential toxicities, it is preferable to use preservative-free TA. In most cases, decantation of preservative prior to injection is considered to be sufficient to avoid potential toxicity. At present, if necessary, benzyl alcohol-free TA is commercially available (Triesence™, Alcon, Ft Worth, Tx, USA) or (Macuaid™, Wakamoto, Tokyo, Japan).

5. Chemovitrectomy in the future: To see is to believe!

Although cataract surgery is one of the safest procedures in ocular surgery, there is always some risk attached. No surgery can be free from risk, thus every effort has to be made to reduce risk in surgery. Vitreous loss is a significant risk of cataract surgery, but proper treatment can prevent further complications ensuing from loss of vitreous. Visualization of vitreous is the key challenge to surgeons trying to provide optimal technical outcomes in such cases, which can be greatly facilitated by chromovitrectomy. Although the present vital dyes or TA may be replaced by better agents in the future, the concept of chromovitrectomy, "visualizing vitreous," will remain as long as vitrectomy is performed.

6. Acknowledgement

Supported in part by a grant from the Research Committee on Chorioretinal Degeneration and Optic Atrophy, Ministry of Health, Labor, and Welfare, Tokyo, Japan; and by a Grant-in-Aid for Scientific Research from the Ministry of Education, Science, and Culture of the Japanese Government, Tokyo, Japan.

7. References

[1] Maerza AA, Ramanathan A, Bidgood P, Horgan S (2009) Visual outcome in cataract surgery complicated by vitreous loss in a district general hospital. Int Ophthalmol. 29:157-160.

[2] Desai P, Minassian D, Reidy A (1999) National cataract surgery survey 1997–8: a report of the results of the clinical outcomes. Br. J. Ophthalmol. 82:1336–1340.

[3] Ionides A, Minassian D, Tuft S (2002) Visual outcome following posterior capsule rupture during cataract surgery. Br. J. Ophthalmol. 85: 222–224.

[4] Ang GA, Whyte IF (2006) Effect and outcomes of posterior capsule rupture in a district general hospital setting. J. Cataract Refract. Surg. 32: 623–627.

[5] Tan JH, Karwatowski WS (2002) Phacoemulsification cataract surgery and unplanned anterior vitrectomy—is it bad news? Eye.16: 117–120.

[6] Chan FM, Mathur R, Ku JJ, Chen C et al (2003) Short-term outcomes in eyes with posterior capsule rupture during cataract surgery. J. Cataract Refract. Surg. 29: 537–541.

[7] Sakamoto T, Miyazaki M, Hisatomi T, Nakamura T, Ueno A, et al (2002) Triamcinolone-assisted pars plana vitrectomy improves the surgical procedures and decreases the postoperative blood-ocular barrier breakdown. Graefes Arch. Clin. Exp. Ophthalmol. 240:4234-4239.

[8] Sakamoto T, Ishibashi T (2009) Visualizing vitreous in vitrectomy by triamcinolone. Graefes Arch.. Clin. Exp. Ophthalmol. 247:1153-1163.

[9] Enaida H, Hata Y, Ueno A, Ishibashi T, Torii H, et al (2004) Visualization of the Cloquet canal during triamcinolone-assisted vitrectomy. Arch. Ophthalmol. 122:1564-1565.

[10] Sonoda KH, Sakamoto T, Enaida H, Miyazaki M, Noda Y, et al (2004) Residual vitreous cortex after surgical posterior vitreous separation visualized by intravitreous triamcinolone acetonide. Ophthalmology. 111:226-230.

[11] Michaels RG (1990) History of retinal detachment surgery. In Retinal detachment, Michaels RG, Wilkinson CP, Rice TA (eds) The CV Mosby Company, St. Louis, pp243-323

[12] Eisner G. Biomicroscopy of the peripheral fundus. NewYork, Springer 1973.

[13] Sebag J, Balazs EA (1989) Morphology and ultrastructure of human vitreous fibers. Invest. Ophthalmol. Vis. Sci. 30:1867-1871.

[14] Takahashi M, Jalkh A, Hoskins J, Trempe CL, Schepens CL (1981) Biomicroscopic evaluation and photography of liquefied vitreous in some vitreoretinal disorders. Arch. Ophthalmol. 99:1555-1559.

[15] Abrams GW, Topping T, Machemer R (1978) An improved method for practice vitrectomy. Arch. Ophthalmol. 96:521-525.

[16] Rodrigues EB, Penha FM, Furlani B, Meyer CH, Maia M, Farah ME (2008) Historical aspects and evolution of the application of vital dyes in vitreoretinal surgery and chromovitrectomy. Dev. Ophthalmol. 42:29-34.

[17] Yao Y, Wang ZJ, Wei SH, Huang YF, Zhang MN (2007) Oral sodium fluorescein to improve visualization of clear vitreous during vitrectomy for proliferative diabetic retinopathy. Clin. Exp. Ophthalmol. 35:824-827.

[18] Ryan EA, Lee S, Chern S (1995) Use of intravitreal autologous blood to identify posterior cortical vitreous in macular hole surgery. Arch. Ophthalmol. 113:822-823.

[19] Melles GR, de Waard PW, Pameyer JH, Houdijn Beekhuis W (1999) Trypan blue capsule staining to visualize the capsulorhexis in cataract surgery. J. Cataract Refract. Surg. 25:7-9.

[20] Cacciatori M, Chadha V, Bennett HG, Singh J (2006) Trypan blue to aid visualization of the vitreous during anterior segment surgery. J. Cataract Refract. Surg. 32:389-391.

[21] Norn MS (1980) Per operative trypan blue vital staining of corneal endothelium. Eight years' follow up. Acta. Ophthalmol. (Copenh) 58:550-555.

[22] Sakamoto T, Hida T, Tano Y, Negi A, Takeuchi S, Ishibashi T, et al (2007) Committee for Triamcinolone Acetonide for Ocular Disease in Japan. Survey of triamcinolone acetonide for ocular diseases in Japan. Nippon Ganka Gakkai Zasshi. 111:936-945.

[23] Jonas JB, Kreissig I, Degenring R (2005) Intravitreal triamcinolone acetonide for treatment of intraocular proliferative, exudative, and neovascular diseases. Prog. Retina. Eye Res. 24:587-611.

[24] Burk SE, Da Mata AP, Snyder ME, Schneider S, Osher RH, et al (2003) Visualizing vitreous using Kenalog suspension. J. Cataract Refract. Surg. 29:645-651.

[25] Yamakiri K, Uchino E, Kimura K, Sakamoto T (2004) Intracameral triamcinolone helps to visualize and remove the vitreous body in anterior chamber in cataract surgery. Am. J. Ophthalmol. 138:650-652.

[26] Wadood AC, Armbrecht AM, Aspinall PA, Dhillon B (2004) Safety and efficacy of a dexamethasone anterior segment drug delivery system in patients after phacoemulsification. J. Cataract Refract. Surg. 30:761-768.

[27] Kaji Y, Hiraoka T, Okamoto F, Sato M, Oshika T (2005) Clinical application of 11-deoxycortisol in visualizing prolapsed vitreous body after posterior capsule rupture in cataract surgery. J. Cataract Refract. Surg. 31:1133-1138.

[28] Yamashita T, Sakamoto T, Yamakiri K, Miura M, Enaida H, et al (2007) Polylactic acid for visualizing the vitreous body during vitrectomy. Invest. Ophthalmol. Vis. Sci. 48:327732-82.

[29] Jacobs PM (2008) Vitreous loss during cataract surgery: prevention and optimal management. Eye 22: 1286–1289.

[30] Ozturk F, Osher RH (2006) Capsular staining: recent developments. Curr. Opin. Ophthalmol. 17:42-44.

[31] Wu L, Velasques R, Montoya O (2008) Non-infectious endophthalmitis associated with trypan blue use in cataract surgery. Int. Ophthalmol. 28: 89-93.

[32] van Dooren BT, Beekhuis WH, Pels E (2004) Biocompatibility of trypan blue with human corneal cells. Arch. Ophthalmol.122:736-742.

[33] Hisatomi T, Enaida H, Matsumoto H, Kagimoto T, Ueno A, et al (2006) Staining ability and biocompatibility of brilliant blue G: preclinical study of brilliant blue G as an adjunct for capsular staining. Arch. Ophthalmol.124:514-519.

[34] Ziakas NG, Boboridis K, Nakos E, Mikropoulos D, Margaritis V, et al (2009) Does the use of trypan blue during phacoemulsification affect the intraocular pressure? Can. J. Ophthalmol. 44:293-296.

[35] Yamakiri K, Sakamoto T, Noda Y, Nakahara M, Ogino N, et al (2007) Reduced incidence of intraoperative complications in a multicenter controlled clinical trial of triamcinolone in vitrectomy. Ophthalmology. 114:289-296.

[36] Moshfeghi DM, Kaiser PK, Scott IU, Sears JE, Benz M, et al (2003) Acute endophthalmitis following intravitreal triamcinolone acetonide injection. Am. J. Ophthalmol. 136:791-796.

[37] Chang YS, Tseng SY, Tseng SH, Wu CL, Chen MF (2006) Triamcinolone acetonide suspension toxicity to corneal endothelial cells. J. Cataract Refract. Surg. 32:1549-1555.

[38] Oh Y, Wee WR, Lee JH, Kim MK (2007) Short-term effect of intracameral triamcinolone acetonide on corneal endothelium using the rabbit model. Eye 21.812–818.

15

Combined Cataract and Glaucoma Surgery

Atilla Bayer
Gulhane Medical Academy, Medical School
Turkey

1. Introduction

The association of cataract with glaucoma has become more frequent because of aging populations and the increased risk of cataract development in the patient with glaucoma. There is an increased risk of cataract in some forms of glaucoma, such as pseudoexfoliative glaucoma. In addition, glaucoma surgery increases the risk for the development of cataract (Hylton et al, 2003; AGIS investigators, 2001). With evolving techniques in both glaucoma and cataract surgery, the optimal management is ever changing in an effort to obtain a higher percentage of perfect results with fever complications and shorter recovery times. It has been widely reported that modern cataract surgery results in a long-term reduction in intraocular pressure (IOP); however, the magnitude and clinical significance of this change continues to be debated. On the other hand, due to the growing armamentarium of medical antiglaucomatous therapy during the past decade, most of these patients are presenting for cataract surgery.

When a visually significant cataract is present and surgery is indicated, clinicians face several challenges. Some anatomical features such as a shallow anterior chamber and a shorter axial length may complicate cataract surgery in eyes with angle closure glaucoma. Conversely, how to successfully control the IOP while managing the cataract may complicate the decision making process in eyes with primary open angle glaucoma (POAG) (Table 1). Glaucoma surgery may be associated with an increased risk of cataract progression (AGIS investigators, 2001).

When glaucoma and cataract coexist, it is logical to think of a combined surgical procedure. This would help reduce surgical trauma and facilitate faster visual and functional recovery. Today's rapidly advancing phacoemulsification techniques, including small incisions and foldable lenses implanted in the bag, as well as the improvements in glaucoma techniques, facilitate safer and more efficient combined surgery. Combined surgery may avoid the occurrence of postoperative IOP spikes following cataract surgery in eyes with advanced glaucoma (Shingleton et al, 2007). In addition, subsequent cataract surgery may compromise the success of an earlier trabeculectomy (Seah et al, 1996).

Combined surgery for glaucoma and cataract is carried out in the presence of a cataract that disturbs function and either:

- a glaucomatous condition that fails to respond to maximally tolerated medical therapy;
- when there is appreciable visual field loss and optic disc damage independent of medical control; or
- when transient IOP elevations might cause further optic nerve damage.

Trabeculectomy First; Cataract Extraction Later	Cataract Extraction First; Trabeculectomy Later if Needed	Combined Cataract and Glaucoma Surgery
When large incision extracapsular cataract extraction is to be employed	Well controlled, mild glaucoma with additional medical options available	Advanced glaucoma
When marked inflammation is present	Ocular hypertension with additional medical options available	Patients on maximally tolerated medical therapy or intolerant to medications
When the risk of surgery is very high	Patients with shallow anterior chamber	Poor compliance to medications
		Low target intraocular pressure
		Patients with coincident glaucoma and cataract requiring two or more medications

Table 1. Options for Surgical Management of Coincident Cataract and Glaucoma

New surgical methods with the potential to significantly reduce IOP, such as ab-interno trabeculotomy and trabecular meshwork bypass stents have recently gained popularity (Godfrey et al, 2009). Many surgeons currently believe the collector system has a better chance to survive if intervention is undertaken earlier, before the distal collector system collapses or before years of topical drug therapy cause outflow scarring.

This chapter attempts to outline the current concepts in the management of cataract and glaucoma by evaluating the evidence in eyes with coincident cataract and glaucoma.

2. Physiopathologic factors: The glaucomatous eye

The glaucomatous eye for some of its characteristics is different from an eye without this pathologic condition. Factors related to glaucoma and other factors associated with its medical treatment are involved (Leske et al, 2002; Lichter et al, 2001; Collaborative Normal-Tension Glaucoma Study Group, 1998a; Collaborative Normal-Tension Glaucoma Study Group, 1998b; Kass et al, 2002). The Glaucoma Treatment Study showed, after 5 years of follow-up, twice the incidence of patients needed cataract surgery when medication was the initial treatment as in patients who underwent glaucoma surgery as the initial treatment (Lichter et al, 2001). The explanation for this finding is unknown. The process seemed to be related to the dynamics of the aqueous and the effect of hypotensive drugs (Lee & Gedde, 2004).

The corneal endothelium is more affected in patients with glaucoma, which explains their higher rate of corneal edema after cataract surgery (Tanihara et al, 1995). Patients with glaucoma have a tendency to have a poor response to pharmacologic pupil dilation and need additional surgical dilation to achieve correct visualization and to avoid the existing hidden cortex masses. Preoperative nonsteroidal anti-inflammatory medications (NSAIDs) in combination with mydriatics may improve intraoperative dilation (Stewart et al, 1999). Ophthalmic viscosurgical devices (OVDs) can be used to increase pupil size. Pupil stretching maneuvers, or the use of iris hooks or rings for pupil dilation are recommended. Lens zonules may also become partially fragmented and disintegrated, especially in patients with pseudoexfoliation syndrome (PES). In advanced cases with PES, the zonular suspension of the lens is weakened to such an extent that phacodonesis occur. The zonular fibers may be separated from their attachments to the lens or ciliary body, causing inferior dislocation of the lens. Loosening of the zonules may induce anterior lens dislocation with an attack of secondary angle-closure glaucoma (ACG), especially with the patient in the prone position (Ritch, 1994). There are a number of methods that can be used to manage zonular weakness. A capsular tension ring (CTR), a circular polymethyl methacrylate (PMMA) device, can be inserted into the capsular bag to manage mild cases of zonular instability, defined as less than or equal to four clock hours of dialysis (Jacob et al, 2003). In cases with more severe zonular weakness, a modified capsular tension ring (mCTR) can be sutured to the sclera (Cionni et al, 2003). Lastly, iris hooks may be used to gently retract the anterior capsule during surgery. As the newer acrylic one-piece intraocular lenses (IOLs) unfold slower when inserted, there may be less trauma to the capsule and zonules. This may be an advantage of these IOLs over three-piece lenses. In glaucomatous eyes, we also see greater alteration of the blood aqueous barrier, indicating a greater incidence of postoperative inflammation.

3. Anesthesia

Combined cataract and glaucoma procedures are generally performed under retrobulbar, peribulbar, or sub-Tenon's anesthesia. Prior to the retrobulbar block, a combination of agents with short-acting sedative and amnesiac properties such as methohexitol 20 to 30 mg, midazolam HCl 1mg, or alfentanil 250µg may be given intravenously to reduce anxiety and pain. The retrobulbar block consists of 2% xylocaine without epinephrine. During the procedure only light sedation or none will be required. The patient's systemic blood pressure must be controlled during the operation for many reasons, but primarily to reduce the risk of suprachoroidal hemorrhage.

In patients with markedly elevated IOP, preoperative administration of intravenous mannitol will minimize the abrupt change in IOP following the incision. Osmotic agents are preferred over aqueous suppressants because they dehydrate the vitreous, thereby reducing vitreous volume. Aqueous suppressants on the other hand, retard aqueous production during the early postoperative period.

4. Preoperative considerations

The preoperative clinical examination is extremely important. Lid position and orbital anatomy should be evaluated to consider superior tunnel incision versus temporal corneal selection. The conjunctiva should be examined carefully. Topical steroids should be administered if the conjunctiva is inflamed. Topical miotics should be discontinued 3 days before the surgery. Pupillary response to pharmacologic dilation should be recorded. If dilation is poor, the patient should be informed of the likely need for pupil stretch or iris manipulation, which may result in anisocoria or pupillary distortion. Patients should be informed preoperatively about the intense character of the postoperative period, which will require frequent visits and prolonged visual recovery, beyond that expected for standard cataract surgery. Finally, the eye should be carefully examined for the presence of pseudoexfoliative material, which can be associated with a more aggressive postoperative inflammatory response, weakened zonular fibers, and poor pharmacologic pupil dilation (Küchle et al, 1996).

5. Intraocular lens choices for patients with glaucoma

Patients with glaucoma have unique functional and structural characteristics that should be considered prior to combined surgery. Decreased contrast sensitivity may be improved with aspheric IOLs; however, if these lenses decenter, they may induce more aberration than spherical IOLs. Patients with glaucoma may have smaller pupils and zonular weakness that may be managed intraoperatively by meticulous surgical technique as well as adjunctive devices including CTRs. In the setting of zonular/capsular instability, there are a number of surgical options to place an IOL in good position including anterior chamber IOLs, iris-sutured posterior chamber IOLs, sclera-sutured posterior chamber IOLs, and iris-claw IOLs, although some may exacerbate glaucoma and should be tailored to the individual patient. Posterior capsule opacification is a common postoperative problem and as it stands, surgical technique, IOL design and potentially IOL material may play a role in decreased incidence. Anterior chamber depth and axial length have been shown to change after glaucoma surgery and should be considered when calculating IOL power (Teichman & Ahmed., 2010). As both glaucoma and multifocal IOLs decrease contrast sensitivity, there has been much debate over whether multifocal IOL implantation into a glaucomatous eye is a reasonable practice (Ahmed & Teichman, 2008).

6. Antimetabolites

Adding pharmacologic adjuncts, such as 5-FU and mitomycin-C (MMC), to the combined procedure has become popular over the past decade. Both drugs act by inhibiting of proliferation of fibroblasts and probably also affect cell migration and extracellular matrix production. With rare exception, use of 5-FU with the procedure fails to demonstrate an advantage over the procedure when this antimetabolite is not used (Grady et al, 1993; Wong et al, 1994; Hurvitz, 1993).

The results with MMC, however, show a reduction in IOP despite appreciable variability in the way in which MMC is applied. Published studies report different MMC concentrations, durations of exposure and techniques of physical application to the eye (Munden & Alward, 1995; Lederer, 1996; Belyea et al, 1997; Carlson et al, 1997).

These data raise the question about whether MMC is required for eyes undergoing primary surgery or whether MMC should be reserved for eyes with failed filtering blebs, eyes that have had previous surgery or eyes with difficult-to-manage secondary glaucomas. As MMC is used so variably and both the short- and long-term consequences of its use in combined surgery are not clearly known, a prospective, randomized, multicentred study merits consideration.

A small piece can be cut from an edge of a triangular Weck-cel sponge using Mayo scissors and trimmed to 1 cm length. When wetted with an antimetabolite it expands to athin porous layer that can be easily tucked beneath the conjunctiva on both sides and posteriorly (Fig. 1). Smooth forceps are used to hold the conjunctival edge away from the sponge during the contact period.

The choice of antimetabolite (if antimetabolite is to be used) and the duration of exposure are individualized, because there is no good evidence favoring any one technique either in general or in specific patient situations. MMC is usually prepared as a solution containing 0.2 to 0.4 mg/ml and placed on the episclera for 2 to 5 minutes. The antimetabolite 5-FU is used in a concentration of 50 mg/ml and left in place for 3 to 5 minutes. Some surgeons apply antimetabolite under the scleral flap also. Contraindications for use of 5-FU and MMC are shown in Table 2.

Contraindications for Use of Antimetabolites
Corneal and conjunctival disorders
Lid function or position abnormalities
Pregnant or nursing women
Young children
Patient contemplating pregnancy

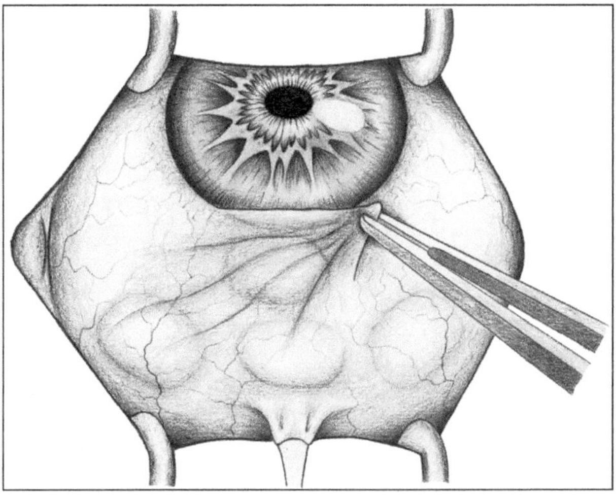

Fig. 1. Intraoperative application of 5-fluorouracil or mitomycin-C on sponge (From Bayer A ed. Glokom Cerrahisi, 1st edition. Ankara:MN Medikal & Nobel; with permission).

7. Pupil management

Glaucoma patients often present with pupils that do not dilate adequately for safe cataract surgery. Pupils may dilate poorly because:

- there are posterior synechiae;
- the iris sphincter is sclerotic;
- an inflammatory membrane involves the iris and anterior lens capsule;
- exfoliation syndrome is present with its consequent affect on the iris and lens capsule (Obstbaum, 2000).

We prefer manipulating the pupil to achieve a diameter of at least 5 mm before beginning cataract curgery. This may result in permanently dilated and poorly reactive pupil during the postoperative period. The basic principle in dealing with a pupil that dilates poorly is to remove the physical adhesions between the iris and lens, such as posterior synechiae or membranes. Synechiae are separated from the anterior lens capsule using a spatula.

Membranes can be peeled using fine forceps. Care is taken not to cause a traumatic iridodialysis. Injecting a high-viscosity viscoelastic agent aids in assessing the extent of pupil dilation (Obstbaum, 2000). If the amount of pupil dilation is not adequate, the pupil is stretched either using two instruments, such as Kuglen hooks (Dinsmore, 1996). The surgeon introduces one Kuglen iris hook through the tunnel incision or a paracenthesis incision and a second Kuglen hook through a paracentehesis incision. The inferior and superior pupillary borders near the 6 and 12 o'clock meridian engaged with the hooks that are oriented in opposite directions (Fig. 2). The surgeon slowly stretches the pupil by pushing each hook toward the anterior chamber angle. The same manevuer is repeated at the 3 and 9 o'clock meridians. After this manevuer, the anterior chamber is filled with additional viscoelastic material to further enlarge the pupil. Alternatively, a single instrument, such as the Beehler pupil dilator can be used (Fine & Hoffman, 1997). If this streching does not result in adequate dilation, the surgeon may perform multiple 0.5 mm radial sphincterotomies using Vannas scissors (Fig. 3). Another option is to use iris retractors (Fig. 4) (Nichamin, 1993). Corneal stab incisions were made at the 1:00, 5:00, 7:00, and 11:00 positions to enlarge the pupil. The angle of the incisions adjacent to the phacoemulsification incision should be made parallel to the iris plane to minimize tenting of the peripheral iris toward the phacoemulsification hand piece entry site.

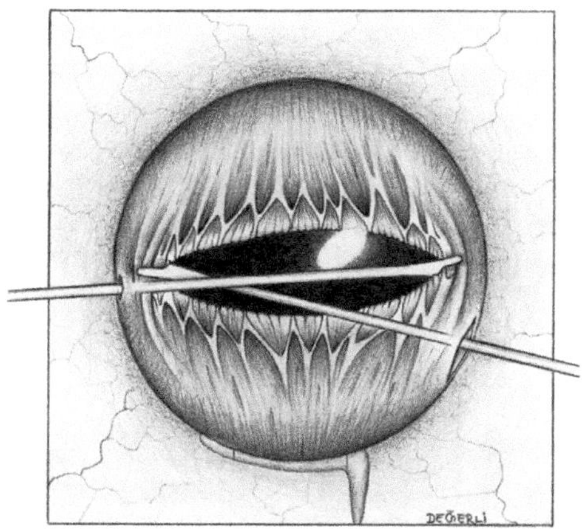

Fig. 2. Pupilary sphincter is stretched in the vertical and horizontal meridians using Kuglen hook (From Bayer A ed. Glokom Cerrahisi, 1st edition. Ankara:MN Medikal & Nobel; with permission).

8. Surgical techniques

Many techniques have been proposed to solve the conflicting problem of a watertight cataract incision and a patent filtering glaucoma procedure. The current combined surgical techniques for cataract and glaucoma include:

- phacoemulsification and trabeculectomy (phacotrabeculectomy);
- extracapsular cataract extraction and trabeculectomy;
- phacoemulsification and trabeculotomy;

- phacoemulsification and non-penetrating surgery;
- phacoemulsification and endocyclophotocoagulation;
- phacoemulsification and canaloplasty

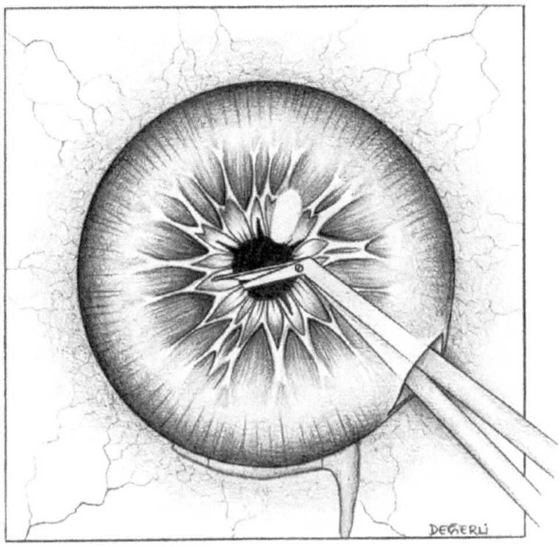

Fig. 3. Fine iris scissors such as Vannas make radial cuts 0.5 to 1 mm in iris sphincter at several locations (From Bayer A ed. Glokom Cerrahisi, 1st edition. Ankara:MN Medikal & Nobel; with permission).

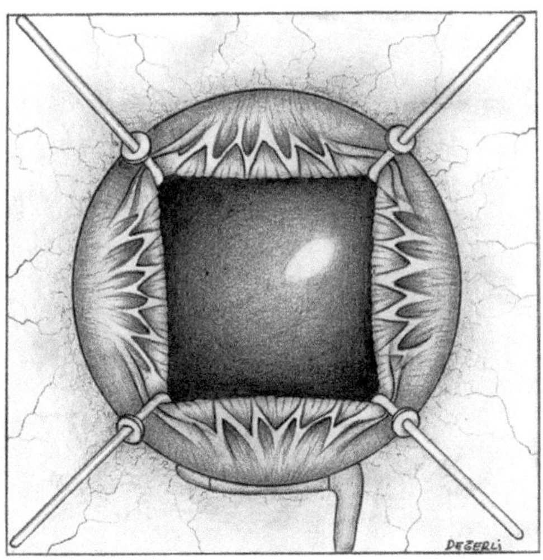

Fig. 4. İris hooks are placed through paracentesis incisions. Pupil is engaged, and hooks are pulled toward periphery (From Bayer A ed. Glokom Cerrahisi, 1st edition. Ankara:MN Medikal & Nobel; with permission).

8.1 Extracapsular cataract extraction and trabeculectomy

Indications for combined extracapsular cataract extraction (ECCE) and trabeculectomy are similar to phacotrabeculectomy. Increased nucleus brunescence, reduced endothelial cell density, and Morgagni's cataracts are factors that favor extracapsular technique rather than phacoemulsification.

Fornix-based conjunctival peritomy is performed and conjunctiva is disinserted from the 10:00 to 2:00 meridian. Cauterization is performed for conjunctiva and episcleral hemostasis. The superficial scleral flap (rectangular, triangular, or circular) is outlined approximately 50% scleral thickness. It is usually placed in the center of the cataract incision, or at either end of it. A crescent knive is used to dissect the scleral flap. A groove is extended along the limbus on both sides at the base of the scleral flap. A stab incision is made to the anterior chamber adjacent to the anterior corner of the scleral flap, and the limbal groove. Anterior capsulotomy is performed using either envelope, or can opener technique. Continuous circular capsulorrhexis, slightly larger than that used for phacoemulsification can also be made. Multiple relaxing incisions may be made in the capsulotomy to facilitate nucleus removal. Cataract incision is extended to adequate width using corneoscleral scissors. After applying light pressure 2mm posteriorly to the incision with a forceps and additional force at the 6:00 meridian, the nucleus slides through the incision (Fig. 5). The lens cortex is removed in the usual fashion and posterior chamber IOL is implanted. The portion of the incision outside the scleral flap is closed with 10-0 nylon suture. The deep block of corneoscleral tissue is excised using either Vannas scissors or a Descemets's punch and peripheral iridectomy is performed. The scleral flap is closed with 2 to 6 interrupted 10-0 nylon sutures. The rate of aqueous outflow is checked by drying the flap area with a sponge as BSS is injected through the paracenthesis. Additional sutures are placed as needed to ensure a formed anterior chamber and moderate aqueous outflow. Finally, the conjunctiva is sutured with interrupted 10-0 nylon sutures in watertight manner.

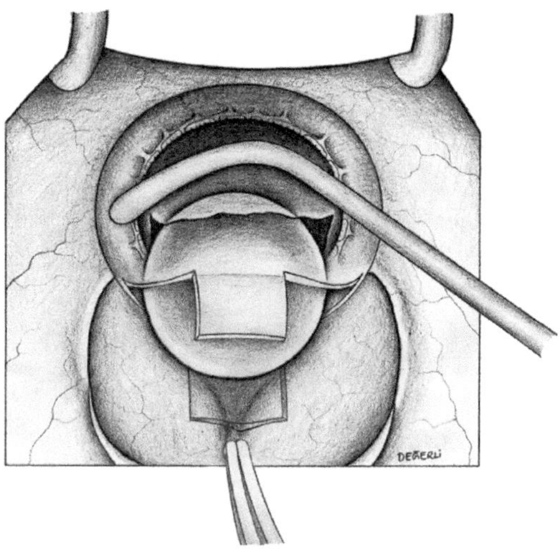

Fig. 5. Extracapsular cataract extraction combined with trabeculectomy. Nucleus removal using a forceps and hook (From Bayer A ed. Glokom Cerrahisi, 1st edition. Ankara:MN Medikal & Nobel; with permission).

8.2 Phacotrabeculectomy

A preferred technique for phacotrabeculectomy is to mimic a standard trabeculectomy procedure. The globe is immobilized with a 4-0 nylon suture beneath the tendon of the superior rectus muscle. Alternatively, corneal traction suture (6-0 or 7-0 silk) can be used. The suture in this case is placed over a length of 3mm through the cornea at 12 o'clock parallel to the limbus at a limbal distance of approximately 0.5 mm.

The conjunctiva is incised using scissors or a blade over a width sufficient to prepare a scleral flap. Either a fornix-based or limbus-based peritomy can be used. Fornix-based or limbus-based conjunctival flaps offer clinical advantages. Two retrospective studies in patients undergoing phacotrabeculectomy showed no difference in IOP control or visual acuity when either fornix-based or limbus-based conjunctival incisions were used (Tezel et al, 1997; Berestka & Brown, 1997). Some surgeons prefer the fornix-based flap is preferred bacause of beter visualization during cataract surgery, but this flap has more leakage and therefore patient follow-up is more complex, especially when antimetabolites have been used (Hoskins & Migliazzo 1994; Cohen et al, 1996).

During 2-site phacotrabeculectomy, a limbus-based, 4X3mm rectangular, half-thickness scleral flap is dissected. The use of cautery should be limited so as to minimize postoperative inflammation. Some surgeons modify the shape and size of this scleral flap. Phacoemulsification is then performed through temporal corneal incision (Fig. 6), and intraocular lens is implanted into the capsular bag. Trabeculectomy opening (2X2 mm) is made using a Kelly Descemet's punch (Bausch & Lomb Surgical) or alternatively using scissors. This is followed by peripheral iridectomy. Scleral flap was closed with 2 to 6 10-0 nylon sutures. Black color is preferable because of the possible need for future suture lysis. The number of the sutures and their tightness should be adjusted during the operation. Injection of balanced salt solution into the anterior chamber permits intraoperative observation of pressure change and seepage of fluid at the edge of the scleral flap. The conjunctival-Tenon's capsule flap is closed with two wing sutures for a fornix-based flap or by a continuous running suture for a limbus-based flap. With the 1-site approach a scleral tunnel incision is made superiorly and the surgeon's preferred technique of phacoemulsification (Fig. 7) and IOL implantation is performed. Two radial incisions are made forward to the limbus and the tunnel incision is converted to a scleral flap. Trabeculectomy, iridectomy, scleral flap closure and conjunctiva closure is performed as mentioned above. Both 1-site and 2-site approaches to phacotrabeculectomy have yielded satisfactory results. In two studies comparing the results of these two techniques, patients who had the 1-site procedure required significantly more medication to maintain IOP control than did the group who had the 2-site procedure (Wyse et al, 1998; El-Sayyad et al, 1999).

Some surgeons have been eliminating the peripheral iridectomy step but there still remains the fear of incarceration and filtration failure. Kaplan-Messas et al randomized 36 patients to phacotrabeculectomy with and without iridectomy, 18 cases in each group. There were 11 additional patients having trabeculectomy alone. IOP lowering success was equal between the groups. There were more hyphemas in the trabeculectomy alone without iridectomy group (Kaplan-Messas et al, 1999). Our preference is to perform iridectomy in all the cases except neovascular glaucoma.

Newer technology has allowed cataract wounds to become smaller (Fig. 8). Whether an even less invasive cataract incision would translate into greater success and safety is unknown. We looked into the question of two-site phacotrabeculectomy compared to bimanual microincisional cataract surgery with trabeculectomy in 58 eyes and found very similar success rates in regards of IOP. Complication rates were similar except for slightly more corneal edema in the two-site phacotrabeculectomy eyes (Bayer et al, 2009).

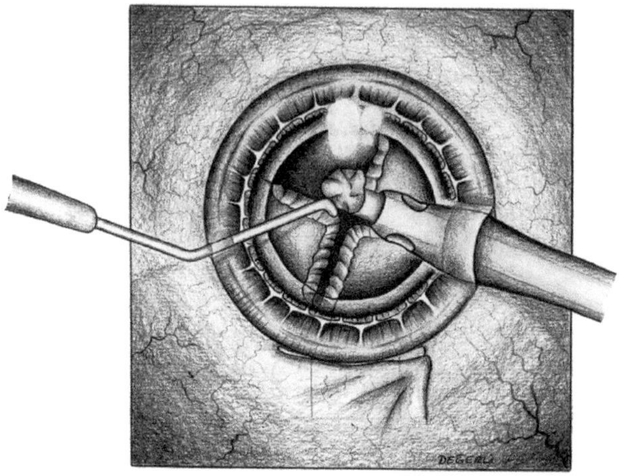

Fig. 6. Two-site phacotrabeculectomy. Phacoemulsification of each quadrant after nuclear cracking (From Bayer A ed. Glokom Cerrahisi, 1st edition. Ankara:MN Medikal & Nobel; with permission).

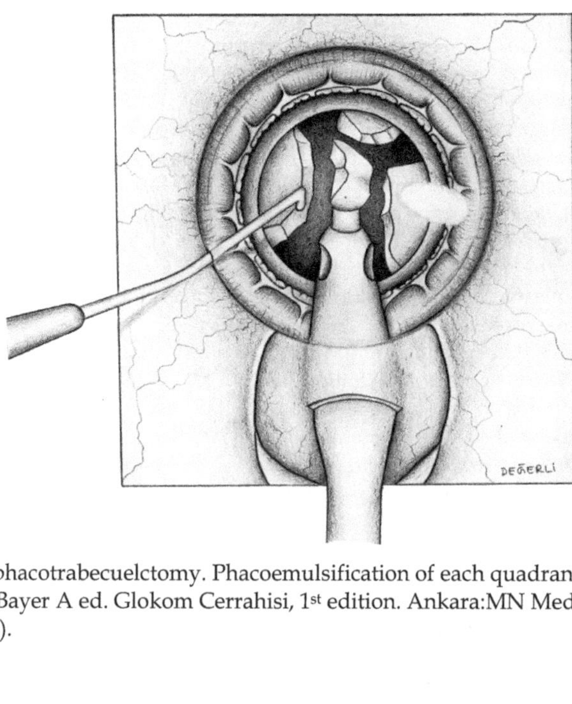

Fig. 7. One-site phacotrabecuelctomy. Phacoemulsification of each quadrant after nuclear cracking (From Bayer A ed. Glokom Cerrahisi, 1st edition. Ankara:MN Medikal & Nobel; with permission).

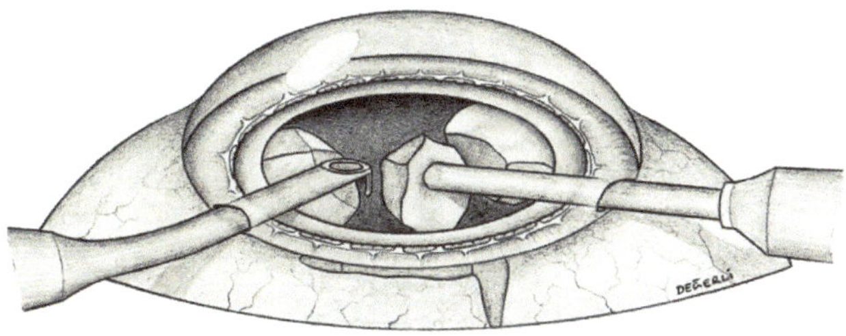

Fig. 8. Microincisional phacotrabeculectomy. Nucleus removal using an irrigating chopper and sleeveless phaco tip (From Bayer A ed. Glokom Cerrahisi, 1st edition. Ankara:MN Medikal & Nobel; with permission).

Careful postoperative follow up after any filtration surgery is vital to the success of the operation. Postoperative care will determine the outcome of surgery in many cases. All glaucoma medications should be discontinued. Aggressive topical steroid use, for example every 2 hours while awake, is recommended during the postoperative week. Topical antibiotics are instilled for 1 week. Topical steroid administration is continued for 2 months postoperatively. Tapering of the steroid dose is based on the amount of inflammation in and around the bleb. The early postoperative period is critical. It is during this time that procedures often fail and complications are most common. If the IOP is high, focal pressure is applied adjacent to the filtration site with a cotton-tip applicator to augment filtration (Traverso et al, 1984). This technique is preferred, because it encourages outflow through the sclerostomy site and can dislodge fibrin or other debris that may be limiting outflow. If the IOP is very low, one would expect to see a huge bleb. Any discrepancy between bleb appearance and IOP should warrant examination of a bleb leak. Once adequate aqueous production is established, by a deep anterior chamber and stable or rising IOP, the surgeon may augment filtration by performing suture lysis (Fig. 9) or release. Finally, part of the routine postoperative regimen should include discussion to educate patients of the potential hazards of blebs such as late leaks or late bleb infections.

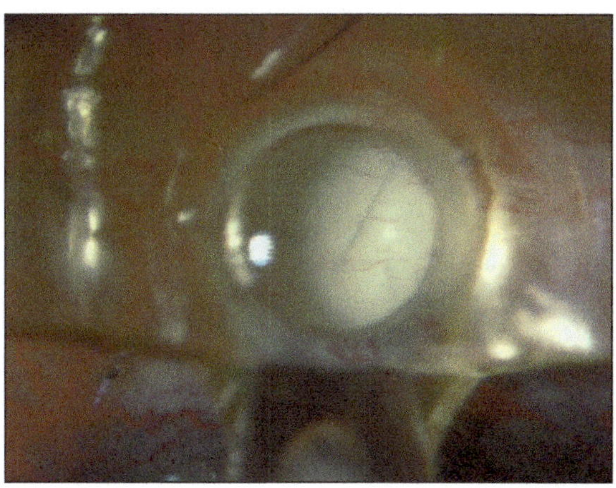

Fig. 9. View of the flap suture under the Hoskins lens during suture lysis.

8.3 Phacotrabeculotomy

Trabeculotomy has been reported to be effective in controlling IOP in eyes with POAG, pseudoexfoliation syndrome, and adult-onset glaucoma (Chihara et al, 1993; Tanihara et al, 1993; Wada et al, 1994).

Phacoemulsification and IOL implantation are performed as mentioned above, before the trabeculotomy ab externo. A clear corneal incision is made, and a corneoscleral incision after limbal peritomy is made in eyes to remove the cataract. After a continuous curvilinear capsulorrhexis, phacoemulsification and IOL implantation are performed. The trabeculotomy ab externo then is performed from a different site. The procedure begins with a limbal peritomy and radial conjunctival incision in the desired quadrant, and a fornix-based conjunctival flap is prepared. Conjunctiva and Tenon's tissue are retracted to expose the sclera. Apart from the site for cataract surgery, a 4 × 4-mm triangular area is marked, and the sclera is incised with a knife. A four-fifth thickness, limbal-based scleral flap is created. The outer wall of Schlemm's canal, which is identified as a dark brown band between the sclera and the scleral spur, is radially incised with a sharp razor blade and removed using modified Vannas scissors. Care is taken not to disrupt the inner wall of Schlemm's canal. Slow leakage of aqueous humor through the trabecular meshwork is confirmed under a surgical microscope. Semicircular trabeculotome probes (right and left) are inserted in both directions into Schlemm's canal, and rotated in to disrupt the inner wall of the canal and the juxtacanalicular tissue of the trabecular meshwork. The scleral flap then is sutured watertight with three 10-0 nylon sutures, and the conjunctival wound is closed with interrupted 10-0 nylon sutures.

Tanito et al. report that combined trabeculotomy and cataract surgery lowers IOP and has a low incidence of surgical complications (Tanito et al, 2001). A significant IOP reduction was observed in the trabeculotomy combined with phacoemulsification and IOL implantation (TPI group) and phacoemulsification and IOL implantation (PI) groups up to 3 years and up to 1 year and 6 months after surgery, respectively; the magnitude of the reduction was significantly larger in the TPI group.The success probabilities of TPI group for IOP control under 21, 17, and 15 mmHg were 95.8%, 58.7%, and 30.0%, respectively, 1 year after surgery. Tanito et al. suggestes that trabeculotomy can be a better option for the older patients.

Lüke et al report that phacotrabeculotomy plus deep sclerectomy offered significant IOP reduction and a success rate that may be comparable with that of the current phacotrabeculectomy (Lüke et al, 2007). Intra- and postoperative complications specific to deep sclerectomy and trabeculotomy were seen in their series, although the overall rate of postoperative complications proved low.

The Trabectome is a surgical device that was cleared by the US Food and Drug Administration in January 2004 for the treatment of adult and juvenile open-angle glaucoma. The concept is similar in principle to ab interno trabeculotomy, the key difference being that a microelectrocautery device is used to ablate a strip of the trabecular meshwork and inner wall of Schlemm's canal, thus allowing direct access of aqueous to the collector channels. This theoretically bypasses the main site of resistance to aqueous outflow and reestablishes the natural drainage passageway out of the eye. Briefly, a 1.7-mm clear corneal incision is made temporally, through which the electrosurgical handpiece is inserted and advanced to the nasal angle under gonioscopic visualization. The tip of the device is inserted into Schlemm's canal through the trabecular meshwork, and the cautery is then activated via a foot pedal. The handpiece is advanced while cautery is activated to ablate an arc of the meshwork, exposing the back wall of Schlemm's canal, usually for 90° to 120°. A modified Swan-Jacob goniolens (Ocular Instruments Inc, Bellevue, Washington) was developed for this procedure. The handpiece is then removed, and a single 10-0 suture is placed through the incision (Mosaed et al, 2009). This procedure has also been combined with microincisional phacoemulsification, and the IOP-lowering effect of the combined procedure has been previously reported to be 30% at 1 year in a study of 304 consecutive eyes (Francis et al, 2008; Minckler et al, 2008).

The main complication reported in the use of the Trabectome is transient hyphema (79% to 100%). There have been no reports of choroidal effusions, infections, or other permanent visual impairment. The potential advantages of this procedure are that it does not involve manipulation of the conjunctiva, the Tenon capsule, or sclera and therefore preserves the option for subsequent standard filtering surgery if necessary. There is also no risk of bleb-related complications such as leaks, blebitis, endophthalmitis, dellen, and dysesthesia, as there is no bleb formation. Hypotony has been rare, most likely if an inadvertent cyclodialysis occurs. The IOP-lowering effect after several months appears to stabilize in the mid-teens through 5 years of follow-up (n = 10).9 After Trabectome, the majority of eyes require a reduced number of IOP-lowering medications. As a brief update on Trabectome, data now include IOP and medication outcomes on a total of 2,012 surgeries, including 1,228 Trabectome-only and 687 combined Trabectome-phacoemulsification surgeries continuing to demonstrate that clinically significant IOP and adjuvant medication reliance decrease follow these surgeries. Updated survival analyses for these two groups are also encouraging, especially for the combined cases.

8.4 Phacoemulsification and non-penetrating surgery

For many years ophthalmic surgeons have tried to find a way of surgically lowering the IOP without creating a filtering bleb and the associated complications. These are bleb dysthesia, bleb leak, hypotony, blebitis, and bleb related endophthalmitis. One current trend in surgery for glaucoma is non-penetrating deep sclerectomy. Although we still do not have the same level of evidence for deep sclerectomy compared with trabeculectomy, some data support a similar efficacy of deep sclerectomy and trabeculectomy with a lower rate of complications. Because of these advantages, support for this technique has increased (Verges C et al, 2002; Gianoli F et al, 1999). By contrast, some reports show that the results of trabeculectomy are superior to those of deep sclerectomy (Chiselita D, 2001).

Deep sclerectomy is aimed at reducing IOP by allowing the filtration of aqeous humor into the subconjunctival space through the trabeculo-descemetic membrane. The surgical technique varies; generally, after carrying out a fornix-based conjunctival peritomy, 5X5 mm superior scleral flap, approximately one-third of scleral thickness is dissected. At this stage, in all lor in selected cases only, sponge soaked with 5-FU or MMC is applied over the sclera. A limbus based deep scleral flap is then prepared leaving a thin layer of sclera over the choroid and the ciliary body. The dissection is carried anteriorly until Schlemm's canal is deroofed and 1-2mm of Descemet's membrane is exposed. At this stage, aqeous humor should be seen percolating through the trabeculo-descemetic membrane (Fig. 10). To increase percolation, some surgeons suggest removing the inner wall of Schlemm's canal. Deep scleral flap is removed and implants are used to avoid postoperative scarring. The superficial flap is the sutured with two 10-0 nylon sutures. Conjunctiva is sutred with interrupted 10-0 nylon sutures.

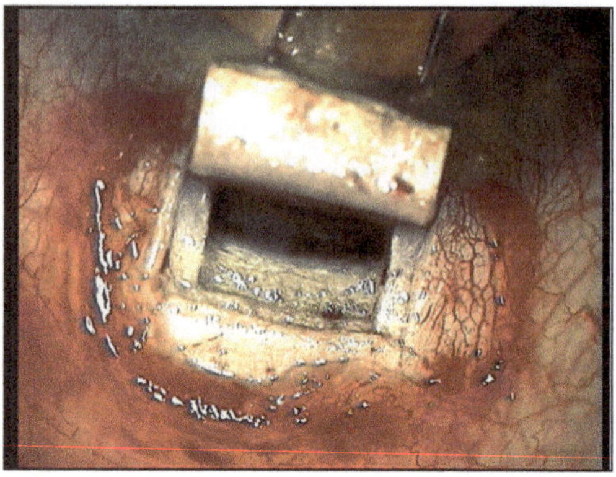

Fig. 10. Title of figure, left justified

Viscocanalostomy is similar to deep sclerectomy and Schlemm's canal is cannulated using a specifically designed 165µm cannula and high molecular weight sodium hyaluronate is slowly injected into the both ostia (Fig. 11). The injection of viscoelastic substance allows progressive atraumatic dilatation of Schlemm's canal.

One advantage of deep sclerectomy is its results in combination with phacoemulsification. D'Eliseo et al. in a randomized prospective work, compared a group of 21 eyes treated with deep sclerectomy with another group of 21 eyes treated with combined phacoemulsification and deep sclerectomy (D'Eliseo D et al, 2003). The IOP values in the group of eyes treated with combined surgery were better (13.1 mm Hg) than in the group treated with deep sclerectomy alone alone (15.2 mm Hg). The authors achieved IOPs lower than 21 mm Hg without medication in 90% of eyes undergoing combined surgery as opposed to 62% of eyes undergoing deep sclerectomy alone. Moreover, the incidence of postoperative hypotony was also reduced in the combined surgery group (20% vs 32%, respectively). Gianoli et al. however, reported similar results when they compared phacotrabeculectomy and phacoemulsification plus deep sclerectomy with a collagen implant, observing the same rate of pressure reduction after 1 year of follow-up (Gionali F et al, 1999).

Rebolleda et al. analyzed Descemet membrane perforations necessary to convert the deep sclerectomy to a trabeculectomy, reporting that in deep sclerectomy cases it was necessary to convert 8.9% after 7 to 28 month follow-up (Rebolleda et al, 2004). IOP values were similar to those obtained in cases not needing perforation. However, their reported complications, although not serious, were significant, with hyphema, choroidal detachment, and fibrinous uveitis.

Viscocanalostomy obtained similar results to those of trabeculectomy during combined phacoemulsification. Park et al. observed IOP reduction and fewer glaucoma medications for IOP control (Park M et al, 2004). Whisart et al. also found similar results, with an IOP decrease of 37% in viscocanalostomy alone compared with 33% when combined with phacoemulsififcation (Park M et al ,2004).Uretmen et al. compared the safety and efficacy of viscocanalostomy and phacoviscocanalostomy in the management of medically uncontrolled open-angle glaucoma. In their study, 20 patients underwent phacoviscocanalostomy and 29 patients underwent viscocanalostomy alone. Significant reduction of IOP and medication occurred in both groups. The mean IOP reduction was 34%

in the eyes that underwent viscocanalostomy alone and 38% in the eyes that underwent phacoviscocanalostomy. The success rates of the two procedures were also comparable. In the combined surgery group, the best corrected visual acuity improved by two or more lines in 90% of the patients. Intraoperative complications did not occur in either group. The authors concluded that combining phacoemulsification with viscocanalostomy does not have a negative effect on the IOP control achieved by viscocanalostomy alone and does not increase the complication rate (Uretmen O et al, 2003).

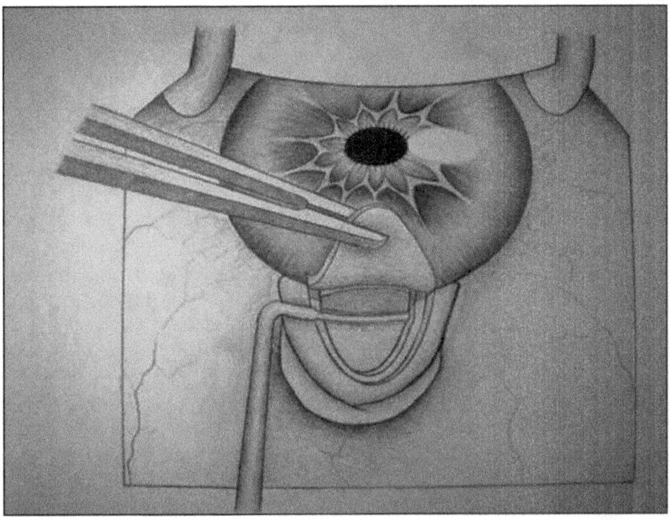

Fig. 11. Cannulation of Schlemm's canal during viscocanalostomy (From Bayer A ed. Glokom Cerrahisi, 1st edition. Ankara:MN Medikal & Nobel; with permission).

8.5 Phacoemulsification and endocyclophotocoagulation

Endoscopic cyclophotocoagulation (ECP) is a new surgical approach which targets the ciliary processes to decrease aqueous humor production thus leading to lower IOP. The use of ECP is becoming more accepted and is no longer reserved for end-stage cases. Previously developed methods targeting the ciliary processes, such as cyclocryotherapy and diode cycloablation, are procedures done without direct visualization of treated tissue and have been reserved for cases with endstage glaucoma after which other medical and surgical modalities have failed to control IOP. The experience with these less precise modalities has led to a degree of apprehension and skepticism about the use of ECP. Still, the use of ECP has increased with more cases performed earlier in the course of treatment (Gayton et al., 1999; Chen et al., 1997; Kahook et al., 2007).

ECP is carried out using a probe attached to a laser unit (Endo Optiks, Little Silver, NJ) which incorporates a diode laser. Pulsed continuous wave energy is emitted at 810 nm, using a 175 W variable xenon light source, a helium-neon laser aiming beam and video camera imaging. All elements are transmitted via fiberoptics within the probe. The 20 gauge probe provides a 70° field of view; the 18 gauge probe provides a 110° field. Power, duration, aiming beam intensity, and illumination are adjustable using controls on the console. A foot pedal controls laser firing; the duration of treatment depends on how long the pedal is depressed. A retrobulbar or subtenons block with lidocaine and bupivicaine is preferred. After orientation of the probe image outside the eye, the probe is inserted intraocularly through a limbal incision. After visualization of the ciliary processes using the video monitor, treatment begins.

The safety and efficacy of ECP has been demonstrated in treating various forms of glaucoma when performed alone or in combination with phacoemulsification (Uram, 1995). ECP procedure is performed following phacoemulsification and IOL implantation and before the viscoelastic removal. Combined phacoemulsification and ECP is commonly practiced with ECP performed, in most cases, through a single clear cornea incision allowing approximately 240 to 300 degrees of treatment (Fig. 12). The remaining 60 to 120 degrees of ciliary processes under the corneal incision are often left untreated with the potential to eventually result in inadequate IOP lowering or frank failure of the procedure. Some surgeons, prefer to perform ECP to 360 degrees through two corneal incisions. Transvitreal approach can also be used for ECP, especially in vitrctomised eyes (Haller JA, 1996).

Complications of ECP include inflammation, hyphema, postoperative IOP spikes, choroidal detachment, choroidal hemorrhage, vitreous hemorrhage, hypotony, phtisis, and preogression to no light perception. ECP appears to be associated with a high rate of development of cataracts.

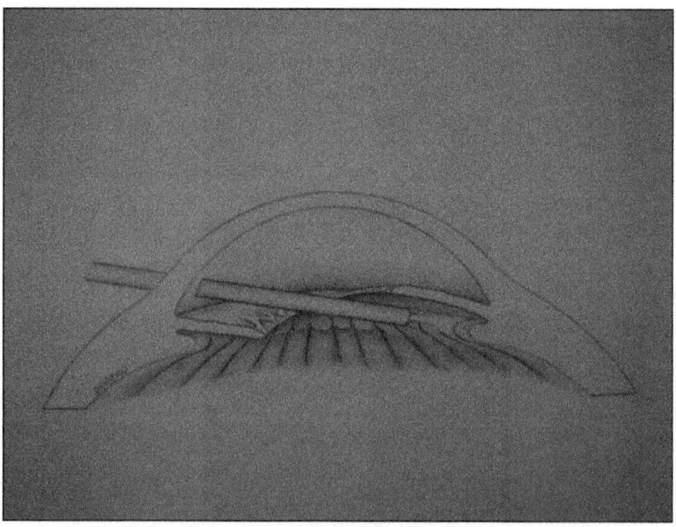

Fig. 12. Position of the probe during endoscopic cyclophotocoagulation from a clear corneal incision (From Bayer A ed. Glokom Cerrahisi, 1st edition. Ankara:MN Medikal & Nobel; with permission).

8.6 Phacocanaloplasty

Canaloplasty is a new angle surgical procedure that involves conjunctival incision, fashioning a trabeculectomy-like scleral flap and a smaller deeper flap (similar to non-penetrating surgery), which is excised to expose Schlemm's canal. A flexible microcatheter with fiber optic illumination at the distal tip is introduced into the canal and advanced for 360° until visible opposite the entrance site. Viscoelastic is continually injected via the catheter lumen. A 10-0 Prolene suture is fastened to the distal catheter tip and then pulled back around the Schlemm's canal while the catheter is withdrawn (Fig. 13). The suture is then tensioned by hand to distend the canal inward. The superficial flap is then closed watertight, followed by secure closure of the conjunctiva. An ultrasound device can be used to verify tensioning and stretching of the canal, if desired.

Canaloplasty has also been successfully combined with phacoemulsification surgery (Lewis RA, 2011; Shingleton B, 2008). Lewis and colleagues have recently reported the 3 year results of combined phacoemulsification and canaloplasty. Eyes with combined cataract-canaloplasty surgery had a mean IOP of 13.6 mm Hg on 0.3 ± 0.5 medications compared with a baseline IOP of 23.5 mm Hg on 1.5 ± 1.0 medications. Intraocular pressure and medication use results in all eyes were significantly decreased from baseline at every time point (Lewis RA, 2011).

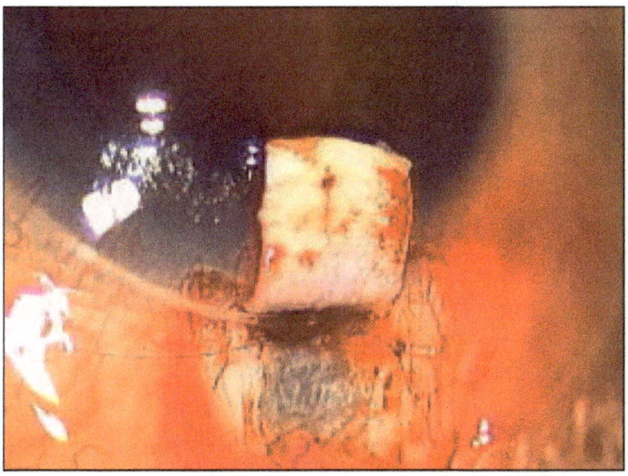

Fig. 13. Canaloplasty. Flexible microcatheter in Schlemm's canal with 10-0 prolene suture fastened to the distal end.

Benefits of this procedure over traditional glaucoma surgery include fewer complications, as it is not intended to create a bleb, therefore minimizing bleb-related complications. The most frequent early complication reported is hyphema. Late postoperative complications included cataract, transient IOP elevation, and partial suture extrusion through the trabecular meshwork. No bleb-related complications were reported so far.

9. Conclusion

Glaucoma surgery, as all the areas of ophthalmology, is changing rapidly. As the issue of cataract and glaucoma touches on two of the major and frequent problems, the choice of optimal care will certainly need to be re-evaluated. We now have new methods to benefit our patients and make a positive impact upon the quality of their lives. No uniform recommendations can be proposed for all cases. Clinicians have to consider a variety of factors before taking important surgical decisions. Greater safety can be provided by considering some of the newer glaucoma procedures. However, the ideal result has not yet been realized. All of these new procedures have their own complications. We need to seek a better understanding of the variables in combined cataract and glaucoma surgery and to strengthen the evidence for adopting specific surgical techniques by designing multicentred, prospective, randomized trial.

10. References

[1] AGIS Investigators (2001): The AdvancedGlaucoma Intervention Study: 8. Risk of cataract formation after trabeculectomy. *Arch Ophthalmol* 2001; 119: 1771–1779.

[2] Ahmed IK, Teichman JC. Multifocal IOLs and glaucoma: how much is too much? In: Chang D, editor. Transitioning to refractive IOLs: the art and science. Thorofare, NJ: Slack Incorporated; 2008, pp. 384–385.

[3] Bayer A, Erdem U¨ , Mumcuoglu T, et al. (2009). Two-site phacotrabeculectomy versus bimanual microincision cataract surgery combined with trabeculectomy. *Eur J Ophthalmol*, Vol.19, No.1, (January-February 2009), pp.46–54, PMID: 19123148.

[4] Belyea DA, Dan JA, Lieberman MF, et al. (1997). Midterm follow-up results of combined phacoemulsification, lens implantation, and mitomycin-C trabeculectomy procedure. J Glaucoma, Vol.6, No.2, (April 1997), pp.90-8, PMID: 9098816.

[5] Berestka JS, Brown SVL. (1996). Limbus- versus fornix-based conjunctival flaps in combined phacoemulsification and mitomycin C trabeculectomy surgery. *Ophthalmology*, Vol.104, No.7, (July 1997), pp.187–196, PMID: 9243657.

[6] Carlson DW, Alward WL, Barad JP, et al. (1997). A randomized study of mitomycin augmentation in combined phacoemulsification and trabeculectomy. Ophthalmology, Vol.104, No.4, (April 1997), pp.719-24, PMID: 9111269.

[7] Chen J, Cohn RA, Lin SC, et al. Endoscopic photocoagulation of the ciliary body for treatment of refractory glaucomas. *Am J Ophthalmol*, Vol.124, No.6, (December 1997), pp.787–796, PMID: 9402825.

[8] Chihara E, Nishida A, Kodo M, et al. (1993). Trabeculotomy ab externo: an alternative treatment in adult patients with primary open-angle glaucoma. *Ophthalmic Surg*, Vol.24, No.11, (November 1993), pp.735-9, PMID:8290211.

[9] Chiselita D.(2001) Non-penetrating deep sclerectomy in primary open angle glaucoma surgery. *Eye*, Vol.15, No.2, (April 2001), pp.197–201, PMID: 11339590.

[10] Cionni RJ, Osher RH, Marques DMV, et al.2003. Modified capsular tension ring for patients with congenital loss of zonular support. *J Cataract Refract Surg*, Vol.29, No.9, (September 2003), pp.1668–1673, PMID: 14522284.

[11] Cohen JS, Greff LJ, Novack G, et al. (1996). A placebo-controlled double-masked evaluation of mitomycin C in combined glaucoma and cataract procedures. *Ophthalmology*, Vol.103, No.11, (November 1996), pp.1934-42, PMID: 8942892.

[12] Collaborative Normal-Tension Glaucoma Study Group (1998). The effectiveness of intraocular pressure reduction in the treatment of normal-tension glaucoma. *Am J Ophthalmol.* Vol.126, No.2, (October 1998), pp.498–505, PMID: 9780094.

[13] Collaborative Normal-Tension Glaucoma Study Group. (1998). Comparison of glaucomatous progression between untreated patients with normal-tension glaucoma and patients with therapeutically reduced intraocular pressures. *Am J Ophthalmol.* Vol.126, No.2, (October 1998), pp.487–497, PMID: 9780094.

[14] D'Eliseo D, Pastena B, Longanesi L, et al.(2003). Comparison of deep sclerectomy with implant and combined glaucoma surgery. *Ophthalmologica,* Vol.217, No.3, (May-June 2003), pp.208-11, PMID: 12660485.

[15] Dinsmore SC. (1996). Modified stretch technique for small pupil phacoemulsification with topical anesthesia. *J Cataract Refract Surg.* Vol.22, No.1, (January-February 1996), pp.27-30, PMID: 8656356.

[16] El-Sayyad F, Helal M, El-Maghraby A, et al.(1997). One-site versus 2-site phacoetrabeculectomy: a randomized study. *J Cataract Refract Surg,* Vol.25, No.1, (January 1999), pp.77–82, PMID: 9888081.

[17] Fine IH, Hoffman RS. (1997). Phacoemulsification in the presence of pseudoexfoliation: challenges and options. *J Cataract Refract Surg,* Vol.23, No.2, (March 1997), pp.160-5, PMID: 9113564.

[18] Francis BA, Minckler D, Dustin L, et al. (2008). Trabectome Study Group Combined cataract extraction and trabeculotomy by the internal approach for coexisting cataract and open-angle glaucoma: initial results. *J Cataract Refract Surg, Vol.34, No.7, (July* 2008), pp.1096–1103, PMID: 18571075.

[19] Gayton JL, Van Der Karr M, Sanders V. (1999). Combined cataract and glaucoma surgery: trabeculectomy versus endoscopic laser cycloablation. *J Cataract Refract Surg,* Vol.25, No.9, (September 1999), pp.1214–1219, PMID: 10476504.

[20] Gianoli F, Schnyder CC, Bovey E, et al. (1999). Combined surgery for cataract and glaucoma: phacoemulsification and deep sclerectomy compared with phacoemulsification and trabeculectomy. *J Cataract Refract Surg,* Vol.25, No.3, (March 1999), pp.343–348, PMID: 10079438.

[21] Godfrey DG, Fellman RL, Neelakantan A. (2009). Canal surgery in adult glaucomas. *Curr Opin Ophthalmol,* Vol.20, No.2, (March 2009), pp.116-21, PMID: 19240543.

[22] Grady JM, Juzych MS, Shin DH, et al. (1993), Trabeculectomy, phacoemulsification, and posterior chamber lens implantation with and without 5-fluorouracil. *Am J Ophthalmol.* Vol.116, No.5, (November 1993), pp.594-9, PMID: 8238220.

[23] Haller JA. (1996). Transvitreal endocyclophotocoagulation. *Trans Am Ophthalmol Soc,* Vol.94, (1996), pp.589-676, PMID: 8981713.

[24] Hoskins HD, Migliazzo C. (1984). Management of failing filtering blebs with the argon laser. *Ophthalmic Surg,* Vol.15, No.9, (September 1984); pp.731-3, PMID: 6493678.

[25] Hurvitz LM. (1993). 5-FU-supplemented phacoemulsification, posterior chamber intraocular lens implantation, and trabeculectomy. *Ophthalmic Surg,* Vol.24, No.10, (October 1993), pp.674-80 PMID: 8259245.

[26] Hylton C, Congdon N, Friedman D, et al. (2003). Cataract after filtration surgery. *Am J Ophthalmol,* Vol.135, No. , pp. 231-232.

[27] Jacob S, Agarwal A, Agarwal A, et al.(2003). Efficacy of a capsular tension ring for phacoemulsification in eyes with zonular dialysis. *J Cataract Refract Surg,* Vol.29, No.2, (February 2003), pp.315–321, PMID: 12648643.

[28] Kahook MY, Lathrop KL, Noecker RJ. (2007). One-site versus two-site endoscopic cyclophotocoagulation. *J Glaucoma,* Vol.16, No.6, (September 2007), pp.527-30, PMID: 17873713.

[29] Kaplan-Messas A, Cohen Y, Blumenthal E, et al.(2009). Trabeculectomy and phacotrabeculectomy with and without peripheral iridectomy. *Eur J Ophthalmol,* Vol.19, No.2, (March-April 2009), pp.231–234, PMID: 19253239.

[30] Kass MA, Heuer DK, Higginbotham EJ, et al. (2002). The Ocular Hypertension Treatment Study: a randomized trial determines that topical ocular hypertensive medication delays or prevents the onset of primary open-angle glaucoma. *Arch Ophthalmol.* Vol.120, No.6, (June 2002), pp.701–713, 12049574.

[31] Küchle M, Vinores SA, Mahlow J, et al. (1996). Blood-aqueous barrier in pseudoexfoliation syndrome: evaluation by immunohistochemical staining of endogenous albumin. *Graefes Arch Clin Exp Ophthalmol,* Vol.234, No.1, (January 1996), pp.12-8, PMID: 8750845 .

[32] Lederer CM Jr.(1996). Combined cataract extraction with intraocular lens implant and mitomycin-augmented trabeculectomy. *Ophthalmology.* Vol.103, No.7, (July 1996), pp.1025-34, PMID: 8684790.

[33] Lee RK, Gedde SJ. (2004): Surgical management of coexisting cataract and glaucoma. *Int Ophthalmol Clin.* Vol. 44, No.2, (Spring 2004), pp.151–166, PMID: 15087734.

[34] Leske MC, Wu SY, Nemesure B, et al. (2002). Risk factors for incident nuclear opacities. *Ophthalmology.* Vol.109, No.7, (July 2002), pp.1303-8. PMID: 12093655.

[35] Lewis RA, von Wolff K, Tetz M, et al. (2011). Canaloplasty: Three-year results of circumferential viscodilation and tensioning of Schlemm canal using a microcatheter to treat open-angle glaucoma. *J Cataract Refract Surg,* Vol.37, No.4, (April 2011), pp.682-90. PMID: 21420593.

[36] Lichter PR, Musch DC, Gillespie BW, et al. (2001). Interim clinical outcomes in the Collaborative Initial Glaucoma Treatment Study comparing initial treatment randomized to medications or surgery. *Ophthalmology,* Vol.108, No.11, (November 2001), pp.1943–1953, PMID: 11713061.

[37] Lüke C, Dietlein TS, Lüke M, et al. (2007). Phaco-trabeculotomy combined with deep sclerectomy, a new technique in combined cataract and glaucoma surgery: complication profile. *Acta Ophthalmol Scand,* Vol.85, No.2, (March 2007), pp.143-8, PMID: 17305727.

[38] Minckler DS, Mosaed S, Dustin L, et al. (2008). Trabectome (trabeculectomy-internal approach): additional experience and extended follow-up. *Trans Am Ophthalmol Soc.* Vol.106, (2008), pp.1–12, PMID:19277230.

[39] Mosaed S, Dustin L, Minckler DS. (2009). Comparative outcomes between newer and older surgeries for glaucoma. Trans Am Ophthalmol Soc, Vol.107, (December 2009), pp.127-33, PMID: 20126489.

[40] Munden PM, Alward WL. (1995). Combined phacoemulsification, posterior chamber intraocular lens implantation, and trabeculectomy with mitomycin C. *Am J Ophthalmol,* Vol.119, No.1, (January 1995), pp.20-9, PMID: 7825686.

[41] Nichamin LD. (1993). Enlarging the pupil for cataract extraction using flexible nylon iris retractors. *J Cataract Refract Surg,* Vol.19, No.6, (November 1993), pp.793-6, PMID:8271181.

[42] Obstbaum SA. Cataract surgery in the glaucoma patient. In: Weinreb RN, Kitazawa Y, Krieglstein GK, editors. Glaucoma in the 21st century. London: Mosby International; 2000. pp. 259-265.

[43] Park M, Tanito M, Nishikawa M, et al. (2004). Combined viscocanalostomy and cataract surgery compared with cataract surgery in Japanese patients with glaucoma. *J Glaucoma,* Vol.13, No.1, (February 2004), pp.55-61, PMID: 14704545.

[44] Rebolleda G, Muñoz-Negrete FJ. (2004) Phacoemulsification-deep sclerotomy converted to phacotrabeculectomy. *J Cataract Refract Surg*, Vol.30, No.7, (July 2004), pp.1597-8, PMID:15210250.

[45] Ritch R. (1994). Exfoliation syndrome and occludable angles. *Trans Am Ophthalmol Soc.* 1994;92:pp, 845-944, PubMed PMID: 7886885.

[46] Seah SK, Jap A, Prata JA Jr, et al. (1996). Cataract surgery after trabeculectomy. *Ophthalmic Surg Lasers*. Vol.27, No.7, (July 1996), pp. 587-94, PMID: 9240775.

[47] Shingleton BJ, Rosenberg RB, Teixeira R, et al. (2007). Evaluation of intraocular pressure in the immediate postoperative period after phacoemulsification. J *Cataract Refract Surg*. Vol.33, No.11, (November 2007), pp.1953-7, PMID: 17964404 .

[48] Shingleton B, Tetz M, Korber N. (2008). Circumferential viscodilation and tensioning of Schlemm canal (canaloplasty) with temporal clear corneal phacoemulsification cataract surgery for open-angle glaucoma and visually significant cataract: one-year results. *J Cataract Refract Surg*, Vol.34, No.3, (March 2008), pp.433-40, PMID: 18299068.

[49] Stewart R, Grosserode R, Cheetham JK, et al. (1999). Rosenthal A. Efficacy and safety profile of ketorolac 0.5% ophthalmic solution in the prevention of surgically induced miosis during cataract surgery. *Clin Ther*, Vol.21, No.4, (April 1999), pp.723–732, PMID :10363737.

[50] Tanihara H, Negi A, Akimoto M, et al. (1993). Surgical effects of trabeculotomy ab externo on adult eyes with primary open angle glaucoma and pseudoexfoliation syndrome. *Arch Ophthalmol*, Vol.111, No.12, (December 1993), pp.1653-61, PMID: 8155036.

[51] Tanihara H, Negi A, Akimoto M, et al. (1995). Long-term surgical results of combined trabeculectomy ab externo and cataract extraction. *Ophthalmic Surg*, Vol.26, No.4, (July-August 1995), pp.316–324, PMID: 8532283.

[52] Tanito M, Ohira A, Chihara E. (2001). Surgical outcome of combined trabeculotomy and cataract surgery. *J Glaucoma*, Vol.10, No.4, (August 2001), pp.302-8, PMID: 11558815.

[53] Teichman JC, Ahmed II. Intraocular lens choices for patients with glaucoma. (2010). *Curr Opin Ophthalmol*. Vol.21, No.2, (March 2010), pp.135-43, PMID: 20040877 .

[54] Tezel G, Kolker AE, Kass MA, et al.: Comparative results of combined procedures for glaucoma and cataract: II: limbus-based versus fornix-based conjunctival flaps. Ophthalmic Surg Lasers 1997, 28:551–557.

[55] Traverso CE, Greenidge KC, Spaeth GL, et al. (1984). Focal pressure: a new method to encourage filtration after trabeculectomy. *Ophthalmic Surg*, Vol.15, No.1, (January 1984), pp.62-5, PMID: 6700947.

[56] Uram M. (1995). Combined phacoemulsification, endoscopic ciliary process photocoagulation, and intraocular lens implantation in glaucoma management. *Ophthalmic Surg*, Vol.26, No.4, (July-August 1995), pp.346-52, PMID: 8532289.

[57] Uretmen O, Ateş H, Güven S, et al. (2003). Comparison of outcomes of viscocanalostomy and phacoviscocanalostomy. *Can J Ophthalmol*, Vol.38, No.7, (December 2003), pp.580-6, PMID: 14740800.

[58] Verges C, Llevat E, Bardavio J.(2002). Laser-assisted deep sclerectomy. *J Cataract Refract Surg*,Vol.28, No.5, (May 2002), pp.758–765, PMID: 11978452.

[59] Wada Y, Nakatsu A, Kondo T. (1994). Long-term results of trabeculotomy ab externo. *Ophthalmic Surg*, Vol.25, No.5, (May 1994), pp.317-20, PMID: 8058264.

[60] Wishart MS, Shergill T, Porooshani H.(2002). Viscocanalostomy and phacoviscocanalostomy: long-term results. *J Cataract Refract Surg,* Vol.28, No.5, (May 2002), pp.745-51, PMID: 11978450.

[61] Wong PC, Ruderman JM, Krupin T, et al. (1994). 5-Fluorouracil after primary combined filtration surgery. *Am J Ophthalmol,* Vol.117, No.2, (February 1994), pp.149-54, PMID: 8116741.

[62] Wyse T, Meyer M, Ruderman JM, et al. (1998). Combined trabeculectomy and phacoemulsification: a one-site versus a two-site approach. *Am J Ophthalmol,* Vol.123, No.3, (March 1998), pp.334–339, PMID: 9512150.

Section 3

Complications

16

Complications Associated with Cataract Surgery

Rehab Ismail[1] and Ahmed Sallam[2]
[1]*University of Aberdeen, Health Services Research Unit, Aberdeen*
[2]*Gloucestershire Hospitals NHS Foundation Trust, Gloucestershire*
UK

1. Introduction

This chapter reviews complications associated wth cataract surgery and includes discussion of their risk factors, clinical presentation, prevention and management strategies. For the sake of discussion these complications are classified into intraoperative, early postoperative and late postoperative complications.

2. Anaesthesia-related complications

Ocular anaesthesia may be complicated by both ophthalmic and systemic factors. There have been reports of potentially life-threatening complications, including optic nerve damage, globe perforation as well as brainstem anaesthesia, dysrhythmias and cardiovascular depression. These complications are mainly seen with sharp needle techniques and are rarely encountered nowadays as cataract surgery is usually performed under topical or sub-Tenon's anaesthesia (1).

2.1 Optic nerve damage

If a sharp needle accidently penetrates the dural sheath of the optic nerve (2), the anaesthetic can track back to the brainstem, causing unconsciousness and severe cardiorespiratory collapse/arrest with a potentially lethal outcome. This complication is rare, with some studies suggesting an incidence of between 0.09% and 0.79% for brainstem depression (3). Needle trauma to the optic nerve tissue can lead to significant loss of vision (4).

2.2 Globe perforation

Globe perforation is a rare complication of sharp needle anaesthesia and has been reported with both retrobulbar and peribulbar approaches with an incidence of 0.009% to 0.13% (3). This complication has potential for causing severe injury to the retina and is more frequently encountered in highly myopic eyes and eyes that underwent scleral buckling for retinal detachment (2).

Globe perforation should be suspected if hypotony is encountered after administering sharp needle anaesthesia. However, this could be absent if a large volume of anaesthetic has been injected intraocularly. Another sign is a dim red reflex and sometimes blood may be seen behind the crystalline lens by the operating surgeon at the start of the operation. Management includes examination of the fundus to assess the extent of retinal damage and to apply argon laser photocoagulation or cryopexy to retinal breaks, if necessary(5). However, in most cases, examination of the fundus is usually difficult due to the presence of vitreous haemorrhage complicating the perforation. B scan ultrasonography is helpful in this context but vitrectomy surgery is usually indicated to remove the haemorrhage and deal with the retinal damage. Of note, in addition to the physical damage that could be caused by the needle injury to the globe, injection of the anaesthetic into the vitreous can also result in retinal toxicity and poor vision (6).

2.3 Retrobulbar haemorrhage

Retrobulbar haemorrhage is an uncommon complication of ocular anaesthesia with an incidence of 0.032 to 3%. The condition is more common with sharp needle techniques (retrobulbar and peribulbar) compared to blunt needle anaesthesia (sub-Tenon's) (1) , and is more common in patients on antiplatelet medications and anticoagulants with elevated an International Normalised Ratio (INR) (5).

Retrobulbar haemorrhage is an emergency condition that needs to be promptly dealt with to save vision. It usually presents shortly after administration of the anaesthetic injection with increasing proptosis, tightness of the lids, subconjunctival haemorrhage and elevated intraocular pressure (IOP) that can lead to occlusion in the central retinal artery or short post ciliary arteries and blindness (5).

Initially mild intermittent compression on the globe can be helpful to stop further bleeding and limit progression of the haemorrhage. If this fails to resolve the condition, then pressure on the globe has to be relieved by performing a lateral canthotomy and cantholysis of the inferior crus of the lateral tarsal ligament. This is usually sufficient to decompress the orbit around the globe in most cases. IOP-lowering medications may be considered but these are usually not sufficient of their own to resolve pressure on the retinal circulation. Elective cataract surgery must be cancelled but may be rescheduled after at least a few weeks. While no immediate laboratory test is essential, patients must be re-assessed to exclude underlying blood dyscrasias. Subsequent cataract surgery is better performed under topical anaesthesia and attention should be given to normalizing the INR level if elevated and stopping antiplatelet medications in liaison with a physician.

3. Surgery-related complications

3.1 Positive vitreous pressure

Positive vitreous pressure can occur due to poor akinesia, inadvertent pressure on the globe from a tight lid speculum, proptosis, retrobulbar haemorrhage, eyelid abnormalities, as well as high hypermetropia. In this situation the iris-lens- diaphragm is pushed forward making surgery difficult and increasing the risk of more serious complications including iris damage, posterior capsule rupture and suprachoroidal haemorrhage (5).

Positive vitreous pressure is best dealt with by early recognition. In many cases a tight lid speculum is the culprit and minor adjustment of the speculum can correct the problem. Should this fail, attention needs to be directed to other causes including retrobulbar haemorrhage that usually manifests before the start of the surgery or aqueous misdirection and suprachoroidal haemorrhage that will present later on during the surgery. In the absence of retrobulbar haemorrhage the surgeon can try to deepen the anterior chamber with a cohesive opthalmic viscosurgical device but should the anterior chamber remain shallow with failure of pushing the iris-lens diagram backwards then the surgeon has to abandon the surgery and examine the fundus with an indirect ophthalmoscope for the presence of suprachoroidal haemorrhage. The absence of suprachoroidal haemorrhage makes the diagnosis of the aqueous misdirection most likely and in this scenario the condition usually resolves after a few hours and surgery can be reconsidered later on. Management of suprachoroidal haemorrhage will be discussed separately in the next section. Less commonly aqueous misdirection will not resolve conservatively and in this case, IOP-reducing agents will need to be given and possible interventions up to and including vitrectomy have to be considered.

3.2 Suprachoroidal haemorrhage

The risk of suprachoroidal haemorrhage is much less common with phacoemulsification and small incision cataract surgery compared to large incision cataract surgery. Data from the most recent national UK-based cataract audit involving 55, 567 operated eyes with phacoemulsification showed an incidence of 0.07% (7). Suprachoroidal haemorrhage results from rupture of the posterior ciliary arteries. The exact pathogenesis is unknown; however, hypertension, generalised arteriosclerosis, glaucoma and high myopia are possible precipitating factors.

Early recognition of suprachoroidal haemorrhage is crucial and cessation of surgery and immediate closure of the wound is necessary to prevent retinal extrusion (expulsive haemorrhage) and permanent loss of vision. This is unlikely to be seen with phacoemulsification surgery as the wound is usually self sealing but could be encountered with ECCE as wound closure is more time consuming but should be undertaken as fast as possible using the most readily available suture (preferably 8-0 but 6-0 sutures can be used). Drainage of the haemorrhage using sclerotomy guided by indirect ophthalmoscopy and / or B scan ultrasound can be considered.

Visual prognosis after suprachoroidal haemorrhage can vary depending on the extent of the haemorrhage. Usually the haemorrhage gradually resolves over a period of time and unless the macula has been affected, good visual recovery is usually achieved. Primary drainage of the suprachoroidal haemorrhage may not be felt to be necessary unless wound closure is not possible due to extreme positive pressure. Postoperatively, attention is given to control IOP and to treat inflammation with topical steroids and cycloplegics. Vitrectomy may be needed to drain a persistent large suprachoroidal haemorrhage but surgery is better to be deferred for 2 weeks to give time for clotted blood to liquefy.

3.3 Descemet's membrane detachment

A small area of Descemet's membrane detachment at the area of the corneal section is not uncommon with phacoemulsification surgery and can be left alone. A wider Descemet's detachment along the section would need full-thickness suturing of the cornea including the Descemet's membrane (8). This is difficult to perform and another option is to inject air or a longer acting gas intracamerally to facilitate opposition of the Descemet's membrane to the stroma. The condition can be avoided by careful attention to wound construction and size as well as by avoiding the use of blunt blades. Extremely rarely the corneal endothelium may become detached during wound manipluations such as wound hydration.

3.4 Posterior capsule rupture and vitreous loss

Posterior capsule rupture is the most common major intraoperative complication observed during cataract surgery. There is wide agreement among ophthalmologists that its incidence can be used as a measure of surgical quality and is an indicator for measuring the quality of surgeons in training and for cataract surgeons' revalidation. The importance of this complication also stems from the fact that patients whose surgery has been complicated by posterior capsule rupture usually require more postoperative follow-up visits and have an increased risk of postoperative complications including endophthalmitis, cystoid macular oedema and retinal detachment.

Several factors could predispose to posterior capsule rupture and vitreous loss during cataract surgery only one of which is the surgeon's experience and skill. Posterior capsule rupture rates in the hands of residents have been reported to vary from 0.5% to 16%, varying according to experience (9). In the United Kingdom, there has been a trend for improvement from the mean benchmark rate of 4.4% defined in the 1997 National Survey to 2.68% in the first Pilot National Electronic Cataract Surgery Survey and 1.92% in a current survey of 55 567 cases (10). The lowest rate found in a major study has been 1.1% on certain supervised training lists in the UK (11). Inadequate mydriasis and a small pupil increase the risk of intraoperative posterior capsule rupture and visual loss because it restricts the surgeon's view during surgery. Pseudoexfoliation (PXF) is another significant risk factor associated with vitreous loss. The risk is increased by several mechanisms including zonular weakness and poor pupil dilatation. Intraoperative floppy iris syndrome (IFIS) in relation to systemic use of tamsulosin is also one of the important causes of a poorly dilated pupil during cataract surgery and could make surgery very difficult due to iris billowing and prolapse to the wound. High myopia is also a well known risk factor for vitreous loss (12). Diabetes mellitus may indirectly influence the rate of posterior capsular rupture through different mechanisms including a rigid pupil and the possibility of the patient having a history of pars plana vitrectomy.

While posterior capsule rupture can occur at any stage of cataract surgery, it commonly occurs in the hands of most surgeons towards the end of the surgery at the time of cortex removal or otherwise while removing the last quadrant of the nucleus mainly because the posterior capsule is more exposed at these stages of the operation. Another cause of posterior capsular tear is an extension of an anterior capsule tear that wraps around the equator - this could occur at the early stage of capsulorrhexis though extension can also occur later on during the surgery. In a large retrospective study of 2646 cases that were operated on by a single experienced surgeon, a tear in the anterior capsule rim was observed in 21 eyes (0.79 %) and extension of the tear into the posterior capsule occurred in almost half the eyes with an anterior capsule tear (13).

Appropriate risk assessment can significantly decrease the risk of intraoperative posterior capsule rupture and vitreous loss. Difficult cases with small pupil, PXF or anticipated IFIS should only be undertaken by senior surgeons or trainees that are at the end of their training programme. Risks inherent to small pupil size or iris billowing could be dealt with intraoperatively with the use of a super-cohesive ophthalmic viscosurgical device (OVD) such as Healon 5 or mechanical measures to dilate and restrain the iris movement such as iris hooks or pupil expansion rings. Posterior capsule rupture can also be avoided by taking extra caution during emulsifying the last nucleus quadrant to protect the posterior capsule through maintaining the anterior chamber depth. Bimanual irrigation aspiration may be safer than coaxial irrigation aspiration as the aspiration port is always directed up and is therefore unlikely to snag the capsule. For anterior capsule tears, the surgeon should be aware of their risk of extension into the posterior capsule and redirection of the tear centrally to the desired circumferential path should be attempted unless the tear has extended into the zonules. This can be achieved with the capsulorrhexis tear-out rescue technique described by Little and associates (14). In this technique the authors recommend first filling the anterior chamber with a cohesive OVD and then folding the progressing anterior capsule flap back on the intact portion of the anterior capsule by forceps and then pulling it centrally to redirect the tear with the force applied in the plane of anterior capsule (14).

If posterior capsule rupture is suspected then the surgeon should stop aspiration and phacoemulsification but maintain irrigation and then inject a cohesive viscoelastic through the side port before withdrawing the handpiece from the eye. Maintaining the anterior chamber depth can prevent extension of the posterior capsule tear and avoid disruption of the anterior vitreous face and vitreous prolapse. Further management depends on the stage at which capsule rupture occurs and whether there is vitreous prolapse into the anterior chamber ('vitreous loss'). If the anterior hyaloid face is intact, removal of residual cortex can be performed using dry aspiration while the anterior chamber is maintained with a cohesive OVD. Another technique is bimanual irrigation aspiration with the irrigation and suction kept to a minimum and the irrigation flow directed away from the tear so as not to disrupt the anterior vitreous face. At all stages of the surgery, the anterior chamber depth should always be maintained.

Vitreous prolapse if it occurs has to be dealt with using anterior vitrectomy. Triamcinolone is increasingly used by surgeons to visualise vitreous. Bimanual vitrectomy through two side ports is the preferred technique as the anterior chamber depth is maintained with this approach limiting the amount of prolapsing vitreous. Trimacinolone serves as a good tool to visualize vitreous fibrils when injected in the anterior chamber and ensures complete anterior vitrectomy.

If there is a small central posterior capsule tear, an experienced surgeon can still implant the lens in the bag preferably after converting it to a posterior capsulorrhexis. In this case, a one-piece lens is much easier to implant. Should this not be feasible then the surgeon can place the intraocular lens in the ciliary sulcus provided that there is sufficient capsular support. Capturing the optic through an intact capsulorrhexis can also be performed to help better centralisation of the lens optic ('optic capture').

Any intraocular lens (IOL) placed in the ciliary sulcus should have sufficient posterior iris clearance and secure fixation. Therefore the choice is between a 3-piece foldable posterior chamber intraocular lens (PCIOL) and a polymethymethacrylate (PMMA) IOL. A 3-piece foldable PCIOL has the advantage of thin, posteriorly angulated C-shaped haptics that do not contact the iris. Ideally, the anterior optic surface should be smooth and have rounded edges to minimize iris chafing and the overall IOL length should be at least 13.5 mm. It is important to reduce the risk of iris chafing that the IOL is inserted with the correct face forwards. Because of the risk of retinal detachment with posterior capsule rupture and vitreous loss, silicone intraocular lenses are better avoided as they may compromise the view should vitrectomy surgery become required. With optic capture, the same IOL power calculated for capsular bag fixation can generally be used. However, should optic capture not be feasible with sulcul IOL, the lens optic will have a more anterior location and the lens power should be reduced by 0.5 to 1.0 D (15). A large diameter (>13.5 mm) PMMA PC IOL is another option but the incision will need to be enlarged to at least 6.5 mm which is not desirable (15). Single piece acrylic lenses are not recommended for ciliary sulcus placement. The haptics are thick and not posteriorly angulated and will therefore contact the posterior surface of the iris when implanted in the sulcus. Furthermore, the overall loop-to-loop dimension of these lenses is only 13.0 mm or less which is short for many eyes. The square edge optic design increases iris chaffing (15).

In eyes with insufficient capsule support, the surgeon has the choice between iris- or scleral-sutured PC IOLs and open loop AC IOLs. In our experience placing an AC IOL is a much easier technique than suturing a PC IOL during the primary surgery (Figure 1).The American Academy of Ophthalmology Technology Assessment study reviewed more than 40 papers that addressed the outcomes of IOLs implanted without adequate capsule support and carried evidence rating of level III or higher. The study was unable to find a significant difference in the safety or efficacy of these 3 methods and therefore use of any of these modalities is appropriate and is left to the discretion of the surgeon (16).

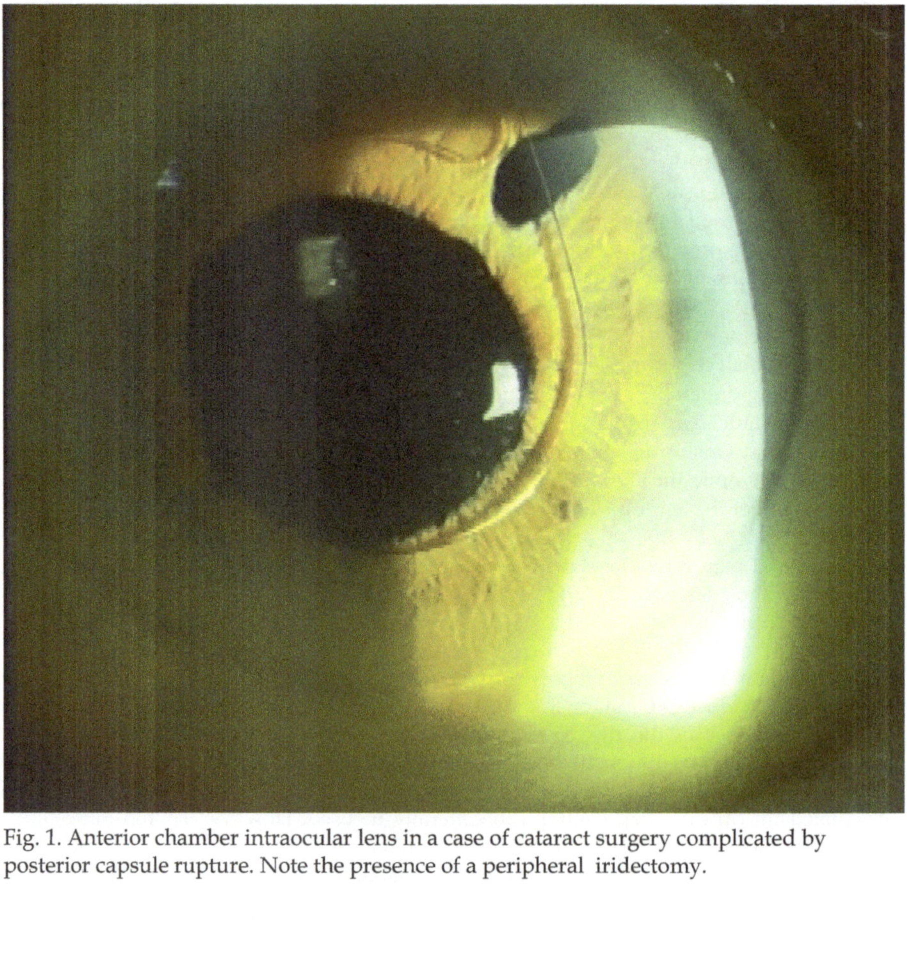

Fig. 1. Anterior chamber intraocular lens in a case of cataract surgery complicated by posterior capsule rupture. Note the presence of a peripheral iridectomy.

3.5 Zonular dialysis

A preoperative zonular dialysis may be the result of pre-existing conditions as traumatic cataract or in association with specific disorders as Marfan Syndrome and Weill-Marchesani Syndrome. Pseudoexfoliation and high myopia are other well recognized causes for zonular weakness and dialysis preoperatively. Signs that could alert the surgeon to the presence of zonular dialysis include phacodonesis, iridodonesis, presence of vitreous in the anterior chamber, or a visible zonular defect. Moreover, the nucleus may appear decentralised (off-centre) with a gap between the iris border and the lens.

Intraoperative zonular dialysis may result from vigorous manoeuvres that traumatise the zonules in one region. These include a traumatic capsulorrhexis, excessive manipulation of the nucleus, or inadvertent aspiration of the capsular bag or anterior capsule. Prompt recognition and early management can decrease the risk of intraoperative vitreous prolapse and postoperative lens decentration or posterior dislocation. Small areas of zonular dialysis (45 degrees or less) recognized at the time of surgery can be dealt with only by maintaining the anterior chamber depth at the time of surgery to limit further progression and prevent vitreous prolapse. A larger defect usually necessitates the use of a capsule tension ring (CTR) to preserve the integrity of the capsular bag and provide the necessary capsular support. It works by reducing asymmetric capsular forces, stabilizing the vitreous base. Moreover, it facilitates phacoemulsification and IOL implantation and decreases postoperative IOL decentration and capsular phimosis. Modified CTR designs are also available and can even be sutured to the sclera to provide additional support to the capsular bag in eyes with very loose zonules.

4. Early postoperative complications

4.1 Shallow anterior chamber (AC)

A shallow anterior chamber after cataract surgery may be associated with low or high IOP. Wound leak is the most common cause of shallow AC with low IOP and therefore, the initial work up aims to check for a wound integrity and perform a Seidel test. Other causes include choroidal effusion or severe uveitis with decreased aqueous formation. Management is directed towards treating the underlying problem in case of a wound leak and uveitis while choroidal effusion is usually self limiting.

Shallow anterior chamber with elevated IOP could be due to pupil block glaucoma, suprachoroidal haemorrhage or malignant glaucoma. Pupil block is an uncommonly encountered complication after cataract surgery where the aqueous humour accumulates under the iris causing the peripheral iris to balloon forward resulting in angle closure glaucoma. The pupillary aperture may be obstructed by complete adhesions between pupillary border of the iris (seclusio pupillae) and lens implant in eyes with severe postoperative uveitis. Other causes include pupil block caused by the anterior hyaloid or lens implant and for this reason it is essential to perform a peripheral iridectomy when implanting an anterior chamber IOL. Retained viscoelastic accumulating behind the lens implant can increase the pressure inside the capsular bag and induce pupil block i.e. capsular distension syndrome. These eyes will have an unexpected degree of myopia which is an important clue to the diagnosis.

Malignant glaucoma is a rare complication after cataract surgery. A blockage of the normal aqueous exchange between the posterior chamber and the anterior vitreous is believed to cause malignant glaucoma. Posterior misdirection of aqueous humor into the vitreous cavity occurs producing a continuous expansion of the vitreous cavity with increased posterior segment pressure. This accumulation of aqueous in the vitreous cavity causes anterior displacement of the lens-iris diaphragm. The resulting shallow or flat AC is believed to exacerbate the condition because of the decreased access of aqueous to the trabecular meshwork. After excluding the presence of pupillary block initial management should be conservative with topical mydriatics and IOP lowering agents including systemic carbonic anhydrase inhibitors and osmotic agents as mannitol. Nd: YAG laser can be performed to disrupt the anterior vitreous face but surgical management in the form of vitrectomy should be performed if conservative treatment and laser fail to resolve the condition. Management of suprachoroidal haemorrhage has been discussed earlier in this chapter.

4.2 Iris prolapse

Iris prolapse can result from inadequate wound closure, accidental postoperative trauma, or raised intraocular pressure. Phacoemulsification wounds are usually self sealing but surgeons should confirm the absence of wound leak at the conclusion of the surgery and not hesitate to suture the wound if needed.

If iris prolapse is of less than 48 hours duration, the iris can be repositioned and the wound is closed. In cases where iris prolapsed has been present for a longer time, iris excision is usually needed to decrease risk of intraocular infection.

4.3 Postoperative uveitis

Mild anterior uveitis is not uncommon after uncomplicated phacoemulsification surgery and usually responds well to routine postoperative corticosteroid drops. Concerns are raised when a patient presents in the early postoperative period with more than a mild postoperative inflammation as this could be endophthalmitis even in the absence of pain and poor vision. As long as the vitreous remains quiet and the anterior chamber inflammation is not worsening, a sensible strategy is to increase the frequency of topical steroids and review the patient after several hours and then the next morning. However, diagnosis of endophthalmitis should be considered if symptoms worsen within 6 to 12 hours and emergency treatment should be commenced without delay.

4.4 Infectious endophthalmitis

Infectious endophthalmitis is the most serious postoperative complication of cataract surgery. Fortunately the incidence is very low and ranges from 1- 3 in 1000 or even less (17). Postoperative endophthalmitis can present as early as the first postoperative day and up to two weeks after surgery. However, most commonly it presents after 3-4 days. Presenting symptoms can include decreased vision and pain although pain is not a constant feature. The anterior chamber inflammation seen is usually significantly greater than that expected after surgery (Figure 2), with extension of inflammation to the vitreous cavity. Other classic signs of endophthalmitis are lid swelling, conjunctival injection, corneal oedema, vitreous abscess and retinitis but these could all be absent in early cases and are not essential for making the diagnosis. The Endophthalmitis Vitrectomy Study (EVS) found that at presentation, 86% of cases of acute postoperative endophthalmitis had hypopyon which can cause an increase in IOP. The majority of these patients complained of progressive pain and reduction in vision and 86% had acuity of 5/200 on initial presentation and 26% had light perception only (18).

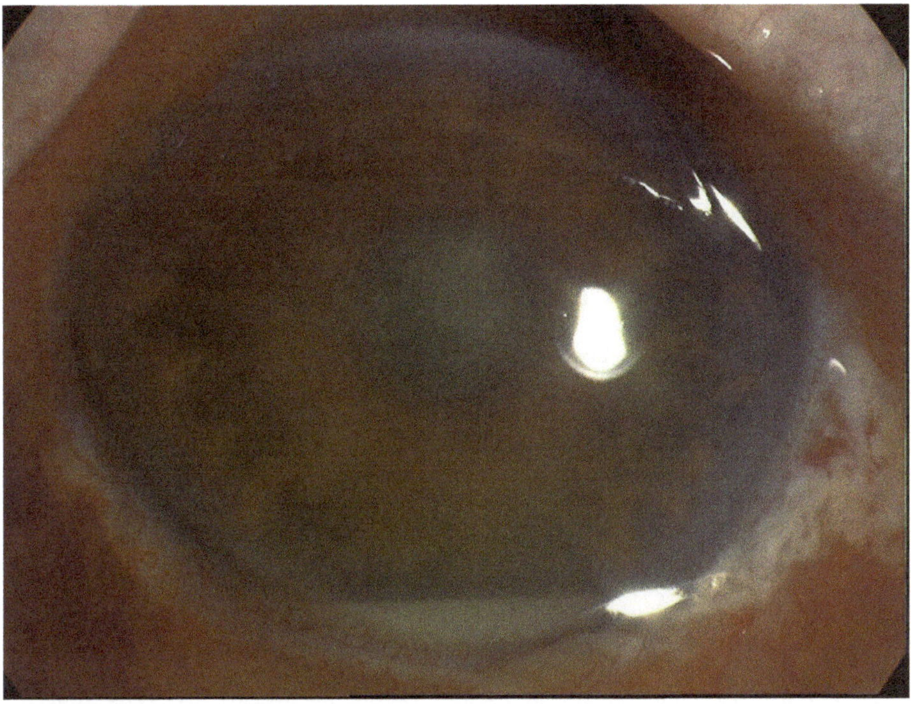

Fig. 2. Marked anterior chamber inflammation and hypopyon in a patient with infective endophthalmitis

The majority of cases of postoperative endophthalmitis result from intraocular microbial contamination from the patient's skin, preocular tear film or ocular adnexa. Posterior capsule rupture is a well known risk factor and it is therefore recommended that the cataract wound is sutured after complicated cases (19). Other risk factors include patient age, intraoperative surgical complications, and poor wound construction. In a case-control study of 10 patients, endophthalmitis after secondary IOL was associated with diabetes, trans-scleral suture fixation of posterior chamber IOLs, polypropylene haptics, and intraocular re-entry through the old wound (20).

The most common pathogens are gram-positive cocci, *Streptococcus epidermidis* and *Staphylococcus (Staph) aureus*. *Staph aureus* endophthalmitis often leads to a more virulent and destructive pattern of visual loss in comparison to that of *Staph epidermidis*. Gram-negative pathogens can also cause severe bacterial endophthalmitis with *Pseudomonas aeruginosa* being the most common casual agent. The normal flora colonising the eyelids and the lashes are the main source of bacteria in endophthalmitis post cataract surgery but other sources of infection include contaminated infusion solutions or instruments and aerosols in the operating theatre (21).

Several antibacterial protocols exist to prevent the occurrence of postoperative endophthalmitis, with topical, intracameral and subconjunctival delivery being the most common approaches. Worldwide, there seems to be significant variation in the methods of delivery of prophylactic antibacterial regimens; for example, topical fluoroquinolones are commonly used in the United States, while intracameral cephalosporins are employed broadly in Europe. The optimal antibacterial strategy for the prevention of endophthalmitis should be the administration of safe, inexpensive antibiotics with a broad spectrum of activity and which also do not require patient compliance for effectiveness (22). In addition, detection and treatment of blepharitis preoperatively as well as preoperative administration of povidine iodine in the conjunctival sac reduces the incidence of postoperative endophthalmitis and are widely employed measures.

Intravitreal injection of antibiotics is the mainstay of treatment for postoperative endophthalmitis and needs to be commenced without delay once the diagnosis is made. Empirical antibiotics to cover gram positive and gram negative organisms are usually used after performing a vitreous tap for culture and sensitivity. With the rising incidence of resistant beta-lactam bacteria, intravitreal injection of vancomycin is the treatment of choice to cover gram-positive organisms. Vancomycin is a bactericidal agent that works by preventing the polymerisation of peptidoglycan in the cell wall and thus causes loss of cell wall integrity with cell lysis. The drug is used at a dose of 1.0-2.0mg/0.1ml and has been reported to have 100% efficacy against gram-positive bacteria but has no efficacy against gram-negative organisms (21). Cover for gram-negative organisms requires an agent with activity against *Pseudomonas aeroginosa.* Ceftazidime at a dose of 2.00-2.25 mg/0.1 ml or amikacin at a dose of 0.4 mg/0.1 ml may be used and have similar success rates close to 90%. Aminoglycosides are also synergistic with vancomycin against gram-positive organisms. However, both gentamicin and amikacin carry a small risk of retinal toxicity and macular infarction when injected intraocularly, but the risk is small and amikacin in particular is widely used (21). The toxic effect can even occur with smaller doses. A localised increase in the concentration may play a part in causing the toxicity. Also, ceftazidime 2.0 mg may be used instead of aminoglycosides in the treatment as well as prophylaxis of gram negative infection (23). Some centres also administer systemic antibiotics alongside intravitreal agents.

Pars plana vitrectomy (PPV) may be necessary for the management of acute endophthalmitis; however the need for vitrectomy in all cases of postoperative endophthalmitis remains questionable. While vitrectomy is expected to decrease the microbial load and increase intraocular diffusion of antibiotics, it carries the potential risk of causing retinal detachment and intraocular haemorrhage in cases of intraocular infection (24). As per the EVS recommendations, patients with only light perception or worse benefit from PPV with a significantly better outcome. However, different centres have different protocols and some centres treat all cases initially with intravitreal antibiotics irrespective of the level of vision and consider vitrectomy for cases that do not respond (24).

Visual prognosis is strongly associated with the type of microorganisms that are cultured. Gram positive coagulase negative cocci are associated with the best prognosis whilst *Streptococci* as well as *enterococci* seem to be associated with the worst visual outcome. Presenting visual acuity is a more powerful predictor of visual prognosis than the microbiological factors. Bacterial growths from vitrectomy cassette specimens have the same prognostic value as specimens taken from other intraocular sources (25).

The chronic form of postoperative endophthalmitis is more insidious and usually manifests after several weeks or even months after the surgery (figure 2).The ratio of acute to chronic cases ranges between 5:1 to 2:1 (17). The organisms responsible tend to be less virulent bacteria or fungi. The inflammation may initially be controlled by postoperative topical steroids but rebound inflammation is common as the steroids are tapered. These cases may be treated with intravitreal antibiotics including vancomycin however in resistant cases treatment directed at surgical removal of the sequestered organisms through removing the intraocular lens and total removal of the capsular bag results in a lower recurrence rate (26).

4.5 Toxic anterior segment syndrome (TASS)

Over the last three decades several authors have reported a non-infectious condition mimicking endophthalmitis following cataract surgery (26). Initially it was termed "sterile postoperative endophthalmitis" however this was a misnomer, as unlike endophthalmitis, the inflammation is limited only to the anterior segment and does not extend to the vitreous cavity. It was later renamed 'toxic anterior segment syndrome' (TASS) (27).

TASS generally presents with severe inflammation that is restricted to the anterior chamber as mentioned before, often resulting in hypopyon. In severe cases of TASS, fibrin may be present in the anterior chamber, on the iris or on the IOL surface. Inflammatory membranes can develop, which result in iris damage and an irregular pupil with impaired pupil function. During the early stages of the condition the IOP is low but the inflammatory membrane can creep over the trabecular meshwork. These changes can result in ocular hypertension or the development of secondary glaucoma and the rise in IOP can be severe.

A number of possible causes have been identified as triggering factors. They include preservatives in drugs or the irrigating solution injected into the anterior chamber during surgery, traces of chemicals used in the sterilization process remaining on the surgical instruments or contamination of these instruments with bacterial endotoxins during sterilisation (28). Because TASS is a toxic insult, it almost always presents as an atypical and unusual form of inflammation one day after surgery.

Differentiation between TASS and infective endophthalmitis is very important but can sometimes be difficult. First, TASS is only an anterior segment inflammation whereas endophthalmitis involves both anterior and posterior segments with extension of the inflammation into the vitreous (29). Second, TASS occurs within the first 24 hours in the postoperative period, however, endophthalmitis is not uncommonly delayed for 4 -7 days and very rarely presents on the first day. Third, patients with infective endophthalmitis are usually more symptomatic than TASS patients who may only complain of mild discomfort. Fourth, limbus-to-limbus corneal oedema is an important differentiating finding strongly suggestive of TASS. If this sign is present on the first postoperative day, a diagnosis of TASS should be strongly considered. Nonetheless, endophthalmitis should never be eliminated as a diagnosis until the therapeutic response is measured and the inflammation remains confined to the anterior segment. Fifth, in an eye with TASS, a fixed dilated pupil, often with mottled or diffuse areas of iris atrophy, is not uncommon. However this is unlikely to be encountered in cases of infective endophthalmitis. Finally, a severe rise of IOP early in the postoperative period is an uncommon finding with endophthalmitis and is more suggestive of TASS (30).

Topical steroids comprise the first line of treatment of TASS. Patients should receive hourly topical steroids and remain in the clinic to be monitored during the day. Steroids can suppress inflammation from endophthalmitis for a short period of time and accordingly the diagnosis of endophthalmitis must be reconsidered if symptoms and signs are getting worse with the use of steroids. For mild or moderate cases of TASS most cases will respond well to topical treatment and recover with time. Severe cases may require the use of oral steroids and visual outcome can be poor due to non resolving corneal oedema or refractory glaucoma.

4.6 Retained Lens Material

Inadequate aspiration of the cortex, especially of the subincisional cortex if the surgeon is using a coaxial irrigation aspiration, is the commonest cause of retained lens material after cataract surgery. This is usually in the form of soft lens matter.
Retained lens material excites an inflammatory reaction in the eye. In cases with minimal cortical matter, the anterior segment inflammation can be controlled medically with topical steroids and cycloplegics until the lens material is absorbed. In cases with significant cortical residue, surgical removal is essential as they can cause significant inflammation with raised IOP and can also move centrally to obstruct the visual axis. There should be a low threshold for intervening quickly with surgery to remove the retained lens matter if intraocular pressure and /or intraocular inflammation is proving difficult to control.

5. Late postoperative complications

5.1 Change in refraction / astigmatism

Corneal topography has been used to evaluate postoperative astigmatism. Topographic analysis has shown a mean flattening of 0.4 to 1.0 dioptre in the temporal region after a sutureless 3 mm temporal corneal incision with no significant vertical steeping or nasal flattening in the majority of patients (31).
In patients with a pre-existing small degree of corneal astigmatism (up to 0.75D), this can be tailored for a favourable outcome by manipulating the incision parameters (size, location and shape). On-axis incisions are the most widely used of these approaches. However cases with more significant amount of astigmatism are unlikely to benefit from incision site modification but could benefit from combined cataract surgery and limbal relaxing incisions or toric intraocular lens implantation.

5.2 Refractive surprises after cataract surgery

Refractive surprises following cataract surgery can be due to inaccurate biometry, insertion of the wrong IOL (either due to manufacturer-associated or surgeon-associated errors) or previous corneal refractive procedures. The best markers of the quality of a biometry service are the percentage of eyes achieving a postoperative spherical equivalent refraction within 0.5 and 1.0D of the target refraction and the total range of refractive error (32). The Royal College of Ophthalmologists (RCOphth) 2004 cataract surgery guidelines state that both optical (partial coherence interferometry (PCI)) and acoustic (ultrasound) methods of axial length measurement can be routinely used (33), although it has been shown that PCI reduces the prediction error of postoperative refractive outcome. The RCOphth guidelines state that each ophthalmology department, if not each surgeon, should personalise the A constant on the basis of continuous audit of the comparison of the predicted and actual spherical equivalent of the postoperative subjective refraction (34).
IOL power calculations in cataract patients who have formerly undergone keratorefractive surgery are often less precise than they are for patients who have not had refractive procedures. This is mainly due to errors in determination of corneal refractive powers and

using wrong keratometry values and is more common in patients who have undergone myopic keratorefractive surgery. As their corneal refractive power may be overestimated, this may lead to a hyperopic postoperative refractive outcome. Several options are available for subsequent correction of refractive surprises, including prescription of spectacles or contact lenses, IOL exchange, keratorefractive surgery, or implantation of a supplementary IOL (i.e., polypseudophakia) (35).

Spectacles may not be ideal for some young self-conscious patients. Likewise contact lenses may not be suitable for older patients. Keratorefractive procedures may not be the best solution due to the inherent risks associated with further corneal surgery. IOL exchange and supplementary IOLs, implanted in the ciliary sulcus anterior to the primary implant, can be an option, especially when capsular changes have firmly fixed the primary implant within the capsular bag making IOL exchange surgically challenging with very significant risks of posterior capsule and zonular rupture (35).

5.3 Posterior capsule opacification (PCO)

A thickened posterior capsule is the most common postoperative cause of decreased vision following cataract surgery with a prevalence of over 40% in many studies within five years of surgery. It is a multi-factorial problem related to patient factors such as age, surgical factors and also factors in the IOL design.

PCO is caused by residual lens epithelial cells, which are left behind after cataract surgery. These residual lens epithelial cells have been shown to produce interleukins (36-38), fibroblast growth factor and transforming growth factor beta in inoculation media. Cytokines may also play a role in the proliferation and development of lens epithelial cells; therefore inhibition of cytokines may lead to prevention of PCO (39). There is also some evidence that the proliferation of lens epithelial cells (Elschnig's pearls) may be linked to the severity and duration of intraoperative or postoperative inflammation.

The IOL implant itself creates a physical barrier between the anterior and posterior lens capsule and IOL designs with square edged optics provide a more effective barrier than round edges thus minimising the risk of PCO. This is usually more effective when the anterior capsulorrhexis is continuous, well centred and overlaps the implant edge by 1-2 mm. Intraocular lens designs have also been improved to reduce trauma and thus decrease the likelihood of epithelial cell proliferation. Together with appropriate aspiration of cortical lens matter and improved surgical experience, these techniques have reduced the prevalence of PCO (40).

PCO is treated with Neodymium:Yttrium Aluminium Garnet (Nd:YAG) laser capsulotomy, preferably six months after surgery after stabilisation of the blood-ocular barrier (Figure 3). Nd:YAG laser capsulotomy should begin with minimal power and an adequate opening should be created, at least encompassing the pupillary area in the undilated position. For patients who require regular fundus examination such as patients with diabetic retinopathy a wider capsulotomy opening is more preferable.

Although Nd: YAG laser capsulotomy is a straightforward procedure, it is not entirely without risk. Iatrogenic complications of Nd:YAG laser capsulotomy include corneal endothelial loss, increase in IOP, uveitis, and retinal detachment. Accidental lens pitting can occur in up to 30% of patients and laser burns on silicone IOLs can resemble pigment deposition (41).

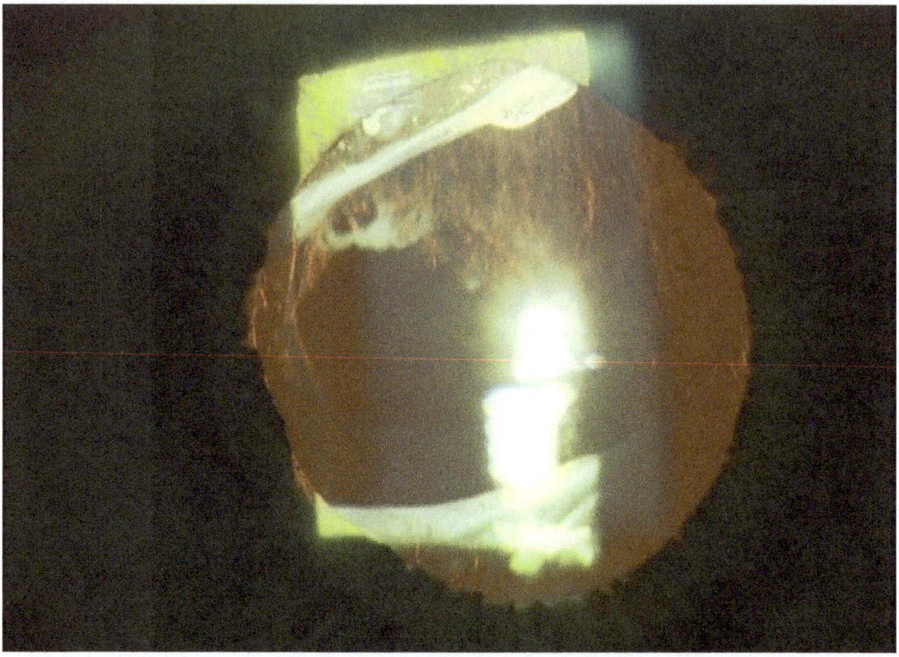

Fig. 3. Nd: YAG posterior capsulotomy laser for posterior capsule opacification

6. Cystoid macular oedema (CMO)

Advances in cataract surgery techniques and increasing awareness of the importance of minimizing vitreous loss have resulted in a marked reduction in the incidence of cystoid macular oedema (CMO) compared with the era of intracapsular cataract surgery (42,43).

Cystoid macular oedema is now considered an infrequent complication and the literature suggests that the incidence of pseudophakic CMO following uncomplicated phacoemulsification of the lens and implantation of an in-the-bag intraocular lens is 0.6–6% (43). The incidence of CMO is higher if the surgery is complicated (e.g., posterior capsule rupture with or without vitreous loss, iris damage and vitreous incarceration through the wound) (44). It is also more common in diabetic eyes and in patients with pre-existing uveitis (45,46).

CMO following cataract surgery results from the maldistribution of intravascular fluid within the macula. Leakage of intravascular contents from the dilated perifoveal capillaries initially causes thickening of the macula, which may progress to cystoid expansions within the outer plexiform (Henle's) layer and inner nuclear layer of the retina (47). Most investigators agree that inflammation is the major aetiologic factor with prostaglandin release being implicated as the possible mediator of inflammation (48).

Pseudophakic CMO is characterized by poor postoperative visual acuity. CMO has a peak incidence of 4-6 weeks following cataract surgery (49) but can occur earlier in complicated cases. Diagnosis is made after slit lamp biomicroscopy but subtle cases can be diagnosed with optical coherence tomography examination (OCT) (Figure 4). Fundus fluorescein angiography could also be helpful in diagnosis of CMO and usually shows perifoveal petaloid staining pattern and late leakage of the optic disc but is not needed in all cases and has been superceded by OCT.

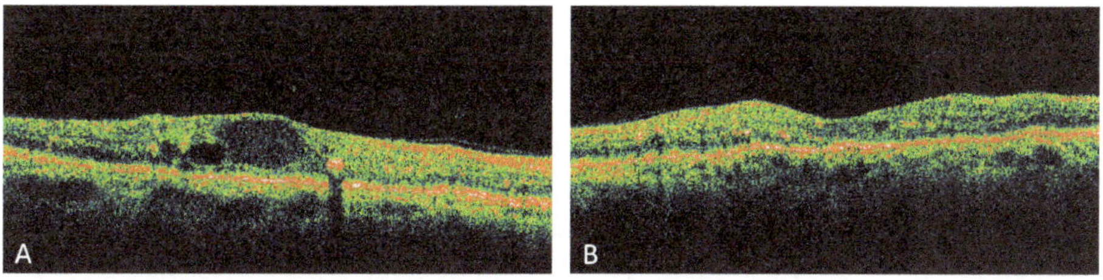

Fig. 4. Optical coherence tomography photographs of chronic cystoid macular oedema before (a) and after (b) treatment with intravitreal triamcinolone.

Most CMO cases (>80%) will resolve spontaneously within weeks to months. The presence of chronic CMO however occurs in a small proportion of patients (1%) leading to chronic or permanent vision loss and hence the argument for early diagnosis and treatment of CMO. Several studies have considered the effect of pharmacologic and surgical treatments for pseudophakic CMO. Most clinicians use a combination of topical corticosteroids and non steroidal anti-inflammatory drugs (NSAIDs) as a first-line treatment in most instances (50). Corticosteroids inhibit several parts of inflammation including prostaglandin synthesis by inhibiting the enzyme phospholipase A2, while NSAIDs interrupt prostaglandin synthesis by inhibiting the enzyme cyclo-oxygenase. A course of 6 weeks treatment is usually tried before a second line treatment is considered. For cases that do not respond, treatment options include periocular or intravitreal steroids and oral acetazolamide. Periocular steroids (sub-Tenon or peribulbar) have the advantageous of being able to reach the posterior segment of the eye in a higher concentration compared to topical application and have less ocular side effects compared to the intravitreal route. Side effects include raised intraocular pressure, cataract, orbital fat prolapse and ptosis but these are less likely to occur after a single injection. Intravitreal triamcinolone injection is an effective treatment option for resistant postoperative CMO, although there are no randomized prospective trials to date. Intravitreal triamcinolone results in a rapid improvement in visual acuity that may be sustained for more than 6 months (51-52). However it is associated with significant ocular morbidity including a high risk of cataract, ocular hypertension and a small risk of infectious or sterile endophthalmitis (Figure 5).

Carbonic anhydrase inhibitors (CAIs), such as acetazolamide, have been used in cases resistant to standard topical treatment with some success (53, 54).They enhance the pumping action of retinal pigment epithelial cells, facilitating the transport of fluid across the retina. However, there are no controlled studies that demonstrated a positive effect of acetazolamide on pseudophakic macular oedema.

Bevacizumab (Avastin) is a monoclonal antibody able to inactivate the effects of vascular endothelial growth factors (VEGF). The role of VEGF in pseudophakic CMO is not clear, yet several authors have reported resolution of CMO after administration of bevacizumab (55) retrospectively. This class of drugs could be of benefit in patients with chronic CMO that have exhibited a steroid hypertensive response to topical or periocular steroids. However, a report by Spitzer et al did not find any beneficial effects with this treatment (56).

When vitreous is incarcerated in the corneal wound following complicated cataract surgery, Nd:YAG laser lysis of vitreous strands has been shown to have a positive effect on restoring the retinal vascular stability and reduction of macular oedema (57). Finally, pars plana vitrectomy (PPV) could be employed in the management of chronic postoperative CMO (58). This helps to remove vitreous strands tracking to the surgical wound after complicated ocular surgery as well as peeling of epiretinal membranes from the surface of the macula when associated with CMO. It also works by removal of inflammatory mediators from the vitreous or retained nuclear lens fragments and possibly by increasing oxygen diffusion to the macula.

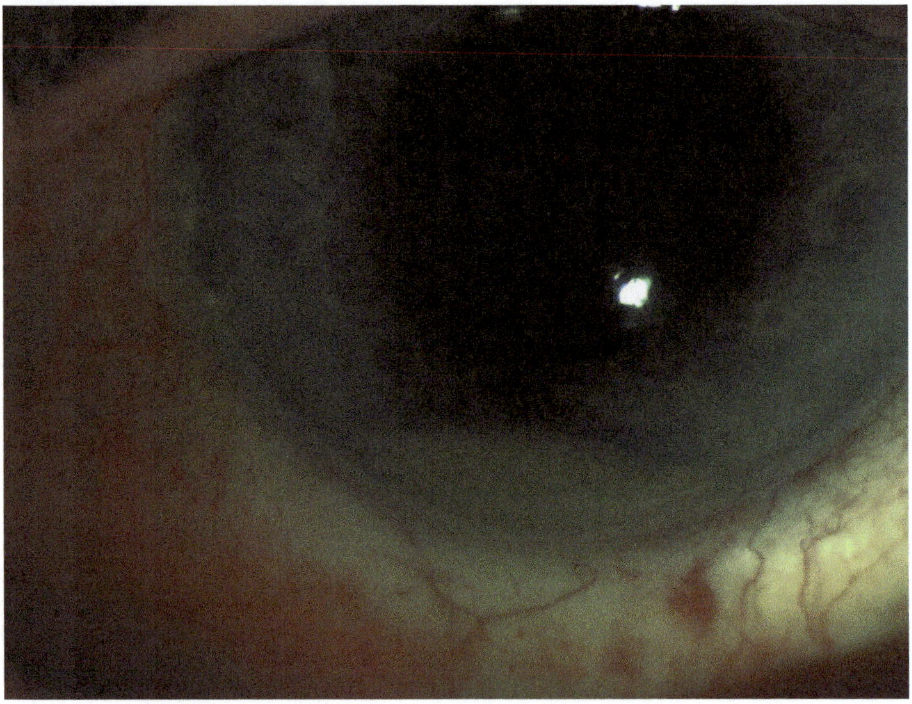

Fig. 5. Sterile endophthalmitis with a pseudohypopyon due to deposition of triamcinolone crystals in the anterior segment after intravitreal triamcinolone treatment.

There is debate whether routine prophylactic treatment of CMO is needed as the cost:benefit ratio of treatment and long term visual benefit are not clear. Unless a patient presented with risk factors for developing CMO—diabetes, previous vein occlusions, uveitis or epiretinal membrane, prophylactic intervention prior to cataract is usually not employed by most clinicians. When indicated, topical NSAIDs are the most widely used class of drugs in the prophylaxis of pseudophakic CMO and several studies have reported that they are effective in this context (59).

6.1 Posterior vitreous detachment and rhegmatogenous retinal detachment

Posterior vitreous detachment (PVD) is considered to be common following cataract surgery and can occur at any time. A published study found a prevalence of PVD in 50.8% of eyes that had undergone cataract surgery compared to 20.8% in the fellow unoperated eye (60). The removal of the crystalline lens and its replacement with a thinner IOL implant leaves more space inside the globe for the vitreous to move forward which may induce a detachment from the posterior pole. The study also found that eyes with an axial length of more than 25mm were at increased risk of developing PVD (60).

Rhegmatogenous retinal detachment (RRD) is rare but is a serious potential complication of cataract surgery. The prevalence is much lower with phacoemulsification and small incision surgery than that found after intra-capsular cataract extraction (ICCE). It is this increased incidence of PVD after cataract surgery that is the main precipitating factor in the development of retinal breaks and subsequent pseudophakic RRD. 75% of retinal detachments occur in the first year while the other quarter may develop within 4 years of surgery (61). The risk of RRD appears to be increased in male patients, myopes and very significantly in those patients who have vitreous loss at the time of cataract surgery. It was also found that scleral-sutured posterior chamber intraocular lenses (PCIOLs) may be associated with a high risk of RD due to pre-existing conditions (myopia, aphakia and vitreous loss) and vitreous disturbances as well as pars plana entry sites during IOL fixation. In addition, retinal breaks may result from traumatic incarceration of the IOL and pre-retinal manipulation of dislocated IOLs (62). Nd:YAG laser posterior capsulotomy may increase the risk of retinal detachment after cataract surgery. The hazard ratio of RD after Nd:YAG laser posterior capsulotomy was 4.9, however, this risk is changed by a factor of 1.3 with an increase of axial length of 1 mm and by a factor of 0.94 for each added year of the patient's age (63).

Pseudophakic retinal detachment can be treated with a number of different approaches including pneumatic retinopexy, scleral buckling and primary pars plana vitrectomy. While choice of surgery remains a matter of personal choice for the surgeon, there is growing popularity in use of pars plana vitrectomy for treatment of retinal detachment particularly because retinal tears in pseudophakic eyes could be multiple and thus difficult to treat successfully with pneumatic retinopexy or a localized buckle. One recent prospective randomized trial that compared primary vitrectomy and scleral buckling in rhegmatogenous retinal detachment showed superiority of the former over the latter in pseudophakic eyes (64).

6.2 Lens dislocation

This is a rare complication with the patient complaining of blurred vision, glare and possibly monocular diplopia. The visual symptoms can be potentially disabling for the patient and requires repositioning of the lens, or IOL exchange. The IOL implant can be displaced by asymmetrical thickening or fibrosis of the lens capsule particularly in cases complicated by zonular dehiscence or patients with pre-existing weakness of the zonules as in pseudoexfoliation syndrome. Lens dislocation can also result from ocular trauma or previous pars plana vitrectomy.

A major problem associated with posteriorly dislocated IOL is retinal damage during the intraocular manipulations. Removal of a posteriorly located IOL through the corneal wound is hazardous and should not be attempted. Pars plana vitrectomy surgery is needed for retrieval of the lens from the vitreous followed by IOL exchange or repositioning in the ciliary sulcus with or without suturing to the sclera (65). However, some patients may be treated conservatively and their aphakia corrected with a contact lens or secondary lens implant.

6.3 Capsular block syndrome

Also known as capsular bag distension, this occurs after cataract removal and placement of a posterior chamber IOL. Typically the patient reports blurring of vision postoperatively, which is usually found to be due to an induced myopic shift, although a hyperopic shift or no refractive change have also been reported(66-68).

The pathogenesis of this condition may be due to a fibrotic reaction with a larger lens optic in the capsular bag allowing enhanced adhesion between the lens and the capsule resulting in sealing of the capsulorrhexis(2). It is postulated that this syndrome may result from osmotic movement of fluid due to various types of collagen and substances produced by the proliferating lens epithelial cells and is associated with lens capsule thickening (69, 70). Nd:YAG posterior capsulotomy laser is usually performed to release the fluid into the vitreous cavity and in most cases this is sufficient to improve the vision. Retained viscoelastic behind the lens can also cause this condition and may have to be removed surgically.

6.4 Ptosis and diplopia

This is an unusual complication of cataract surgery and usually occurs several months later. It is important to take a thorough ocular history, as it is possible that the ptosis may have been present prior to cataract surgery but went unnoticed.

This form of ptosis is often transient and does not require intervention, although persistent ptosis may require surgical intervention. Causes of persistent ptosis usually involve damage to the levator muscle due to the toxic effects of anaesthesia, prolonged oedema, and trauma from direct injection into the muscle, or from the lid speculum during cataract surgery.

Persistent diplopia is an uncommon complication after cataract surgery. Some cases are due to vertical or less commonly horizontal muscle imbalance which is thought to be due to direct surgical trauma or due to an anaesthetic myotoxic effect (71). Patients with pre-operative diplopia should also be counselled about this risk as the deviation may be unstable in a quite large proportion of these patients and some cases may need surgical treatment to correct their diplopia (72). Another cause of postoperative diplopia is aniseikonia due to surgically induced anisometropia.

6.5 Corneal oedema and pseudophakic bullous keratopathy (PBK)

Postoperative corneal oedema is not a rare complication of phacoemulsification. Epithelial oedema (that is not associated with stromal oedema) is usually due to increased IOP and is reversible when the cause is treated. Presence of corneal stromal oedema postoperatively is a sign of endothelial damage. This may result from pre-existing endothelial pathology as in Fuch's Endothelial Dystrophy or intraoperative endothelial trauma particularly after phacoemulsification of dense nuclei and in complicated cases with posterior capsular rupture and vitreous loss. Postoperative uveitis can also lead to endothelial cell loss and corneal oedema as in TASS.

Postoperatively, corneal stromal oedema can be localized or diffuse and is usually associated with underlying Descemet's membrane folds, hence the name striate keratopathy. Clinically, this could also be associated with epithelial oedema and in severe cases epithelial bullae may be seen. Vision is usually significantly affected in patients with striate keratopathy although mild cases can manifest with blurred vision early in the morning which improves later in the day. Chronic unresolved corneal oedema (decompensated corneal oedema) can lead to progressive scarring with severe decline in visual acuity.

Mild stromal oedema secondary to intraoperative trauma usually settles with time. While topical steroids can help decrease associated intraocular inflammation and limit further insult to the endothelium from inflammation, steroids have no direct effect on the corneal endothelium. Reduction of raised IOP can also help the cornea to recover by decreasing further damage to the endothelium and while most IOP-lowering drops may be used it is better to avoid topical CAIs as they can adversely affect recovery of corneal endothelium. Hypertonic saline drops can help improve the symptoms until the cornea recovers but does not change the outcome. Bandage contact lenses can also be helpful in decreasing pain from ruptured epithelial bullae and recurrent corneal erosions in eyes with advanced corneal oedema. Penetrating keratoplasty (PKP) would be the definitive treatment for eyes with decompensated corneal oedema to improve the vision. More recently, Descemet's stripping endothelial keratoplasty (DSEK) is becoming more popular and has the advantage of more rapid visual recovery and less corneal astigmatism.

For hard nuclei or in cases with borderline corneal endothelial function, a dispersive ophthalmic viscosurgical device (OVD) is of benefit to protect the cornea and decrease the severity of postoperative corneal oedema. The best dispersive OVD in our experience is Viscoat (40 mg sodium chondroitin sulphate and 30 mg sodium hyaluronate). In this context the authors inject the dispersive OVD first and then place the cohesive OVD underneath it to form a soft shell as described by Arshinoff (73). Healon5 is a viscoadaptive OVD that combines cohesive with dispersive properties and therefore can be used in both routine and complex cataract surgery and provides corneal protection (74). However, caution is needed when using Healon5 as overfilling the anterior chamber can result in difficult manipulation of the anterior capsule and can also predispose to phaco burn (74). Creating a fluid space around the phaco tip before phacoemulsification should circumvent these problems. This can be performed by partially filling the anterior chamber with the OVD and injecting balanced salt solution (BSS) underneath, as described by Arshinoff in his ultimate soft-shell technique (74, 75).

7. Conclusion

Cataract surgery is the commonest surgical operation performed in the world. Perioperative complications can be reduced by training and reflective surgical practice. Adequate preventive measures, timely diagnosis and early recognition as well as appropriate management of complications can decrease ocular morbidity. Posterior capsule rupture and vitreous loss is the most common intraoperative complication and is regarded as the benchmark of the quality of a surgeons' training and experience. Anticipation of the likelihood of complications before, during and after surgery is the most important way to reduce complications.

8. References

[1] El-Hindy N, Johnston RL, Jaycock P, Eke T, Braga AJ, Tole DM, et al. The Cataract National Dataset Electronic Multi-centre Audit of 55,567 operations: anaesthetic techniques and complications. Eye (Lond) 2009 Jan; 23(1):50-55.

[2] Karampatakis V, Natsis K, Gigis P, Stangos NT. The risk of optic nerve injury in retrobulbar anesthesia: a comparative study of 35 and 40 mm retrobulbar needles in 12 cadavers. Eur J Ophthalmol 1998 Jul-Sep; 8(3):184-187.

[3] Eke T, Thompson JR. Serious complications of local anaesthesia for cataract surgery: a 1 year national survey in the United Kingdom. Br J Ophthalmol 2007 Apr; 91(4):470-475.

[4] Rodriguez-Coleman H, Spaide R. Ocular complications of needle perforations during retrobulbar and peribulbar injections. Ophthalmol Clin North Am 2001 Dec; 14(4):573-579.

[5] Reddy MK. Complications of cataract surgery. Indian J Ophthalmol 1995 Dec; 43(4):201-209.

[6] Wadood AC, Dhillon B, Singh J. Inadvertent ocular perforation and intravitreal injection of an anesthetic agent during retrobulbar injection. J Cataract Refract Surg 2002 Mar; 28(3):562-565.

[7] Jaycock P, Johnston RL, Taylor H, Adams M, Tole DM, Galloway P, et al. The Cataract National Dataset electronic multi-centre audit of 55,567 operations: updating benchmark standards of care in the United Kingdom and internationally. Eye (Lond) 2009 Jan; 23(1):38-49.

[8] Stainer L. Cataract surgery complicatins1. Intraoperative complications. Continuing education & training. On line publication; course code C-11440. 2009:23-29.

[9] Zare M, Javadi M-A, Einollahi B, Baradaran-Rafii A-R, Feizi S, Kiavash V. Risk factors for posterior capsule rupture and vitreous loss during phacoermulsification.*J Ophthalmic Vis Res*. 2009; 4(4):208-212.

[10] Johnston RL, Taylor H, Smith R, Sparrow JM. The Cataract National Dataset electronic multi-centre audit of 55,567 operations: variation in posterior capsule rupture rates between surgeons. Eye (Lond) 2010 May; 24(5):888-893.

[11] Zaidi FH, Corbett MC, Burton BJ, Bloom PA. Raising the benchmark for the 21st century--the 1000 cataract operations audit and survey: outcomes, consultant-supervised training and sourcing NHS choice. Br J Ophthalmol 2007 Jun; 91(6):731-736.

[12] Kuchle M, Schonherr U, Dieckmann U. Risk factors for capsular rupture and vitreous loss in extracapsular cataract extraction. The Erlangen Ophthalmology Group. Fortschr Ophthalmol 1989; 86(5):417-421.

[13] Marques FF, Marques DM, Osher RH, Osher JM. Fate of anterior capsule tears during cataract surgery. J Cataract Refract Surg 2006 Oct; 32(10):1638-1642.

[14] Little BC, Smith JH, Packer M. Little capsulorhexis tear-out rescue. J Cataract Refract Surg 2006 Sep; 32(9):1420-1422.

[15] Chang DF, Masket S, Miller KM, Braga-Mele R, Little BC, Mamalis N, et al. Complications of sulcus placement of single-piece acrylic intraocular lenses: recommendations for backup IOL implantation following posterior capsule rupture. J Cataract Refract Surg 2009 Aug; 35(8):1445-1458.

[16] Wagoner MD, Cox TA, Ariyasu RG, Jacobs DS, Karp CL, American Academy of Ophthalmology. Intraocular lens implantation in the absence of capsular support: a

report by the American Academy of Ophthalmology. Ophthalmology 2003 Apr; 110(4):840-859.
[17] Rogers NK, Fox PD, Noble BA, Kerr K, Inglis T. Aggressive management of an epidemic of chronic pseudophakic endophthalmitis: results and literature survey. Br J Ophthalmol 1994 Feb; 78(2):115-119.
[18] Han DP, Wisniewski SR, Wilson LA, Barza M, Vine AK, Doft BH, et al. Spectrum and susceptibilities of microbiologic isolates in the Endophthalmitis Vitrectomy Study. Am J Ophthalmol 1996 Jul; 122(1):1-17.
[19] Oxford KW, Abbott RL, Fung WE, Ellis DS. Aspergillus endophthalmitis after sutureless cataract surgery. Am J Ophthalmol 1995 Oct; 120(4):534-535.
[20] Scott IU, Flynn HW, Jr, Feuer W. Endophthalmitis after secondary intraocular lens implantation. A case-report study. Ophthalmology 1995 Dec; 102(12):1925-1931.
[21] Sallam A, Jayakumar S, Lightman S. Intraocular delivery of anti-infective drugs-bacterial, viral, fungal and parasitic. Recent Pat Antiinfect Drug Discov 2008 Jan; 3(1):53-63.
[22] Fintelmann RE, Naseri A. Prophylaxis of postoperative endophthalmitis following cataract surgery: current status and future directions. Drugs 2010 Jul 30; 70(11):1395-1409.
[23] Campochiaro PA, Lim JI. Aminoglycoside toxicity in the treatment of endophthalmitis. The Aminoglycoside Toxicity Study Group. Arch Ophthalmol 1994 Jan; 112(1):48-53.
[24] Theelen T TM. Treatment of acute bacterial endophthalmitis after cataract surgery without vitrectomy. In: Kirchhof B, Wong D. Vitreo-retinal Surgery (Essentials in Ophthalmology) 1st ed. Springer Press, 2007:70–81. Vitreo-retinal Surgery. 1st ed. ed.: Springer Press; 2007. p. 70-81.
[25] Durand M. Microbiologic factors and visual outcome in the Endophthalmitis Vitrectomy Study. Am J Ophthalmol 1997 Jul; 124(1):127-130.
[26] Winward KE, Pflugfelder SC, Flynn HW, Jr, Roussel TJ, Davis JL. Postoperative Propionibacterium endophthalmitis. Treatment strategies and long-term results. Ophthalmology 1993 Apr; 100(4):447-451.
[27] Monson MC, Mamalis N, Olson RJ. Toxic anterior segment inflammation following cataract surgery. J Cataract Refract Surg 1992 Mar; 18(2):184-189.
[28] Choi JS, Shyn KH. Development of toxic anterior segment syndrome immediately after uneventful phaco surgery. Korean J Ophthalmol 2008 Dec; 22(4):220-227.
[29] Holland SP, Morck DW, Lee TL. Update on toxic anterior segment syndrome. Curr Opin Ophthalmol 2007 Feb; 18(1):4-8.
[30] Olson RJ. TASS versus endophthalmitis. Cataract and Refractive Surgery Today Journal. 2006:51-52.
[31] Vass C, Menapace R. Computerized statistical analysis of corneal topography for the evaluation of changes in corneal shape after surgery. Am J Ophthalmol 1994 Aug 15; 118(2):177-184.
[32] Gayton JL, Sanders VN. Implanting two posterior chamber intraocular lenses in a case of microphthalmos. J Cataract Refract Surg 1993 Nov; 19(6):776-777.
[33] Gills JP, Gayton JL, Raanan M. Multiple intraocular lens implantation. In: Gills JP, Fenzel R, Martin RG, eds. Cataract Surgery: The State of the Art. Slack; Thorofare, NJ. ; 1998. p. 183-195.

[34] Gale RP, Saldana M, Johnston RL, Zuberbuhler B, McKibbin M. Benchmark standards for refractive outcomes after NHS cataract surgery. Eye (Lond) 2009 Jan; 23(1):149-152.
[35] Fenzl RE, Gills JP, 3rd, Gills JP. Piggyback intraocular lens implantation. Curr Opin Ophthalmol 2000 Feb; 11(1):73-76.
[36] Sundelin K, Sjostrand J. Posterior capsule opacification 5 years after extracapsular cataract extraction. J Cataract Refract Surg 1999 Feb; 25(2):246-250.
[37] Garston MJ. Three cases of late Cataract Surgery Complications. Rev of Optom. 2008; 145(04):85.
[38] Neuhann IM, Neuhann TF, Heimann H, Schmickler S, Gerl RH, Foerster MH. Retinal detachment after phacoemulsification in high myopia: analysis of 2356 cases. J Cataract Refract Surg 2008 Oct; 34(10):1644-1657.
[39] Duncan G. Lens cell growth and posterior capsule opacification: in vivo and in vitro observations. Br J Ophthalmol 1998 Oct; 82(10):1102-1103.
[40] Schmidbauer JM, Escobar-Gomez M, Apple DJ, Peng Q, Arthur SN, Vargas LG. Effect of haptic angulation on posterior capsule opacification in modern foldable lenses with a square, truncated optic edge. J Cataract Refract Surg 2002 Jul; 28(7):1251-1255.
[41] Auffarth GU, Newland TJ, Wesendahl TA, Apple DJ. Nd:YAG laser damage to silicone intraocular lenses confused with pigment deposits on clinical examination. Am J Ophthalmol 1994 Oct 15; 118(4):526-528.
[42] Gass JDM. Stereoscopic Atlas of Macular Diseases Diagnosis and Treatment, 4th edition. St. Louis: MO: MosbyYearbook. ; 1997. p. 478-81.
[43] Flach AJ. The incidence, pathogenesis and treatment of cystoid macular edema following cataract surgery. Trans Am Ophthalmol Soc 1998; 96:557-634.
[44] Frost NA, Sparrow JM, Strong NP, Rosenthal AR. Vitreous loss in planned extracapsular cataract extraction does lead to a poorer visual outcome. Eye (Lond) 1995; 9 (Pt 4)(Pt 4):446-451.
[45] Bonnet S. Repercussions of cataract surgery on the development of cystoid macular edema in the diabetic patient. Bull Soc Belge Ophtalmol 1995;256:127-129.
[46] Foster RE, Lowder CY, Meisler DM, Zakov ZN. Extracapsular cataract extraction and posterior chamber intraocular lens implantation in uveitis patients. Ophthalmology 1992 Aug; 99(8):1234-1241.
[47] Ray S, D'Amico DJ. Pseudophakic cystoid macular edema. Semin Ophthalmol 2002 Sep-Dec; 17(3-4):167-180.
[48] Hee MR, Puliafito CA, Wong C, Duker JS, Reichel E, Rutledge B, et al. Quantitative assessment of macular edema with optical coherence tomography. Arch Ophthalmol 1995 Aug; 113(8):1019-1029.
[49] Jaffe NS, Luscombe SM, Clayman HM, Gass JD. A fluorescein angiographic study of cystoid macular edema. Am J Ophthalmol 1981 Dec; 92(6):775-777.
[50] Heier JS, Topping TM, Baumann W, Dirks MS, Chern S. Ketorolac versus prednisolone versus combination therapy in the treatment of acute pseudophakic cystoid macular edema. Ophthalmology 2000 Nov; 107(11):2034-8; discussion 2039.
[51] Conway MD, Canakis C, Livir-Rallatos C, Peyman GA. Intravitreal triamcinolone acetonide for refractory chronic pseudophakic cystoid macular edema. J Cataract Refract Surg 2003 Jan; 29(1):27-33.
[52] Koutsandrea C, Moschos MM, Brouzas D, Loukianou E, Apostolopoulos M, Moschos M. Intraocular triamcinolone acetonide for pseudophakic cystoid macular edema:

optical coherence tomography and multifocal electroretinography study. Retina 2007 Feb; 27(2):159-164.
[53] Cox SN, Hay E, Bird AC. Treatment of chronic macular edema with acetazolamide. Arch Ophthalmol 1988 Sep; 106(9):1190-1195.
[54] Marmor MF, Maack T. Enhancement of retinal adhesion and subretinal fluid resorption by acetazolamide. Invest Ophthalmol Vis Sci 1982 Jul; 23(1):121-124.
[55] Rotsos TG, Moschos MM. Cystoid macular edema. Clin Ophthalmol 2008 Dec; 2(4):919-930.
[56] Spitzer MS, Ziemssen F, Yoeruek E, Petermeier K, Aisenbrey S, Szurman P. Efficacy of intravitreal bevacizumab in treating postoperative pseudophakic cystoid macular edema. J Cataract Refract Surg 2008 Jan; 34(1):70-75.
[57] Steinert RF, Wasson PJ. Neodymium: YAG laser anterior vitreolysis for Irvine-Gass cystoid macular edema. J Cataract Refract Surg 1989 May; 15(3):304-307.
[58] Fung WE. Vitrectomy for chronic aphakic cystoid macular edema. Results of a national, collaborative, prospective, randomized investigation. Ophthalmology 1985 Aug; 92(8):1102-1111.
[59] Rossetti L, Chaudhuri J, Dickersin K. Medical prophylaxis and treatment of cystoid macular edema after cataract surgery. The results of a meta-analysis. Ophthalmology 1998 Mar; 105(3):397-405.
[60] Hilford D, Hilford M, Mathew A, Polkinghorne PJ. Posterior vitreous detachment following cataract surgery. Eye (Lond) 2009 Jun; 23(6):1388-1392.
[61] Tielsch JM, Legro MW, Cassard SD, Schein OD, Javitt JC, Singer AE, et al. Risk factors for retinal detachment after cataract surgery. A population-based case-control study. Ophthalmology 1996 Oct; 103(10):1537-1545.
[62] Shakin EP, Carty JB, Jr. Clinical management of posterior chamber intraocular lens implants dislocated in the vitreous cavity. Ophthalmic Surg Lasers 1995 Nov-Dec; 26(6):529-534.
[63] Ninn-Pedersen K, Bauer B. Cataract patients in a defined Swedish population, 1986 to 1990. V. Postoperative retinal detachments. Arch Ophthalmol 1996 Apr; 114(4):382-386.
[64] Heimann H, Bartz-Schmidt KU, Bornfeld N, Weiss C, Hilgers RD, Foerster MH, et al. Scleral buckling versus primary vitrectomy in rhegmatogenous retinal detachment: a prospective randomized multicenter clinical study. Ophthalmology 2007 Dec; 114(12):2142-2154.
[65] Lewis H, Sanchez G. The use of perfluorocarbon liquids in the repositioning of posteriorly dislocated intraocular lenses. Ophthalmology 1993 Jul; 100(7):1055-1059.
[66] Chee SP, Jap A, Theng JT. Induced myopia associated with capsular bag distension syndrome. Ophthalmology 2001 Sep; 108(9):1517.
[67] Theng JT, Jap A, Chee SP. Capsular block syndrome: A case series. J Cataract Refract Surg 2000 Mar; 26(3):462-467.
[68] Wendrix G, Zeyen T. Late-onset capsular bag distention syndrome after cataract surgery: 2 case-reports. Bull Soc Belge Ophtalmol 2006;(301) (301):67-69.
[69] Sugiura T, Miyauchi S, Eguchi S, Obata H, Nanba H, Fujino Y, et al. Analysis of liquid accumulated in the distended capsular bag in early postoperative capsular block syndrome. J Cataract Refract Surg 2000 Mar; 26(3):420-425.

[70] Cheung D, James N. Late-onset capsular block syndrome: an occult cause of decreased vision in a 63-year-old pseudophakic Asian woman. Eye (Lond) 2001 Feb; 15(Pt 1):107-108.

[71] Capo H, Guyton DL. Ipsilateral hypertropia after cataract surgery. Ophthalmology 1996 May; 103(5):721-730.

[72] Wylie J, Henderson M, Doyle M, Hickey-Dwyer M. Persistent binocular diplopia following cataract surgery: aetiology and management. Eye (Lond) 1994; 8 (Pt 5) (Pt 5):543-546.

[73] Arshinoff SA. Dispersive-cohesive viscoelastic soft shell technique. J Cataract Refract Surg 1999 Feb; 25(2):167-173.

[74] Arshinoff SA. Using BSS with viscoadaptives in the ultimate soft-shell technique. J Cataract Refract Surg 2002 Sep; 28(9):1509-1514.

[75] Sallam A, Kashani S, Sherafat H. Healon5 and corneal wound burn during phacoemulsification. J Cataract Refract Surg 2007 May; 33(5):754; author reply 754-5.

17

Post-Operative Infections Associated with Cataract Surgery

Baseer U. Ahmad[1], Igor Estrovich[1] and Thomas Steinemann[2]
[1]*Department of Ophthalmology, Cole Eye Institute, Cleveland Clinic Foundation, Cleveland, Ohio*
[2]*Department of Ophthalmology, MetroHealth Medical Center, Cleveland, Ohio*
USA

1. Introduction

Post-operative surgical infection represents an uncommon but potentially devastating complication of cataract surgery. In the past several decades, cataract surgery has made major advances with the introduction of small-incision phacoemulsification, viscoelastic substances, and improved lens designs, as well as refinement of surgical techniques. As a result, post-operative care has become simpler and visual recovery has become much faster. Due to these factors, the incidence of post-operative infectious complications has also generally declined. In fact, the incidence of post-operative endophthalmitis has decreased since the mid-1900s from 0.5% to 0.04%-0.41% in the early 21st century (Kattan, et al, Ravindran, et al). In the past decade, however, these rates appear to have increased due to the greater use of clear corneal incision techniques. As such, it is fundamentally important for the cataract surgeon to be familiar with recognition, etiology, and management of post-operative endophthalmitis.

2. Epidemiology

By most accounts, the incidence of post-operative endophthalmitis is consistently less than 1 in 1000 cases. There appears to be little geographic variability in the incidence of acute post-operative endophthalmitis. When comparing the largest incidence studies of respective countries, the risk in developed countries such as the United States (0.09%), Canada (0.043%), and Great Britain (0.099%) is comparable to the risk in less developed countries like India (0.09%) and Greece (0.08%) (Kalpadakis, et al, Kattan, et al, Lloyd&Braga-Mele, Mollan, et al, Ravindran, et al).

3. Clinical presentation

Post-operative infections related to cataract surgery primarily include endophthalmitis and corneal suture infection. Endophthalmitis may present acutely or in a more chronic form, depending on the causative organism. Symptoms of endophthalmitis include decreased vision, mild to severe ocular pain, photophobia, and floaters. The characteristic finding in endophthalmitis is vitreous inflammation, but it is often accompanied by other signs including anterior chamber cell and flare, hypopyon, ciliary injection, and corneal edema.

Chronic cases may be more indolent with smoldering anterior chamber reaction, vitritis, and no significant external inflammation or pain. If the source of infection is suture-related, focal corneal infiltrate, anterior chamber reaction, and hypopyon may be early signs of a suture abscess and may develop into endophthalmitis if not treated promptly adequately.

4. Etiology

Using techniques of molecular identification, it has been demonstrated that an organism isolated from the vitreous was genetically indistinguishable from an isolate recovered from the patient's eyelid, conjunctiva, or nose in over 80% of cases. Speaker et al found an association between the external bacterial flora and the bacteria isolated from vitrectomy specimens in 82% of the patients with postoperative endophthalmitis (Speaker, et al). Similarly, the Endophthalmitis Vitrectomy Study (EVS) group found that the intraocular isolates were indistinguishable from conjunctival and lid specimens in 68% of the bacterial postoperative endophthalmitis cases. These and other similar series have supported the hypothesis that most cases of post-surgical endophthalmitis are caused by introduction of microorganisms from the conjunctiva and eyelid during operative manipulation and during the perioperative period.

However, intraocular contamination appears to be relatively common after uneventful cataract surgery; the rate of culture positivity in anterior chamber aspirate ranges from 0-46% and has shown that bacteria routinely enter the anterior chamber during cataract surgery (Dickey, et al, Leong, et al, Sherwood, et al, Srinivasan, et al). They may be carried into the eye by irrigation or may adhere to the intraocular lens or instruments as they are inserted through the incision. It is thought that the host reaction can overcome and prevent a bacterial infection in its initial phases as evidenced by the discrepancy between the high incidence of aqueous humor contamination and and the low incidence of postoperative endophthalmitis. The integrity of the lens capsule may also play a role in the prevention of infection (Dickey, et al).

Another potential cause of post-operative infection is the chronic colonization or adherence of bacteria to biomaterial. This tendency of relatively easy adherence can lead the development of a biofilm on the surface of the intraocular lens. Vafidis et al conducted a study in which an intraocular lens was placed across the conjunctival flap and section for 5 seconds during cataract surgery, and this resulted in a bacterial contamination rate of 26%, demonstrating the ability of bacteria (mainly *S. epidermidis*, 87%) to adhere instantaneously to intraocular lenses (Vafidis, et al). *Propionibacterium acnes* has also been commonly reported to form biofilms in orthopedic settings upon hardware (Holmberg, et al), and this bears similarity to the white, film-like deposits on intraocular lens surfaces that have been described in chronic endophthalmitis cases.

A rare category of post-operative surgical infection associated with cataract surgery is represented by suture complications. These have been described as early as weeks and as late as years after cataract surgery. Such abscesses can occur if the knots are unburied, broken, exposed, or loosely placed. Such sutures can accumulate mucus and act as a wick allowing a route for bacteria to penetrate the eye. Of note, another rare etiology described by a small case series has been of scleral flap necrosis and infectious endophthalmitis after cataract surgery, in which the scleral tunnels may have acted as abscess cavities (Ormerod, et al).

From a microbial standpoint, acute cases (occurring <6 weeks) are most commonly caused by gram-positive bacteria, of which coagulase-negative Staphylococcus (CoNS) is most often encountered (Table 1) (Kodjikian, et al). Chronic post-operative endophthalmitis (occurring >6 weeks) is usually due to lower virulence microorganisms, particularly *P. acnes* (Table 2)

(Al-Mezaine, et al, Haapala, et al). Suture-related infection may occur at any time, but the inoculating organisms generally resemble those in acute post-surgical cases and case reports have described *Streptococcus pneumoniae, staphylococcus aureus,* and *staphylococcus epidermidis* growth from positive cultures.

Endophthalmitis-Vitrectomy Study (1995, n=420)		Endophthalmitis National Survey, France (2009, n=95)	
No growth	17.9%	No growth	52.6%
Equivocal growth	12.9%	Not precisely identified	3.1%
Gram +ve, coagulase -ve	46.9%	Coagulase -ve Staphylococcus	27.4%
Other Gram +ve	15.5%	Staphylococcus aureus	6.3%
		Streptococcus	7.4%
Gram -ve	4.7%	Gram -ve	3.2%
Polymicrobials	3.8%		

Table 1. Etiology of Acute Endophthalmitis

Haapala, et al (2005, n=8)		Al-Mezaine, et al (2009, n=17)	
Propionibacterium acnes	75%	Propionibacterium acnes	41.2%
S. epidermidis	12.5%	Coagulase -ve Staphylococcus	17.6%
Other Gram -ve	12.5%	Polymicrobial	17.6%
		Fungal infection	17.6%
		Other Gram -ve	6%

Table 2. Etiology of delayed-onset, culture proven endophthalmitis

5. Treatment

The landmark study in current treatment of acute postcataract endophmitis was the Endophthalmitis Vitrectomy Study (EVS) , a multicenter prospective randomized study that compared the effectiveness of immediate vitrectomy to vitreous tap with injection of intravitreal anbiotics.

In the EVS, patients with clinical evidence of acute postoperative endophthalmitis were randomly assigned to emergent vitreous tap or vitrectomy, with both groups receiving injection of intravitreal antibiotics (0.4 mg amikacin and 1.0 mg vancomycin). Patients were also given subconjunctival injections of antibiotics (25 mg vancomycin, 100 mg ceftazidime) and steroid (6 mg dexamethasone phosphate), topical fortified antibiotics (50 mg/ml vancomycin and 20 mg/ml amikacin) and steroid (prednisolone acetate), as well as oral steroids (prednisone 30 mg bid x 5-10 days). Patients were also randomly assigned to receive systemic IV antibiotics (2 g ceftazidime IV Q8h and 7.5 mg/kg amikacin IV followed by 6 mg/kg Q12h) or no systemic antibiotics. Intravitreal steroids were not used.

Results and conclusions of the EVS included:

i. On average, signs and symptoms occurred 6 days after surgery (75% presented within 2 weeks of surgery).
ii. Positive cultures were obtained in 69%, of which 94% were Gram positive bacteria.
iii. Intravenous antibiotics were of no benefit and do not improve final outcome.
iv. Immediate vitrectomy had significant benefits only when patients presented with light perception vision or worse. Otherwise, emergent treatment with tap and intravitreal anbiotics should be given if presenting vision is better than light perception.

v. Roughly half of patients in both the tap and vitrectomy groups achieved final visual acuity of 20/40 or better (52.3% versus 53.7% respectively).

As a result of the EVS, acute endophthalmitis with vision better than light perception is usually treated with an anterior chamber/vitreous tap and intravitreal injection of vancomycin for Gram positive coverage, and amikacin or ceftazidime for Gram negative coverage.

For chronic endophthalmitis, no clear treatment strategies have been established. Propionibacterium acnes, the major causative organism, often forms capsular plaques and therapy with intravitreal antibiotics alone is associated with very high rates of recurrence. Instead, pars-plana vitrecomy with capsulectomy appears to be the most effective strategy based on studies involving relative large numbers of patients with delayed-onset P. acnes endopthalmitis (Aldave, et al, Clark, et al). Fungal etiologies are much rarer, more difficult to manage, and often treated with varying success using intravitreal antifungals such as amphotericin or voriconazole.

For suture-related infections, topical fortified antibiotic therapy may be adequate if the presentation is mild and if treated early in the course when the infection is confined to the cornea and anterior chamber. Appropriate initial therapy may include vancomycin (25-50 mg/ml) for gram-positive organisms, in combination with ceftazidime (50 mg/ml) or tobramycin (15 mg/ml) as frequently as every hour depending on the severity of presentation. In any suspected case of endophthalmitis or if progression is noted, early intravitreal antibiotics should be administered.

6. Recent trends and advice on prevention

Interestingly, the large variability in institutional methods such as sterilization of surgical instruments and patient flow in surgical suites seems to minimally impact the rate of infection. For instance, at the Aravind Eye Hospital in India, surgical instruments are sterilized using a short-cycle method, the surgeon alternates between two operating table in the same operating room, and uses the same sterile gloves for multiple cases. These studies collectively suggest that increasing facility efficiency and optimizing patient flow does not come at the expense of outcomes.

Preoperatively, recognition of blepharitis or predisposing risk factors is important. Case reports have described possibly inadequately treated blepharitis and rosacea associated with cases of endophthalmitis despite the use of good surgical technique. It is therefore prudent to treat significant cases of blepharitis, rosacea, and related disorders prior to surgery.

During the immediate perioperative period, commonly employed methods to reduce the risk of endophthalmitis include placing povidone-iodine 5% drops in the conjunctival sac as part of the preoperative preparation of the eye, using adhesive drapes to isolate the lashes and lid margins from the operative field, and maintaining appropriate intraoperative aseptic technique (Ciulla, et al, Ou&Ta). The effectiveness of perioperative topical antibiotics has been controversial. Topical therapy for 3 days prior to surgery can reduce bacterial counts but has not been shown to reduce the incidence of infection. In 2006, a preliminary report from a large European prospective multicenter randomized clinical trial indicated that injection of 1 mg cefuroxime into the anterior chamber at the conclusion of cataract surgery can reduce the incidence of endophthalmitis fivefold . The validity of generalizing these results to all cataract procedures awaits publication of the final report. The use of vancomycin in infusion fluid during phacoemulsification has been proposed but remains controversial (Ciulla, et al, Ou&Ta). Given the difficulty of obtaining preservative-free antibiotics that are commercially available in doses appropriate for intracameral prophylaxis, surgeons need to weigh these results against the risk of dilutional errors or preservative toxicity.

Paradoxically, recent surgical advances such as the use of sutureless clear corneal incisions and sutureless surgery have shown an increase in rates of endophthalmitis over the past decade (Lundstrom, et al, Taban, et al). While this small incidence represents a modest risk for individuals undergoing cataract extraction, the global volume of the most common surgery worldwide magnifies the burden of this risk. Meticulous attention to watertight incision closure is critical in the prevention of endophthalmitis, particularly when clear corneal incisions are employed.

Finally, corneal sutures should be removed as soon as possible after wound integrity has been restored, and may be done at the one week post-operative visit. The will help ensure that that even an adequate suture does not break or become loose over time and act as a nidus of infection even years later.

While cataract surgery remains one of the most successful and safe procedures in ophthalmology, rare but serious infectious complications can arise. Proper preoperative preparation, sterile perioperative surgical technique, proper wound construction, post-operative removal of sutures, vigilance of early signs of infection, and aggressive early treatment of infection are keys to prevention of devastating post-surgical infections.

7. Disclaimer

The authors declare that they have no conflicts of interest or proprietary interests to disclose.

8. References

Results of the Endophthalmitis Vitrectomy Study. A randomized trial of immediate vitrectomy and of intravenous antibiotics for the treatment of postoperative bacterial endophthalmitis. Endophthalmitis Vitrectomy Study Group. Arch Ophthalmol, 1995. 113(12): p. 1479-96.

Prophylaxis of postoperative endophthalmitis following cataract surgery: results of the ESCRS multicenter study and identification of risk factors. J Cataract Refract Surg, 2007. 33(6): p. 978-88.

Al-Mezaine, H.S., A. Al-Assiri &A.A. Al-Rajhi, Incidence, clinical features, causative organisms, and visual outcomes of delayed-onset pseudophakic endophthalmitis. Eur J Ophthalmol, 2009. 19(5): p. 804-11.

Aldave, A.J., J.D. Stein, V.A. Deramo, G.K. Shah, D.H. Fischer, et al., Treatment strategies for postoperative Propionibacterium acnes endophthalmitis. Ophthalmology, 1999. 106(12): p. 2395-401.

Ciulla, T.A., M.B. Starr &S. Masket, Bacterial endophthalmitis prophylaxis for cataract surgery: an evidence-based update. Ophthalmology, 2002. 109(1): p. 13-24.

Clark, W.L., P.K. Kaiser, H.W. Flynn, Jr., A. Belfort, D. Miller, et al., Treatment strategies and visual acuity outcomes in chronic postoperative Propionibacterium acnes endophthalmitis. Ophthalmology, 1999. 106(9): p. 1665-70.

Dickey, J.B., K.D. Thompson &W.M. Jay, Anterior chamber aspirate cultures after uncomplicated cataract surgery. Am J Ophthalmol, 1991. 112(3): p. 278-82.

Haapala, T.T., L. Nelimarkka, J.M. Saari, V. Ahola &K.M. Saari, Endophthalmitis following cataract surgery in southwest Finland from 1987 to 2000. Graefes Arch Clin Exp Ophthalmol, 2005. 243(10): p. 1010-7.

Holmberg, A., R. Lood, M. Morgelin, B. Soderquist, E. Holst, et al., Biofilm formation by Propionibacterium acnes is a characteristic of invasive isolates. Clin Microbiol Infect, 2009. 15(8): p. 787-95.

Kalpadakis, P., I. Tsinopoulos, G. Rudolph, K. Schebitz &S.J. Froehlich, A comparison of endophthalmitis after phacoemulsification or extracapsular cataract extraction in a socio-economically deprived environment: a retrospective analysis of 2446 patients. Eur J Ophthalmol, 2002. 12(5): p. 395-400.

Kattan, H.M., H.W. Flynn, Jr., S.C. Pflugfelder, C. Robertson &R.K. Forster, Nosocomial endophthalmitis survey. Current incidence of infection after intraocular surgery. Ophthalmology, 1991. 98(2): p. 227-38.

Kodjikian, L., A. Salvanet-Bouccara, S. Grillon, F. Forestier, J.L. Seegmuller, et al., Postcataract acute endophthalmitis in France: national prospective survey. J Cataract Refract Surg, 2009. 35(1): p. 89-97.

Leong, J.K., R. Shah, P.J. McCluskey, R.A. Benn &R.F. Taylor, Bacterial contamination of the anterior chamber during phacoemulsification cataract surgery. J Cataract Refract Surg, 2002. 28(5): p. 826-33.

Lloyd, J.C. &R. Braga-Mele, Incidence of postoperative endophthalmitis in a high-volume cataract surgicentre in Canada. Can J Ophthalmol, 2009. 44(3): p. 288-92.

Lundstrom, M., G. Wejde, U. Stenevi, W. Thorburn &P. Montan, Endophthalmitis after cataract surgery: a nationwide prospective study evaluating incidence in relation to incision type and location. Ophthalmology, 2007. 114(5): p. 866-70.

Mollan, S.P., A. Gao, A. Lockwood, O.M. Durrani &L. Butler, Postcataract endophthalmitis: incidence and microbial isolates in a United Kingdom region from 1996 through 2004. J Cataract Refract Surg, 2007. 33(2): p. 265-8.

Ormerod, L.D., J.E. Puklin, J.G. McHenry &M.L. McDermott, Scleral flap necrosis and infectious endophthalmitis after cataract surgery with a scleral tunnel incision. Ophthalmology, 1993. 100(2): p. 159-63.

Ou, J.I. &C.N. Ta, Endophthalmitis prophylaxis. Ophthalmol Clin North Am, 2006. 19(4): p. 449-56.

Ravindran, R.D., R. Venkatesh, D.F. Chang, S. Sengupta, J. Gyatsho, et al., Incidence of post-cataract endophthalmitis at Aravind Eye Hospital: outcomes of more than 42,000 consecutive cases using standardized sterilization and prophylaxis protocols. J Cataract Refract Surg, 2009. 35(4): p. 629-36.

Sherwood, D.R., W.J. Rich, J.S. Jacob, R.J. Hart &Y.L. Fairchild, Bacterial contamination of intraocular and extraocular fluids during extracapsular cataract extraction. Eye (Lond), 1989. 3 (Pt 3): p. 308-12.

Speaker, M.G., F.A. Milch, M.K. Shah, W. Eisner &B.N. Kreiswirth, Role of external bacterial flora in the pathogenesis of acute postoperative endophthalmitis. Ophthalmology, 1991. 98(5): p. 639-49; discussion 650.

Srinivasan, R., S. Tiroumal, R. Kanungo &M.K. Natarajan, Microbial contamination of the anterior chamber during phacoemulsification. J Cataract Refract Surg, 2002. 28(12): p. 2173-6.

Taban, M., A. Behrens, R.L. Newcomb, M.Y. Nobe, G. Saedi, et al., Acute endophthalmitis following cataract surgery: a systematic review of the literature. Arch Ophthalmol, 2005. 123(5): p. 613-20.

Vafidis, G.C., R.J. Marsh &A.R. Stacey, Bacterial contamination of intraocular lens surgery. Br J Ophthalmol, 1984. 68(8): p. 520-3.

18

Early Post-Operative Complications in Cataract Surgery

Emin Kurt[1,*] and Hüseyin Mayalı[2]
[1]Department of Ophthalmology, Celal Bayar University, Manisa,
[2]Eye Clinic, Buca Gynaecology and Paediatric Hospital, İzmir,
Turkey

1. Introduction

To date a number of techniques have been used for cataract surgery. However phacoemulsification is the most common method. Other methods such as intra- and extracapsular cataract extraction, mini-nuc, phacosection, sandwich and phaconit have also been used by many surgeons. Over the years, the techniques of cataract surgery have evolved into a safe and successful procedure for visual rehabilitation. The incidence of most complications has significantly decreased with better instrumentation and affordable high quality intraocular lens implants. Better pre-operative evaluation has helped. This has also reduced the number of poor results owing to the presence of other eye diseases in a patient. However some risk factors are intrinsic to the patient and, short of avoiding surgery altogether, very little can be done to eliminate them. In the event of surgery, high-risk cases should be operated on in an appropriate setting, by a surgeon who has the right level of experience. Although cataract surgery is safe for the majority of patients, some complications that involve the anterior and the posterior segment can occur. Cataract surgery complications can be divided into intraoperative complications, and postoperative complications. These complications are anaesthesia-related complications, posterior capsular rupture and vitreous loss, vitreous prolapse, expulsive haemorrhage, Descemet's membrane detachment, intraocular haemorrhage, wound malapposition, shallow anterior chamber, iris prolapse, infectious endophthalmitis, corneal oedema, dropped nucleus or retained nuclear fragments, suture-induced astigmatism, cystoid macular oedema, retinal detachment, posterior capsule opacification, and bullous keratopathy. The most important of these complications are often associated with posterior capsular rupture and infectious endophthalmitis. The incidence of posterior capsule tear during cataract surgery ranges from 0.2% to 16.0%. A higher incidence of posterior capsule tear and vitreous loss is associated with pseudoexfoliation, diabetes mellitus, trauma, hard or brunescent nuclei, and white cataract. Postoperative endophthalmitis remains a devastating outcome after cataract surgery, despite improved methods of prophylaxis, surgical technique, and treatment. This complication causes significant morbidity and distress and often severe visual impairment or blindness. The reported incidence of endophthalmitis after cataract surgery varies considerably around the world. Occurring about once every 500 operations worldwide, the relatively low incidence of endophthalmitis makes it

* Corresponding Author

difficult to identify the risk factors clearly. If the posterior capsule tear causes occur vitreous loss and dropped fragments or nucleus drop it can lead to long-standing uveitis, vitritis, cystoid macular oedema, and secondary glaucoma. In the late period it is important to be vigilant in terms of posterior capsular opacification and retinal detachment. In this review, the diagnosis, treatment and prevention of early postoperative complications of cataract surgery are discussed. Early recognition and prompt treatment of these problems can minimize the risk of ocular morbidity.

2. Endophthalmitis

Infectious endophthalmitis following cataract surgery is still a devastating condition, despite major improvements in surgical techniques in the last decades. Most series report on an incidence rate ranging from 0.05% to 0.4% in different studies worldwide (Melo et al., 2010; Taban et al., 2005).

Infectious endophthalmitis is defined as infection causing severe inflammation involving both the anterior and posterior segments of the eye after intraocular surgery. It is a serious intraocular inflammatory condition that also results in infection of the vitreous cavity (Lemley & Han, 2007). Although it is rare, it has the potential to have a severe impact on vision and may even lead to a loss of the eye. Fortunately a number of factors including increased knowledge of the pathogenesis of the condition, improved surgical and diagnostic techniques, and a wider choice of management options have led to a decrease in the incidence of post-surgical cases.

Typically, postoperative endophthalmitis is caused by the peri-operative introduction of microbial organisms into the eye. The primary source of this intraocular infection is considered to be bacteria from the patient's ocular cornea, conjunctiva, lacrimal glands, blepharitis, and extraocular muscles (Maguire, 2008). However, contamination of sterilized instruments, disposable supplies, prepared solutions, the surgical field, or the intraocular lens, have been reported. Epidemic clusters of endophthalmitis have resulted from these types of external contaminations (Cruciani et al., 1998; Gibb et al., 2006).

The bacteria most frequently isolated are Gram-positive coagulase-negative cocci which account for 70% of culture-positive cases. Gram-negative bacteria account for just 6% of culture-positive cases; however, an infection with these bacteria, particularly with Pseudomonas aeruginosa, can lead to a devastating visual outcome (Eifring et al., 2003; Mamalis et al., 2002).

Once organisms gain access to the vitreous cavity, overwhelming inflammation is likely to occur, making rapid recognition, diagnosis and treatment critical in optimizing final outcomes. Although most cases of postoperative endophthalmitis occur within 6 weeks of surgery, infections seen in high-risk patients or infections caused by slow-growing organisms may occur months or years after the procedure (Cruciani et al., 1998; Eifrig et al., 2002; Taban et al., 2005).

The most common risk factors are posterior capsular rupture, retained lens material, the specific surgical procedure, wound leak and less experienced surgeons. Published studies have demonstrated an increased risk of endophthalmitis after placement of a secondary intraocular lens, possibly due to prolonged surgical time or ocular manipulation (Eifrig et al., 2002). Prolene haptic sutures have also been implicated as a possible risk factor. Other factors that are more controversial include increased patient age, corneal incision site and wound configuration (Chan et al., 2010).

Cataract patients with an acute postoperative form of infectious endophthalmitis may present as early as the day after surgery or up to two weeks later. Common clinical ocular associations include injection, conjunctival chemosis, purulent discharge, corneal oedema, anterior chamber cell and flare reaction, hypopyon, vitreous opacification, choroidal swelling, periphlebitis, and retinal haemorrhages. Adnexal swelling may also be present. Symptoms classically include pain and decreased vision (Kamalarajah et al., 2004; Kressloff et al., 1998; Lemley & Han, 2007; Mamalis et al., 2002). The inflammation seen is significantly greater than that otherwise expected post cataract surgery (Kamalarajah et al., 2004).

Taking appropriate measures to prevent endophthalmitis is crucial. Many different factors in cataract surgery have been investigated extensively for their role as a risk factor for endophthalmitis. Currently, the three most accepted methods of reducing the risk are to use an appropriate antiseptic solution (povidone-iodine), adequate draping of the surgical field to exclude the eyelashes and the use of intracameral antibiotics, such as cefuroxime at the conclusion of surgery (Chan et al., 2010).

A definitive approach to treatment of postoperative endophthalmitis is not uniformly agreed upon by many vitreoretinal surgeons. Therapeutics generally involves administration of intravitreal broad spectrum antibiotics with associated vitreous tap/biopsy (VTB) or pars plana vitrectomy (PPV). The choice of topical, peri-ocular, and even systemic antibiotics is increasingly controversial compared with 10 years ago (Maguire, 2008).

Most cases are caused by Gram-positive and Gram-negative micro-organisms. The antibiotics selected should cover the broad range of Gram-positive and Gram-negative organisms causing clinical endophthalmitis. Antibiotics can be delivered into the eye by several routes, including direct intraocular injection, systemic administration, peri-ocular injection, and topical application (Table 1). Out of all the available antimicrobial agents evaluated for intraocular injection only a few are used regularly in clinical practice. Intraocular vancomycin in combination with an aminoglycoside has been a commonly used regimen for the initial empiric treatment of presumed bacterial endophthalmitis (Flynn et al., 1991).

An alternative to the aminoglycosides for coverage of Gram-negative organisms is the use of intraocular ceftazidime, a third-generation cephalosporin (Campochiaro & Green, 1992; Jay et al., 1987; Stonecipher et al., 1991). These antibiotic combinations will theoretically provide broad coverage for nearly all of the organisms causing bacterial endophthalmitis (Stonecipher et al., 1991).

Intravitreal administration is used in order to deliver a high concentration of antibiotic directly in the eye. However, repetitive injections of intraocular antibiotics may cause significant retinal toxicity. In a rabbit model, eyes treated with a second or third intraocular vancomycin/aminoglycoside injection at 48-hour intervals showed progressive toxicity (Oum et al., 1989). Topical and subconjunctival antibiotics are often prescribed in addition to intravitreal antibiotics in order to increase the concentration of antibiotics within the anterior segment of the eye. Aqueous and vitreous solution samples are usually taken and sent to the laboratory for cultures. Vitreous samples are more likely to yield positive cultures. A smear placed on a glass slide and stained with a variety of chemicals provides a rapid result but it is not as sensitive or specific as results obtained from culture growth on different types of media. However, the latter can take up to a fortnight and therefore broad spectrum treatment must be provided until this is done (Barza et al., 1997).

Owing to concern as to whether intraocular antibiotics with or without vitrectomy are sufficient to treat infectious endophthalmitis, local ocular therapy is commonly supplemented with systemic antibiotics. Intraocular inflammation and/or performing a PPV alter the blood-retina barrier in a manner that allows better intravitreal penetration of systemically administered antibiotics (Meredith, 1993).

PPV may be necessary depending on level of vision. As a result of the EVS it is generally felt that in patients with light perception only or worse vision, PPV should be performed as the results of the study showed that these patients had a significantly better outcome compared with other modes of treatment (Endophthalmitis Vitrectomy Study Group [EVSG], 1995). The question arises whether PPV should be applied more frequently to patients presenting with vision of hand movements (HM) or better (Altan et al., 2009). The advantage of this procedure is that it enables the removal of a significant amount of the infecting organism, exo- and endotoxins, inflammatory agents, and any opacities and vitreous membranes that could result in retinal detachment (EVSG, 1995; Lemley & Han, 2007; Maguire, 2008).

Detractors of this approach have pointed to potential complications of surgery in severely inflamed eyes with poor visibility, a more rapid turnover of intravitreal antibiotics and the risks of delayed therapy (Maguire, 2008). Vitreal samples can easily be taken at the same time and subsequent intravitreal antibiotic distribution is greatly improved. However, significant inflammation may make visualisation difficult when performing the vitrectomy. Patients may also require multiple PPV procedures (Lemley & Han, 2007).

Intravenous Abs		
	Ceftazidime	2 g q 8 h (ciprofloxacin 750 p.o. bid)[a]
	Amikacin	6.0 mg/kg 12 h
Intravitreal Abs		
	Vancomycin	1.0 mg
	Amikacin	0.4 mg
Subconjunctival Abs		
	Vancomycin	25mg in 0.5 cc
	Ceftazidime	100mg in 0.5 cc
	Dexamethasone	6.0mg
Topical Abs		
	Vancomycin	50 mg/ml gtts q h
	Amikacin	20 mg/ml gtts q h
Steroids		
	Prednisone	30mg BID for 5–10 days

Abbreviations: Abs, antibiotics; bid, twice a day.
[a]In penicillin allergic patients.

Table 1. Standard pharmacological agents utilized in the Endophthalmitis Vitrectomy Study

3. Dropped nucleus

Loss of nuclear material into the vitreous cavity carries a major risk of loss of sight. This complicates 0.1% to 1% of cases of cataract extractions (Figure 1.) (Hoeve & Stilma, 2010). It can happen in even experienced hands, and can be a worry as corrective action requires intervention in the posterior segment (Lu et al., 1999). Removing a dropped nucleus or even nuclear fragments is essential as it can either lead to long-standing uveitis, vitritis, cystoid macular oedema, and secondary glaucoma (Kaputsa et al., 1996; Lu et al., 1999).

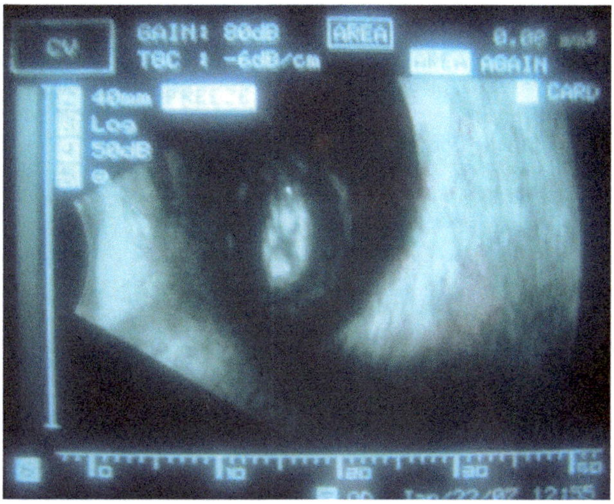

Fig. 1. Dropped nucleus

Clinical studies implicate posterior extension of breaks in the capsulorrhexis as a common cause of this complication. Congenital posterior polar cataract, which predisposes to posterior capsular dehiscence, is another risk factor for dropped nucleus (Kim & Miller, 2002). A higher incidence of posterior capsule tear and vitreous loss is associated with pseudoexfoliation, diabetes mellitus, trauma, hard or brunescent nuclei, and white cataract (Browning & Cobo, 1985; Guzek et al., 1987).

Management of these tears is especially difficult when the nucleus begins to drop into the vitreous. Rapid intervention is crucial to prevent the nucleus from dropping completely into the posterior vitreous. Manoeuvres performed through the anterior segment to retrieve the nuclear fragments can worsen the situation. Vitreous will prolapse through the surgical incision and, as a consequence, the partially dropped nuclear fragments might sink further back. Moreover, these manoeuvres can lead to serious late posterior segment complications and the risk for peripheral tears and retinal detachment (Gilliland et al., 1992; Lambrou & Stewart, 1992).

A dropped nucleus can lead to various problems that require additional treatment (Horiguchi et al., 2003). The surgeon should be familiar with the option of temporary aphakia or a sulcul lens and might also consider views of local surgeons performing PPV. Outcomes are typically excellent when there is minimal vitreous manipulation and traction and the residual lens material is removed in a controlled fashion by three-port PPV with phacofragmentation. It is recommended that PPV be performed within one to two weeks after cataract extraction (Hoeve & Stilma, 2010).

4. Raised intraocular pressure

Elevated intraocular pressure is a common problem following cataract surgery. An increase in intraocular pressure frequently occurs after otherwise uneventful phacoemulsification cataract surgery. The exact mechanism responsible for the acute rise in intraocular pressure after phacoemulsification is not known but is probably multifactorial (Unal & Yücel, 2008). The first report of ocular hypertension one day after cataract surgery was documented by Gormaz in 1962 (Gormaz, 1962).

In most patients, postoperative increase in intraocular pressure following cataract surgery is transient and benign (Tranos et al., 2004). Nearly all patients' pressures returned to baseline with or without treatment. Some individuals, however, may experience pain, corneal oedema, glaucomatous nerve damage, or anterior ischemic optic neuropathy (Ermis et al., 2005).

Elevated pressure is the most frequent postoperative complication demanding treatment following phacoemulsification (Hildebrand et al., 2003). As many as 18% to 45% of patients may experience an intraocular pressure greater than 28 mm Hg following phacoemulsification, but most pressures will return to normal by 24 hours postoperatively (Tranos et al., 2004). The peaks most commonly occur 8 to 12 hours after surgery, and only 1.3% to 10.0% of cases record an intraocular pressure higher than 30 mm Hg 24 hours postoperatively. After uneventful phacoemulsification in eyes without glaucoma, however, intraocular pressure spikes may reach 68 mm Hg (Hildebrand et al., 2003). The causes of the elevated intraocular pressure are likely multifactorial (Table 2). Causes of elevated intraocular pressure are numerous (Bomer et al., 1995; Hildebrand et al., 2003; Tanaka et al., 1997; Thorofare & Slack, 2007).

Retained lens debris
Retained viscoelastic
Hyphaema or red blood cells
Watertight wound closure
Use of corneoscleral sutures vs. non-sutured incision
Steroid response (3 to 6 weeks after surgery)
Iris pigment release
Pre-existing glaucoma
Degree of surgical trauma
Secluded/occluded pupil with iris bombe
Uveitis or inflammatory cells
Expulsive haemorrhage
Aqueous misdirection
Epithelial down growth

Table 2. Causes of increased intraocular pressure following cataract surgery

It is well accepted that retained viscoelastic material inhibits aqueous outflow through the trabecular meshwork resulting in a higher incidence and degree of postoperative increase in intraocular pressure (Tanaka et al., 1997). Higher molecular weight viscoelastics have been shown to result in a higher rise in post-operative intraocular pressure (Borazan et al., 2007).

When considering the various causes of pressure elevation, topical steroids are often suspected. However, steroids in the immediate postoperative period are rarely a cause of pressure rise. Typically, a steroid-induced glaucoma requires 3 to 6 weeks of continuous use to elicit an intraocular pressure response (Thorofare & Slack, 2007).

The rise in intraocular pressure in the latter group will settle after discontinuation of topical steroids but those in the former group will often require anti-glaucoma medication or even surgery in more extreme cases (Chan et al., 2010). Surgical trauma, watertight wound closure, retained lenticular debris, the release of iris pigment, hyphaema, and inflammation are also thought to contribute to elevations in intraocular pressure (Hildebrand et al., 2003).

Patients at risk for a known increase in intraocular pressure and vision loss should be pretreated. There are several classes of drugs used to treat postoperative increases in intraocular pressure including: oral and topical carbonic anhydrase inhibitors (acetazolamide, brinzolamide, dorzolamide, and methazolamide), prostaglandin analogues (latanoprost, bimatoprost, and travoprost), alpha agonists (apraclonidine and brimonidine), beta blockers (timolol and levobunolol), and miotics (intracameral carbachol, pilocarpine, and intracameral acetylcholine). Although several drugs lower intraocular pressure after cataract surgery, none of them consistently prevents pressure increases from occurring (Browning et al., 2002; Byrd & Singh, 1998).

5. Iris prolapse

Iris prolapse can result from inadequate wound closure, accidental trauma, or raised intraocular pressure. Iris prolapse is extremely rare following small incision surgery but may occur after extracapsular cataract extraction (Figure 2) (Reddy, 1995). Complications include defective wound healing, chronic anterior uveitis, excessive astigmatism, endophthalmitis, cystoid macular oedema and epithelial ingrowth (Wright et al., 1988). Peribulbar or retrobulbar anaesthesia is necessary for iris manipulation. Treatment depends on the time interval between cataract surgery and identification of the prolapse. In cases of iris prolapse of less than 48 hours duration, the iris tissue can be reposited. If however, the prolapse is of longer duration, the risk of infection mandates that the prolapsed section of iris is excised (Byrd & Singh, 1998).

6. Corneal oedema

Postoperative corneal oedema can be localized or diffuse. Postoperative localized stromal and/or epithelial oedema (Figure 3), especially in the half of the cornea near the main section indicates intraoperative trauma. Factors that predispose to corneal oedema following cataract surgery include the following: intraoperative mechanical endothelial trauma, prior endothelial disease or cell loss, excessive postoperative inflammation, and prolonged postoperative elevation of intraocular pressure (Reddy, 1995).

Raised intraocular pressure manifests as diffuse microcystic epithelial oedema, which is best visualized by retro-illumination. Postoperative corneal stromal oedema could also indicate pre-existing endothelial pathology as in Fuchs' endothelial dystrophy. Pre-operatively patients should be carefully examined for evidence of Fuchs' dystrophy or other conditions that produce a low endothelial cell count (Reddy, 1995; Wright et al., 1988; Yanoff & Duker, 2004).

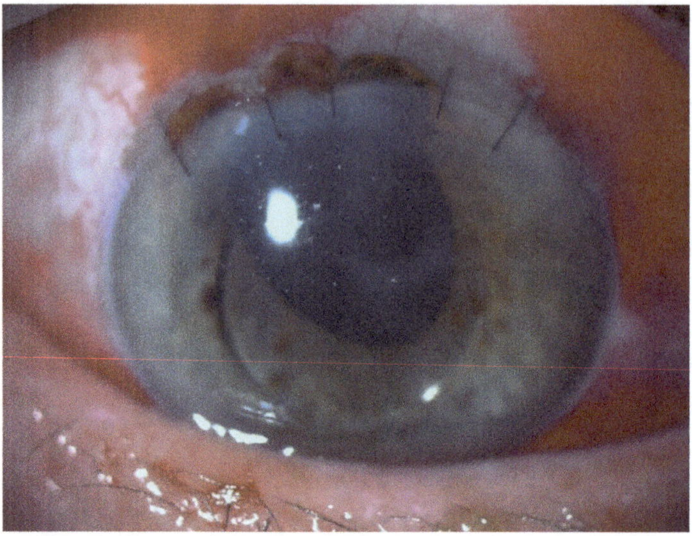

Fig. 2. Iris Prolapse (courtesy of Mehmet Baykara, Uludağ University, Bursa)

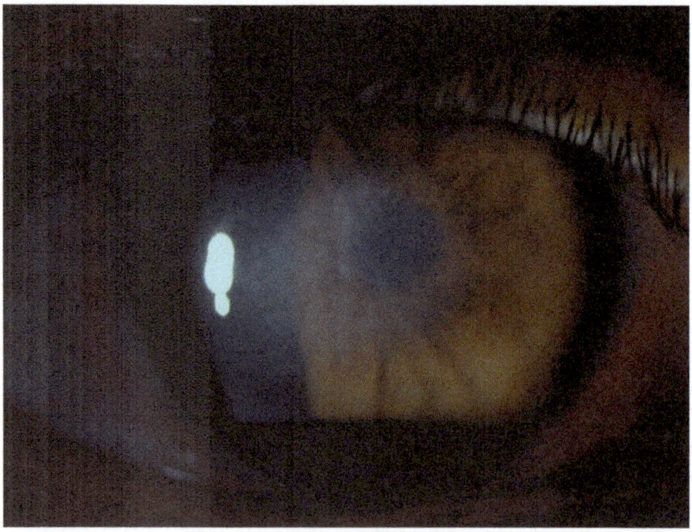

Fig. 3. Corneal Oedema

Previous studies have found that at birth the corneal endothelial cell density is approximately 5,000 cells/mm^2 and until the age of 20 years there is a significant decline in this number. Subsequently this decrease plateaus to a rate of 0.6% per year. In normal circumstances the reserves of endothelial cells mean that there are enough to last a lifetime (Edelhauser, 2000). The role of the corneal endothelium is to maintain the correct level of corneal hydration. It forms a physical barrier between the corneal stroma and aqueous humour and acts as an ion pump. Injury of a significant number of cells results in significant decrease in endothelial cell density and this can impair the ability of the endothelium to maintain corneal clarity, resulting in irreversible corneal oedema. The patient will experience permanent blurring in their vision and ocular pain. There are a number of factors that could lead to endothelial damage during phacoemulsification (Takahashi, 2005).

Localised temperature increases associated with the phacoemulsification probe can lead to thermal damage to adjacent corneal tissue. Some types of phaco probes are now available with cooling functions to counteract this effect. High irrigation or aspiration rates can result in turbulent flow and air bubbles or lens particles connecting with and causing damage to the endothelium. It may be possible to adjust irrigation and aspiration flow rates to minimise this. Excessive duration of phacoemulsification may also result in endothelial cell damage. The ultrasound energy utilised in phacoemulsification is also associated with the production of free radicals (Holst et al., 1993). Free radicals are reactive species with one or more unpaired electrons in their outer orbits. Such chemicals can cause damage to the corneal endothelium known as oxidative stress (Yanoff & Duker, 2004).

Pseudophakic bullous keratopathy describes the irreversible oedema and endothelial cell damage that occurs after cataract surgery. The advent of phacoemulsification techniques and the use of IOLs and ophthalmic viscosurgical devices have helped to reduce the number of cases of pseudophakic bullous keratopathy following cataract surgery (Kang et al., 2005). The most common cause of corneal endothelial decompensation is surgical trauma (Narayanan et al., 2006).

Postoperatively corneal oedema and inflammation should be aggressively treated with topical corticosteroids, and intraocular pressure should be controlled below 20 mmHg. In patients with diffuse epithelial oedema, tonometry should be performed and if intraocular pressure is raised, the condition should be treated with topical and/or systemic anti-glaucoma medication. Reduction of intraocular pressure is important for reducing the corneal oedema because increased intraocular pressure can compromise endothelial cell function, lead to epithelial oedema, and cause further endothelial damage (Narayanan et al., 2006; Yanoff & Duker, 2004).

Therapy for pseudophakic corneal oedema and aphakic corneal oedema is aimed at reducing discomfort and/or increase visual acuity. The corneal oedema associated with phacoemulsification is chronic and usually non-inflammatory. Several medical treatment options are available. Epithelial oedema can often be managed with topical hypertonic agents such as sodium chloride (5%) ointment or drops. Hypertonic eye ointment at night is particularly useful because the oedema tends to be more severe on waking in the morning because of lack of evaporation during the night when the eyes are closed (Narayanan et al., 2006).

7. Toxic anterior segment syndrome

Toxic anterior segment syndrome is an acute, sterile, anterior segment inflammation that can occur after any anterior segment surgery. Early and intense postoperative inflammation after anterior segment surgery accompanied by minimal or no pain, fibrin formation, corneal oedema and the absence of vitreous involvement are the diagnostic criteria for toxic anterior segment syndrome. It almost always occurs as a complication of uneventful cataract surgery or anterior segment surgery and can result in damage to the intraocular tissues (Huang et al., 2010).

Toxic anterior segment syndrome most commonly occurs acutely following anterior segment surgery, typically 12-72 h after cataract extraction. Anterior segment inflammation is usually quite severe with hypopyon. Endothelial cell damage is common, resulting in diffuse corneal oedema. Most patients are asymptomatic with the exception of blurred vision; others may complain of mild discomfort. No bacterium is isolated from ocular samples. The causes of toxic anterior segment syndrome are numerous and difficult to isolate (Cornut & Chiquet, 2011).

The primary differential diagnosis is infectious endophthalmitis (Table 3). Development of new techniques such as polymerase chain reaction may prove more useful in the differentiation of sterile endophthalmitis and early infectious endophthalmitis (Holland et al., 2007; Van Gelder, 2001). Fibrinous uveitis of its own does not usually cause corneal clouding but can also enter the differential diagnosis.

Characteristics	Infectious endophthalmitis	Toxic anterior segment syndrome
Onset	3–7 days	1–3 days
Symptoms	Pain, blurred vision	Blurred vision
Cornea	Oedema 2 +	Oedema 1 +
Anterior chamber	Cells 3 +, Fibrin variable, Hypopyon 3 +	Cells 1–3 +, Fibrin 1–3 +, Hypopyon 1 +
Vitreous	Vitritis	Clear
Response to steroids	Negative	Positive

Table 3. Diagnosis: infectious endophthalmitis versus toxic anterior segment syndrome

Anterior segment findings include fibrin formation with occasional hypopyon and, in later stages, inflammatory membranes that can cause pupil distortion and glaucoma. Severe disease can lead to permanent endothelial damage, profound cystoid macular oedema, a permanently dilated pupil, and even permanent damage to the trabecular meshwork leading to resistant glaucoma that requires multiple operations (Holland et al., 2007; Parikh & Edelhauser, 2003).

Toxic anterior segment syndrome has numerous causes, and most cases are attributed to 1) contaminants on surgical instruments, resulting from improper or insufficient cleaning; 2) products introduced into the eye during surgery, such as irrigating solutions or ophthalmic medications; or 3) other substances that enter the eye during or after surgery, such as topical ointments or talc from surgical gloves (Mamalis et al., 2006).

Gram-negative bacteria may proliferate if the water reservoir in the phaco machine or inside the autoclave is not replaced on a regular basis. Gram-negative bacteria are typically destroyed during the autoclaving procedure; however, heat-stable lipopolysaccharide endotoxin may remain behind. Endotoxin deposits are removed only by acetone or alcohol if operating instruments are dry. If heat-stable lipopolysaccharide endotoxin gets into the eye during the operation, it may cause severe anterior segment inflammation. Prevention of Toxic anterior segment syndrome primarily depends on using appropriate protocols for cleaning and sterilizing surgical equipment and paying careful attention to all solutions, medications and ophthalmic devices used during anterior segment surgery (Avisar & Weinberger, 2010; Mamalis et al., 2006).

Management of toxic anterior segment syndrome involves use of topical steroids every hour and non-steroidal anti-inflammatory drugs (NSAIDs) every 6 hours. Milder cases will resolve from within a few days to 1 to 3 weeks, but if persisting for more than 6 weeks more dire consequences are likely (Parikh & Edelhauser, 2003).

8. References

Altan T, Acar N, Kapran Z, Unver YB, Yurttaser S, Küçüksümer Y, & Eser I. Acute-onset endophthalmitis after cataract surgery: success of initial therapy, visual outcomes, and related factors. Retina, vol. 29, pp. 606-612, 2009.

Avisar R, & Weinberger D. Corneal endothelial morphologic features in toxic anterior segment syndrome. Cornea, vol. 29, pp. 251-3, 2010.

Barza M, Pavan PR, Doft BH, Wisniewski SR, Wilson LA, Han DP, & Kelsey SF. Evaluation of microbiological diagnostic techniques in postoperative endophthalmitis in the Endophthalmitis Vitrectomy Study. Archives of Ophthalmology vol. 115,pp. 1142–1150, 1997.

Bomer TG, Lagreze W-DA, & Funk J. Intraocular pressure rise after phacoemulsification with posterior chamber lens implantation: effect of prophylactic medication, wound closure, and surgeon's experience. British Journal of Ophthalmology, vol. 79, pp.809-813. 1995.

Borazan M, Karalezli A, Akman A, & Akova YA. Effect of antiglaucoma agents on postoperative intraocular pressure after cataract surgery with Viscoat. Journal of Cataract and Refractive Surgery, vol. 33, pp. 1941-1945, 2007.

Browning DJ, & Cobo LM. Early experience in extracapsular cataract surgery by residents, Ophthalmology, vol. 92, pp. 1647-1653, 1985.

Browning AC, Alwitry A, Hamilton R, Rotchford A, Bhan A, & Amoaku WM. Role of intraocular pressure measurement on the day of phacoemulsification cataract surgery. Journal of Cataract and Refractive Surgery, vol. 28, pp. 1601-1606, 2002.

Byrd S, & Singh K. Medical control of intraocular pressure after cataract surgery. Journal of Cataract and Refractive Surgery, vol. 24, pp. 1493-1497, 1998.

Campochiaro PA, & Green WR. Toxicity of intravitreous ceftazidime in primate retina. Archives of Ophthalmology, vol. 110, pp. 1625-1629, 1992.

Chan E, Mahroo AR, & Spalton DJ. Complications of cataract surgery. Clinical & Experimental Optometry vol. 93,pp. 379–389, 2010.

Cornut PL, & Chiquet C. Toxic anterior segment syndrome. Journal de Français d'Ophtalmologie, vol. 34, pp. 58-62, 2011.

Cruciani M, Malena M, Amalfitano G, Monti P, & Bonomi L. Molecular epidemiology in a cluster of cases of postoperative Pseudomonas aeruginosa endophthalmitis. Clinical Infectious Disease, vol. 26, pp. 330-333, 1998.

Edelhauser HF. The Resiliency of the Corneal Endothelium to Refractive and Intraocular Surgery. Cornea, vol. 19, pp. 263-273, 2000.

Eifrig CW, Flynn HW Jr, Scott IU, & Newton J. Acute-onset postoperative endophthalmitis: review of incidence and visual outcomes (1995-2001). Ophthalmic Surgery and Lasers, vol. 33, 373-378, 2002.

Eifrig CWG, Scott IU, Flynn HW Jr, & Miller D. Endophthalmitis caused by Pseudomonas aeruginosa. Ophthalmology vol. 110, pp. 1714–1717, 2003.

Endophthalmitis Vitrectomy Study Group. Results of the endophthalmitis vitrectomy study (1995) a randomized trial of immediate vitrectomy and of intravenous antibiotics for the treatment of postoperative bacterial endophthalmitis. Archives of Ophthalmology, vol. 113, pp. 1479-1496, 1995.

Ermis SS, Ozturk F, & Inan UU. Comparing the effects of travoprost and brinzolamide on intraocular pressure after phacoemulsification. Eye, vol. 19, pp. 303-307, 2005.

Flynn HW Jr, Pulido JS, Pflugfelder SC, Davis JL, Culbertson WW, Roussel TJ, & Miller D. Endophthalmitis therapy: changing antibiotic sensitivity patterns and current therapeutic recommendations. Archives of Ophthalmology, vol. 109, pp. 175-176, 1991.

Gibb AP, Fleck BW, & Kempton-Smith L. A cluster of deep bacterial infections following eye surgery associated with construction dust. The Journal of Hospital Infection, vol. 63, pp. 197-200, 2006.

Gilliland GD, Hutton WL, & Fuller DG. Retained intravitreal lens fragments after cataract surgery, Ophthalmology, vol. 99, pp. 1263–1267, 1992.

Gormaz A. Ocular tension after cataract surgery. American Journal of Ophthalmology, vol. 53, pp. 832-841, 1962.

Guzek JP, Holm M, Cotter JB, Cameron JA, Rademaker WJ, Wissinger DH, Tonjum AM, & Sleeper LA. Risk factors for intraoperative complications in 1000 extracapsular cataract cases, Ophthalmology, vol. 94, pp. 461–466, 1987.

Hildebrand GD, Wickremasinghe SS, Tranos PG, Harris ML, & Little BC. Efficacy of anterior chamber in controlling early intraocular pressure spikes after uneventful phacoemulsification. Journal of Cataract and Refractive Surgery, vol. 29, pp. 1087-1092, 2003.

Hoeve M, & Stilma J. Dropped nucleus' on cataract extraction. Nederlends Tijdschrift voor Geneeskunde, vol. 154, pp;154, A1797, 2010.

Holland SP, Morck DW, & Lee TL. Update on toxic anterior segment syndrome. Current Opinion in Ophthalmology, vol. 18, pp. 4-8, 2007.

Holst A, Rolfsen W, Svensson B, llinger K, & Lundgren B. Formation of free radicals during phacoemulsification, Current Eye Research, vol. 12, pp. 359–365, 1993.

Horiguchi M, Kojima Y & Shimada Y. Removal of lens material dropped into the vitreous cavity during cataract surgery using an optical fiber-free intravitreal surgery system. Journal of Cataract and Refractive Surgery, vol. 29,pp. 1256-1259, 2003.

Huang Y, Dai Y, Wu X, Lan J, & Xie L. Toxic anterior segment syndrome after pediatric cataract surgery. Jornal of American Association for Pediatric Ophthalmology and Strabismus, vol. 14, pp. 444-446, 2010.

Jay WM, Fishman P, Aziz M, & Shockley RK. Intravitreal ceftazidime in a rabbit model: Dose- and time-dependent toxicity and pharmacokinetic analysis. Journal of Ocular Pharmacology, vol. 3, pp. 257-262, 1987.

Kamalarajah S, Silvestri G, Sharma N, Khan A, Foot B, Ling R, Cran G, & Best RM. Surveillance of endophthalmitis following cataract surgery in the UK. Eye, vol. 18, pp. 580–587, 2004.

Kang PC, Klintworth GK, Kim T, Carlson, AN, Adelman R, Stinnett S,& Afshari NA. Trends in the indications for penetrating keratoplasty,1980–2001. Cornea, vol. 24, pp. 801–803, 2005.

Kapusta MA, Chen JC & Lam WC. Outcomes of dropped nucleus during phacoemulsification, Ophthalmology, vol. 103, pp. 1184–1187, 1996.

Kim IK & Miller JW. Management of dislocated lens material. Seminars in Ophthalmology, vol. 17, pp 162-166, 2002.

Kressloff MS, Castellarin A, & Zarbin MA. Endophthalmitis. Survey of Ophthalmology, vol. 43, pp. 193–224, 1998.

Lambrou FH, & Stewart MW. Management of dislocated lens fragments during phacoemulsification, Ophthalmology, vol. 99, pp. 1260–1262, 1992.

Lemley C A, Han, D P. Endophthalmitis A Review of Current Evaluation and Management. Retina, vol. 27, pp. 662-680, 2007.

Lewis RA. What is the best way to prevent and manage postoperative intraocular pressure spikes? In: Chang DF (ed). Curbside Consultation in Cataract Surgery. Thorofare, NJ, Slack, 2007; 187-189.

Lu H, Jiang YR, & GrabowHB. Managing a dropped nucleus during the phacoemulsification learning curve, Journal of Cataract and Refractive Surgery, vo. 25, pp. 447–450, 1999.

Maguire JI. Postoperative endophthalmitis: optimal management and the role and timing of vitrectomy surgery. Eye , vol. 22, pp 1290-3000, 2008.

Mamalis N, Kearsley L, & Brinton E. Postoperative endophthalmitis. Current Opinion in Ophthalmolology, vol. 13, pp. 14–18, 2002.

Mamalis N, Edelhauser HF, Dawson DG, Chew J, LeBoyer RM, & Werner L. Toxic anterior segment syndrome. Journal of Cataract and Refractive Surgery, vol. 32, pp. 324-333, 2006.

Melo GB, Bispo PJ, Regatieri CV, Yu MC, Pignatari AC, & Höfling-Lima AL. Incidence of endophthalmitis after cataract surgery (2002-2008) at a Brazilian university-hospital. Arquivos Brasileiros de Oftalmologia, vol. 73, pp. 505-507, 2010.

Meredith TA. Antimicrobial pharmacokinetics in endophthalmitis treatment: Studies of ceftazidime. Transactions of the American Ophthalmological Society, vol. 91, pp. 653-699, 1993.

Narayanan R, Gaster RN, & Kenney MC. Pseudophakic corneal edema: A review of mechanisms and treatments. Cornea, vol. 25: pp. 993-1004, 2006.

Oum BS, D'Amico DJ, & Wong KW. Intravitreal antibiotic therapy with vancomycin and aminoglycoside: An experimental study of combination and repetitive injections. Archives of Ophthalmology, vol. 107, pp. 1055-1060, 1989.

Parikh CH, & Edelhauser HF. Ocular surgical pharmacology: corneal endothelial safety and toxicity. Current Opinion in Ophthalmology, vol. 14, pp. 178-185, 2003.

Reddy MK. Complications of cataract surgery. Indian Journal of Ophthalmology, vol. 43, pp. 201-209, 1995.

Stonecipher KG, Parmley VC, Jensen H, & Rowsey JJ. Infectious endophthalmitis following sutureless cataract surgery. Archives of Ophthalmology, vol. 109, pp. 1562-1563, 1991.

Taban M, Behrens A, Newcomb RL, Nobe MY, Saedi G, Sweet PM, & McDonnell PJ. Acute endophthalmitis following cataract surgery: a systematic review of the literature. Archives of Ophthalmology, vol. 123, pp. 613-620, 2005.

Takahashi H. Free Radical Development in Phacoemulsification. Cataract Surgery Jornal of Nippon Medical School, vol. 72, pp. 4-12, 2005.

Tanaka T, Inoue H, Kudo S, & Ogawa T. Relationship between postoperative intraocular pressure elevation and residual sodium hyaluronate following phacoemulsification and aspiration. Journal of Cataract and Refractive Surgery, vol. 23, pp. 284-288,1997.

Tranos P, Bhar G, & Little B. Postoperative intraocular pressure spikes: the need to treat. Eye, vol. 18, pp.673-679, 2004.

Unal M, Yücel I. Effect of bimatoprost on intraocular pressure after cataract surgery. Canadian Journal of Ophthalmology, vol. 43, pp. 712-716, 2008.

Van Gelder RN. Applications of the polymerase chain reaction to diagnosis of ophthalmic disease. Survey of Ophthalmology, vol. 45, pp. 248–258, 2001.

Wright PL, Wilkinson CP, Balyeat HD, Popham J, & Reinke M. Angiographic cystoid macular edema after posterior chamber lens implantation. Archives of Ophthalmology, vol. 106, pp. 106: 740–744, 1988.

Yanoff M, & Duker J. Complications of Cataract Surgery. 2 nd ed. St. Louis: Mosby, 2004, pp.381-390.

19

Endophthalmitis, Prevention and Treatment

Elvis Ojaimi and David T. Wong
University of Toronto, Vitreoretinal Department, St Michael's Hospital
Canada

1. Introduction

Endophthalmitis is a devastating eye condition that can lead to permanent visual loss or even loss of the eye. It can occur from an immune mediated response to an antigen (sterile endophthalmitis) or most commonly from an infectious cause. Infectious endophthalmitis can be classified broadly into endogenous and exogenous. Endogenous endophthalmitis occurs from hematological spread in the setting of bacteremia or fungemia and is seen in the setting of immunosuppression, intravenous drug use, chronic indwelling urinary catheterization or remote infection. Exogenous endophthalmitis refers to an intraocular infection caused by the introduction of organisms from the external environment. This can occur in the setting of trauma (traumatic endophthalmitis) or surgery (acute & chronic postoperative endophthalmitis, filtering bleb-associated, intravitreal injections and secondary to extension of infection). Acute postoperative endophthalmitis can occur following any surgery that involves penetration of the eye including cataract, glaucoma, corneal and vitrectomy surgery. Endophthalmitis has also been reported in external ocular surgeries such as strabismus and scleral buckle surgery. These are probably associated with inadvertent perforation, infected explant material, and intraocular spread of external pathogens. Table 1 describes a classification for endophthalmitis. This chapter will be limited to exogenous endophthalmitis.

Endophthalmitis	
Exogenous	**Endogenous**
Acute onset postoperative • Cataract surgery • Glaucoma filtering surgery (penetrating) • Penetrating keratoplasty • Vitrectomy surgery • External ocular surgery (rarely)	
Delayed (chronic) onset postoperative	
Posttraumatic	
Filtering bleb-associated	
Other: • Intravitreal injections • Infectious spread from keratitis or scleritis	

Table 1. Endophthalmitis categories

2. Epidemiology

2.1 Exogenous endophthalmitis

2.1.1 Cataract surgery

The incidence of endophthalmitis following cataract surgery was described in a recent review as ranging from <0.05% to >0.3%.[1] In our study we reported a rate of suspected endophthalmitis of 0.14% from more than 440,000 cataract surgeries in Ontario, Canada over a 4 year period.[2] In Europe, the results of a recent, large, randomized multicentre study of antibacterial prophylaxis revealed an incidence of endophthalmitis ranging from 0.049% to as high as 0.345% seen in the control group.[3] In an article by West et al.[4], a 5% sampling of Medicare beneficiary data files revealed an increase in the rate of endophthalmitis from the time period 1994– 1997 when compared with 1998–2001. The pooled rate over the entire 8-year period (which corresponds to the rise in clear corneal cataract surgery) was also high at 2.15 per 1000 surgeries (0.2%). Taban et al.[5] performed a systematic review of the English literature and concluded that endophthalmitis rates were rising. Using a regression analysis model and excluding case reports, the authors found the rate of pooled endophthalmitis to be 0.265% from 2000 to 2003. Rates as high as 0.49% were also described in a study from Dublin.[6]

The rate of chronic post-operative endophthalmitis is less clear but less common than the acute type.

2.1.2 Glaucoma surgery

Bleb-associated endophthalmitis has been classified into early onset and late (delayed) onset, with 4 weeks after surgery being the arbitrary cut-off.[7] Rates of endophthalmitis following non-augmented trabeculectomy surgery have been reported to occur between 0.2 - 1.5%.[7] The rate increases significantly with intraoperative 5-FU or MMC. A recent US based retrospective study, utilizing the US medicare database reported the rate of endophthamitis to be between 0.3-0.7% following trabeculectomy surgery.[8] For glaucoma drainage devices, the study found an endophthalmitis rate of 2.0%.[8] The rate of endophthalmitis following non penetrating glaucoma surgery is probably rare, with one case reported in the literature.[9]

2.1.3 Vitreoretinal procedures

2.1.3.1 Vitrectomy surgery

Internationally published rates of endophthalmitis for 20G vitrectomy range from 0.018% to 0.07%.[10-12] The incidence of endophthalmitis following 23G vitrectomy in the UK has been estimated at around 0.04%.[12] A higher rate of endophthalmitis has been suggested for 25G vitrectomy. However, in a recent meta-analysis the evidence was found to be tentative. [13] The reported increase in risk of postoperative endophthalmitis after 25G was due to mainly two studies. Kunimoto et al[14] identified 7 cases of endophthalmitis among 3103 25-gauge PPV surgeries (0.23%, or roughly 1 in 400), and Scott et al[15] identified 11 cases in 1307 PPV surgeries (0.84%, or 1 in 119). In each series, this incidence was significantly higher than that observed after 20-gauge PPV during the same period among the same group of vitreoretinal surgeons. Most of the postoperative endophthalmitis cases that were reported involved both straight incision technique and were left fluid-filled at the end of the case.[13]

2.1.3.2 Intravitreal injections

Retrospective reports of eyes receiving triamcinolone indicate a per-injection endophthalmitis risk between zero and 0.87%.[16] There was one case of endophthalmitis out of 3159 injections of triamcinolone (0.03%) performed in the SCORE and DRCR.net trials.[16] Interestingly, in the DRCR.net trials 3 cases of endophthalmitis from 3226 receiving intravitreal Ranibizumab were reported.

ANCHOR and MARINA studies demonstrated a low rate of endophthalmitis in eyes receiving intravitreal Ranibizumab. At 2 years there were only three cases of endophthalmitis out of 5921 injections (0.05%) in ANCHOR. MARINA and the pivotal trial for pegaptanib (VISION) each reported a 0.05% per-injection rate of presumed endophthalmitis. The PACORES Trial utilized Bevacizumab and reported a higher incidence of 0.16%, whereas other large, retrospective trials reported rates ranging from a 0.019–0.07%.[16]

Immunocompromised patients may be at greater risk of developing endophthalmitis. Data from several studies suggest a 0.11% per-injection risk associated with intravitreal antivirals.[16]

2.1.4 Other

In a systematic review of the literature, the overall pooled estimate (1972-2002) of the incidence of acute endophthalmitis after penetrating keratoplasty (PK) was 0.382% based on 90,549 PK's. The rate of endophthalmitis from 1972 to 1999 was 0.392%, whereas the rate from 2000 to 2003 was 0.200%, representing an almost 2-fold decrease in the incidence.[17]

After sustaining open globe injury, the chance of developing endophthalmitis is estimated to be approximately 7% with studies ranging between 0% and 13%. Injuries including intraocular foreign bodies may have higher rates of endophthalmitis, ranging from 11% to 30%, highest in a study of rural penetrating trauma.[18]

2.2 Endogenous endophthalmitis

This infection occurs when microorganisms in the bloodstream cross the blood-ocular barrier to infect the intraocular tissues. It is relatively rare, accounting for only 2–8% of endophthalmitis cases and these patients usually have underlying diseases such as diabetes, human immunodeficiency virus infection, intravenous drug abuse, renal failure on dialysis, cardiac disease, malignancy, immunosuppressive therapy, or indwelling catheters that predispose them to infection.[18]

3. Clinical

3.1 History and symptoms

Acute postoperative endophthalmitis refers to infectious endophthalmitis that occurs shortly after ocular surgery or intravitreal injection. Patients usually present within 1–2 weeks of surgery and often within a few days. A history of complicated cataract surgery, including posterior capsular rupture may be identified. Symptoms of acute post-operative endophthalmitis include pain, visual loss, eye redness and swollen eyelid. Almost all subjects had symptoms in the Endophthalmitis Vitrectomy Study (EVS), with 94.3% of patients reporting blurred vision, 82.1% reporting red eye, 74.3% reporting pain, and 34.5% reporting a swollen lid.[19]

Chronic postoperative endophthalmitis is characterized by insidious inflammation occurring usually weeks to months after intraocular surgery. It consists of recurrent episodes of low-grade inflammation and pain may or may not be present. It may rarely be precipitated by YAG-laser capsulotomy. Patients may describe visual symptoms including progressive visual loss and floaters. Inflammation may initially respond to steroids but usually recurs following steroid taper.

Endophthalmitis following bleb-surgery can occur in the early postoperative period, but occurs more often months to years after filter surgery. One recent large study showed a mean time between glaucoma filtering surgery and endophthalmitis of 19.1 months, with a range of 3 days to 9 years.[20] A history of anti-metabolite use is relevant because these can promote a thin, cystic bleb that becomes vulnerable to infection and leakage. Presentation is similar to acute postoperative endophthalmitis and is usually with redness, reduced vision and pain.

Diagnosing posttraumatic endophthalmitis immediately after the ruptured globe injury can be difficult because of trauma-induced inflammation and the disruption of normal anatomy. Traumatic endophthalmitis may occur within a few days or up to several weeks between injury and onset. Symptoms include decreasing vision, increasing pain, or a greater than expected degree of pain. The course of posttraumatic endophthalmitis can be affected by factors including, the type of injury, the presence or absence of an intraocular foreign body (IOFB) and the time between injury and treatment.

3.2 Signs

Table 2 outlines the signs of endophthalmitis according to classification. Common signs of acute postoperative endophthalmitis include decreased visual acuity, lid swelling, conjunctival and corneal edema, anterior chamber cells and fibrin, hypopyon, vitreous inflammation, retinitis, and blunting of red reflex.[18] Retinal periphlebitis may be an early sign. Bleb-associated endophthalmitis has similar features. It is characterized by sudden intraocular inflammation in an eye that has been quiet for months or years following filtering surgery. Bleb purulence is noted is most patients, with an appearance of a milky white bleb. In the absence of vitritis and hypopyon, the term blebitis is given. This tends to respond to conservative measures with fortified topical antibiotics and systemic therapy. Endophthalmitis following intravitreal injections also follows a similar course to acute postoperative endophthalmitis. However, distinction from sterile endophthalmitis is sometimes possible. This may represent inflammation resulting from reaction to the drug, components of the drug vehicle, or sterile microbial toxins in the formulation. Additionally, triamcinolone acetonide crystals can migrate into the anterior chamber and mimic a hypopyon.[18] Gravity induced shifting of this material may distinguish it from a true hypopyon, as well as the absence of anterior chamber flare or fibrin.

Delayed (chronic) endophthalmitis can occur in the early postoperative period but usually manifests weeks to months after surgery, with a chronic low grade inflammation that is initially responsive to topical steroids but rebounds following taper. There is usually the absence of a hypopyon. The uveitis may be granulomatous with large keratic precipitates on the cornea or precipitates on the intraocular lens. A white intracapsular plaque is commonly observed with Propionibacterium infection, often associated with retained lens particles and sequestration of organisms. The plaques can also be seen less frequently with other bacteria and fungal infections. Stringy white infiltrates and "fluff balls" or "pearls-on-a-string" near the capsular remnant are characteristic but not pathognomonic of fungal infection. Vitreous cellular reaction is usually mild, but dense, diffuse vitritis can be seen in some infections, notably with S epidermidis.[18]

Acute postoperative endophthalmitis

- Reduced visual acuity (<5/200 in 86%*)
- Afferent papillary defect (11.7%*)
- Lid edema
- Conjunctival injection and swelling
- Conjunctival discharge (+/- purulent)
- Corneal edema
- Anterior chamber inflammation - cells, flare, fibrin, hypopyon
- Vitreous inflammation - anterior vitreous cells, haze (unable to see retinal vessel 79.1%*)
- Signs of intraocular surgery
- +/- signs of complicated cataract surgery- wound leak, abscess, vitreous incarceration etc.
- Retinal and choroidal involvement
- Signs of extraocular extension in advanced cases

Delayed (chronic) postoperative endophthalmitis

- Low-grade anterior chamber inflammation (granulomatous)
- +/- mutton-fat keratic precipitates
- Vitritis (common)
- Fibrin, hypopyon
- Enlarging capsular plaque (may require maximal dilation or even gonioscopy to visualize)
- Signs that may suggest fungal cause - persistent corneal edema, a corneal infiltrate, a mass in the iris or ciliary body, necrotizing scleritis, "pearls -on-a-string" in the anterior chamber, paradoxical worsening of the inflammatory course after steroid therapy

Filtering bleb-associated endophthalmitis

- White milky bleb containing pus
- Severe anterior chamber inflammation +/- hypopyon
- Vitritis

Posttraumatic endophthalmitis

- Intraocular foreign body
- Lid edema & Chemosis
- Greater than expected anterior chamber cell inflammation, fibrinoid response
- Hypopyon
- Vitritis, vitreous opacification
- Retinal involvement if the view allows - retinitis, vasculitis
- Extension of exudate from a wound
- Purulence

Intravitreal injection

- Similar to acute postoperative endophthalmitis
- Differentiate from sterile endophthalmitis (Triamcinolone acetonide crystals in the anterior chamber, gravity-induced shifting of material, absence of anterior chamber flare or fibrin)

Extension from infection

- Corneal abscess or infective scleritis

* Endophthalmitis Vitrectomy Study Table.1 Baseline characteristics by treatment group[19]

Table 2. Signs of exogenous endophthalmitis

4. Etiology

Endophthalmitis type	%
Acute postoperative endophthalmitis[19]	
Gram positive coagulase negative growth	46.9 (67% of positive cultures)
Other gram positive growth	15.5 (22.4% of positive culures)
Gram negative growth	4.1 (5.8% of positive cultures)
Polymicrobial	2.9
No growth	30.7
Chronic postoperative endophthalmitis[18]	
Propionibacterium species	63
Staph epidermidis	16
Candida parapsilosis	16
Corynebacterium species	5
Other: Actinomyces, Nocardia, Achromobacter, Cephalosporium, Acremonium, Paecilomyces, and Aspergillus species	
Filtering bleb-associated endophthalmitis[22]	80% positive culture (several cases had more than one species of strep or staph)
Streptococcus species	41 % of positive culture
Staphylococcus species	28 % of positive culture
Enterococcus species	23 % of positive culture
Gram negative	
Post traumatic endophthalmitis	
Gram positive organisms	~75 (~20% due to Bacillus)
Gram negative organisms	
Fungal	
Intravitreal injection	
Similar to acute postoperative with coagulase-negative staphylococcus	
Other: Streptobacillus parasanguis, Mycobacterium chelonae, Streptobacillus species	

Table 3. Causative organisms

4.1 Organisms

Table 3 outlines the organisms involved in exogenous endophthalmitis. Gram-positive bacteria cause the majority of exogenous endophthalmitis cases. Coagulase-negative staphylococcal isolates are the most common cause of postoperative endophthalmitis cases. Other species involved include Staphylococcus aureus, streptococci, enterococci, and Gram-positive rods such as Bacillus. Gram-negative bacteria were isolated from a relatively low number of post-operative endophthalmitis cases. According to the Endophthalmitis Vitrectomy Study (EVS), around 69% had culture positive result, and of those around 70% were gram-positive coagulase negative organisms and only 2.2% enterococcus species. The literature suggests that the spectrum of organisms may be shifting with the introduction of prophylactic antibiotics. Enterococcus spp. were found to cause 25.3% of all cases of endophthalmitis, suggesting an increased proportion of cases of enterococcal endophthalmitis. This relative increase in the proportion of endophthalmitis cases due to Enterococcus spp. was attributed to the introduction of intracameral cefuroxime as a means of anti- bacterial prophylaxis. Although intracameral cefuroxime was quite effective in reducing the overall number of endophthalmitis infections, enterococci are relatively resistant to cefuroxime.[1]

Both Gram-positive and Gram- negative organisms can cause post-traumatic endophthalmitis. Polymicrobial infections and fungal infections also have been reported. Gram-positive organisms constitute the majority of pathogens in post-traumatic endophthalmitis. Among Gram-positive microbes, Staphylococcus epidermis is isolated most commonly. Although Bacillus cereus may not be as common as Staphylococcus epidermis, it is relatively frequently associated with IOFBs and is associated with a very poor visual prognosis. The incidence of post-traumatic endophthalmitis caused by Pseudomonas species as the only isolate ranges from 0% to 23.1%[21]

The spectrum of causative organisms associated with bleb-associated endophthalmitis has been reported to differ from that of acute-onset endophthalmitis after cataract surgery. The more virulent streptococcal species and gram-negative organisms are more common causes of delayed-onset bleb-associated endophthalmitis. In a study at Bascom Palmer Eye Institute between 1996 and 2001, streptococcal species and gram-negative organisms, followed by staphylococcal species were found to be the commonest organisms. Gram-negative organisms and Haemophilus influenzae are also commonly isolated.[22]

The spectrum of organisms isolated in chronic postoperative endophthalmitis is quite different to other categories of exogenous endophthalmitis, with Propionibacterium species accounting for the majority of cases and fungal organisms comprising a significant proportion. A review of endophthalmitis cases presenting more than 4 weeks after cataract surgery found 63% Propionibacterium species, 16% S epidermidis, 16% Candida parapsilosis, and 5% Corynebacterium species.[18]

5. Differential diagnosis

5.1 Retained lens fragment

Retention of lens cortex or nucleus may cause significant intraocular inflammation in an acute or chronic setting. Operative details from the cataract surgeon and visualizing the fragments may aid in differentiating this condition from endophthalmitis.

5.2 TASS, toxic anterior segment syndrome

This condition is due to marked inflammation due to noninfectious substances that enter the eye, such as bacterial toxins, preservatives, cleaning compounds or intraocular solutions. This condition can sometimes be differentiated from endophthalmitis by its rapid onset (within 12-24hrs following surgery or intravitreal injection), lack of pain or redness, diffuse corneal edema and lack of isolated organisms by gram stain or culture.

6. Prevention

6.1 Risk factors

The risk of developing acute postoperative endophthalmitis is associated with a number of factors such as the presence of eyelid or conjunctival disease, the patient's general condition including, diabetes, skin disease, the use of immunosuppressive drugs, the type of intraocular surgery performed, and intraoperative complications. Table 4 outlines risk factors associated with endophthalmitis according to the category.

Endophthalmitis category	Risk factors
Acute postoperative endophthalmitis	**Preoperative** Age, diabetes, chronic bacterial blepharitis, active conjunctivitis, lacrimal drainage system obstruction, eyelid pathology such as ectropion **Operative** Wound abnormalities, vitreous loss, prolonged surgery, contaminated irrigation solutions, polypropylene haptics **Postoperative** Wound leak, vitreous incarceration, contaminated eye drops
Chronic postoperative endophthalmitis	Unclear
Traumatic endophthalmitis	Retained IOFB, lens rupture, delayed timing of primary repair, age greater than 50 years, female gender, large wound size, location of wound, ocular tissue prolapse, placement of primary intraocular lens (IOL), and rural locale
Bleb-associated endophthalmitis	Antimetabolites (5-FU, MMC), inferior bleb location, tube exposure after conjunctival erosion in drainage devices, younger age in drainage devices, blepharitis, diabetes, limbus-based conjunctival flaps, silk conjunctival sutures, early postoperative complications and bleb manipulation from revision or needling

Table 4. Risk factors for endophthalmitis

Traumatic endophthalmitis has been associated with retained IOFB, lens rupture, delayed timing of primary repair, age greater than 50 years, placement of primary intraocular lens (IOL), and rural locale. The composition of IOFB may play a role with infection, with non-metallic objects having a higher risk of infection. These foreign bodies may be contaminated with infectious material and intuitively, may increase the risk of infection. Treatment delay has been shown to be an important factor in the development of post-traumatic endophthalmitis. Delayed primary repair, especially more than 24 hours, is considered to be a risk factor for post-traumatic endophthalmitis in the absence of an IOFB. Contaminated injuries can be significant risk factors for the development of infection. For example, penetrating globe injuries by a cat claw, contaminated utensils, or injuries sustained during dental procedures are all considered highly contaminated. Also, the likelihood of injury with a contaminated object is increased in rural settings where trauma frequently occurs after farm-related accidents. The increased risk of infection with organic matter may be due to an increased microbial inoculum, greater extent of injury, and possibly more virulent organisms that may be resistant to antibiotics.

Bleb-associated endophthalmitis has been associated with antimetabolites (5-FU, MMC), inferior bleb location, tube exposure after conjunctival erosion in drainage devices, younger age in drainage devices, blepharitis, diabetes, limbus-based conjunctival flaps, silk conjunctival sutures, early postoperative complications and bleb manipulation from revision or needling. In a study at Bascom Palmer, potential risk factors and clinical features among the study population included history of bleb leak, bleb manipulations (needling, compression sutures, laser suture lysis, bleb revision, and autologous blood injection), bleb defects, inferior bleb location, and nasolacrimal duct obstruction.[22]

6.2 Prophylaxis

6.2.1 Pre-operative

Treatment of local ocular factors, such as blepharitis, conjunctivitis, eyelid pathology (ectropion or entropion) and nasolacrimal duct obstruction is imperative before elective intraocular surgery. Systemic risk factors such as diabetes and immunosuppression should be optimized. Figure 1 is an outline of one approach for prophylaxis against endophthalmitis following cataract surgery.

The low incidence of endophthalmitis makes the study of risk factors and preventative measures difficult. Pre-operative application of topical antbiotics is becoming common practice in the USA and Canada. In a recent survey of Canadian ophthalmologists we found preoperative topical antibiotics were routinely used by 78% of respondents.[23] There are studies that suggest the use of preoperative late-generation fluoroquinolones decreases the incidence of infection,[24] but at this stage there are no large, prospective, randomized controlled trials that demonstrate this. Despite the lack of level I evidence, pre-operative topical antibiotics probably have a role. They have been shown to decrease bacterial load and penetrate the anterior chamber to achieve significant intraocular concentration.

In terms of prophylaxis for traumatic endophthalmitis, prophylactic perioperative systemic antibiotics are commonly administered for ruptured globes, but no prospective evidence for its benefit has been established. Despite this it is common practice to give systemic antibiotics either broad spectrum intravenous or oral.

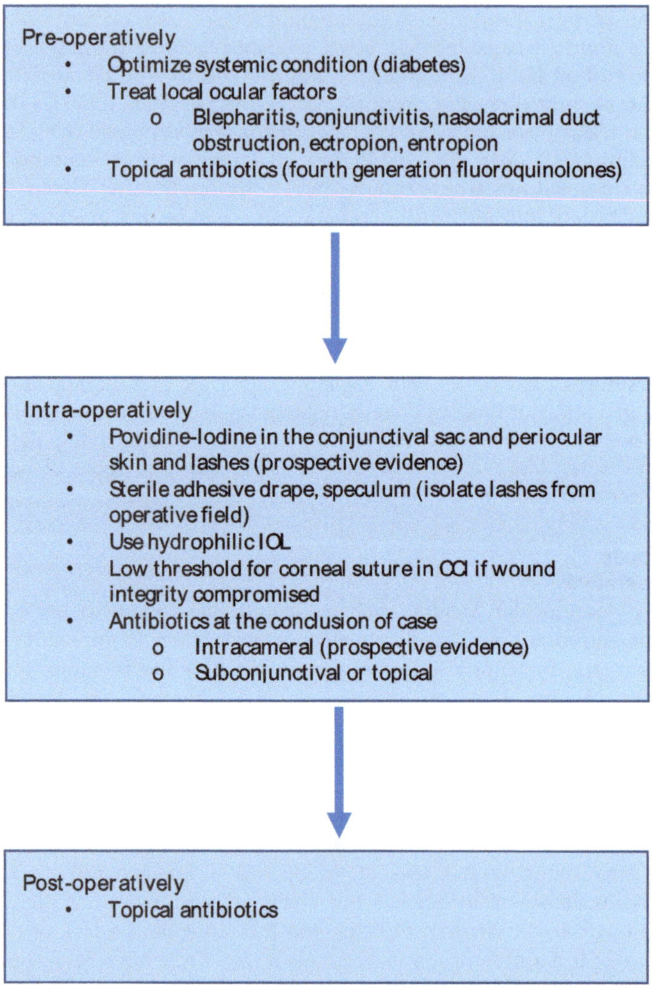

Fig. 1. Guide for prophylaxis against acute postoperative endophthalmitis following cataract surgery

6.2.2 Intraoperative

A review of the literature by Ciulla et al. supported the role of Povidine-Iodine in prophylaxis against endophthalmitis.[25] Povidine-Iodine as a prophylactic technique has been demonstrated to reduce the risk of endophthalmitis in a prospective study. Instillation of Povidine-Iodine should be instilled into the conjunctival sac and incorporate the lashes and surrounding periocular skin within the surgical field. Cutting of the eyelashes is not considered necessary, however, modern drapes with a speculum should exclude lashes from the surgical field.

The European Society of Cataract and Refractive Surgery conducted the first prospective, randomized, multicentre clinical trial concerning antibacterial prophylaxis of postoperative endophthalmitis.[3] They investigated the use of intracameral antibiotics (cefuroxime 1 mg /0.1 cc) following phacoemulsification. In the absence of cefuroxime administration there was a 5- to 6-fold increased risk for endophthalmitis, which was in line with retrospective results reported from Sweden. In addition to the administration of intracameral cefuroxime at the time of surgery, other factors in that study that were associated with a reduction in the risk for endophthalmitis were the use of acrylic material for the IOL optic and the choice of scleral tunnel as the site of incision. It is conceivable that hydrophilic polymer surfaces may be useful in avoiding the development of bacterial colonies by possibly inhibiting or delaying bacterial colonization. Well-constructed clear corneal incisions are necessary to prevent microleaks and the risk of intraocular contamination. To eliminate these risks, a single interrupted 10-0 nylon suture should be applied across an incision where the structural integrity is in question.

Other drugs are also being investigated for intracameral use, including fluoroquinolones, and some centres utilize Vancomycin.[26] Caution needs to be taken when using these drugs for prophylaxis because of the potential for resistant strains, which can become problematic in the treatment of established cases. There is evidence in the literature to suggest a change in the spectrum of pathogens that cause postoperative endophthalmitis and growing resistance to certain prophylactic antibiotics.[27] There are also other issues with intracameral antibiotics including, dosing errors and potential toxicity.

Some ophthalmologists utilize intraoperative subconjunctival antibiotics but the evidence is tentative. There are reports that demonstrate a reduced incidence of endophthalmitis with subconjunctival antibiotics. Experimental models have shown adequate anterior chamber concentrations following the administration possibly making it a valid prophylactic option. Antibiotic soaked collagen shields placed in the eye at the conclusion of surgery are also utilized but the evidence is limited at this stage.

Intravitreal antibiotic administration in the setting of trauma is controversial. Some authors advocate this in all cases of penetrating eye injuries, while others recommend it in the presence of risk factors.[21] Suggested regimen includes Vancomycin 1mg/0.1cc and Ceftazidime 2.25mg/0.1cc.

6.2.3 Post-operative

The use of topical antibiotics postoperatively is common practice despite limited evidence. Topical antibiotics such as the fourth generation fluoroquinolones have good penetration and can achieve therapeutic concentrations in the anterior chamber. However, these concentrations are not achieved in the vitreous cavity. It has been suggested that post-operative antibiotics may be more appropriately used in high dose and short duration to reduce the risk of emergent resistant strains.

7. Management

7.1 Workup & treatment of acute postoperative endophthalmitis

Figure 2 outlines a management algorithm for suspected acute postoperative endophthalmitis. In the early stage, a diagnosis of endophthlamitis can be difficult to make because signs can be mild. Close observation (every 6 hrs) is recommended for a patient presenting with symptoms suggestive of endophthalmitis but not enough signs to confirm because inflammatory signs can escalate rapidly. In patients with signs suggestive of endophthalmitis, including significant anterior chamber and vitreous inflammation, +/- hypopyon and reduced visual acuity, urgent management is required. Visual acuity should be obtained to determine whether VA ≥ HM or PL, as this would influence treatment. A thorough ocular examination must be performed and post-operative complications such as wound leak should be detected. An ultrasound should be done if the view precludes a good posterior segment examination. Retinal and/or choroidal detachment can be ruled out, and signs such as vitreous opacities and/or chorioretinal thickening (severe cases) provide further support for a diagnosis of endophthalmitis.

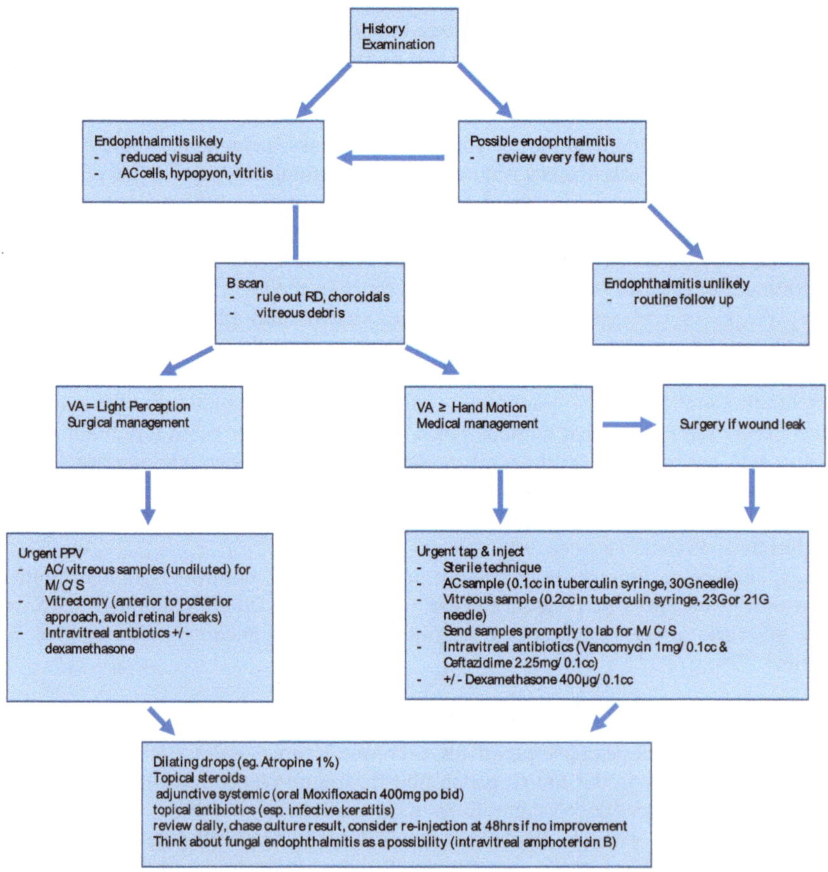

Fig. 2. Management algorithm in acute postoperative cataract endophthalmitis

The EVS addressed the relative efficacy of immediate PPV versus vitreous tap in the treatment of postoperative endophthalmitis. Patients presenting with light perception only visual acuity had a threefold-improved chance of obtaining 20/40 vision after immediate vitrectomy (33%) compared to vitreous tap or biopsy (11%). There was a 56% chance of obtaining 20/100 or better vision after immediate PPV compared to 30% chance after vitreous tap or biopsy. In patients presenting with vision of hand motions or better, there was no significant difference between the two treatment groups in final visual acuity. Based on the EVS, aqueous and vitreous samples can be obtained at the time of PPV, if it is indicated. It is worth mentioning that the EVS excluded patients presenting with no light perception visual acuity or significant opacification of the anterior chamber to the point of obscuring iris tissue, so that more virulent organisms may have been excluded. Also, the EVS studied endophthalmitis in post cataract surgery, and these results may not apply to other intraocular surgeries.

An anterior chamber tap, vitreous tap and intravitreal antibiotic injection should be done aseptically. Povidine-iodine, surgical drape, lid speculum, and an operating microscope may be used. A 30-gauge needle attached to a 1cc tuberculin syringe is inserted through the limbus into the anterior chamber and an aqueous specimen is aspirated without collapsing the anterior chamber. A quantity of approximately 0.1 cc can usually be obtained. Outside the operating room, a vitreous specimen may be obtained either by vitreous needle tap (23G or 21G in a non-vitrectomized eye) or by vitreous biopsy with a cutting/aspirating probe such as The Intrector® portable vitrectomy instrument (Insight Instruments, Inc.). A dry vitreous specimen can be obtained with the cutter in the operating room (before the infusion is turned on). Samples should be obtained for Gram stain, culture (aerobic, anaerobic, and fungal), as well as antibiotic sensitivities. Culture inoculation by the surgeon or the laboratory within minutes of obtaining specimens is ideal to maximize recovery of organisms. Anaerobic cultures should be kept for at least 14 days to recover slow-growing species (for example, P acnes) and fungal cultures should be kept for several weeks. There may be a role for PCR in the detection of fastidious organisms.

Current recommendations for empirical therapy are vancomycin 1.0 mg/0.1cc and ceftazidime 2.25 mg/ 0.1cc. Amikacin 400 μg/0.1cc can be considered in exchange for ceftazidime in β-lactam sensitive patients. Retinal toxicity is a potential complication of intravitreal antibiotic therapy. Toxicity has not been studied well for most antibiotics and it is possible that toxicity may develop with repeat injections. Most studies have been in animal models and application to humans may not be ideal. Gentamicin retinal toxicity is a well-known phenomenon, with macular infarction described even with lower doses (0.1mg). Retinal toxicity is less common but also reported with amikacin. Intravitreal ceftazidime appears safer than aminoglycosides, but it can cause retinal toxicity when given at doses higher than the recommended 2.25 mg/0.1 cc. A study in squirrel monkeys (vitreous cavity volume of $1/5^{th}$ to $1/7^{th}$ the human volume) showed retinal toxicity with a ceftazidime dose of 10 mg in 0.1cc and no retinal toxicity with 2.25mg.[28] The dose of intravitreal antibiotic is particularly relevant in eyes that have had an air-fluid exchange or patients that have silicone oil or gas filled eyes, so that dose adjustment should be considered.[29,30] Vancomycin has been nontoxic in intravitreal doses up to 2mg in pigmented rabbits.[31] The role of fourth generation fluoroquinolones as intravitreal therapy remains unclear and optimal dosage in the human eye is not known. Experimental data suggests a Moxifloxacin dose of ≤160ug/0.1cc is probably safe.[32]

The major limitation of intraocular antimicrobials is the short duration of action. Reinjection should be considered if the infection fails to stabilize or improve more than 48 hours after the first injection. Based on consensus view, the EVS protocol recommended reinjection if the infection was worsening at 36 - 60 hours after initial injection. The rationale for reinjection is based on the observation of rapid half-life elimination of some intravitreal antibiotics in animal eyes.[33,34] In addition, 48 hours after treatment, culture results become available. If cultured organisms are likely to be resistant to the initially injected antibiotics and the infection is not improving, alternative antibiotics could be used.

Most antimicrobials penetrate the vitreous cavity poorly after intravenous injection because of the blood-eye barrier. The EVS showed no difference in visual acuity or media clarity with or without intravenous antibiotics when given in addition to intravitreal antibiotics. These results led many physicians to avoid intravenous antibiotics in post- operative endophthalmitis. However, recent evidence demonstrates the intraocular penetration of oral moxifloxacin and gatifloxacin.[35,36] Ninety percent minimal inhibitory concentrations (MIC90) were achieved after two 400 mg oral doses against many Gram-positive and Gram-negative pathogens implicated in postoperative endophthalmitis. Given their favorable characteristics of broad coverage, good tolerability, and ease of oral administration, these agents are promising adjunct therapies for all forms of exogenous endophthalmitis.

Currently, there is no consensus regarding the use of intraocular steroids in the management of endophthalmitis. There are theoretical advantages including modulation of the host inflammatory response to minimize ocular damage. Some retinal physicians advocate systemic steroids. The EVS used oral steroids, but the benefit was not evaluated. An advantage was found with systemic steroids in a retrospective study compared to only topical or no steroids.[37] Das et al evaluated the efficacy of intravitreal dexamethasone in the management of exogenous endophthalmitis and reported an early reduction in inflammation, but with no influence on final visual outcome.[38] In another prospective, randomized trial of 29 patients with endophthalmitis after cataract surgery, Gan et al showed a trend towards better visual acuity with adjuvant intravitreal dexamethasone. In contrast, a retrospective study found patients that received intravitreal corticosteroids had a reduced likelihood of achieving a 3-line improvement in visual acuity.[39] At this stage, the use of intravitreal dexamethasone and timing is dependent upon surgeon preference.

Topical antibiotic therapy is indicated when there is concurrent infective keratitis. Dilating drops such as atropine 1% bid are beneficial to minimize posterior synechiae and reduce ciliary spasm.

7.2 Surgical approach

Figure 3 outlines an approach to vitrectomy surgery in endophthalmitis. If the patients systemic condition allows, general anesthesia may be the anesthetic of choice because obtaining adequate local anesthesia for an inflamed painful eye can be difficult. Following the application of povidine-iodine solution, draping and lid speculum, the corneal or scleral wound should be closed with 10-0 nylon suture. An attempt should be made to aspirate anterior chamber fluid (around 0.1cc) with a 30G needle and 1cc tuberculin syringe. An infusion cannula (25G or 23G or 20G 6mm) is inserted pars plana if the view allows. If anterior segment opacity precludes view of the infusion cannula, an anterior chamber maintainer can be utilized initially. The infusion is kept off to allow for an undiluted vitreous sample, which is obtained with manual aspiration of a tuberculin syringe connected to a 3-way stopcock, connected to the aspiration tubing of vitrectomy probe. Both samples are either sent quickly to the microbiology laboratory for urgent gram stain, culture and sensitivities or the material is plated directly onto blood agar, chocolate agar, Sauboraud's media, thioglycolate broth and placed on two glass slides for Gram and Giemsa stains.

- Consider general anesthesia
- Prep & drape
- Suture the corneal wound with a 10-0 nylon
- Insert 3 ports (25 or 23G) pars plana & place plugs
- Anterior chamber tap (27 or 30G needle, tuberculin syringe)
- Place the infusion line in the anterior chamber when the view is very poor, but keep the infusion off. Alternatively consider a 20G 6mm infusion line pars plana
- Vitreous sample (undiluted) - connect cutter/aspiration line to a 3-way stop cock connected to a tuberculin syringe and manually aspirate 0.2-0.3cc of vitreous fluid
- Send anterior chamber and vitreous samples for urgent M/C/S or inoculate onto appropriate plates and slides
- Methodical approach from anterior to posterior
- Clear anterior chamber of fibrin/inflammatory debris/membrane using cutter/aspiration via a limbal approach
- Switch the infusion to pars plana port once the view allows to confirm position
- Consider endoscopic approach in the presence of a very poor view if available
- Core vitrectomy
- Peripheral vitrectomy if visualization allows
- Measures to avoid retinal breaks
    - Refrain from inducing PVD or shaving the vitreous base if the retina is necrotic and severely inflamed
- No air-fluid exchange is done unless indicated
- Check sclerotomies & ensure sealed
- Inject intravitreal antibiotics ceftazidime 2.25mg/0.1cc and vancomycin 1mg/0.1cc
    - Consider reducing the antibiotic dose in gas/air filled eyes or silicone oil filled eyes to reduce the risk of retinal toxicity. Especially for ceftazidime.
- Consider intravitreal dexamethasone 400μg/0.1cc

Fig. 3. Surgical approach in acute post-operative (cataract surgery) endophthalmitis

Infusion is then started and the anterior chamber is cleared to enable visualization. This includes careful removal of membranes and avoiding trauma to the iris with resultant hyphema. A core vitrectomy is then performed and the vitrectomy is carried posteriorly. Attempts were made to clear ≥ 50% of the vitreous with no aim of inducing a posterior vitreous detachment in the EVS to avoid secondary complications.[19] Aggressive removal of vitreous in the vicinity of inflamed and necrotic retina has the potential risk of creating retinal tears and detachment. Eyes with a posterior vitreous detachment allow for a more complete vitrectomy. These eyes may have inflammatory debris over the posterior pole that can be gently aspirated. In situations where visibility is too poor to adequately define posterior vitreous, attempts to clear reformed anterior chamber debris/membrane should be performed. Membranes can also develop on the posterior aspect of the intraocular lens and this should be cleared. If the opacity precludes adequate view following core vitrectomy, the procedure can be discontinued rather than risk retinal/choroidal trauma with the cutter. Intraoperative complications in this setting include retinal breaks and hemorrhage as well as choroidal hemorrhage, which can be devastating. Retinal breaks can be treated with laser photocoagulation or cryotherapy and gas or silicone oil tamponade. However, this poses dosing issues when injecting intravitreal antibiotics. One step to avoid choroidal hemorrhage includes maintaining a steady intraocular pressure during surgery. If this complication develops, the bottle height should be raised to occlude the source, but in severe cases it can lead to loss of the eye. Intravitreal antibiotics should be injected pars plana at the conclusion of the case, once the sclerotomy sites are sealed. Modification in the dose of ceftazidime may be required in eyes with gas or oil fill to account for the reduction in vitreous fluid. Intravitreal dexamethasone is optional and given at the surgeons discretion.

Kuhn and Gini recommended an approach not based on presenting acuity alone, but on the overall clinical picture and course.[40,41] In the presence of a poor reflex or absent retinal detail at presentation, or no improvement within 24 h of initial conservative therapy with intravitreal injections, PPV was offered to the patient. Their vitrectomy technique differed significantly from that of the EVS. They defined a 'complete' PPV as that starting at the anterior segment and working posterior which included, utilizing temporary keratoprosthesis if necessary, evacuating the AC of fibrin and cellular material, and then working purposely posterior towards the retina with engagement and removal of the posterior hyaloids and irrigation of any macular hypopyon and debris. Conservative shaving of the vitreous base was recommended depending on limitations in visualization. Silicone oil was an option for necrotic or detached retina or those otherwise having multiple tears. In their non-randomized consecutive series of 47 patients, 91% achieved a visual acuity of 20/40 or better compared to 53% in the EVS. In this limited report, no retinal detachments developed (8.3% EVS), there were no lost eyes from phthisis, and no additional PPV was required. The authors base these positive results on advances in vitrector technology and the development of wide-angle viewing systems since the EVS. The development of the endoscope in vitrectomy surgery has likewise increased the amount of patients, previously excluded by the EVS inclusion criteria, to more aggressive management.[42]

7.3 Treatment in other causes of exogenous endophthalmitis

Application of the EVS to traumatic endophthalmitis may not be appropriate because of differences in organisms and potential for concurrent posterior injury with trauma. In severe cases, vitrectomy should be strongly considered to clear infected vitreous and manage coexisting injury including vitreous hemorrhage and retinal breaks. However, significant challenges are encountered due to altered anatomy and visualization difficulties.

Vancomycin (1 mg/0.1 cc) has been the treatment of choice for bacterial infection, with broad coverage of Gram-positive bacteria implicated in chronic postoperative endophthalmitis.[43] If fungi are implicated, intravitreal amphotericin B (5-10 μg/0.1 mL) should be considered. Voriconazole or miconazole can be considered if organisms are resistant to amphotericin B. PPV is often advocated for treatment of chronic postoperative endophthalmitis. Removal of vitreous infiltrates with total capsulectomy, intravitreal antibiotic and intraocular lens removal or exchange has the lowest recurrence rate.[43] Even with these interventions, recurrent inflammation may still occur. The effectiveness of orally administered fourth-generation quinolones, such as gatifloxacin and moxifloxacin, may obviate the need for such aggressive procedures in the future.

- Insert infusion line infero-temporal 3.5mm from the limbus
- Create superonasal and superotemporal transconjunctival scleral tunnel sclerotomies for the light pipe and vitrector
- Create a limbal paracentesis and inject viscoelastic into the bag and anterior chamber
- Place iris hooks to allow better visualization of the zonular apparatus
- Create a superior corneal wound
- Rotate the IOL out of the bag
- Cut the optic of the foldable IOL with an intraocular scissors about ¾ of its length and remove in one piece
- Insert an intraocular forceps through the clear corneal incision between the sutures to grasp the anterior capsule and stretch it to expose the zonules
- Use the vitrector through the pars plana cannula to cut the zonules 360°
- The entire capsular bag is then removed with the intraocular forceps and sent for gram stain and inoculation onto bacterial and fungal media
  - At least 2 medias for anaerobic culture should be used
- Suture the corneal wound
- Perform core vitrectomy
- Posterior hyaloid detachment, vitreous base shaving and aspiration of deposits can be carried out
- Aspirate remaining viscoelastic
- Inject intravitreal Vancomycin 1mg/0.1cc

Fig. 4. Technique for vitrectomy in eyes with chronic endophthalmitis and a foldable acrylic IOL

Many retinal surgeons extrapolate from EVS data and apply this to the treatment of bleb-associated endophthalmitis. However, this may not be appropriate and a lower threshold for PPV may be warranted given the more virulent organisms involved. However, insertion of sclerotomies should be away from the infected bleb. Also, intensive fortified topical antibiotics should be utilized where blebitis is also present.

Our future challenges will be staying ahead of the constant evolution of bacterial resistance. Bacteria have survived the primordial soup at the dawn of life and somewhere in the bacterial plasmids are the genetic codes to all forms of antibiotics that we may develop. Despite the power of bacterial evolution, future advancements in antibiotic pharmacology, surgical and prophylactic techniques will be necessary to keep us one step ahead.

8. References

[1] Fintelmann RE, Naseri A. Prophylaxis of postoperative endophthalmitis following cataract surgery. Current status and future directions. Drugs 2010;70(11):1395-1409

[2] Hatch WV, Cernat G, Wong D et al. Risk Factors for Acute Endophthalmitis after Cataract Surgery: A population-based Study. Ophthalmology 2009;116:425-430

[3] Endophthalmitis Study Group, European Society of Cataract & Refractive Surgeons. Prophylaxis of postoperative endophthalmitis following cataract surgery: results of the ESCRS multicenter study and identification of risk factors. J Cataract Refract Surg 2007 Jun; 33 (6): 978-88c

[4] West ES, Behrens A, McDonnell PJ, et al. The incidence of endophthalmitis after cataract surgery among the U.S. Medicare population increased between 1994 and 2001. Ophthalmology 2005; 112:1388–1394.

[5] Taban M, Behrens A, Newcomb RL, et al. Acute en- dophthalmitis following cataract surgery: a systematic re- view of the literature. Arch Ophthalmol 2005 May; 123 (5): 613-20

[6] Khan RI, Kennedy S, Barry P. Incidence of presumed postoperative endophthalmitis in Dublin for a 5-year period (1997–2001). J Cataract Refract Surg 2005; 31:1575–1581.

[7] Ang GS, Varga Z, Shaarawy. Postoperative infection in penetrating versus non-penetrating glaucoma surgery. Br J Ophthalmol 2010;94:1571-1576

[8] Stein JD, Ruiz D Jr, Belsky D, et al. Longitudinal rates of postoperative adverse outcomes after glaucoma surgery among medicare beneficiaries 1994 to 2005. Ophthalmology 2008;115:1109e1116.e7.

[9] Chiselita D, Danielescu C. Postoperative endophthalmitis asfter non-penetrating deep sclerectomy. Oftalmologia 2010;54(1):36-40

[10] Kunimoto DY, Kaiser RS, Wills Eye Retina Service. Incidence of endophthalmitis after 20- and 25-gauge vitrectomy. Ophthalmology 2007; 114(12): 2133–2137

[11] Cohen SM, Flynn Jr HW, Murray TG, Smiddy WE. Endophthalmitis after pars plana vitrectomy. The Postvitrectomy Endophthalmitis Study Group. Ophthalmology 1995; 102: 705–712

[12] Patel KC, Rahman R. Incidence of post-operative endophthalmitis following 23-gauge transconjunctival sutureless vitrectomy in the United Kingdom: a survey. Eye 2011 [epub ahead of print]

[13] Bahrani HM, Fazelat AA, Thomas M et al. Endophthalmitis in the Era of Small Gauge Transconjunctival Sutureless Vitrectomy-MetaAnalysis and Review of Literature. Sem Ophthalmol 2010;25(5-6):275-282

[14] Kunimoto DY, Kaiser RS, Wills Eye Retina Service. Inci- dence of endophthalmitis after 20- and 25-gauge vitrectomy. Ophthalmology 2007;114:2133–7

[15] Scott IU, Flynn HW Jr, Dev S, et al. Endophthalmitis after 25-gauge and 20-gauge pars plana vitrectomy: incidence and outcomes. Retina 2008;28:138–42

[16] Sampat KM, Garg SJ. Complications of intravitreal injections. Curr Opin Ophthalmol 2010;21(3):178-183
[17] Taban M, Behrens A, Newcomb RL et al. Incidence of Acute Endophthalmitis Following Penetrating Keratoplasty - A Systematic Review. Arch Ophthalmol 2005;123:605-609
[18] Lemley CA, Han DP. Endophthalmitis: a review of current evaluation and management. Retina 2007;27(6):662-680
[19] Endophthalmitis Vitrectomy Study Group. Results of the Endophthalmitis Vitrectomy Study. A randomized trial of immediate vitrectomy and of intravenous antibiotics for the treatment of postoperative bacterial endophthalmitis. Arch Ophthalmol 1995;113:1479–1496
[20] Busbee BG, Recchia FM, Kaiser R, et al. Bleb-associated endophthalmitis: clinical characteristics and visual out- comes. Ophthalmology 2004;111:1495–1503
[21] Bhagat N, Nagori S, Zarbin M. Post-traumatic Infectious Endophthalmitis. Surv Ophthalmol 2011.[Epub ahead of print]
[22] Song A, Scott IU, Flynn HW et al. Delayed-onset Bleb-associated endophthalmitis. Clinical Features and Visual Acuity Outcomes. Ophthalmology 2002;109:985-991
[23] Hammoudi DS, Abdolell M, Wong DT. Patterns of perioperative prophylaxis for cataract surgery in Canada. Can J ophthalmol 2007;42:681-8
[24] DeCroos FC, Afshari NA. Perioperative antibiotics and anti-inflammatory agents in cataract surgery. Curr Opin Ophthalmol 2008;19:22-26
[25] Ciulla TA, Starr MB, Masket S. bacterial endophthalmitis prophylaxis for cataract surgery: an evidence-based update. Ophthalmology 2002;109:13-24
[26] Anijeet DR, Palimar P, Peckar CO. Intracameral vancomycin following cataract surgery: An eleven year study. Clin Ophthalmol 2010;4:321-326
[27] Recchia FM, Busbee BG, Pearlman RB et al. Changing trends in the microbiologic aspects of postcataract endophthalmitis. Arch Ophthalmol 2005;123:341-346
[28] Campochiaro PA, Green WR. Toxicity of intravitreous ceftazidime in primate retina. Arch Ophthalmol 1992;110:1625-9
[29] Hegazy HM, Kivilcim M, Peyman GA et al. Evaluation of toxicity of intravitreal ceftazidime, vancomycin, and ganciclovir in a silicone oil-filled eye. Retina 1999;19:553-7
[30] Mieler WF, Glazer LC, Bennett SR et al. favourable outcome of traumatic endophthalmitis with associated retinal breaks or detachment. Can J Ophthalmol 1992;27:348-52
[31] Pflugfelder SC, Hernandez E, Fliesler Sj et al. Intravitreal vancomycin. Retinal toxicity, clearance, and interaction with gentamicin. Arch Ophthalmol 1987;105:831-7
[32] Thompson AM. Ocular toxicity of fluoroquinolones. Clin Experiment Ophthalmol 2007;35:566-77
[33] Aguilar HE, Meredith TA, el-Massry A et al. Vancomycin levels after intravitreal injection. Effects of inflammation and surgery. Retina 1995;15:428-32
[34] Barza M, Lynch E, Baum JL. Pharmacokinetics of newer cephalosporins after subconjunctival and intravitreal injection in rabbits. Arch Ophthalmol 1993;111:121-5
[35] Hariprasad SM, Mieler WF, Holz ER. Vitreous and aqueous penetration of orally administered gatifloxacin in humans. Arch Ophthalmol 2003;121:345–350

[36] Hariprasad SM, Shah GK, Mieler WF, et al. Vitreous and aqueous penetration of orally administered moxifloxacin in humans. Arch Ophthalmol 2006;124:178–182
[37] Koul S, Phillpson BT, Phillpson A. Visual outcome of endophthalmitis in Sweden. Acta Ophthalmol (Copenh) 1989;67:504-9
[38] Das T, Jalali S, Gothwal VK et al. Intravitreal dexamethasone in exogenous bacterial endophthalmitis: results of a prospective randomized study. Br J Ophthalmol 1999;83:1050-5
[39] Shah GK, Stein JD, Sharma S et al. Visual outcomes following the use of intravitreal steroids in the treatment of postoperative endophthalmitis. Ophthalmology 2000;107:486-9
[40] Kuhn F, Gini G. Vitrectomy for endophthalmitis. Ophthalmology 2006;113:714
[41] Kuhn F, Gini G. Ten years after...are findings of the Endophthalmitis Vitrectomy Study still relevant today? Graefes Arch Clin Exp Ophthalmol 2005;243:1197-9
[42] De Smet MD, Carlborg EA. Managing severe endophthalmitis with the use of an endoscope. Retina 2005;25:976-80
[43] Deramo VA, Ting TD. Treatment of propionibacterium acnes endophthalmitis. Curr Opin Ophthalmol 2001;12:225-9

20

Endophthalmitis Following Cataract Surgery: Clinical Features, Treatment and Prophylaxis

Avinash Pathengay, Stephen G. Schwartz,
Harry W. Flynn Jr. and Darlene Miller
*Department of Ophthalmology, Bascom Palmer Eye Institute, University of Miami,
Miller School of Medicine, Miami, Florida
USA*

1. Introduction

Acute-onset postoperative endophthalmitis is characterized by marked inflammation of intraocular fluids and tissues. Despite appropriate therapeutic intervention, endophthalmitis may result in severe visual loss. Postoperative endophthalmitis has been reported following every type of ocular surgery but because cataract surgery is the most commonly performed type of ocular surgery, this setting is the most frequent cause in clinical practice.

2. Incidence

The incidence of acute-onset postoperative endophthalmitis **(Table 1)** after cataract surgery has steadily declined from 2% in the first half of the twentieth century to current levels ranging from 0.03% to 0.21% (Leopold, 1971; Allen & Mangiaracine, 1964; Aaberg et al., 1998; West et al., 2005; Jensen et al., 2008; Moshirfar et al., 2007; Freeman et al., 2010; Ravindran et al., 2009; Wykoff et al., 2010). The reported rate of delayed-onset (chronic) postoperative endophthalmitis following cataract surgery in one single-center series was 0.017% (Mezaine et al., 2009).

	Author	Years	No. of cases	Incidence %
1	Leopold	(1920-1940)	Meta-analysis	2.00
2	Allen & Mangiaracine	(1958-1962)	22/20,000	0.09
3	Aaberg et al.	(1984-1994)	34/41,654	0.07
4	West et al.	(1994-2001)	1026/4,77,627	0.21
5	Jensen et al.	(1997-2007)	40/29,276	0.14
6	Moshirfar et al.	(2003-2005)	14/20,013	0.07
7	Freeman et al.	(1996-2005)	754/4,90,690	0.15
8	Ravindran et al.	(2007-2008)	38/42,426	0.09
9	Wykoff et al.	(1995-2009)	8/28,568	0.03

Table 1. Reported incidence of acute-onset postoperative endophthalmitis

3. Risk factors

There are concerns that clear corneal sutureless temporal incision cataract surgery may increase the risk of endophthalmitis (Nichamin et al., 2006). In a nosocomial survey (2002-2009) at a university teaching hospital involving resident, fellow, and faculty surgeons, there was no increase in the incidence of endophthalmitis in the era of sutureless clear corneal cataract surgery (Wykoff et al., 2010). Other more established risk factors for developing acute-postoperative endophthalmitis include patients with diabetes mellitus, cases with posterior capsular rupture and advanced age (Hatch et al., 2009; Doft et al., 2001). A range of risk factors for acute-onset postoperative endophthalmitis is summarized in **Table 2**.

A. Preoperative:

1. Diabetes mellitus.
2. Immune compromise.
3. Chronic blepharitis.
4. Infection of the lacrimal drainage system.
5. Contaminated eye drops.
6. Contact lens wear.
7. Contralateral ocular prosthesis.

B. Intraoperative:

1. Application of 2% Xylocaine gel before povidone-iodine instillation.
2. Prolonged surgery.
3. Secondary IOL.
4. Posterior capsular rupture.
5. Vitreous loss.
6. Contaminated irrigating solution.
7. Clear corneal incision (controversial).

C. Post operative

1. Wound leak.
2. Vitreous incarceration.

Table 2. Risk Factors for Acute-onset Postoperative Endophthalmitis

4. Classification, isolates and clinical features

The diagnosis of endophthalmitis is made by the constellation of clinical symptoms and signs. The symptoms and signs vary according to time of presentation (acute-onset postoperative endophthalmitis (APE) (occurring within six weeks of cataract surgery) and chronic postoperative (CPE) endophthalmitis (presenting 6 weeks or more after the surgery) (Johnson et al., 1997).

APE is associated with rapid onset of visual loss, pain, marked intraocular inflammation usually with hypopyon **(Figure 2)** and caused by rapidly growing bacteria with coagulase-negative Staphylococci **(Figure 2)** being the most common isolated organism (followed by other Gram positive organisms like *Staphylococcus aureus, Streptococcus* species and Gram negative bacteria) (Han et al., 1996). Endophthalmitis caused by the coagulase-negative staphylococci may have less severe inflammatory signs, often creating difficulty in distinguishing between an infectious and a noninfectious etiology on clinical grounds.

APE, when caused by more virulent organisms such as other Streptococcus species and Gram negative organisms, may be associated with corneal infiltrate, cataract wound abnormalities, afferent pupillary defect, loss of red reflex, initial light perception-only vision, and symptom onset within 2 days of surgery. (Johnson et al., 1997). In CPE caused by less virulent bacteria and fungi, the inflammation is often low-grade and slowly progressive **(Table 3).** *Propionibacterium acnes* is the most common organism isolated in CPE (Mezaine et al., 2009; Clark et al., 1999). Other less virulent organisms include Gram positive organisms (coagulase negative *Staphyloccocus, Corynebacterium* species) (Fox et al., 1991), Gram negative organisms (*Alcaligenes xylosoxidans, Acinetobacter calcoaceticus, Ochrobactrum anthropi*) (Aaberg et al., 1997; Gopal et al., 2000) and fungi (*Candida* species, *Aspergillus* species, and *Curvularia* species) (Pflugfelder et al., 1988; Pathengay et al., 2006a). Mild to moderate vitritis, white posterior capsular plaque **(Figure 3)** and keratic precipitates are common clinical signs in CPE (Mezaine et al., 2009; Johnson et al., 1997). Hypopyon is less frequently seen as compared to acute-onset postoperative endophthalmitis (Johnson et al., 1997). The presence of a white plaque inside the capsular bag has been reported in a large series of patients with *P. acnes* endophthalmitis (Nichamin et al., 2006). However, this plaque is not unique to *P. acnes* and has been described in CPE caused by other microorganisms as well (Mezaine et al., 2009; Pathengay et al., 2006a).

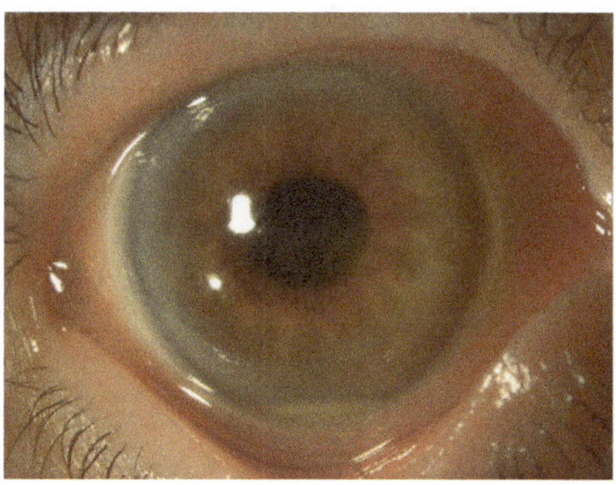

Fig. 1. Acute-onset postoperative endophthalmitis.

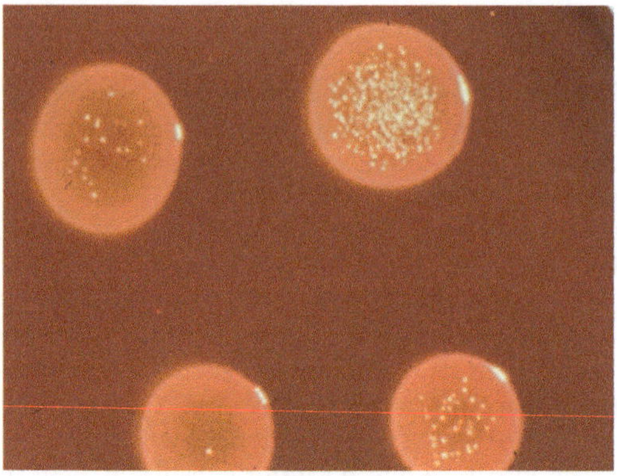

Fig. 2. Coagluase negative Staphylococci isolates from vitreous growing on blood agar.

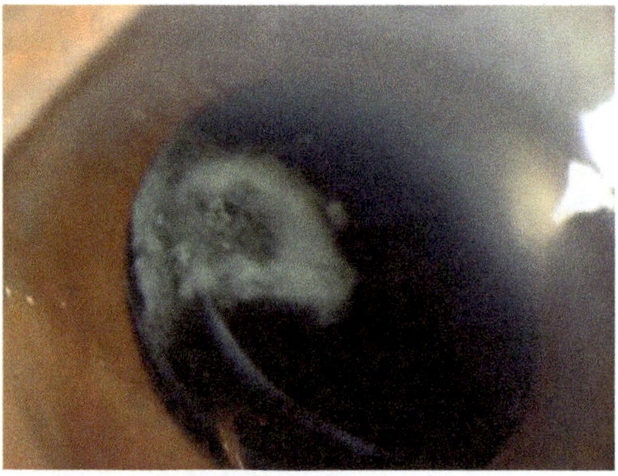

Fig. 3. Delayed-onset postoperative endophthalmitis.

Bacteria	**Fungi**
P. acnes	*Candida parapsilosis*
S. epidermidis	Other *Candida* species
Corynebacterium species	*Paecilomyces* species
Xanthomonas maltophilia	*Aspergillus* species
Alcaligenes xylosoxidans	*Acremonium* species

Table 3. Bacteria and Fungi commonly associated with delayed postoperative endophthalmitis.

5. Differential diagnosis

The differential diagnosis of endophthalmitis following cataract surgery is summarized in **Table 4.** Toxic anterior segment syndrome (TASS) can mimic infectious endophthalmitis and is often associated with various toxins entering the eye at the time of surgery (Doshi et al., 2010; Cutler Peck et al., 2010).

The inflammatory response is usually seen with in the first 24 hours after surgery and there is little or no pain. In TASS, corneal edema can be severe and extending "wall to wall". It can be associated with a hypopyon and fibrin formation in the anterior chamber and the vitreous is typically not involved, as is the case with an infectious endophthalmitis. Dehemoglobinized red blood cells in the vitreous cavity can also be confused with endophthalmitis (Nguyen et al., 2006). Retained lens fragments have been reported to cause a marked inflammatory reaction with hypopyon, which may also clinically resemble infectious endophthalmitis (Irvine et al., 1992).

A. Toxic anterior segment syndrome (TASS).

B. Retained lens material.

C. Flare-up of pre-existing uveitis.

D. Dehemoglobinized vitreous hemorrhage.

Table 4. Differential Diagnosis of Endophthalmitis after Cataract Surgery.

6. Management

It is important to examine the surgical wound for leakage and vitreous incarceration which may need to be addressed at the time of treatment. If visualization of the posterior segment is limited by either inflammatory material or corneal edema, B-scan echography may help assess the degree of vitreous opacification and determine the presence of either choroidal or retinal detachment.

The treatment of endophthalmitis is usually performed using topical, peribulbar, or retrobulbar anesthesia. A vitreous tap is more commonly utilized but pars plana vitrectomy (PPV) is considered in more advanced cases. The goals of PPV include the following:

1. Obtain intraocular fluid for microbiological analysis (the vitreous specimen generally yields higher culture positivity rates compared to aqueous) (Han et al., 1996);
2. Debulk vitreous of toxins, microorganisms and inflammatory debris.

Although postoperative endophthalmitis is a clinical diagnosis, confirmation by culture of intraocular fluid specimens is an important step in the management. Vitreous can be obtained using a needle (vitreous tap) or by PPV. If a vitreous tap is employed, the use of a 23-gauge butterfly needle **(Figure 4)** may offer better stability than a straight needle attached directly to a syringe (Raju & Das, 2004). The undiluted vitreous specimen is then inoculated onto the culture media. The Endophthalmitis Vitrectomy Study reported no significant differences between 3-port PPV versus needle tap/biopsy with respect to microbiologic yield, operative complications, short-term (9-12 months) retinal detachment risk, or visual outcomes (Han et al., 1999).

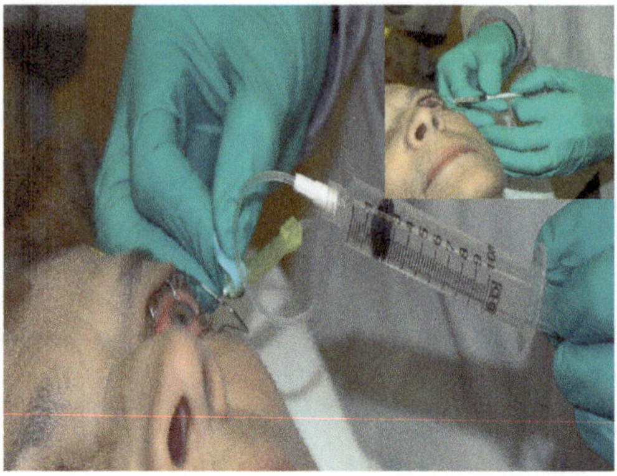

Fig. 4. Butterfly needle used for vitreous tap (upper right: injection of intravitreal antibiotics in separate syringes).

PPV may be performed using small-gauge sutureless (Tan et al., 2008) **(Figure 5)** or 20-gauge vitrectomy techniques and instrumentation. In the Endophthalmitis Vitrectomy Study (EVS), a goal of PPV was the removal of approximately 50% of the formed vitreous. If the cornea is clear and the pupil dilates well, a more complete PPV can be considered. In typical APE, it is not generally necessary to remove the IOL. In some patients, visibility may be improved by stripping fibrin from the iris or the surface of IOL (Friberg, 1991). In selected cases of delayed postoperative endophthalmitis caused by *Propionobacterium acnes* or fungi which are not responsive to initial treatment, or when there is recurrence of inflammation, IOL explantation may be considered along with the removal of entire capsular bag (Clark et al., 1999).

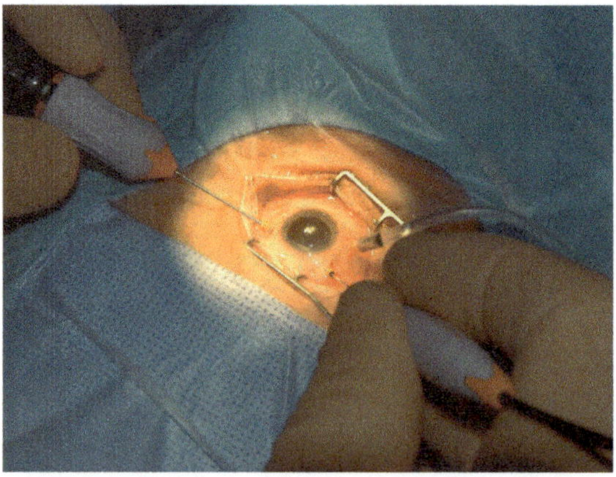

Fig. 5. 23-gauge PPV performed in a patient with acute-onset postoperative endophthalmitis.

Intravitreal antibiotic therapy **(Figure 6)** is standard treatment of presumed bacterial postoperative endophthalmitis **(Table 5)**. When endophthalmitis is initially suspected, the pathogen is not known therefore the choice of antimicrobial agent must be made empirically. The EVS reported that the combination of vancomycin (1 mg/0.1 cc) and amikacin (0.4 mg/ 0.1 cc) were usually effective against the broad spectrum of bacteria causing APE (Endophthalmitis Vitrectomy Study Group, 1995). In the EVS, 100% of the Gram positive bacteria were susceptible to vancomycin, 89% of the Gram negative bacteria were susceptible to both amikacin and ceftazidime, and the remaining 11% were resistant to both amikacin and ceftazidime (Han et al., 1996). However, there are multiple reports of toxicity following administration of intravitreal aminoglycosides, including macular infarction (Campochiaro & Lim, 1994). An alternative to the aminoglycosides for coverage of Gram negative organisms is the use of intravitreal ceftazidime 2.25 mg, a third-generation cephalosporin (Jay et al., 1987; Roth & Flynn, 1997). Although ceftazidime may precipitate when mixed with vancomycin, this has not been reported to alter its effectiveness in the clinical setting (Kwok et al., 2002). It is generally recommended to use a separate needle and syringe for each antibiotic.

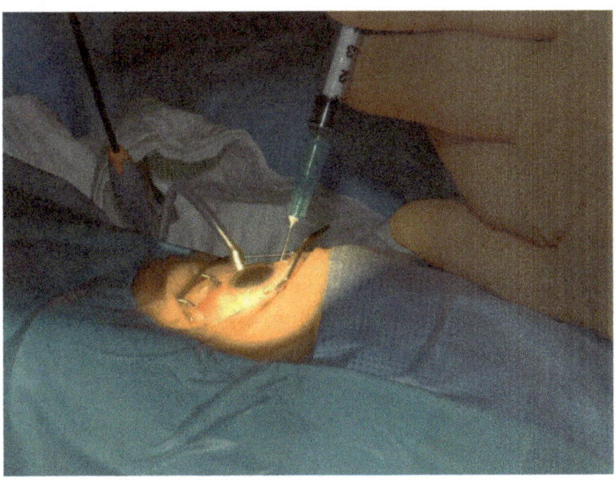

Fig. 6. Intravitreal antibiotics administered at the end of PPV.

A. Seidel test for potential wound leak

B. Use topical, peribulbar or retrobulbar anesthesia for either vitreous tap or vitrectomy

C. Obtain intraocular specimen

1. 30-gauge needle for anterior chamber tap (optional)
2. 25 or 23-gauge needle for vitreous tap
3. Pars plana vitrectomy (PPV)

D. Preparation of intravitreal antibiotics (usually by pharmacist)

E. Dosages for intravitreal injection

1. Vancomycin 1 mg
2. Ceftazidime 2.25 mg or amikacin 0.4 mg
3. Dexamethasone 0.4 mg (Optional)

Table 5. Suggested Endophthalmitis Treatment In The Setting Of A Clear Corneal Incision

Intravitreal corticosteroids reduce inflammation-induced ocular damage associated with presumed bacterial endophthalmitis. In a prospective randomized clinical trial of 63 bacterial endophthalmitis cases, intravitreal dexamethasone was reported to reduce inflammation scores early in the course of treatment but had no independent influence on the final visual outcome (Das et al., 1999). In a series of endophthalmitis caused by virulent bacteria such as Gram negative organisms and *Staphylococcus aureus,* better visual acuity outcomes were reported after adjunctive treatment with intravitreal dexamethasone (Irvine et al., 1992). Intravitreal triamcinolone acetonide has also been reported to reduce inflammation without exacerbating the infection in a small series of endophthalmitis cases (Pathengay et al., 2006b).
Postoperative fungal endophthalmitis more commonly presents as a delayed-onset (chronic) case. Fungi should be suspected in patients that fail to respond to standard intravitreal antibiotic therapy. Traditionally, intravitreal amphotericin B was used commonly to treat suspected fungal endophthalmitis, but intravitreal voriconazole (with or without adjunctive oral therapy) is becoming more frequently employed (Vasconcelos-Santos & Nehemy, 2009).

7. Endophthalmitis vitrectomy study

The EVS was a large multicenter randomized clinical trial comparing vitreous tap to PPV in patients presenting with endophthalmitis within 6 weeks of cataract surgery or secondary IOL implantation **(Table 6).** A total of 420 patients with APE after cataract surgery was randomly assigned to undergo 3-port PPV or tap/biopsy. They were also randomized to receive either systemic antibiotics (ceftazidime and amikacin) or no systemic antibiotics. At the end of 9 months, patients were assessed for final visual acuity and media clarity.

7.1 Primary results

In patients who presented with hand motions (HM) visual acuity or better, there were no statistically significant differences between eyes assigned to vitreous tap versus PPV. In patients who presented with light perception (LP) visual acuity, PPV was associated with significantly more favorable outcomes. The usage of systemic antibiotics was not associated with significant improvements in either visual acuity or media clarity outcomes. (Doft & Barza, 1996; Barza et al., 1997)

A. Background - largest series of endophthalmitis after cataract surgery (N=420)

1. EVS enrolled endophthalmitis patients after extracapsular cataract extraction, scleral tunnel phacoemulsification, or secondary IOL within 6 weeks of surgery.
2. Initial results were reported in 1995 and subsequent reports were published in the following years.

B. EVS primary results

1. Patients with LP vision fared better with initial PPV.
2. When patients presented with HM or better vision, equal visual acuity outcomes were reported in the PPV and vitreous tap groups.
3. There was no apparent benefit from the use of systemic antibiotics (amikacin and ceftazidime) compared to controls (no IV antibiotics).

C. EVS secondary results

1. Gram positive bacteria were isolated from 94.2% patients and Gram negative bacteria in 6.5%. Coagulase-negative micrococci were the most common bacteria isolated in 70% of patients. Diabetes mellitus was associated with a higher yield of Gram positive, coagulase-negative micrococci.
2. Patients with diabetes mellitus and visual acuity better than LP achieved better visual outcomes with initial PPV (not statistically significant).
3. Additional procedures (as a result of worsening intraocular inflammation or infection or for complications) after the initial treatment: 8% of PPV eyes and 13% of tap eyes.
4. There was no statistical difference between PPV and tap groups in terms of microbiological yield, operative complications, retinal detachment (8.3%) or visual acuity outcomes (overall, 53% equal to or better than 20/40 in EVS).
5. In the EVS the incidence of retinal detachment (RD) was 8.3% and there was no difference in frequency of RD based on whether initial management was PPV or tap.

Table 6. Summary of the Endophthalmitis Vitrectomy Study (EVS)

7.2 Other results

Confirmed microbiologic growth was demonstrated in 69.3% of EVS patients. Undiluted vitreous produced a higher percentage of confirmed positive cultures when compared with aqueous (Barza et al., 1997). Gram positive bacteria were isolated from 94.2% patients and Gram negative bacteria from 6.5%. Coagulase-negative micrococci were the most common bacteria isolated in 70% of patients. An additional procedure (as a result of worsening intraocular inflammation or infection or for complications) after the initial treatment was performed in 8% of PPV eyes and 13% of tap eyes. (Doft et al., 1998). In the EVS the incidence of retinal detachment (RD) was 8.3% and there was no difference in frequency of RD based on whether initial management was PPV or tap. (Doft et al., 2000).

Although patients in the EVS derived no demonstrable benefit from these systemic antibiotics, the study made no recommendations regarding treatment with other systemic antibiotics (eg, systemic fluoroquinolones) or systemic antimicrobial agents for other types of endophthalmitis (eg, chronic, bleb-associated, traumatic, fungal, and endogenous forms) (Flynn & Scott, 2008).

Endophthalmitis patients with significant opacification of the anterior chamber precluding the use of PPV, or without light perception visual acuity, were excluded from the EVS. Because these eyes with more severe infection or involving more virulent organisms were

excluded from the EVS, the effect might have shifted the EVS outcomes to more favorable results. Although the EVS provides general guidelines, the clinician ultimately must decide on the best treatment strategy for the individual patient (Flynn & Scott, 2008).
The EVS, conducted during 1991-1994, enrolled patients with scleral tunnel incisions. A follow-up retrospective study of patients recruited during 1996-2005 with clear corneal incisions reported generally similar outcomes compared with the EVS (Lalwani et al., 2008).

8. The European Society of Cataract and Refractive Surgeons (ESCRS) Endophthalmitis Study

The European Society of Cataract and Refractive Surgeons (ESCRS) Endophthalmitis Study was conducted at 24 centers in 9 European countries from 2003 to 2006. It was a partially masked, randomized, placebo-controlled study evaluating the prophylactic effect of intracameral cefuroxime injection and/or perioperative levofloxacin eye drops on the incidence of endophthalmitis after cataract surgery. A total of 16,603 patients was recruited in the four arms of the study.
The ESCRS Study reported that the use of intracameral cefuroxime was associated with a significant reduction in the incidence of postoperative endophthalmitis compared to instillation of topical antibiotics. The rate of endophthalmitis was 4.92 times higher in the control group than the cefuroxime-treated group. Perioperative topical levofloxacin was associated with a reduced incidence of endophthalmitis but this difference did not achieve statistical significance. In this study, reported risk factors included clear corneal incisions, silicone IOLs, and surgical complications (Barry et al., 2006; Endophthalmitis Study Group, European Society of Cataract & Refractive Surgeons, 2007)

9. Prophylaxis

The presumed source of the causative organism in the EVS and ESCRS Study was the ocular surface of study patients (Bannerman et al., 1997; Seal et al., 2008). In a systematic review of all prophylactic methods for cataract surgery, instillation of 5% povidone-iodine on the conjunctiva 3 minutes before the surgery received the highest rating and was the only measure that gained a Grade B rating based on evidence from randomized clinical trials (Ciulla et al., 2002).

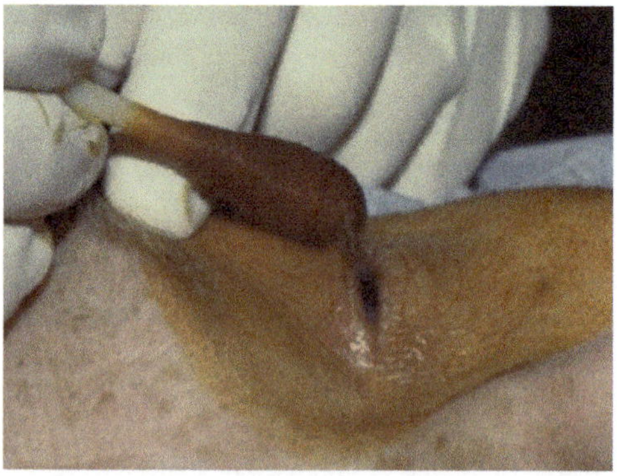

Fig. 7. Povidone-iodine used as prophylaxis preoperatively.

Povidone-iodine **(Figure 7)** has reported efficacy in reducing the bacterial load in the conjunctival fornices and is more effective than silver protein solution (Speaker & Menikoff, 1991). A recent study reported that repeated irrigation of the operative field with povidone-iodine 0.25% achieved an extremely low bacterial contamination rate in the anterior chamber at the completion of cataract surgery (Shimada et al., 2011).

Preoperative antibiotic administration is associated with a significant decrease in conjunctival bacterial colony counts after the use of certain antibiotics but has not shown superiority to antisepsis with povidone-iodine (Isenberg et al., 1985). A prospective study demonstrated that the addition of moxifloxacin drops had no significant effect in the preoperative reduction of conjunctival bacterial colonization above the effect of povidone-iodine 5% alone (Halachimi-Eyal et al., 2009).

Antibiotics in the irrigating fluid for cataract surgery have been reported to reduce anterior chamber bacterial contamination rates significantly but their effect on endophthalmitis prevention is less convincing (Sobaci et al., 2003; Srinivasan et al., 2008). The reported lack of effectiveness of both vancomycin and gentamicin in the irrigation fluid may be due to the requirement of more than 140 minutes to exhibit bactericidal effect, whereas the half-life of antibiotics in the anterior chamber is only 51 minutes (Gritz et al., 1996). Intracameral antibiotics have many negative consequences including potential toxicity, increased cost, and the potential for more rapid emergence of resistant bacteria. At least 10 patients in the EVS developed endophthalmitis in spite of receiving antibiotics in the irrigating fluid for cataract surgery.

Other antibiotics which have been used intracamerally include vancomycin, cefazolin and moxifloxacin. Although the safety of moxifloxacin has been reported, there are no published reports about its usage in routine clinical cases (Arbisser, 2008).

Intracameral vancomycin has been reported to significantly reduce the incidence of postoperative endophthalmitis after cataract surgery in a large series from the UK (Anijeet et al., 2010). Since vancomycin is generally reserved for the treating severe life-threatening or organ-threatening infections, such as endophthalmitis, the United States Centers for Disease Control and Prevention guidelines recommended that this drug should not be used for prophylaxis. Similarly, a study from Spain has reported prophylactic efficacy of intracameral cefazolin, in diminishing the rate of postoperative endophthalmitis without toxic effects on the cornea or retina (Romero et al., 2006). Concerns about the intracameral antibiotic include lack of commercial availability, problems with dosing, pH, and improper constituents within the injection that could lead to postoperative TASS, possible fungal or bacterial contamination during mixing or cystoid macular edema.

Traditionally, subconjunctival antibiotics were commonly administered after intraocular surgery but are less often utilized today. The rationale for subconjunctival antibiotic administration at the completion of the procedure is to inhibit growth of bacteria that may gain entry into the eye. Studies performed evaluating the effectiveness of prophylactic subconjunctival antibiotics in reducing the incidence of postoperative endophthalmitis reported conflicting results (Iyer et al., 2004).

The use of povidone-iodine to reduce the intraoperative bacterial load and the creation of reliably self-sealing incisions to reduce ingress of contaminants are probably the most important of all these factors in reducing the risk of acute postoperative bacterial endophthalmitis. **Table 7** summarizes techniques in the reduction of the risk of endophthalmitis after cataract surgery.

A. Proposed Methods

1. Preoperative povidone-iodine antisepsis
2. Preoperative topical antibiotics
3. Properly sized and constructed incision
4. Antibiotics in irrigating solution
5. Antibiotics injected into AC
6. Postoperative subconjunctival antibiotics
7. Postoperative topical antibiotics

B. Current Choices for Intracameral Antibiotics

1. Vancomycin
2. Cefuroxime
3. Moxifloxacin

C. Potential Complications of Intracameral Antibiotics

1. Microbial contamination during mixing
2. Incorrect preparation and dosage
3. Allergy
4. Cystoid macular edema
5. Corneal edema

Table 7. Prophylaxis For Endophthalmitis After Cataract Surgery.

10. Conclusion

The incidence of endophthalmitis after cataract surgery is variable from about 0.03%-0.15%. Povidone-iodine prophylaxis is generally recommended for cataract surgery. Blepharitis, vitreous loss and wound leak are major potential preoperative, intraoperative and postoperative risk factors for endophthalmitis. The significance of clear corneal incisions as a potential risk factor for endophthalmitis remains controversial. The differential diagnosis of endophthalmitis include TASS, retained lens fragments, uveitis and chronic vitreous hemorrhage. The most common organisms causing post-operative endophthalmitis are coagulase negative staphylococci. In the treatment of presumed bacterial endophthalmitis, intravitreal vancomycin and ceftazidime are commonly used for empiric coverage of both Gram positive and Gram negative bacteria. In about 50% of patients, 20/40 or better visual acuity can be achieved after treatment.

11. References

Aaberg, T.M. Jr.; Rubsamen, P.E.; Joondeph, B.C.; & Flynn, H.W. Jr. Chronic postoperative gram-negative endophthalmitis. *Retina*. 1997;17:260-2.

Aaberg, T.M. Jr.; Flynn, H.W. Jr.; Schiffman, J.; & Newton, J. Nosocomial acute-onset postoperative endophthalmitis surgery: a ten-year review of incidence and outcomes. *Ophthalmology* 1998; 105: 1004-1010.

Allen, H.F.; & Mangiaracine, A.B. Bacterial endophthalmitis after cataract extraction: a study of 22 infections in 20,000 operations. *Arch. Ophthalmol.* 1964; 72: 454-462.

Anijeet, D.R.; Palimar, P.; & Peckar, C.O. Intracameral vancomycin following cataract surgery: An eleven-year study. *Clin. Ophthalmol.* 2010;4:321-6.

Arbisser, L.B. Safety of intracameral moxifloxacin for prophylaxis of endophthalmitis after cataract surgery. *J. Cataract Refract. Surg.* 2008;34:1114-20.

Bannerman, T.L.; Rhoden, D.L.; McAllister, S.K.; Miller, J.M.; & Wilson, L.A. The source of coagulase-negative staphylococci in the Endophthalmitis Vitrectomy Study: a comparison of eyelid and intraocular isolates using pulsed-field gel electrophoresis: the Endophthalmitis Vitrectomy Study Group. *Arch. Ophthalmol.* 1997;115:357–361.

Barry, P.; Seal, D.V.; Gettinby, G.; Lees, F.; Peterson, M.; & Revie, C.W. ESCRS study of prophylaxis of postoperative endophthalmitis after cataract surgery: preliminary report of principal results from a European multicenter study: the ESCRS Endophthalmitis Study Group. *J. Cataract Refract. Surg.* 2006; 32:407–410.

Barza, M.; Pavan, P.R.; Doft, B.H.; Wisniewski, S.R.; Wilson, L.A.; Han, D.P.; & Kelsey, S.F. Evaluation of microbiological diagnostic techniques in postoperative endophthalmitis in the Endophthalmitis Vitrectomy Study. *Arch. Ophthalmol.* 1997;115:1142-50.

Campochiaro, P.A. & Lim, J.I. Aminoglycoside toxicity in the treatment of endophthalmitis. The Aminoglycoside Toxicity Study Group. *Arch. Ophthalmol.* 1994; 11:248-53.

Ciulla, T.A.; Starr, M.B.; Masket, S. Bacterial endophthalmitis prophylaxis for cataract surgery: an evidence-based update. *Ophthalmology* 2002;109:13–24.

Clark, W.L.; Kaiser, P.K.; Flynn, H.W. Jr.; Belfort, A.; Miller, D.; & Meisler, D.M. Treatment strategies and visual acuity outcomes in chronic postoperative *Propionibacterium acnes* endophthalmitis. *Ophthalmology* 1999;106;1665-1670.

Cutler Peck, C.M.; Brubaker, J.; Clouser, S.; Danford, C.; Edelhauser, H.E.; & Mamalis, N. Toxic anterior segment syndrome: common causes. *J Cataract Refract Surg.* 2010;36:1073-80.

Das, T.; Jaleli, S.; Gothwal, V.K.; Sharma, S.; & Naduvilath, T.J. Intravitreal dexamethasone in exogenous bacterial endophthalmitis: results of a prospective randomised study. *Br. J. Ophthalmol.* 1999;83:1050–5.

Doft, B.H. & Barza, M. Optimal management of postoperative endophthalmitis and results of the Endophthalmitis Vitrectomy Study. *Curr. Opin. Ophthalmol.* 1996;7:84-94.

Doft, B.H.; Kelsey, S.F.; & Wisniewski, S.R. Additional procedures after the initial vitrectomy or tap-biopsy in the Endophthalmitis Vitrectomy Study. *Ophthalmology* 1998;105:707-16.

Doft, B.M.; Kelsey, S.F.; & Wisniewski, S.R. Retinal detachment in the Endophthalmitis Vitrectomy Study. *Arch. Ophthalmol.* 2000 Dec;118:1661-5.

Doft, B.H.; Wisniewski, S.R.; Kelsey, S.F.; & Groer-Fitzgerald, S. Endophthalmitis Vitrectomy Study Group. Diabetes and postoperative endophthalmitis in the Endophthalmitis Vitrectomy Study. *Arch. Ophthalmol.* 2001;119:650-656.

Doshi, R.R.; Arevalo, J.F.; Flynn, H.W. Jr.; & Cunningham, E.T. Jr. Evaluating exaggerated, prolonged, or delayed postoperative intraocular inflammation. *Am. J. Ophthalmol.* 2010 ;150:295-304.

Endophthalmitis Study Group, European Society of Cataract & Refractive Surgeons. Prophylaxis of postoperative endophthalmitis following cataract surgery: results of the ESCRS multicenter study and identification of risk factors. *J. Cataract Refract. Surg.* 2007;33:978-88.

Endophthalmitis Vitrectomy Study Group. Results of the Endophthalmitis Vitrectomy Study. A randomized trial of immediate vitrectomy and of intravenous antibiotics for the treatment of postoperative bacterial endophthalmitis. *Arch. Ophthalmol.* 1995;113:1479–96.

Flynn, H.W. Jr. & Scott, I.U. Legacy of the endophthalmitis vitrectomy study. *Arch Ophthalmol.* 2008;126:559-61.

Fox, G.M.; Joondeph, B.C.; Flynn, H.W. Jr.; Pflugfelder, S.C.; & Roussel, T.J. Delayed-onset pseudophakic endophthalmitis. *Am. J. Ophthalmol.* 1991;111:163-73.

Friberg, T.R. En bloc removal of inflammatory fibrocellular membranes from the iris surface in endophthalmitis. *Arch. Ophthalmol.* 1991;109:736-737.

Freeman, E.E.; Roy-Gagnon, M.H.; Fortin, E.; Gauthier, D.; Popescu, M.; & Boisjoly, H. Rate of endophthalmitis after cataract surgery in Quebec, Canada 1996-2005. *Arch Ophthalmol.* 2010; 128: 230-234.

Gopal, L.; Ramaswamy, A.A.; Madhavan, H.N.; Saswade, M.; & Battu, R.R. Postoperative endophthalmitis caused by sequestered *Acinetobacter calcoaceticus. Am. J. Ophthalmol.* 2000;129:388-90.

Gritz, D.C.; Cevallos, A.V.; Smolin, G.; & Whitcher, J.P. Jr. Antibiotic supplementation of intraocular irrigating solutions. An in vitro model of antibacterial action. *Ophthalmology* 1996;103:1204 -1208.

Halachimi-Eyal, O.; Lang, Y.; Keness, Y.; & Miron, D. Preoperative topical moxifloxacin 0.5% and povidone–iodine 5.0% versus povidone–iodine 5.0% alone to reduce bacterial colonization in the conjunctival sac. *J. Cataract Refract. Surg.* 2009; 35:2109–2114.

Han, D.P.; Wisniewski, S.R.; Wilson, L.A.; Barza, M.; Vine, A.K.; Doft, B.H.; & Kelsey, S.F. Spectrum and susceptibilities of microbiologic isolates in the Endophthalmitis Vitrectomy Study. *Am J Ophthalmol.* 1996;122:1-17.

Han, D.P.; Wisniewski, S.R.; Kelsey, S.F.; Doft, B.H.; Barza, M.; & Pavan, P.R. Microbiologic yields and complication rates of vitreous needle aspiration versus mechanized vitreous biopsy in the Endophthalmitis Vitrectomy Study. *Retina* 1999;19:98-102.

Hatch, W.V.; Cernat, G.; Wong, D.; Devenyi, R.; & Bell, C.M. Risk factors for acute endophthalmitis after cataract surgery: a population-based study. *Ophthalmology* 2009;116:425-430.

Irvine, W.D.; Flynn, H.W. Jr.; Murray, T.G.; & Rubsamen, P.E. Retained lens fragments after phacoemulsification manifesting as marked intraocular inflammation with hypopyon. *Am. J. Ophthalmol.* 1992;15;114:610-4.

Isenberg, S.L.; Apt, L.; Yoshmori, R.; Khwarg, S. Chemical preparation of the eye in ophthalmic surgery: IV: comparison of povidone-iodine on the conjunctiva with a prophylactic antibiotic. *Arch. Ophthalmol.* 1985; 103:1340-42.

Iyer, M.N.; Han, D.P.; Yun, H.J.; Eastwood, D.; Kim, J.E.; Connor, T.B.; Wirostko, W.J.; & Dev, S. Subconjunctival antibiotics for acute postcataract extraction endophthalmitis: is it necessary? *Am. J. Ophthalmol.* 2004;137:1120-1121.

Jay, W.M.; Fishman, P.; Aziz, M.; & Shickley, R.K. Intravitreal ceftazidime in a rabbit model: dose and time dependent toxicity and pharmacokinetic analysis. *J. Ocul. Pharmacol.* 1987;3:257.

Jensen, M.K.; Fiscella, R.G.; Moshirfar, M.; & Mooney, B. Third- and fourth-generation fluoroquinolones: retrospective comparison of endophthalmitis after cataract surgery performed over 10 years. J. Cataract Refract. Surg. 2008;34:1460-7.

Johnson, M.W.; Doft, B.H.; Kelsey, S.F.; Barza, M.; Wilson, L.A.; Barr, C.C.; & Wisniewski, S.R. The Endophthalmitis Vitrectomy Study. Relationship between clinical presentation and microbiologic spectrum. *Ophthalmology*. 1997 Feb;104(2):261-72.

Kwok, A.K.; Hui, M.; Pang, C.P.; Chan, R.C.; Cheung, S.W.; Yip, C.M.; Lam, D.S.; & Cheng, A.F. An in vitro study of ceftazidime and vancomycin concentrations in various fluid media: implications for use in treating endophthalmitis. *Invest. Ophthalmol. Vis. Sci.* 2002;43:1182-1188.

Lalwani, G.A.; Flynn, H.W. Jr.; Scott, I.U.; Quinn, C.M.; Berrocal, A.M.; Davis, J.L.; Murray, T.G.; Smiddy, W.E.; & Miller, D. Acute-onset endophthalmitis after clear corneal cataract surgery (1996-2005): Clinical features, causative organisms, and visual acuity outcomes. *Ophthalmology*. 2008 ;115(3):473-6.

Leopold, I. Incidence of endophthalmitis after cataract surgery. *Trans. Ophthalmol. Soc. U.K.* 1971; 191: 575-609.

Mezaine, H.S.; Al-Assiri, A.; & Al-Rajhi, A.A. Incidence, clinical features, causative organisms, and visual outcomes of delayed-onset pseudophakic endophthalmitis. *Eur J Ophthalmol*. 2009;19: 804-811 .

Moshirfar, M.; Feiz, V.; Vitale, A.T.; Wegelin, J.A.; Basavanthappa, S.; & Wolsey, D.H. Endophthalmitis after uncomplicated cataract surgery with the use of fourth-generation fluoroquinolones: a retrospective observational case series. *Ophthalmology* 2007; 114: 686-691.

Nichamin, L.D.; Chang, D.F.; Johnson, S.H.; Mamalis, N.; Masket, S.; Packard, R.B.; & Rosenthal, K.J. American Society of Cataract and Refractive Surgery Cataract Clinical Committee. ASCRS White Paper: What is the association between clear corneal cataract incisions and postoperative endophthalmitis? *J. Cataract Refract. Surg*. 2006 ; 32:1556-9.

Nguyen, J.K.; Fung, A.E.; Flynn, H.W. Jr.; & Scott, I.U. Hypopyon and pseudoendophthalmitis associated with chronic vitreous hemorrhage. *Ophthalmic Surg. Lasers Imaging*. 2006;37:317-9.

Pathengay, A.; Shah, G.Y.; Das, T.; & Sharma, S. *Curvularia lunata* endophthalmitis presenting with a posterior capsular plaque. *Indian J. Ophthalmol*. 2006a;54:65-6.

Pathengay, A.; Shah, G.Y.; Das, T.; & Sharma, S. Intravitreal triamcinolone acetonide in the management of exogenous bacterial endophthalmitis. *Am. J. Ophthalmol.* 2006;141:938-940.

Pflugfelder, S.C.; Flynn, H.W. Jr.; Zwickey, T.A.; Forster, R.K.; Tsiligianni, A.; Culbertson, W.W.; & Mandelbaum, S. Exogenous fungal endophthalmitis. *Ophthalmology*. 1988;95:19-30.

Raju, B. & Das, T. Hyderabad Endophthalmitis Research Group. Simple and stable technique of vitreous tap. *Retina*.2004; 24: 803-805.

Ravindran, R.D.; Venkatesh, R.; Chang, D.F.; Sengupta, S.; Gyatsho, J.; & Talwar, B. Incidence of post-cataract endophthalmitis at Aravind Eye Hospital: outcomes of more than 42,000 consecutive cases using standardized sterilization and prophylaxis protocols. *J. Cataract Refract. Surg*. 2009: 35:4; 629-636.

Roth, D.B. & Flynn, H.W. Jr. Antibiotic selection in the treatment of endophthalmitis: the significance of drug combinations and synergy. *Surv. Ophthalmol*. 1997;41:395-401.

Romero, P.; Méndez, I.; Salvat, M.; Fernández, J.; & Almena, M. Intracameral cefazolin as prophylaxis against endophthalmitis in cataract surgery. *J. Cataract Refract. Surg.* 2006;32:438-41.

Seal, D.; Reischl, U.; Behr, A.; Ferrer, C.; Alió, J.; Koerner, R.J.; & Barry, P. ESCRS Endophthalmitis Study Group. Laboratory diagnosis of endophthalmitis: comparison of microbiology and molecular methods in the European Society of Cataract & Refractive Surgeons multicenter study and susceptibility testing. *J. Cataract Refract. Surg.* 2008;34:1439-50.

Shimada, H.; Arai, S.; Nakashizuka, H.; Hattori, T.; & Yuzawa, M. Reduction of anterior chamber contamination rate after cataract surgery by intraoperative surface irrigation with 0.25% povidone-iodine. *Am. J. Ophthalmol.* 2011;151:11-17.

Sobaci, G.; Tuncer, K.; Tas, A.; Ozyurt, M.; Bayer, A.; & Kutlu, U. The effect of intraoperative antibiotics in irrigating solutions on aqueous humor contamination and endophthalmitis after phacoemulsification surgery. *Eur. J. Ophthalmol.* 2003;13:773–778.

Speaker, M.G. & Menikoff, J.A. Prophylaxis of endophthalmitis with topical povidone-iodine. *Ophthalmology* 1991; 98:1769–1775.

Srinivasan, R.; Gupta, A.; Kaliaperumal, S.; Babu, R.K.; Thimmarayan, S.K.; & Belgode, H.N. Efficacy of intraoperative vancomycin in irrigating solutions on aqueous contamination during phacoemulsification. *Indian J. Ophthalmol.* 2008;56:399–402.

Tan, C.S.; Wong, H.K.; Yang, F.P.; & Lee, J.J. Outcome of 23-gauge sutureless transconjunctival vitrectomy for endophthalmitis. *Eye* 2008; 22:150-151.

Vasconcelos-Santos, D.V. & Nehemy, M.B. Use of voriconazole in the surgical management of chronic postoperative fungal endophthalmitis. *Ophthalmic Surg. Lasers Imaging* 2009:40,425-431.

West, E.S.; Behrens, A.;, McDonnell, P.J.; Tielsch, J.M.; & Schein, O.D. The incidence of endophthalmitis after cataract surgery among U.S. Medicare population increased between 1994 and 2001. *Ophthalmology* 2005; 112: 1388-1394.

Wykoff, C.C.; Parrott, M.B.; Flynn, H.W. Jr.; Shi, W.; Miller, D.; & Alfonso, E.C. Nosocomial acute-onset postoperative endophthalmitis at a university teaching hospital (2002-2009). *Am. J. Ophthalmol.* 2010 Sep;150(3):392-398.

21

Macular Edema and Cataract Surgery

Miltiadis K Tsilimbaris, Chrysanthi Tsika,
Vasilios Diakonis, Aleksandra Karavitaki and Ioannis Pallikaris
University of Crete Medical School, Department of Ophthalmology
Greece

1. Introduction

Macular edema (macular oedema) is the accumulation of fluid within the retinal spaces, among the several layers of the tissue due to mechanical factors (anatomic failure, traction) or chemical factors (inflammation, drugs). The macular edema causes thickening of the retina and it may be diffuse or local. Cystoid macular edema (CME) also spelled as cystoid macular oedema (CMO) is the local form of the condition when it accumulates into cystic spaces mainly in the outer layers of the central retina (macula). CME is a painless condition. The effect on visual function depends on the severity of the condition and is usually associated with blurred or distorted vision. CME can be recognized by visual acuity reduction, characteristic appearance of the macula during fundoscopy, fluorescein angiography or ocular coherence tomography (OCT). It is important to distinguish the different varieties of CME that can range from fluorescein angiography findings only (angiographic CME) to symptomatic CME. Chronic cystoid macular edema refers to clinically significant CME that persist for more than six months (Gass & Norton, 1969; Berkow et al., 1997).

The cause of CME depends on the underlying disease process. It has been reported in association with local ocular conditions (epiretinal membrane, subretinal neovascularization), ocular or systemic vascular diseases (central and branch retinal vein obstruction, diabetic retinopathy), inflammatory conditions (pars planitis), conditions that lead to mechanical/tractional stress of the retina (vitreomacular traction syndrome), use of medications (epinephrine, latanoprost), and inherited diseases (retinitis pigmentosa). Rare causes of CME such as juvenile retinoschisis, Goldmann-Favre disease and nicotinic acid maculopathy are characterized by different pathogenesis, positive family history and different patterns in the fluorescein angiography.

Postoperative CME represents a well-known distinct entity associated with a variety of intraocular operations. Operations such as scleral buckling, pneumatic retinopexy or combined PKP and transscleral sutured posterior chamber IOL implantation can be complicated by postoperative CME (Notage et al., 2009; Van der Schaft et al, Tunc et al., 2007). CME following cataract surgery is currently the most commonly encountered postoperative CME. Post-cataract or Pseudophakic CME was initially described by Irvine SR in 1953 and Gass & Norton in 1966; this is why this entity is also known as Irvine-Gass syndrome (Irvine, 1953, 1976; Gass & Norton, 1966). Although most patients with CME after cataract surgery are visually asymptomatic, demonstrating only CME findings on angiography and on OCT, clinically significant CME still occurs even after an uncomplicated cataract extraction using phacoemulsification.

2. Incidence, epidemiology, risk factors

CME is the most common cause for sub-optimal visual outcome after cataract extraction procedures and represents today the most common cause of unexpected visual loss after uneventful cataract surgery (Ray & D'Amico, 2002). CME may occur after both complicated and uncomplicated cataract surgery, with no significant gender or race predilection.

Angiographic CME is detected in fluorescein angiography as a capillary perifoveal leakage with a petaloid appearance while in clinical CME biomicroscopic findings together with significant visual impairment are also present. Older reports on angiographic CME after intracapsular cataract extraction (ICCE) mention rates as high as 50-70% while after extracapsular cataract extraction (ECCE) the rate has been reported to be close to 18% ranging from 16 to 40% (Ray & D'Amico, 2002, Nagpal et al., 2001). Ursell et al. (1999) investigated the existence of angiographic CME after phacoemulsification the 60th day after surgery; they reported 19% of angiographic CME in 103 eyes, with no development of clinical CME in any of these eyes.

The incidence of clinically significant CME has been reported to be from 1% to 12% depending on factors such as surgical technique, selection of IOL, intra-operative complications and post-operative management. In 1998, Flach performed fluorescein angiograms in all cases with VA lower than 20/40 after ECCE with PC-IOL implantation and revealed a 7% incidence of post-operative clinical CME. The lack of use of post-operative steroids may have contributed to that high rate in this particular study. Following an uncomplicated phacoemulsification with an intact posterior capsule, the rate for CME has been reported to be as low as 0-2%. (Mentes et al., 2003; Flach et al., 1998). Recently, Loewenstein & Zur (2010) reported a rate of 0.1-2.35% for clinical CME following modern cataract surgery techniques.

Risk factors responsible for the development of CME after cataract extraction include several intraoperative complications such as posterior capsular rupture, vitreous loss and vitreous incarceration into the incision site and anterior chamber. Advanced age has been also reported as a risk factor for the development of the syndrome (Rossetti & Autelitano , 2000). Percival (1998) studied the effect of different factors on CME development after lens implantation. He reported a 13% incidence of CME after ECCE with intact posterior capsule, while if the capsule was ruptured the rate increased to 27%. Moreover, vitreous in the anterior chamber resulted in the appearance of CME in 33% of cases. Other authors have also shown the relationship between posterior capsule rapture and postoperative CME (Nikica et al., 1992; Chambless et al., 1979). The same positive correlation with postoperative CME has been reported by several authors for vitreous loss (Ah-Fat et al., 1998; Iwao et al., 2008). In a 2000 review by Rosetti & Autelitano, vitreous loss was correlated with an overall increase in CME by 10-20%. The use of iris supported IOLs is also associated with increased incidence and late onset of CME, which has been attributed to the chronic irritation of the iris. Iris is a tissue that responds to injury with secretion of inflammatory mediators. Gulkilik et al. (2006) found the presence of CME in 70% of patients after iris trauma compared to 20,5% of patients without iris injury. In general, the incidence of CME in complicated cases of cataract extraction has been reported to range from 1.5% to 35.7%

(Nikica et al. 1992). The type of intraocular lens (IOL) implanted may also play some role in postoperative CME formation. Kraff et al. (1985) reported that the use of ultraviolet (UV)-filtering IOLs might reduce the formation of angiographic CME. Finally, Ferrrari et al. (1999) reported an association between macular edema formation and the amount of energy during phacoemulsification; in their study, a higher incidence of CME was associated with energies that exceeded one joule. On the other hand several other factors do not seem to play any significant role. In a study performed by Gulkilik et al (2006) no correlation was found between postoperative CME and cataract type, iris colour or pseudoexfoliation; in the same study no correlation between phacoemulsification time and CME development was found.

The risk of visually significant CME has decreased with the development of advanced surgical techniques, such as modern phacoemulsification with micro-incisional techniques and foldable intraocular lenses (IOLs), when compared to older techniques, especially intra-capsular cataract extraction (Wetzig et al, 1979; Sorr et al, 1979). If the diagnosis of visually significant ME is based on visual loss to the 20/40 level or worse, the incidence is 2 - 10% following ECCE or ICCE and 0 - 2% following phacoemulsification with an intact posterior capsule. However, in at least one large series comparing postoperative CME after ECCE and phacoemulsification in patients with no underlying systemic disease, no significant differences were found between the two techniques. Even though the angiographic CME was slightly higher for ECCE, the clinical incidence was similar (0-6% for phacoemulsification compared to 0-7.6% for ECCE) (Powe et al., 1994).

The risk of CME formation after cataract surgery may increase in the presence of several ocular or systemic diseases when compared with history free patients. In a review study by Rotsos et al it was suggested that cataract surgery in diabetic patients might accelerate pre-existing diabetic macular edema leading to poor visual outcome. Even in the absence of diabetic macular edema, diabetic patients tend to have a higher risk of developing CME after uncomplicated cataract extraction (Dowler et al., 1995, 2000; Dowler & Hykin, 2001; Schatz, 1994; Pollack, 1992). In addition to diabetes, uveitis is also a significant pre-operative condition predisposing to CME. The rates reported in the literature may reach 56% while in most case it is recurrent (Krishna et al., 1998; Estafanous et al., 2001).). For this reason a careful selection of patients with uveitis has been suggested as a way to decrease the frequency of postoperative CME development (Suresh et al., 2001). Preoperative steroids may be given, topically and/or systemically in uveitis patients. The presence of epiretinal membrane also predisposes to increase of macular thickness and macular edema after cataract extraction. Finally, patients under local therapy with prostaglandin analogues have been reported to have a higher incidence of CME after cataract extraction. Agange et al presented a case report of a glaucomatic patient who developed recurrent CME with three separate trials of three different prostaglandins after uncomplicated cataract surgery. Other studies have also reported same findings (Yeh & Ramanathan, 2002; Altintaş et al., 2005; Panteleontidis et al., 2010).

In a study conducted in our institution, we prospectively examined macular thickness alterations after uncomplicated phacoemulsification in four different groups of patients. One group consisted of otherwise fit patients while the others included patients with diabetes, epiretinal membrane and glaucoma. We concluded that regardless of group, a statistically significant mean foveal thickness (MFT) increase occurs one month after surgery, while this increase regresses six months after surgery. Even though MFT regressed during the follow up period, in patients with diabetes mellitus and epiretinal membrane it remained significantly higher even six months after cataract surgery. With regard to diabetic patients, these showed the greatest difference between postoperative and preoperative macular thickness, indicating that the underlying pathophysiology is influenced significantly by the cataract extraction process. Despite these macular alterations, visual acuity improved significantly after cataract surgery in all patients in this study, while none of the patients demonstrated clinical CME (M. Eleftheriadou et al., 2010).

3. Pathogenesis, pathophysiology

The formation of CME is due to leakage of perifoveal capillaries, which if severe enough, leads to pooling in the outer layers of the central retina. Cystoid spaces are formed in the foveal area, in the outer plexiform layer and Henle's layer while some fluid accumulates in the nerve fiber layer, inside thin-walled cysts (Gass & Norton, 1966). Recently, histological findings have proved that the cysts may form also in the inner plexiform layer. The rod and cone photoreceptors in the area under the cysts are consistently found to be decreased in number.

Although the exact pathogenesis of post cataract CME is unknown, the main mechanism involved is considered to be inflammation. Inflammation in the vitreous, as described by Gass, represents a consistent finding in eyes with postoperative CME. This has been also documented in specimens of vitreous aspiration, where inflammatory cells were identified (Tso et al., 1982; Flach et al., 1998). In general, intraocular surgery seems to trigger the accumulation of macrophages and neutrophils that are further activated by circulating inflammatory agents, including cyclooxygenase and lipooxygenase metabolites, proteolytic agents and more, leading to the appearance of clinical signs of inflammation (perilimbal injection and anterior chamber flare). Cytokines such as interferon-γ, interleukin-2 and tumor necrosis factor-α also participate in the proccess inducing the production of cycloxygenase. (Wakefield & Lloyd, 1992; Miyake et al., 2000). Experimental studies of lens implantation in animal models have confirmed that trauma of the lens epithelial cells leads to the secretion of inflammatory mediators (Miyake et al., 1990). Other factors such as nitric oxide, complement and platelet-activating factor secreted by different cell types are believed to play important role in triggering inflammation postoperatively (Lightman & Chan, 1990). The induced inflammation has been also suggested to affect the function of Bito's pump, which is located in the ciliary epithelium and is responsible for the removal of inflammatory mediators from the eye (El-Harazi et al., 2001). Furthermore, the procedure of cataract surgery itself has been suggested recently to induce pro-inflammatory gene expression and protein secretion (Xu et al., 2011).

After a cataract operation, posterior diffusion of inflammatory factors is supposed to lead to blood-retina barrier (BRB) breakdown. The BRB is responsible for restricting movement of plasma constituents into the retina and in maintaining retinal homeostasis. A BRB breakdown leads to increased capillary permeability of the perifoveal network, and results in cyst formation and intraretinal fluid accumulation both intra- and extracellularly (Yanoff et al., 1984). Fluid accumulation disturbs cell function and retinal configuration. Müller cells are thought to act as metabolic pumps, which keep the macula dry. The accumulation of fluid in the outer plexiform layer is considered to be a late phenomenon following breakdown of the Muller cells. This produces the characteristic petaloid pattern of CME on fluorescein angiography (Figure 1).

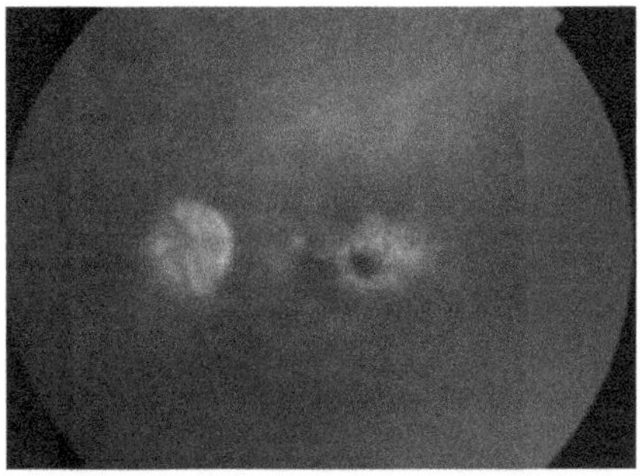

Fig. 1. Late phase of fluorescein angiography demonstrating the characteristic petaloid pattern of CME.

It is still not clear why the fluid that leaks from the perifoveal capillaries accumulates in the foveal region despite the massive production and distribution of the inflammatory agents throughout the retina. The relative avascularity of the avascular zone in combination with the high metabolic activity of the foveal area may explain in part the reduced reabsorption of leaking fluid in this area. Moreover, the thinner constitution of the inner limiting membrane (ILM) in the macula, may allow the diffusion of inflammatory agents in greater extent in this area than elsewhere. Even if all the aforementioned is crucial to the formation of CME, the fact that the majority of cases resolve spontaneously suggests that the more important question is what factors prolong its existence.

4. Clinical presentation, symptoms, diagnosis

4.1 Clinical presentaion & symptoms

Macular edema developing after cataract surgery does not necessarily imply a reduction of visual acuity. Thus, CME can appear either as an angiograpic or tomographic entity without visual impairment or as a condition with significant visual impairment. Angiographic CME is reported to occur in 3% to 70 % of patients whereas clinically significant CME appears in 0.1% to 12%. This means that an important percentage of CME remains asymptomatic.

The definition of clinical CME is slightly different amongst authors but generally involves a visual acuity worse than 20/40 with a parallel biomicroscopic observation and angiographic documentation of perifoveal leakage. It usually occurs 3-12 weeks postoperatively (peek incidence 6-10 weeks), but in some instances its onset may be delayed for months or years after surgery (Mao & Holland, 1988). Unlike diabetic macular edema, which can be an important diffferential diagnosis, it does not usually occur less than two weeks after cataract surgery.

When visually significant, the CME can induce a reduction of visual acuity that ranges, down to 20/65 or 20/80 (Chan et al., 2010). It can also impair other visual functions such as contrast sensitivity (Ibanez et al. 1993). Metamorphopsia and micropsia may be reported by patients suffering from CME, while a hyperopic shift is often observed (Quillen & Blodi, 2002).

4.2 Diagnosis

Several diagnostic modalities provide important information about macular status and can assist ophthalmologists in diagnosing CME. The main diagnostic techniques used in everyday practice include biomicroscopy, fluorescein angiography and optical coherence tomography.

4.2.1 Slit-lamp biomicroscopy

In patients suffering from CME after cataract operation, anterior chamber findings may sometimes be present such as limbal ciliary flush, mild iritis and vitritis. The signs of surgical complications may also be observed such as a vitreous strand(s) to the iris or the wound, a dislocated IOL or a disrupted posterior capsule. Retinal biomicroscopy (Figure 2) reveals loss of the normal foveal reflection, thickening of the retina and multiple cystoid areas in the sensory retina that are better observed through a red free filter. A thorough biomicroscopic examination should always be performed in order to exclude other causes of post-operative loss of visual acuity such as macular holes, branch vascular occlusions and epiretinal membranes.

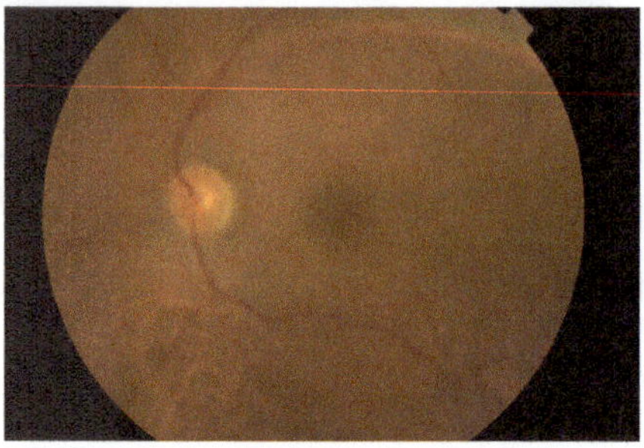

Fig. 2. Biomicroscopic appearance of a macula with cystoid macular edema. The findings may be minimal requiring careful observation and confirmation with imaging techniques such as OCT and fluorescein angiography

4.2.2 Flouorescein angiography

Flouoreoscein angiography (FA) is the gold standard for the diagnosis of macular edema (Figure 3). Macular edema is characterized by small hyperflouorescent spots (due to early leakage) in the arteriovenous phase and by the development of a 'flower petal' pattern ('petaloid') of hyperfluorescence in the late phase, caused by accumulation of fluorescein dye within the microcystic spaces in the outer plexiform layer of the retina, with a radial arrangement around the center of the foveola (corresponding to the arrangement of Henle's

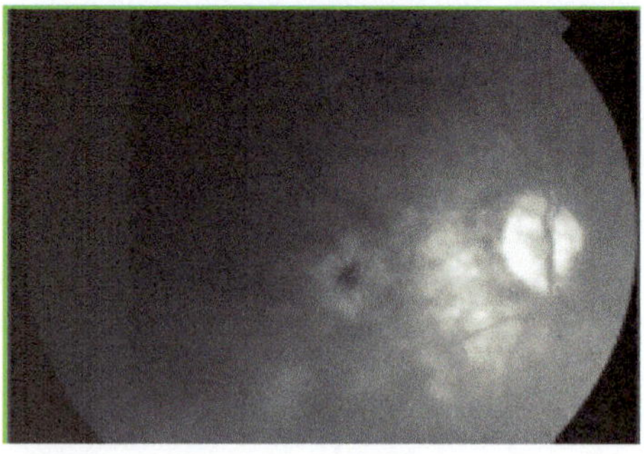

Fig. 3. Late phase of fluorescein angiography demonstrating the characteristic petaloid pattern of CME.

layer). Another common angiographic finding of cystoid macular edema, especially after cataract surgery, is the hyperfluorescence of the optic disc; this feature may predict a better response to anti-inflammatory medications.

It has been reported extensively that after cataract operation, patients will develop angiographic macular edema (flouorescein dye leakage), in a larger percentage when compared to the incidence of CME detected biomicroscopically. Nevertheless, both findings are not directly associated with visual acuity alterations.

4.2.3 Optical coherence tomography (OCT)

Since the introduction of OCT, the diagnosis and follow up of macular edema has been greatly facilitated (Figure 4). This modality offers a non-invasive imaging technique that provides high resolution cross sectional images of the macula. CME in OCT appears as a collection of hyporeflective spaces within the retina, with an overall macular thickening and loss of the foveal depression. OCT is as effective as FA at detecting ME, while it produces highly reproducible measurements so that serial examination may be used for follow up. A macular thickness change that is equal or more than 40 μm has been described as an index of OCT-significant macular edema (Wittpenn et al., 2008). The amount of macular thickening has not been well-correlated with visual loss. Small pachymetric macular changes seem not to influence visual acuity but when macular pachymetry alterations are in the 100μm or more range, visual acuity may be influenced. (Kim & Bressler, 2007). This inability to directly correlate macular thickness and visual acuity is probably related to the fact that extracellular edema may cause mechanical stress on the retina, while the visual pathways remain intact. Finally, OCT is extremely valuable in following a patient's response to treatment and determining whether or not further treatment is necessary. There is no consensus yet on whether OCT should be done in all patients after cataract surgery to detect CME.

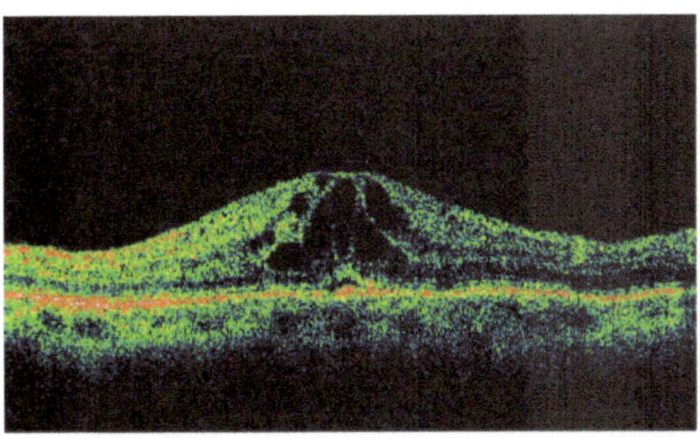

Fig. 4. Postoperative cystoid macular edema in OCT. Notice the collection of hyporeflective spaces within the retina, the increased macular thickness and the loss of the foveal depression.

5. Treatment

Most cases of pseudophakic CME, resolve spontaneously. This is why the value of prophylactic treatment remains doubtful. However, a large meta-analysis study that reviewed 16 randomized Clinical Trials (RCTs) involving 2898 eyes, concluded that there is some prophylactic effect against both angiographic and clinical CME when using topical NSAIDs or steroids pre-operatively (Ross et al., 1998).

Today, there is no standard approach for treating CME occurring after cataract extraction. In addition to any pharmacological treatment, the overall confrontation should also include the correction of the underlying cause, if possible.

First-line treatment of postsurgical CME includes topical administration of anti-inflammatory agents, such as nonsteroidal anti-inflammatory drugs (NSAIDs) and corticosteroids. The ophthalmic NSAIDs are non-selective inhibitors of cyclooxygenase (COX) - ketorolac, nepafenac, diclofenac etc - which inhibit the formation of prostaglandins from arachidonic acid. The steroids (including prednisolone, dexamethasone etc) act by blocking prostaglandin activity through the inhibition of the formation of arachidonic acid. Both categories can be provided as eye drops immediately after the CME is diagnosed (clinically and/or angiographically) or after a short period of attendance due to the self-limiting character of the condition. The effectiveness of topically administered NSAIDs is proved by several studies (Miyake et al., 1980; Yannuzzi et l., 1981; Flach et al., 1991; Italian Diclofenac Study Group, 1997) and their use is suggested as alternative to steroids when possible (Warren & Fox, 2008) due to the well-known side effects after long-term administration of steroids (eg. elevation of IOP).

The combination of the two categories is also proposed in the literature. In 2000, Heier et al. investigated the use of ketorolac versus prednisolone versus their combination for treating acute post-operative CME. The combination was proved to be the most effective, while between monotherapies, ketorolac surpassed prednisolone. Furthermore, in the study of Henderson et al. in 2007, a faster resolution of the edema was noticed in patients that received NSAIDs plus steroids. Whitpenn et al. (2008) also reported a lower incidence of CME in a group of low-risk patients that received ketorolac plus prednisolone preoperatively and 4 weeks postoperatively versus patients that received prednisolone alone.

The postoperative CME seems to respond well to topical anti-inflammatory agents even when it becomes chronic. Weisz et al. in 1998, in a study concerning 10 eyes of 9 patients with CME lasting more than 24 months, administered topical ketorolac for at least three months. The CME improved or resolved during treatment but recurred after the interruption of the administration. As far as the relative effectiveness of the different NSAIDs is concerned, no significant evidence is provided by the literature to support superiority of any of them over the others (Rho, 2003; Maca, 2010).

Recently, there has been a discussion on the benefit of initiation of anti-inflammatory treatment immediately after surgery. It is suggested that in patients belonging in high-risk groups for developing CME (DR, RVO, ERM), the direct application of such agents can reduce the frequency of appearance to the levels of patients who are not in high risk (Henderson et al., 2007).

Many experts administer topical steroids intensively such as 2-hourly and non-steroidal anti-inflammatory agents 6-hourly and assess response after a trial period of two weeks. When the CME does not respond to topical therapy, systemic therapy may be considered by some authorities. Oral carbonic anhydrase inhibitors are the most usual agents administered complementary to the topical treatment - acetazolamide is the most frequent choice (Ismail et al., 2008). However their benefit in postoperative CME is still debated and they are not used by many authorities. The carbonic anhydrase inhibitors should be given with caution and not for a prolonged period, due to the loss of potassium that they cause and the consequent systematic risks (Kaur et al., 2002). The systemic use of steroids is not indicated for postoperative CME, because of the disproportionate benefit compared to their systemic side effects. Recently, the oral administration of a COX-2 inhibitor (valdecoxib) has been suggested to have therapeutic effect on the post-operative CME (Reis et al., 2007). In this study, 10 patients with post-operative CME received 10mg/day of valdecoxib for 3 weeks. All but one increased the BCVA and remained stable for at least 15 months.

However, there are cases where the CME doesn't respond to any topical or systemic treatment or it regresses every time the treatment is ceased. In such cases, periocular or intraocular corticosteroids represent an option. The most commonly used steroid is triamcinolone, which is administered by injection either in the area of the orbital floor (periocularly) or as a posterior sub-Tenon's injection or, failing this with no improvement after a period of time (typically a further two weeks observation), intravitreally (Karacorlu et al., 2003; Boscia et al., 2005; Koutsandrea et al., 2007). Recently, the preference of intravitreal administration has increased considerably because it is much more effective with lesser dosage of the drug. It is important to note, however, that the intravitreal route is accompanied with some risk for complications such as endophthalmitis (Tao & Jonas, 2011). Moreover, elevation of IOP is always likely to occur after several repetitions of the intravitreal injection although, as with topical administration, the effect is often transient, even if it lasts longer (Sobrin & D'Amico, 2005; Tao & Jonas, 2011).

For the refractory cases some investigators have tried the use of anti-VEG agents intravitreally such as bevacizumab with encouraging results (Diaz-Llopis et al., 2007; Barone et al., 2008). The pathophysiological mechanism for this action of antiangiogenics is not clear but it is probably related to the stabilization of the BRB that they induce. The frequency of the injection repetition as well as the dosage, are only few of the questions regarding the intravitreous administration of anti-VEGFs in CME.

Since the mid 2000's a few studies have appeared concerning the intravitreal administration of NSAIDs in CME. Ketorolac and diclofenac have been administered intravitrealy in CME of a variety of aetiologies including cases of postoperative persistent CME (Wafapoor & McCluskey, 2006; Tsilimbaris et al., 2008; Masoud et al., 2010). The results are contradictory but not discouraging for the consideration of the IVT use of the NSAIDs for certain indications.

Last treatment options when all the aforementioned has failed, is the surgical treatment. Surgical intervention should be reserved for special indications. The iatrogenic induction of posterior vitreous detachment during standard pars plana vitrectomy (PPV) is believed to ameliorate the supply of oxygen to the affected retinal area and to relieve the macula from any possible traction that could contribute to the formation of the CME. A few studies have shown improvement after PPV alone (Pendergast et al., 1999), PPV combined with ILM peeling (Peyman et al., 2002) or PPV combined with IVT triamcinolone (Bencić et al., 2006). Likewise, in cases of vitreous incarceration in the anterior segment, anterior vitrectomy or YAG laser disruption of vitreous adhesions may have therapeutic effect. Finally, in rare cases it may be necessary to remove an anterior chamber IOL.

To conclude, the treatment of CME post cataract surgery is not always obvious. Even though the topical anti-inflammatory agents have in the majority of cases a reasonable effect especially if combined with topical steroids, there maybe times that the CME is refractory to any treatment and persists resulting in low visual acuity and eventually in atrophy of the adjacent retinal structures. Intravitreal agents such as corticosteroids, anti-VEGFs and NSAIDs have been tried for refractory cases with various results. Surgical treatment is the last choice for nonresponsive cases of chronic and clinically significant pseudophakic CME.

6. Prognosis

Pseudophakic CME typically has a good prognosis. Spontaneous resolution with subsequent visual improvement may occur within 3-12 months in 80% of the patients (Bonnet, 1995). Similarly in 90% of eyes the edema resolves over a two years period (Benitah & Arroyo, 2010). Persistent macular edema or multiple remissions and exacerbations can result in foveolar photoreceptor damage with permanent impairment of vision. (Gass & Norton, 1969).

7. References

Agange N. & Mosead S. (2010). Prostaglandin-induced cystoid macular edema following routine cataract extraction. J Ophthalmol, Vol. 2010, No. 690707 (published on line)

Ah-Fat F.G., Sharma M.K., Majid M.A. & Yang Y.C. (1998). Vitreous loss during conversion from conventional extracapsular cataract extraction to phacoemulsification. J Cataract Refract Surg, Vol. 24, pp. (801-805).

Altintaş O., Yüksel N., Karabaş V.L. & Demirci G. (2005). Cystoid macular edema associated with latanoprost after uncomplicated cataract surgery. Eur J Ophthalmol, Vol. 15, No. 1, pp. (158-161).

Barone, A., Prascina, F., Russo, V., Iaculli, C., Primavera, V., Querques, G., Stella, A. & Delle Noci,

N. (2008). Successful treatment of pseudophakic cystoid macular edema with intravitreal bevacizumab. J Cataract Refract Surg, Vol. 34, pp. (1210-1212).

Bencić, G., Vatavuk, Z. & Mandić, Z. (2006). Pars plana vitrectomy and intravitreal triamcinolone for chronic pseudophakic cystoid macular edema. Acta Med Croatica, Vol. 60, No. 2, pp. (93-96).

Benitah N.R. & Arroyo J.G. (2010). Pseudophakic cystoid macular edema. Int Ophthalmol Clin, Vol. 50, pp. (139-153).

Berkow J.W., Flower R.W., Orth D.H. et al. Fluorescein and Indocyanine Green Angiography: Technique and Interpretation. 2nd ed. Ophthalmology Monograph 5. San Francisco: American Academy of Ophthalmology:1997: 117-8

Bonnet S. (1995). Repercussions of cataract surgery on the development of cystoid macular edema in the diabetic patient. Bull Soc Belge Ophtalmol, Vol. 256, pp (127-129).

Boscia F., Furino C., Dammacco R., Ferreri P., Sborgia L. & Sborgia C. (2005). Intravitreal triamcinolone acetonide in refractory pseudophakic cystoid macular edema: functional and anatomic results. Eur J Ophthalmol, Vol.15, No. 1, pp (89-95).

Chambless W.S. (1979). Phacoemulsification and the retina: cystoid macular edema. Ophthalmology, Vol. 86, pp. (2019-2022).

Chan E., Mahroon O.A.R. & Spalton D.J. (2010). Complications of cataract surgery. Clin Exp Optom, Vol. 93, No. 6, pp. (379-389).

Diaz-Llopis M., Amselem L., Cervera E., Garcia-Delpech S., Torralba C. & Montero J. (2007). Intravitreal

injection of bevacizumab for pseudophakic cystoid macular edema resistant to steroids. Arch Soc Esp Ophthalmol, Vol. 82, pp. (447-450)

Dowler J.G.F., Hykin P.G., Lightman S.L. & Hamilton A.M. (1995). Visual acuity following extracapsular cataract extraction in diabetes: a meta-analysis. Eye, Vol. 9, pp. (313-317).

Dowler J.G., Hykin P.G. & Hamilton A.M. (2000). Phacoemulsification versus extracapsular cataract extraction in patients with diabetes. Ophthalmol, Vol. 107, pp. (457–462).

Dowler J. & Hykin P.G. (2001). Cataract surgery in diabetes. Curr Opin Ophthalmol, Vol. 12, pp. (175–178).

Eleftheriadou M., Fragiskou S., Kymionis G, Panteleontidis V, Papadaki T. & Tsilimbaris M.K. (2010). Cystoid Macular Edema and Macular Thickness Alterations After Cataract Surgery Determined by Optical Coherence Tomography (OCT). Invest Ophthalmol Vis Sci, Vol. 51: E-Abstract 4727

El-Harazi S.M., Feldman R.M. (2001). Control of intra-ocular inflammation associated with cataract surgery. Curr Opin Ophthalmol, Vol. 12, pp. (4–8).

Estafanous M.F., Lowder C.Y., Meisler D.M. & Chauhan R. (2001). Phacoemulsification cataract extraction and posterior chamber lens implantation in patients with uveitis. Am J Ophthalmol, Vol. 31, pp. (620–625).

Ferrari M.T., Cavallo M., Minnino L., Cardascia N. (1999). Macular edema induced by phacoemulcification. Doc Ophthalmol, Vol. 97, pp. (325-327).

Fishman G.A., Fishman M. & Maggiano J. (1977). Macular Lesions Associated With Retinitis Pigmentosa. Arch Ophthalmol, Vol. 95, No. 5, pp. (798-803).

Flach A.J., Jampol L.M., Weinberg D., Kraff M.C., Yannuzzi L.A., Campo R.V., Neumann A.C., Cupples H.P. & Lefler W.H. (1991). Improvement in visual acuity in chronic aphakic and pseudophakic cystoid macular edema after treatment with topical 0.5% ketorolac tromethamine. Am J Ophthalmol, Vol. 112, pp. (514–519).

Flach A.J. (1998). The incidence, pathogenesis and treatment of cystoid macular edema following cataract surgery. Trans Am Ophthalmol Soc, Vol. 96, pp. (557-634).

Gass J.D., Norton E.W. (1966). Cystoid macular edema and papilledema following cataract extraction. A fluorescein fundoscopic and angiographic study. Arch Ophthalmol, Vol. 76, pp. (646–661).

Gass J.D., Norton E.W. (1969). Follow-up study of cystoid macular edema following cataract extraction. Trans Am Acad Ophthalmol Otolaryngol, Vol. 73, No. 4, pp. (665-682).

Gulkilik G., Kocabora S., Taskapili M. & Engin G. (2006). Cystoid macular edema after

phacoemulsification: risk factors and effect on visual acuity. Can J Ophtalmol, Vol. 41, pp. (699-703).

Heier, J.S., Topping, T.M., Baumann, W., Dirks, M.,S. & Chern, S. (2000). Ketorolac versus Prednisolone versus Combination Therapy in the Treatment of Acute Pseudophakic Cystoid Macular Edema. Ophthalmology, Vol. 107, pp. (2034 -2039).

Henderson, B.A., Kim, J.Y., Ament, C.S., Ferrufino-Ponce, Z.K., Grabowska, A. & Cremers, S.L. (2007). Clinical pseudophakic cystoid macular edema Risk factors for development and duration after treatment. J Cataract Refract Surg, Vol. 33, pp. (1550–1558).

lbanez H.E., Lesher M.P., Singerman L.J., Rice T.A. & Keep G.F. (1993). Prospective Evaluation of the

Effect of Pseudophakic Cystoid Macula Edema on Contrast Sensitivity. Arch Ophthalmol, Vol. 111, pp. (1635-1639).

Irvine, S.R. (1953). A newly defined vitreous syndrome following cataract surgery. Am J Ophthalmol, Vol. 36, No. 5, pp. (499-619).

Irvine A.R. (1976). Cystoid maculopathy. Surv Ophthalmol, Vol. 21, pp. (1-17).

Ismail R.A., Sallam A. & Zambarakji H.J. (2008). Pseudophakic macular edema and oral acetazolamide: an optical coherence tomography measurable, dose-related response. Eur J Ophthalmol, Vol. 18, No. 6, pp. (1011-1013).

Italian Diclofenac Study Group. (1997). Efficacy of diclofenac eye drops in preventing postoperative inflammation and long-term cystoid macular edema. J Cataract Refract Surg, Vol. 23, pp. (183–189). Karacorlu, M., Ozdemir, H. & Karacorlu, S. (2003). Intravitreal triamcinolone acetonide for the treatment of chronic pseudophakic cystoid macular oedema. Acta Ophthalmol Scand, Vol. 81, pp. (648–652).

Kaur I.P., Smitha R., Aggarwal D., Kapil M. (2002). Acetazolamide: future perspective in topical glaucoma therapeutics. Int J Pharm, Vol. 248, No. 1-2, pp. (1–14).

Kim SJ & Bressler NM. (2007). Analysis of macular edema after cataract surgery in patients with diabetes using optical coherence tomography. Ophthalmol, Vol. 114, No. 5, pp. (881-889).

Koutsandrea, C.C., Moschos, M.M., Brouzas, D., Loukianou, E., Apostolopoulos M. & Moschos, M. (2007). Intraocular triamcinolone acetonide for cystoid macular edema. Optical Coherence Tomography and multifocal electroretinography study. Retina, Vol. 27, pp. (159 –164).

Kraff M.C., Sanders D.R., Jampol L.M. & Lieberman H.L. (1985). Factors affecting pseudophakic cystoids macular edema: five randomized trials. J Am Intraocular Implant Soc, Vol. 11, pp. (380-385).

Krishna R., Meisler D.M., Lowder C.Y., Estafanous M. & Foster R.E. (1998). Long-term follow-up of extracapsular cataract extraction and posterior chamber intraocular lens implantation in patients with uveitis. Ophthalmology, Vol. 105, pp. (1765–1769).

Lightman S. & Chan C.C. (1990). Immune mechanisms in choroido-retinal inflammation in man. Eye, Vol. 4, pp. (345–353).

Loewenstein A. & Zur D. (2010). Postsurgical Cystoid Macular Edema. Dev Ophthalmol, Vol. 47, pp. (148–159).

Maca S.M., Amon M., Findl O., Kahraman G. & Barisani-Asenbauer T. (2010). Efficacy and tolerability of preservative-free and preserved diclofenac and preserved ketorolac eye drops after cataract surgery. Am J Ophthalmol, Vol. 149, No. 5, pp. (777-784).

Mao L.K. & Holland P.M. (1988). "Very late onset" cystoid macular edema. Ophthalmic Surg, Vol. 19,

pp. (633–635).

Masoud S., Saee K., Azireza R. & Peyman, G.A. (2010). Pilot study of intravitreal injection of diclofenac for treatment of macular edema of various etiologies. Retina, Vol. 30, No. 3, pp. (509-515).

Mentes J., Erakgun T., Afrashi F. & Kerci G. (2003). Incidence of cystoid macular edema after uncomplicated phacoemulsification. Ophthalmologica, Vol. 217, pp. (408-412).

Miyake K., Sakamura S. & Miura H. (1980). Long-term follow-up study on prevention of aphakic cystoid macular oedema by topical indomethacin. Br J Ophthalmol, Vol. 64, pp. (324–328).

Miyake K., Mibu H., Horiguchi M. & Shirasawa E. (1990). Inflammatory mediators in postoperative aphakic and pseudophakic baboon eyes. Arch Ophthalmol, Vol. 108, pp. (1764–1767).

Miyake K., Masuda K., Shirato S., Oshika T., Eguchi K., Hoshi H., Majima Y., Kimura W. & Hayashi F. (2000). Comparison of diclofenac and fluorometholone in preventing cystoid macular edema after small incision cataract surgery: a multicentered prospective trial. Jpn J Ophthalmol, Vol. 44, pp. (58–67).

Miyake K., Sakamura S., Miura Iwao M., Inatani M., Iwao K. & Kawaji T. (2008). Cystoid macular edema caused by intraocular lens dislocation after trabeculectomy. Can J Ophthalmol, Vol. 43, No. 6, pp. (728-729).

Nagpal M., Nagpal K. & Nagpal P.N. (2001). Postcataract cystoid macular edema. Ophthalmol Clin North Am, Vol. 14, pp. (651-659).

Nikica G., Ljerka HP., Jelena P., Metez-Soldo K. & Mladen B. (1992). Cystoid macular edema in anterior chamber lens implantation following posterior capsule rupture. Doc Ophthalmol, Vol. 81, pp. (309-315). Nottage J.M., Bhasin V. & Nirankari V.S. (2009). Long-term safety and visual outcomes of transscleral

sutured posterior chamber IOLs and penetrating keratoplasty combined with transscleral sutured posterior chamber IOLs. Trans Am Ophthalmol Soc, Vol. 107, pp. (242-250).

Panteleontidis V., Detorakis E.T., Pallikaris I.G., Tsilimbaris M.K. (2010). Latanoprost-dependent

cystoid macular edema following uncomplicated cataract surgery in pseudoexfoliative eyes. Ophthalmic Surg Lasers Imaging, Vol. 9, pp. (1-5).

Pendergast S.D., Margherio R.R., Williams G.A. & Cox M.S. (1999). Vitrectomy for chronic pseudophakic cystoid macular edema unresponsive to medical treatment. Am J Ophthalmol, Vol. 128, pp. (317-323). Percival P. (1981). Clinical factors relating to cystoid macular edema after lens implantation. J Am Intraocul Implant Soc, Vol. 7, pp. (43-45).

Peyman G.A., Canakis C., Livir-Rallatos C. & Conway M.D. (2002). The effect of internal limiting membrane peeling on chronic recalcitrant pseudophakic cystoid macular edema: a report of two cases Brief report. Am J Ophthalmol, Vol. 133, No. 4, pp. (571-572).

Pollack A., Leiba H., Bukelman A. & Oliver M. (1992). Cystoid macular oedema following cataract extraction in patients with diabetes. Br J Ophthalmol, Vol. 76, pp. (221-224).

Powe N.R., Schein O.D., Gieser S.C., Tielsch J.M., Luthra R., Javitt J. & Steinberg E.P. (1994). Synthesis of the literature on visual acuity and complications following cataract extraction with intraocular lens implantation. Cataract Patient Outcome Research Team. Arch Ophthalmol, Vol. 112, pp. (239-252).

Quillen D.A. & Blodi B.A. (2002). Clinical Retina, AMA Press, ISBN 1-57947-284-2, USA.

Ray S & D'Amico DJ. (2002). Semin Ophthalmol, Vol. 17, No. 3-4, pp. (167-180).

Reis A., Birnbaum F., Hansen L.L. & Reinhard T. (2007). Successful treatment of cystoid macular edema with valdecoxib. J Cataract Refract Surg, Vol. 33, pp. (682-685).

Rho, D.S. (2003). Treatment of acute pseudophakic cystoid macular edema: Diclofenac versus ketorolac. J Cataract Refract Surg, Vol. 29, pp. (2378-2384).

Ross L., Chaudhwi J. & Dickersin K. (1998). Medical prophylaxis and treatment of cystoid macular edema after cataract surgery. The Results of a Meta-analysis. Ophthalmol, Vol. 105, No. 3, pp. (397-405).

Rossetti L. & Autelitano A. (2000). Cystoid macular edema following cataract surgery. Curr Opin Ophthalmol, Vol. 11, pp. (65-72).

Rotsos T.G. & Moschos M.M. (2008). Cystoid Macular Edema. Clin Ophthalmol, Vol. 2, No. 4,pp. (919-930).

Schatz H., Atienza D., McDonald H.R. & Johnson R.N. (1994). Severe diabetic retinopathy after cataract surgery. Am J Ophthalmol, Vol. 117, pp. (314-321).

Sobrin L. & D'Amico D.J. (2005). Controversies in Intravitreal Triamcinolone Acetonide Use. Int Ophthalmol Clin, Vol. 45, No. 4, pp. (133-141).

Sorr E.M., Everett W.G., Hurite F.G. (1979). Incidence of fluorescein angiographic subclinical macular edema following phacoemulsification of senile cataracts. Trans Am Acad Ophthalmol, Vol. 86, pp. (2013-2018).

Suresh P.S. & Jones N.P. (2001). Phacoemulsification with intraocular lens implantation in patients with uveitis. Eye, Vol. 15, pp. (621–628).

Tao Y. & Jonas J.B. (2011). Intravitreal triamcinolone. Ophthalmologica, Vol. 225, No. 1, pp. (1-20).

Thomas J.V., Gragoudas E.S., Blair N.P. & Lapus J.V. (1978). Correlation of epinephrine use and macular edema in aphakic glaucomatous eyes. Arch Ophthalmol, Vol. 96, pp. (625-628).

Tsilimbaris MK, Panagiotoglou TD, Tsika C, Pandeleondidis V, Kymionis G. (2008). Intravitreal Injection of Ketorolac Tromethamine in Postoperative Cystoid Macular Edema. Invest Ophthalmol Vis Sci, 49: E-Abstrac 2693

Tso M.O. (1982). Pathology of cystoid macular edema. Ophthalmol, Vol. 89, pp. (902–915).

Tunc M., Lahey J.M., Kearney J.J., Lewis J.M. & Francis R. (2007). Cystoid macular oedema following pneumatic retinopexy vs scleral buckling. Eye, Vol. 21, No. 6, pp. (831-834).

Ursell P.G., Spalton D.J., Whitcup S.M. & Nussenblatt R.B. (1999). Cystoid macular edema after phacoemulsification: relationship to blood-aqueous barrier damage and visual acuity. J Cataract Refract Surg. Vol. 25, No. 11, pp. 1492-1497.

Van der Schaft T.L., van Rij G., Renardel de Lavalette J.G. & Beekhuis W.H. (1989). Results of penetrating keratoplasty for pseudophakic bullous keratopathy with the exchange of an intraocular lens. Br J Ophthalmol, Vol. 73. No. 9, pp. (704-708).

Wafapoor H. & McCluskey J. (2006). Intravitreal Ketorolac as a Treatment of Diabetic and Non–Diabetic Macular Edema. Invest Ophthalmol Vis Sci, Vol.47: E-Abstract 4252.

Wakefield D. & Lloyd A. (1992). The role of cytokines in the pathogenesis of inflammatory eye disease. Cytokine, Vol. 4, pp. (1–5).

Warren K.A. & Fox J.E. (2008). Topical Nepafenac as an alterant treatment for cystoid macular edema in steroid responsive patients. Retina, Vol. 28, pp. (1427–1434).

Wetzig P.C., Thatcher D.B. & Christiansen J.M.(1979). The intracapsular versus the extracapsular cataract technique in relationship to retinal problems. Trans Am Ophthalmol Soc, Vol. 77, pp. (339-347).

Weisz, J.M., Bressler, N.M., Bressler, S.B. & Schachat, A.P. (1999). Ketorolac treatment of pseudophakic cystoid macular edema identified more than 24 months after cataract extraction. Ophthalmology, Vol. 106, pp. (1656 -1659).

Wittpenn J.R., Silverstein S., Heier J., Kenyon K.R., Hunkeler J.D. & Earl M., on behalf of the Acular LS for Cystoid Macular Edema (ACME) Study Group. (2008). A randomized, masked comparison of topical ketorolac 0.4 plus steroid vs steroid alone in low-risk cataract surgery patients. Am J Ophthalmol, Vol.146, pp. (554 -560).

Xu H., Chen M., Forrester J.V. & Lois N. (2011). Cataract Surgery Induces Retinal Pro-inflammatory Gene Expression and Protein Secretion. Invest Ophthalmol Vis Sci, Vol. 52, pp. (249 -255).

Yanoff M., Fine B.S., Brucker A.J. & Eagle R.C. Jr. (1984). Pathology of human cystoid macular edema. Surv Ophthalmol, Vol. 28(Suppl), pp. (505–511).

Yannuzzi L.A., Landau A.N. & Turtz A.I. (1981). Incidence of aphakic cystoid macular edema with the use of topical indomethacin. Ophthalmology, Vol. 88 ,pp. (947–953).

Yeh P.C. & Ramanathan S. (2002). Latanoprost and clinically significant cystoid macular edema after uneventful phacoemulsification with intraocular lens implantation. J Cataract Refract Surg, Vol. 28, No. 10, pp. (1814-1818).

22

Toxic Anterior Segment Syndrome (TASS) and Prophylaxis Against Postoperative Endophthalmitis

Rosario Díez, Lourdes Jordano and César Hita
Hospital Universitario de Getafe
Spain

1. Introduction

Cataract surgery with intraocular lens (IOL) implantation is the most frequently performed operation in people over 65 years old. It has high success rates and complications are rare, but they do occur and can be either infectious or non infectious. Since the 1980s cases have been reported, usually as series of cases, of important inflammation in the anterior segment of the eye sometimes even with hypopyon and tissue damage after cataract surgery due to the entrance into the eye of toxic substances. They were first referred to as sterile endophthalmitis even if only the anterior segment was involved. In 1992, Monson et al (Monson et al., 1992) termed it Toxic Anterior Segment Syndrome (TASS).

2. Incidence

TASS can present as sporadic cases or in outbreaks. Many eyes with TASS are never diagnosed and many are not reported because they are not severe or they represent a very low percentage of the total cataract surgeries performed, thus the real incidence rates for TASS are unknown. But when a few cases accumulate in a short period of time, specially if they are severe, surgical centres search for information so as to prevent future cases.

3. Clinical spectrum

TASS is an acute and sterile anterior segment inflammatory reaction which usually presents after anterior segment surgery. Its incidence is unknown and it is due to the entrance of toxic but non infectious substances into the eye. It typically starts within 12 to 48 hours of intraocular surgery, but it can also occur even later. Symptoms include blurry vision and minimal to moderate ocular pain. Signs such as inflammatory cells or flare or even fibrin in aqueous humour, and diffuse (limbus to limbus) corneal oedema without vitreous involvement are characteristic (Figure 1). Most of the cases are reported after uneventful cataract surgery. Recently, TASS after phakic IOL surgery or vitrectomy has also been reported. Although many symptoms and signs are similar to those of endophthalmitis, TASS characteristically affects the anterior segment and is Gram stain and culture negative and improves with steroid treatment.

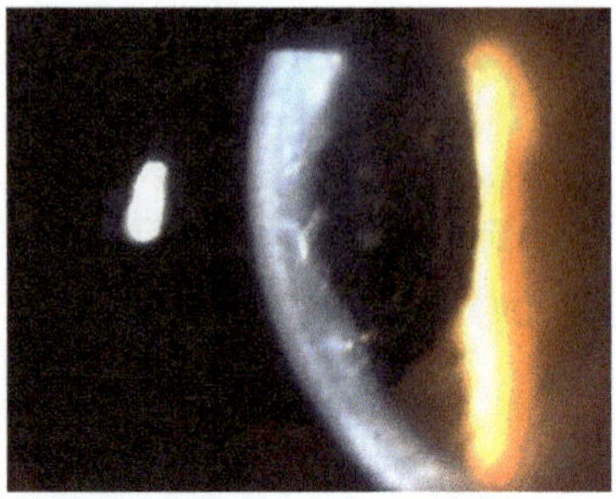

Fig. 1. Cornea oedema and fibrin on the IOL

Inflammation can be very severe resulting in hypopyon and fibrin formation due to the leakage of the blood-aqueous barrier. Limbus-to-limbus corneal oedema is a very typical sign resulting from diffuse endothelial damage. In some cases, severe tissue damage can lead to corneal decompensation requiring Descemet´s Stripping Automated Endothelial Keratoplasty or Penetrating Keratoplasty. Epithelial downgrowth over Descemet´s membrane has also been reported as a complication of TASS by Wallace, which required surgical treatment (Wallace et al., 2007). In early stages of TASS patients can present with low intraocular pressure. Permanent damage to the trabecular meshwork may cause ocular hypertension or secondary glaucoma which may require filtering procedures or tube shunt devices. Iris damage may cause a fixed irregular and/or dilated pupil.

4. Differential diagnosis

The differential diagnosis of (infectious) endophthalmitis can be challenging but there are some clues which can be helpful to diagnose TASS. TASS starts in the early postoperative period, usually within the first 24 hours. Inflammation is limited to the anterior structures of the eye and responds to either topical or oral steroids which can be given as a trial under strict monitoring as a steroid can improve TASS but unfortunately can theoretically exacerbate endophthalmitis if given too early in the course of treatment of the latter. There is a diffuse limbus to limbus oedema in TASS, pain is minimal or absent, and usually there is no lid swelling, conjunctival chemosis or discharge.

Unfortunately, none of the above mentioned symptoms and signs totally rule out the possibility of postoperative endophthalmitis. Gram stain and cultures from aqueous and vitreous taps are always negative in TASS but this could also happen in endophthalmitis when either the sample is too scarce or the bacterial count is too low. Pijla et al and the Endophthalmitis Vitrectomy Study reported that only 65 to 70% of all infectious endophthalmitis cultures were positive (Pijla et al., 2010) (Endophthalmitis Vitrectomy Study Group, 1995). Therefore, it should be remembered that the primary objective if suspecting TASS in a patient is to rule out postoperative infectious endophthalmitis, because postponing its diagnosis and treatment could be blinding for the eye´s functionality and cause severe permanent damage to the anatomy of the eye.

5. Aetiology

As mentioned above, the aetiology of TASS is not infectious. It has been associated with many entities that reach the interior of the eye at any time during the surgery in the operating theatre. They can be divided into extraocular substances which penetrate in the anterior chamber during or after surgery (topical antiseptics, glove powder or topical ointment), substances associated with the surgical procedure (anaesthetics, preservatives, inadequately reconstituted balanced solutions, ocular viscoelastic devices, mitomicin C or intraocular lenses) and irritants on the surface of intraocular surgical devices due to insufficient cleaning/flushing (detergents, gram-negative endotoxins in ultrasonic bath water, metal degradation in the surgical instruments or impurities in autoclave vapour). Many of the later are associated with reusable instruments.

TASS is usually reported as outbreaks which cause great concern in the surgical team. The broad spectrum of aetiologies mentioned above makes it very hard to know the real cause when TASS is present. Endothelial toxicity has been associated with many intraocular drugs and may be influenced by chemical composition, the concentration, the pH, or the osmolality of the medication or vehicle or the addition of preservatives.

Breebart et al and Parikh et al studied the effect of intraocular irrigating solutions, instrument related contaminants and intraocular drugs on corneal endothelium (Breebaart et al., 1990) (Parikh & Edelhauser, 2003) (Parikh et al., 2002). They concluded that the initial rupture of endothelial cell junctions and the acute lost of its barrier function was the cause of the corneal oedema seen with TASS. Whether the cornea returns to its preoperative status in absence of oedema depends on the remaining endothelial cells and their capacity to cover the damaged area where cells where lost.

The main factors involved in TASS are described in further detail as follows.

5.1 Preservatives

It is of capital importance that drugs injected in the anterior chamber are preservative-free. Benzalkonium chloride (BAK) was involved in several TASS cases (Liu et al., 2001) (Eleftheriadis et al., 2002). Topical benzalkonium chloride rarely affects the endothelium when used properly. Sodium metabisulphite has also been involved in TASS (Avisar & Weinberger, 2010). It is used mixed with epinephrine when the latter is used in irrigating solutions to maintain good intraoperative pupil dilation (Data from Spain).

5.2 Intracamerular anaesthetics

Preservative free 0.5% bupivacaine and preservative free 2% lidocaine were reported to increase corneal thickness and opacification (Kadonoso et al, 1998). Conversely, the use of preservative-free 1% lidocaine has proved to be safe during phacoemulsification cataract surgery as it rapidly gets diluted to less significant concentrations in the anterior chamber so is washed off the cornea and iris to non-toxic level during phacoemulsification (Heuermann et al., 2002).

5.3 Balanced saline solution (BSS) and endotoxines

Kutty et al found that the existence of endotoxines in balanced saline solution (BSS) was responsible for an outbreak of TASS (Kutty et al., 2008). Further more, medications added to BSS can be another potential source of TASS.

5.4 Maintenance of surgical materials

Proper cleaning of surgical material is of cardinal importance in TASS prophylaxis as inadequate cleaning of phacoemulsification and irrigation/aspiration (I/A) handpieces is the most frequently identified practice associated with TASS. Residual ophthalmic viscoelastic devices (OVD), debris or chemical substances used in the cleaning protocol can deposit in the inner and outer surfaces of reusable instruments if they are not properly removed. This is more likely to happen with reusable surgical materials such as cannulas, phacoemulsification handpieces and I/A tips. Both Parikh and Jun concluded that both enzymatic and non-enzymatic detergents used in instrument cleaning can eventually be deposited in the lumen of these and damage endothelium of rabbit and human eyes (Parikh et al., 2002) (Jun & Chung, 2010). Using detergents in wrong concentrations is another cause of TASS. Instruments processed with detergents should be rinsed with abundant sterile distilled or sterile deionized water. Needless to say, disposable material should never be reused. When instruments are sterilized they can also get contaminated. Ultrasonic baths dislodge dried debris from instruments, especially OVDs. Gram-negative bacteria can be found in water baths, ultrasound baths and autoclave reservoirs. This bacteria are destroyed during heat sterilization but their heat-stable bacterial wall endotoxines remain intact and can deposit on instruments (Kreisler et al., 1992) (Holland & Morck, 2007) (Andonegui et al., 2009). Another author (Hellinger et al., 2006) found sulphate, copper, zinc or silica impurities in the autoclave steam moisture.

5.5 Denatured ophthalmic viscoelastic devices

OVD can remain adherenet to the lumen of cannulas and reusable I/A tips when these are not correctly flushed after surgery. During sterilization OVD are denatured becoming hazardous in the anterior segment (Mathys et al., 2008).

5.6 Antibiotics

Administration of intraocular antibiotics during surgery is a very common practice. Gills recommended vancomycin and gentamicin in the irrigating solution during cataract surgery for postoperative endophthalmitis prophylaxis (Gills, 1991). There is increasing concern about the development of vancomycin-resistant bacterial strains, especially because this antibiotic is used as a last-step drug for gram-positive bacteria. Even more, macular toxicity has been associated with gentamicin use in irrigating solutions and when injected intravitreally even though Ball did not find a macular thickness increase with the use of a combination of these two antibiotics in cataract surgery (Ball & Barret, 2006). Furthermore, the concentration of these antibiotics used in irrigating solutions and the duration that they are in contact with bacteria responsible for endophthalmitis are not enough to be effective, based on their bactericidal or bacteriostatic characteristics (Peck et al., 2010). Other authors described the use of intracameral cefotaxime (Kramann et al., 2001), cefazolin (Garat et al., 2005) (Romero et al., 2006), and cefuroxime (Montan et al., 2002) (Díez et al., 2009), but no toxicity has been reported. Nevertheless, there is always a possibility that these antibiotics could result in TASS due to an error in drug concentration or pH. This highlights the role of specially trained pharmacy staff.

5.7 Autoclave

Autoclaves must be periodically checked for preventive maintenance as recommended by manufacturer´s direction. Even more, it is mandatory to check for this daily or, at least, weekly. Hellinger reported a case of TASS due to the quality of the water and vapour of a vapour generator autoclave (Hellinger et al., 2006). Sulphate, nickel, copper or zinc in vapour condensations can cause TASS outbreaks, which are specially severe with copper and zinc particles. When maintenance of the autoclave is poor this can result in an important source of debris. Thus, water composition used in autoclaves should be checked and substituted, if necessary, by deionized and ultrafiltered water. Glutaraldehide should not be used for sterilization as it is extremely toxic when insufficiently rinsed instruments contact cells of the anterior segment of the eye. Plasma gas sterilization promotes metal degradation in cannuled instruments and secondarily can cause TASS (Duffy et al., 2000).

5.8

Even though TASS is defined as an acute inflammation, it is not rare to find TASS delayed days after surgery. It is usually caused by **intraocular lenses** (chemicals used in packaging, polishing, cleaning or sterilization of the lens) or even **ocular ointments** (Figure 2). An outbreak was reported by Werner when ocular ointment containing petroleum was associated to tight ocular postoperative patching (Werner et al., 2006).

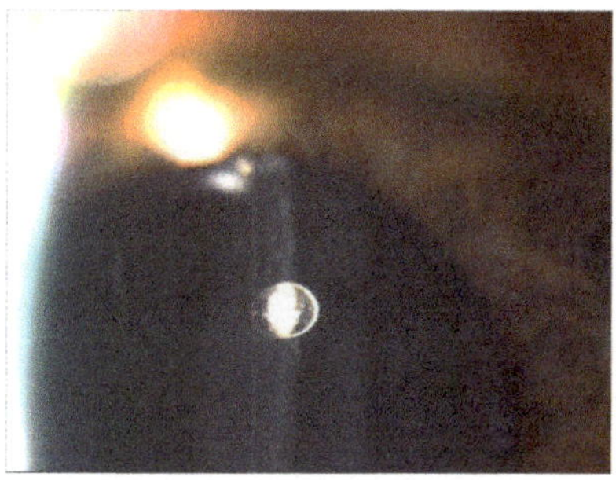

Fig. 2. Intraocular ointment drop in the anterior chamber

5.9 Glove powder

When powder enters the eye it can result in TASS. But some powder-free gloves release a compound that causes TASS even if gloves merely touch the IOL during surgery.

5.10 Others drugs

Five cases of severe intraocular inflammation that developed after an intravitreal injection of the same lot of bevacizumab have recently been reported. Taking all observations together, the authors suggest that the cause of the sterile endophthalmitis associated with lot B3003B01 of bevacizumab was the result of some toxic byproduct whose concentration may not be high enough when bevacizumab is given systemically. The degeneration during the storage may increase its toxicity, and the eyes sensitized by repeated intravitreal bevacizumab may respond to the increased antigenicity (Sato et al., 2010). Also, two cases of TASS have been reported resulting from impurities in generic trypan blue that was administered intracamerally to improve visualization of the capsule. The corneal oedema persisted and the patients developed endothelial and trabecular meshwork damage. Penetrating keratoplasty was performed in both cases (Buzard et al., 2010).

6. Management of TASS

The treatment of TASS is centred on dampening the inflammation because once the toxic agent penetrates the anterior segment of the eye it causes immediate damage and unfortunately washing out the toxins is not effective in reducing the intense inflammatory reaction.

When an acute postoperative inflammatory reaction is present, the first thing to do is to rule out infectious endophthalmitis. Once this has been done hourly topical 1% prednisolone acetate should be started. Close follow-up is mandatory in order to detect worsening inflammation or stabilization of the patient´s condition. Of course, should the inflammation increase, even if cultures or gram stain results are negative, it is strongly recommended to initiate treatment for infectious endophthalmitis given the potentially catastrophic consequences of failing to treat the later condition quickly. Slit lamp evaluation is useful to document corneal oedema and fibrin or cells in the anterior chamber.

Intraocular pressure can initially decrease secondary to trabeculitis and in later stages can increase secondary to permanent trabecular meshwork damage. The eye should undergo gonioscopic exploration if corneal oedema allows it so as to inspect for the development of peripheral anterior synechias. Confocal microscopy, where available, allows determination of endothelial cell lost and study if permanent corneal damage is present. The final result will depend on the type of toxic, its concentration and the time it remains in the anterior chamber, and how long treatment was delayed. Mild cases of inflammation will recover corneal transparency in a few days or weeks, whilst moderate cases can exhibit a certain level of corneal oedema and/or ocular hypertension. The most severe cases will associate prolonged corneal oedema, corneal opacity, ocular hypertension or glaucoma, chronic anterior uveitis, cystoid macular oedema secondary to chronic inflammation and a fixed midriatic pupil secondary to iris damage. Ocular rehabilitation may include queratoplasty, trabeculectomy or tube shunt devices.

7. What to do in TASS outbreaks? TASS prevention

The most important thing to do is to create a team where all surgical staff are represented: surgeons, nurses, sterilization area staff, pharmacists, and ideally preventive medicine or public health doctors. The medical records from patients who developed TASS should be available for the team who should document the surgical procedure, clinical presentation, the first time the inflammatory process was diagnosed, therapeutic approach and follow up. Furthermore, data recording the names of everyone in the surgical team, anaesthetics, intraocular drugs or viscoelastic devices, intraocular lenses and surgical incidences should be registered and ready to be reviewed. It is important that lot or batch numbers of drugs, substances and intraocular lenses are documented. Practice protocols must be reviewed to detect any mistakes during their application. This is very important for those members of staff responsible for cleaning and sterilization (Mammalis et al., 2006).

The authors believe that reusable instruments should be replaced regularly, specially cannulas and I/A tips, even though lumen surface irregularities or deposits are not evident. Of extreme importance is to rinse with sterile deionized water both the irrigation and aspiration ports and the I/A tips of the phacoemulsifier. Because gram-negative bacteria growth is frequent in ultrasound water baths this water should be replaced daily.

To learn more about instrument cleaning, disinfection and sterilization measures we recommend the Recommended Practices for Cleaning and Sterilizing Intraocular Instruments (Hellinger et al, 2007).

On the other hand, both irrigating solutions and any kind of intraocular medication should be correctly reconstituted. The authors believe that the operating room nurse in charge of intraocular drugs should repeat in a firm, loud voice the name of the substances he or she handles to the surgeon. It is also important to make sure that every intraocular medication is preservative-free and is of the proper concentration. This is specially important for epinephrine (adrenaline), which is frequently added to irrigating solutions, and intracamerular anaesthetics or antibiotics. It is important to note that lidocaine, indocyanine green, trypan blue and acetylcholine chloride are mixed with BSS instead of sterile water.
As most of the reported outbreaks of TASS are related to cleaning, disinfection and sterilization or reusable intraocular material, these should be the most thoroughly reviewed steps (Holland et al., 2007). Therefore, when an outbreak of TASS is detected the maintenance of autoclave should be emphasised as well as improving cleaning, disinfection and sterilization practices. Of great importance is following the directions for management of equipment provided by the manufacturers.
It is mandatory to report TASS cases to Regional or National Public Health Departments depending on each country´s organization.

8. Conclusions

Toxic Anterior Segment Syndrome is a challenging postsurgical inflammatory process both as isolated case or as outbreak. Today its clinical evolution is well-known. It is of capital importance to rule out infectious endophthalmitis because prompt diagnosis and treatment ensures better functional results. The low incidence or mild intraocular inflammation due to TASS or the fact that it is a sterile inflammation should not make clinicians underestimate this complication.
Unfortunately, it can be as destructive as infectious postoperative endophthalmitis. This fact highlights that either cleaning, disinfection or sterilization protocols should be improved or that some kind of intraocular medication has been used which is inadequate for this route. Thus, all the surgical team should be aware of this clinical entity, that any substance that is introduced into the eye is a possible cause of TASS and the different policies that can be incorporated to prevent it.

9. Overview of Postoperative Endophthalmitis (POE) Prophylaxis

Postoperative endophthalmitis (POE) is an uncommon but devastating intraocular surgical complication (Figure 3). As cataract surgery is by far the most frequently performed intraocular operation in the anterior segment, it is also the most frequent cause of POE and this has very important clinical, economic and legal consequences (Khan et al., 2005). Of note intraocular operations in which large amounts of the vitreous are removed are less likely to cause endophthalmitis as vitreous acts as a broth for the microorganisms involved. Although it is a rare complication POE is an important public health issue due to the progressive aging of the population and the millions of cataract surgery procedures done in a year all around the world. It is greatly feared as it can lead to severe and permanent visual loss. Over the years the phacoemulsification technique has improved with the use of smaller clear corneal incisions, faster surgical times, lens implantation, intraocular antibiotics, topical anaesthesia and sutureless wounds but endophthalmitis rates have not decreased as much as expected (Melo et al., 2010) (Barry et al., 2006) (Miller et al., 2005).

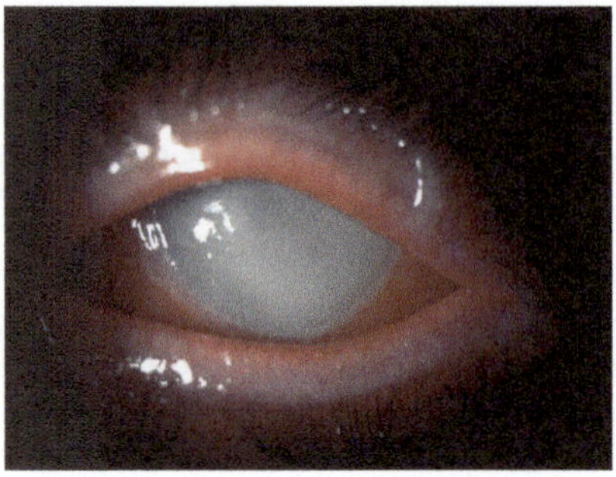

Fig. 3. Postoperative endophthalmitis with severe inflammation.

POE is an unexpected severe intraocular inflammation which affects both the anterior and posterior segments of the eye and is associated with vitreous echoes in both A and B modes with ocular ultrasound echography. A differential diagnosis of TASS and retained lens material is mandatory to consider. Diagnosis is based on the clinical features but cultures from aqueous and vitreous should be done. The most frequent cause is gram positive bacteria (Endophthalmitis Vitrectomy Study Group, 1995). Incidence has varied in the past decades- in the 1970´s it was 0.32%, in the 1980´s 0.16% and in the 1990´s 0.08%. In the first years of the 21st century the incidence increased to 0.26%. Different authors suggest that the cause may be non-sutured corneal incisions or postoperative hypotony. Incidence varies between series from 0.07% to 0.5% (Díez et al, 2009) (Miller et al., 2005).

The aims of prophylaxis in cataract surgery are to prevent postoperative endophthalmitis or surgical wound infection. Although the need for prophylactic antibiotics in clean surgical cases is debated among general surgeons, there is almost uniform agreement among ophthalmic surgeons on the need for antibiotic prophylaxis in the clean cataract surgical case because of the serious adverse effects associated with endophthalmitis. Some argue that antibiotics are not needed for clean surgical cases; however, because of the devastating effects of endophthalmitis, antibiotics are almost universally used for elective cataract surgery, even in healthy patients. Potential pathogens must be determined as well as local resistance patterns. An effective antibiotic must be selected, although no antibiotic is effective against all potential pathogens (Liesegang et al., 2001). It is not necessary to cover all potential pathogens or to sterilize the operative site, but it is necessary to eliminate most bacteria from the site. The least toxic and least expensive antibiotic should be selected; older antibiotics are not necessarily obsolete. The antibiotic must be administered at an appropriate time and dose. The antibiotic must be in the wound or anterior chamber at the time of introduction of organisms if the antibiotic is being used to clear an inoculation of introduced organisms. If the objective is to eliminate the bacteria from the surface, then topical antibiotics must be given time to work. It is not effective to administer the topical antibiotic only at the start of surgery, and it is minimally effective to administer the topical antibiotic after the wound is closed. The antibiotic should be administered for the shortest time possible and is usually not effective as a prophylactic in the postoperative period.

It is a general principle in infectious disease to avoid potent antibiotics for prophylaxis, as these should be reserved for therapy. If the patient gets a postoperative infection, generally a different antibiotic is selected for therapy. There are two approaches to prophylaxis. One is to reduce the number of organisms on the surface of the eye by using topically applied antisepsis and/or antibiotics. The other involves diffusion of antibiotics into the ocular tissues during the perisurgical period by topical, subconjunctival, systemic, or intracameral route.

10. Effects on costs and quality of life

Complications of endophthalmitis affect the patient´s quality of life. These include: loss of vision, corneal opacity (21,3%), secondary cataract (40,4%), intraocular pressure increase (29,8%), residual vitreous opacity (63.8%), macular epirretinal membrane, retinal detachment (6.4%) or even enucleation (Miller et al., 2005). The patient will likely undergo intraocular injections, some times vitrectomy, and requires close follow-up. Secondarily, the patient may need other operations for the complications mentioned above. All of these involve an important decrease in the patient´s quality of life and a significant economic cost.

11. Risk factors

11.1 Local risk factors

Any infectious or even inflammatory local process may be considered as a risk factor for POE. Some authors found that chronic use of topical medication, contact lens wear, blepharitis, chronic dacriocystitis, and chronic eyelid or conjunctival inflammation were associated to higher conjunctival contamination rates and multiresistant bacteria (Miño de Kaspar et al., 2003, 2009). Therefore these conditions should be treated prior to elective cataract surgery. It is known that external ocular microorganisms are responsible for intraocular infection after surgery (Speaker et al., 1991) and presurgical protocols for treating bacterial endophthalmitis are not effective to guarantee sterility (Ciulla et al., 2002). When preoperative topical drugs for unusual conjunctival bacteria such as coagulase-negative Staphylocci or Corynebacteria species were used, the organisms grew back 48 hours after the treatment was interrupted (Fernández Rubio et al., 2004). It was suggested that these bacteria had some kind of reservoir from where they colonized the conjunctiva. Thus, if more aggressive bacteria remain in the conjunctiva for a long period of time this would increase the risk for intraocular contamination after cataract surgery.

There is a strong association between atopic dermatitis and Staphylococcus (S.) aureus conjuntival colonization increasing the risk of intraocular infection due to this organisms (Nakata et al., 2000). In patients with chronic blefaritis S. aureus, S. epidermidis, P. acnes and corinebacteria were found more frequently (Groden et al., 1991). Gram-positive cocci, S. aureus and Streptococcus pneumonaie are associated with acute forms of dacriocystitis whilst gram-negative bacteria like Haemophilus influenzae, Pseudomonas species and enterobacteria are more frequent in the chronic form (Mills et al., 2007).

11.2 Senior versus training surgeons

There is not enough evidence to presume that senior surgeons have lower incidence rates of endophthalmitis than residents or fellows (Hollander et al., 2006) (Kamalarajah et al., 2007). Training surgeons may have more posterior capsule ruptures whilst senior surgeon may not suture as many corneal incisions arising from cataract surgery as the former.

11.3 Intraocular lens (IOL)

The role of intraocular lenses in endophthalmitis has not been fully established. Infections have been reported with both injectable and non-injectable IOLs. The trend is to use injectable lenses which allow smaller incisions and avoid contact and colonization with ocular surface bacteria, thus reducing the risk of an endophthalmitis. There is no difference between 1-piece and three-piece IOLs, but there are differences suggesting that silicone IOLs are more prone to intraocular infection due to surface factors (ESCRS Endophthalmitis Study Group, 2007). The most important factor may be the site of the clear corneal incision, in particular, when the incision is temporal (Schauersberger, et al.) (Baillif et al., 2009). Cusumano (Cusumano et al., 1994) and Ng (Ng et al., 1996) compared plymethilmethacrylic acid (PMMA) and hidrogel IOLs and found statistically significant differences in the adhesion of bacteria on the lens surface on non hidrogel lenses. Hidrogel IOLs are foldable, highly biocompatible and have a hydrophilic surface leading to a lower risk of endophthalmitis.

IOLs may also have their surface covered in heparine or fluor thus reducing bacteria adhesion and therefore inflammation and endophthalimtis (Arciola et al., 1994) (Eloy et al., 1993). Recently other authors have investigated drug delivery with intraocular lenses suggesting that antibiotic-soaked IOLs have potential to become a clinically significant technique in the prevention of postoperative endophthalmitis (Shaw et al., 2010).

11.4 Surgical complications

Intraoperative complications may increase the risk of POE. Posterior capsule tears with or without vitreous loss increases the risk of POE (Driebe et al., 1986) (Menikoff et al., 1991) (Kelkar et al., 2008) (Kim et al., 2007). The eye finds it easier to defend against bacteria when there is no vitreous in the anterior chamber, in fact, aqueous humour is contaminated in up to 20% of all patients at the end of cataract surgery, but only a very low percentage develops POE.

12. Prophylaxis

12.1 Presurgical prophylaxis

12.1.1 Topic antibiotics

Based on heterogeneous evidence, topical antibiotic agents are used worldwide as adjuvant of povidone-iodine for postoperative prophylaxis. The goals of prophylactic antibiotics in cataract surgery are to reach an optimal concentration in the aqueous humour and cornea and to reduce bacterial flora in the lids and conjunctiva sac. To do so, prophylactic treatment is started a few days before surgery or the day of surgery or using a combination of these strategies.

Gram-positive species are very common in conjunctival and lid flora. Vasavada et al (Vasavada et al., 2008) reported Staphylococcus species as the most prevalent of all being cultured in up to 90,4% to 94,4% of asymptomatic people. Of the Staphylococcus species isolated, 71% were S. epidermidis. Gram-negative organisms included Pseudomonas aeruginosa, Pseudomonas stutzeri, Enterobacter cloacae, Enterobacter hormaechei, Proteus vulgari, and Acinetobacter species. The anaerobic cultures mainly consisted of Propionibacterium acnes and Peptostreptococcus species. Streptococcus species was present in 2% of all specimens.

The fourth-generation fluoroquinolones moxifloxacin and gatifloxacin achieve high anterior chamber concentrations and have a broad bactericidal spectrum. They have similar killing rates in vitro studies and appear to be more effective than earlier quinolones (Kowalsky et al, 2006). Thus, they are adequate to obtain an effective antibiotic concentration before the anterior chamber is penetrated to allow bacteria inside it. But it should be noted that the drug is rapidly washed out once phacoemulsification of the cataract begins.

12.1.2 Systemic antibiotics

Prior studies of intravenous antibiotics revealed poor intravitreous penetration. Antibiotics that reached significant levels may not reach minimum inhibitory concentration (MIC) for many hours. Vancomycin or aminoglycosides failed to reach MIC in phakic human eyes with intact vitreous cavities. Some authors consider that fourth generation fluoroquinolones should be considered as oral prophylaxis in high-risk patients such as those undergoing vitreous loss during cataract surgery, chronic blepharitis, lacrimal drainage obstruction or relative inmunocompromise although the authors do not.

12.2 Surgical prophylaxis in the operating theatre

12.2.1 Operating room

POE outbreaks have been reported associated to operating theatre/room air conditioning systems, and they are usually caused by Aspergillus rather than bacteria. These outbreaks are often related to repairs in the operating theatre. Antiseptic solutions (povidone-iodine, clorhexidine), BSS, OVDs, mydriatic and antibiotic drops are also a source of contamination. Eye drops can be contaminated with Pseudomonas aeruginosa (Pinna et al., 2009) or Fusarium species (Cakir et al., 2009). Where possible, single dose eye drops should be used. If not available, a different bottle should be used in every different patient.

Correct cleaning and sterilization of the instruments is of critical importance and therefore, periodic monitoring of protocols and cleaning and sterilization systems are mandatory. The authors recommend following the manufacturers' practice guides focusing on cannulated instruments.

Antisepsia measures of the surgical team are also of chief importance, specially those related to hand scrubing.

12.2.2 Povidone-iodine

It is know that the most important sources of bacteria responsible for postoperative endophthalmitis are those in the conjunctiva and eyelids. One of the measures that have proven to be effective in postoperative prophylaxis is to decrease the amount of bacterial flora or occasional pathogens. Ciulla et al (Ciulla et al., 2002) describes several prophylactic methods concluding that 5% povidone-iodine irrigation before surgery was the most strongly recommended prophylactic measure.

It has proved to be effective against a wide range of bacteria, including methicillin-resistant Staphylococcus (MRSA) (Guzel et al., 2009), as well as fungi, protozoa and viruses. It has very rapid cytotoxic activity on prokaryotic cells once it reaches the cell wall (Lacey& Catto, 1993).

Conjunctival irrigation with 5% povidone-iodine preoperatively is more effective eliminating bacteria from the ocular surface than the instillation of 2 drops (Miño de Kaspar et al., 2005). Irrigation has a mechanical effect as it washes bacteria away from the surface and crypts. A period of time ranging from one to three minutes should be waited for before washing povidone-iodine from the ocular surface. The skin of the eye lids and eye lashes should be cleaned with 10% povidone-iodine, but note that total sterilization cannot be achieved-approximately 20% of the resident flora are resistant to surgical scrubs and antiseptics.

5% povidone-iodine has been shown to be effective and safe. Its toxicity is limited to conjunctival irritation, keratitis and contact dermatitis. The entry of povidone-iodine in the anterior chamber should be avoided as it is toxic for the endothelium. Therefore, whenever used at the end of the surgery it should only be applied on the surface of the eye once the surgeon has made sure the incisions are sealed and the ocular pressure is not low.

0.5% clorhexidine is safe and effective as an alternative skin disinfectant when the patient is allergic to povidone-iodine. It is also safe and effective in diminishing skin colonization with Staphylococci in patients before operation. It is not clear though if it is in practice as effective as povidone-iodine.

12.2.3 Draping and topical anaesthesia

Careful draping of the eyelid margins is of critical importance to reduce the incidence of anterior chamber contamination (Masket, 2007). Topical anaesthesia allows the patient to blink, which may increase the difficulty to properly retract the eyelids and carefully drape the lid margins. Hence, poor draping may be associated with the use of topical anaesthesia. There is no clear evidence to suggest topical anaesthesia as a risk factor for postoperative endophthalmitis. However, some retrospective studies concluded there was a higher incidence of endophthalmitis with topical anaesthesia compared to peribulbar or retrobubar anaesthesia (García-Arumi et al., 2007). On the other hand, Greenbaum (Greenbaum, 2007) considers the role of more frequent postoperative patching on eyes having retrobulbar anaesthesia as the factor which explains the lower incidence of endophthalmitis in these patients.

12.2.4 Corneal incisions

Two of the most important factors to consider under this topic are postoperative square corneal tunnel incisions and ocular hypotony. An entry wound that is distorted during surgery is more likely to permit the entrance of fluid from the ocular surface during and after the surgery. The width of the incision is also important as it is more dangerous to work through a 3.5 mm tunnel than a 2.5 mm tunnel. Another factor is wound localization, where temporal localization has been associated with a higher risk of endophthalmitis. Furthermore, a low intraocular pressure results in a poor apposition of the edges of the wound. The authors routinely hydrate the corneal stroma - this forces the apposition of the wound edges. Many critics believe this is a too temporary measure as they believe it lasts for 1 or 2 hours. Stromal swelling can persist 24 hours or more after the surgery (Fine et al., 2007). This can be proven with ultrasound.

Any incision suspected of incompetence should be considered for suturing as it increases the risk for potential infection. In the last few years tissue adhesives are gaining popularity. There are three possibilities: cyanoacrylate, polymerizing liquid hydrogel and fibrin glue. Their role in cataract surgery and in endophthalmitis prophylaxis has not been fully established.

12.2.5 Antibiotics employed in the operating room

In recent years there has been great controversy on the use of vancomycin as a prophylactic agent against endophthalmitis rather than a therapeutic agent. It is a bactericidal antibiotic. It is effective against gram-positive pathogens, including methicillin-resistant Staphylococcus species and Bacillus cereus.

There is fear that its overuse as a prophylactic agent will permit the development of multidrug resistant bacteria. To prevent this from occurring, the Centers for Disease Control and Prevention (CDC) of the United States, in the year 1995, discouraged the use of vancomycin in irrigation solutions or as routine surgical prophylaxis (Centers for Disease Control, 1995). Despite these guidelines, many Ophthalmologists continue using it. Surgeons who use vancomycin in irrigating solutions justify its use based on the fact that there is a potential effect on residual bacteria in the anterior chamber after cataract surgery. Ferro, Feys and Mendivil and Mendivil (Ferro et al., 1997) (Feys et al., 1997) (Mendivil A. & Mendivil M.P., 2000) failed to demonstrate a bactericidal effect following vancomycin in the bottle. In fact, the presence of S. epidermidis was the same in both the prophylaxis and the control arms.

Gordon (Gordon, 2001) believed that vancomycin should not be used as prophylaxis. Endophthalmitis has been reported despite its use, it is rapidly washed out from the anterior chamber in less than 4 hours and its concentration rapidly falls below MICs of gram-positive bacteria. Potentially, bacterial growth could be resumed once the antibiotic is washed-out of the anterior chamber. The authors agree with Gordon that there is no scientific evidence to use "in the bottle" vancomycin as a routine prophylaxis regimen and therefore do not recommend this measure.

Prophylactic antibiotic bolus injections into anterior chamber were described in the 1970´s. In the early 1990´s Gimbel (Gimbel et al., 1994) described a protocol to reduce endophthalmitis rates using intracameral vancomycin. After that, Montan (Montan et al., 2002) chose cefuroxime for endophthalmitis prophylaxis based on the ethiological spectrum of their previous endophthalmitis cases. They assumed that gram-negative bacteria would account for an insignificant amount of future cases. Thus, this regimen would effectively prevent infections due to gram-positive bacteria. They therefore concluded that cefuroxime was a valid alternative to vancomycin as a prophylactic agent even though enterococcal infections and some gram-negative bacteria were not covered. Vancomycin should be a last-resort antibiotic agent for treatment and not for prophylaxis, as recommended by the U.S. Centers for Disease Control and Prevention, Atlanta, Georgia. (Hospital Infection Control Practices Advisory Committee, 1995)

The European Society of Cataract and Refractive Surgeons (ESCRS) designed a multicentre prospective randomized partially masked study to investigate whether the incidence of endophthalmitis could be reduced using antibiotics (Barry et al., 2006) (ESCRS Endophthalmitis Study Group, 2007). Initially they were to recruit 35.000 patients having cataract surgery across several countries in Europe. Treatment effects were so marked that 16.603 patients were enough to halt the study and reach significant findings. One of the most interesting of them was that patients not receiving cefuroxime injection after the surgery were 4.92 times more likely to develop endophthtalmitis than patients receiving it. Intracameral injection of 1 mg of cefuroxime in 0.1 ml of saline had a statistically significant effect in reducing the risk of endophthalmitis after cataract phacoemulsification surgery. Previously, a Swedish report had advised of a 5-fold to 6-fold increased risk for endopththalmitis in patients not receiving intracameral cefuroxime (Montan et al., 2002). Two groups from Spain (Díez et al., 2009) (García-Sáenz et al., 2010) proved cefuroxime to be effective and safe in preventing endophthalmitis. Intracamerular cefuroxime proved to be more effective than subconjunctival cefuroxime in a paper published in 2008 (Yu-Wai-Man et al., 2008). Intracameral cefuroxime has a good safety profile and does not result in anterior segment toxicity (Montan et al., 2002) (Díez et al., 2009) (Gupta et al., 2005) (Yoeruek et al., 2008). Once in the anterior chamber, levels of cefuroxime over the MIC are maintained approximately 4 hours after the injection.

Despite the evidence supporting intracameral cephalosporins many surgeons in the United States prefer topical fourth-generation fluoroquinolones. They argue that intracameral cefuroxime must be prepared in a pharmacy department as it is not commercially available thus there is always a certain risk of errors in the dosage, pH, stability or sterility of the drug. When prepared in a laminar flux cabin and stored in single patient doses these risks can be decreased significantly. Only a relatively small percentage of patients allergic to beta-lactams are allergic to cephalosporins too. Nevertheless, the authors recommend sending them to have allergy tests done before surgery is performed as the benefits of been able to use these on patients outweigh many-fold the risk of delaying elective surgery of the eye.

It has been suggested that moxifloxacin would be preferable to cefuroxime because of its broader spectrum of action, better MIC levels and lower bacterial resistance. (O´Brien et al., 2007) (Scoper, 2008) (Jensen et al., 2008). Moxifloxacin is available as a self-preserved commercial ophthalmic formulation and requires no special preparation for intracameral therapy. It has a pH of 6.8 and an osmolality of 290 mOsm/kg (compatible with human anterior chamber fluid) (Lane et al., 2008). It is diluted from the commercially available drops to a 1 mg/0.1 ml solution as described by Arshinoff (Arshinoff, 2007). Intraocular toxicity was shown to be equivalent to standard vancomycin and saline control in a study in rabbit eyes by Kowalski (Kowalski et al., 2005). Retinal safety of intravitreal moxifloxacin up to 100 μg/ml in mice or 150 μg in rabbits has been shown and caused no electroretinogram (ERG) or retinal histologic anormalities. Another study showed the safety of moxifloxacin in a concentration of 1 mg/ml and a dose of 100 μg/0.1 ml evaluated by OCT and a retrospective review of clinical records (Arbisser, 2008). Lane observed that moxifloxacin in an intracameral dose of 250 μg/0.05 ml was as safe as BSS in a 3 month follow up (Lane et al., 2008).

Once injected into the aqueous humour, high initial levels are achieved (710 μg/ml) and remained at 6 μg/ml or greater for 4 hours after the injection. This is well above the minimum bactericidal concentration against ocular isolates such as Staphylococcus aureus (0.13 μg/ml) or Staphylococcus epidermidis (0.25 μg/ml).

A recent cost-effectiveness analysis published in 2009 revealed that none of the fluoroquinolone antibiotics would have theoretical cost-effectiveness ratios superior to intracameral cefuroxime. Moreover, to achieve a threshold cost equivalence with intracameral cefuroxime, gatifloxacin or moxifloxacin should have an efficacy 9-fold to 30-fold greater (Sharify et al., 2009).

Intracameral cefazoline been reported to be used in several papers mainly from Spain. Its choice as a prophylactic agent for postoperative endophthalmitis is based on the bacteria cultures and antibiograms from their own cases and data published (Garat et al., 2005) (Romero et al., 2006). These authors believe that the first-generation cephalosporin cefazoline 1 mg in 0.1 ml of saline injected in anterior chamber has a broader spectrum of activity against gram-positive bacteria than the second-generation cefuroxime. In fact, both cefuroxime and cefazolin have similar physicochemical and pharmacokinetic characteristics. Cefazolin is bactericidal against gram-positive cocci, specially Staphylococcus (except for methicilin-resistant Staphylococci) and Streptococcus. Garat et al (Garat et al., 2005) use 2.5 mg/0.1 ml bolus which has proved to be effective reducing endophthalmitis rates from 0.422% to 0.047% and to be safe. Unfortunately, cefazoline-resistant bacteria such as Enterococcus constitute an important gap in the coverage of gram-negative bacteria with this antibiotic. Endophthalmitis due to anaerobic bacteria is not prevented by cefazolin. These authors also suggest that cefazolin is easier to obtain and less expensive resulting in a very good option for developing countries. Cefazolin is used almost exclusively for surgical prophylaxis whereas cefuroxime is used systemically as a therapeutic option potently increasing pathogen resistance to the latter.

12.2.6 Patching

The use of an eye patch after cataract surgery is part of the postoperative routine in many hospitals. So-called "no stitch, no-patch" cataract surgery has become popular in the last few years because of modern surgical techniques. There is no clear evidence suggesting an influence of patching on the incidence of endophthalmitis. Patients tend to feel safer when the operated eye is patched, but it delays the beginning of postoperative antibiotic treatment. An alternative procedure may be patching the eye for a few hours and then initiating postoperative drop treatment.

12.3 Postoperative prophylaxis

12.3.1 Postoperative antibiotics

Although most ophthalmic surgeons apply an antibiotic ointment or solution at the end of the procedure, there is no literature to support the continued use of postoperative antibiotics. Several papers have been published on different ophthalmologists´s practices worldwide after cataract surgery. Ninety six percent of the ophthalmologists in the United States (Masket, 1998) and ninety five percent in Australia (Morlet et al., 1998) answered positively when asked if they used postoperative antibiotics to prevent endophthalmitis.

If antibiotics are prescripted immediately after surgery the authors recommend that their use is prolonged until the incisions are sealed and to halt their instillation quickly to minimise the risk of development of resistant strains (Guías de Práctica Clínica de la Sociedad Española de Retina y Vítreo, 2011)

13. Conclusions

As previously discussed, some prophylactic measures have proved to be essential because there is scientific evidence to support them whilst others can be incorporated into clinical practice although their relevance is yet to be established.

To summarize, prior to surgery risk factors, especially those which are local, must be diagnosed in order to be adequately treated before the patient is booked for surgery. Preoperative antibiotics in the absence of risk factors have not been shown to reduce the incidence of endophthalmitis. When in the operating theatre proper draping is mandatory to ensure lid margin and eye lash isolation from de operating field. Disposable operating materials might reduce the risk of contamination and thus may be better than reusable material which should be monitored for adequate cleaning and sterilization. 10% povidone-iodine should be used to clean the skin and 5% should be used in conjunctival fornices for 3 minutes (grouped evidence rating IIA, clinical recommendation B). In patients who are allergic to iodine, clorhexidine is a possible alternative. Care should be taken during corneal incision construction. The authors consider that corneal hydration and checking of wounds to assess if they are watertight are very useful measures and when there are any doubts concerning the wound´s archithecture it should be sutured. There is not enough scientific evidence to recommend the use of subconjunctival or "in the bottle" antibiotics for the prophylaxis of endophthalmitis. In a clinical trial promoted by the ESCRS, intracameral cefuroxime (1mg in 0.1ml) in the bag and when the anterior chamber was not full, achieved a 5-fold decrease in the risk of postoperative endophthamitis (grouped evidence rating IB, clinical recommendation A). Its use also has a very good cost-effectiveness ratio. As of the present there are no double-masked, randomised clinical trials that recommend intracameral moxifloxacin at the end of phacoemulsification for postoperative endophthalmitis prophylaxis. Finally, there is no scientific evidence to support antibiotic use in the postoperative period to decrease the incidence of POE, but it seems reasonable to use them until the incisions are sealed- this normally means a week of topical antibiotics. Sharp suspension of the treatment and not tapering of these drops is recommended.

14. References

Andonegui J., Jiménez-Lasanta L., Alisadea D., & Lameiro F. (2009). Brote de síndrome tóxico del segmento anterior después de cirugía vítrea. *Arch Soc Esp Oftalmol, 2009,* 84:403-406. ISSN: 0365-6691

Arbisser L.B. (2008). Safety of intracameral moxifloxacin for prophylaxis of endophthalmitis after cataract surgery. *J Cataract Refract Surg* 2008, 34: 1114-1120. ISSN: 0886-3350

Arciola C.R., Caramazza R., & Pizzoferrato A. (1994). In vitro adhesion of Staphylococcus epidermidis on heparin-surface modified intraocular lenses. *J Cataract Refract Surg,* 1994, 20: 158-161. ISSN: 0886-3350

Arshinoff S.A. (2007). "Advantages and Use of Intracameral Moxifloxacin for Bacterial Prophylaxis in Cataratact Surgery", poster presented at the ASCRS Symposium on Cataract, IOL and Refractive Surgery, San Diego, California, USA, April 2007

Avisar R., & Weinberger D. (2010). Corneal endotelial morphologic features in toxic anterior segment syndrome. *Cornea,* 2010, 29: 251-153. ISSN: 0277-3740

Baillif S., Ecochard R., Hartmann D., Freney J., & Kodjikian L. (2009). Intraocular lens and cataract surgery: comparison between bacterial adhesion and risk of postoperative endophthalmitis according to intraocular lens biomaterial. *J Fr Ophtalmol,* 2009, 32: 515-28. ISSN: 0181-5512

Ball J.L, Barrett G.D. (2006). Prospective randomized controlled trial of the effect of intracameral vancomycin and gentamicin on macular retinal thickness and visual function following cataract surgery. *J Cataract Refract Surg,* 2006, 32:789–794. ISSN: 0886-3350.

Barry P., Seal D.V., Gettinby G., Lees F., Peterson M., & Revie C.W. (2006). ESCRS study of prophylaxis of postoperativeendophtalmitis after cataract surgery: Preliminary report of principal results from a European multicenter study. *J Cataract Refract Surg,* 2006, 32: 407-410. ISSN 0886-3350

Breebaart A.C., Nuyts R.M.M.A., Pels E., Edelhauser H.F., & Verbraak F.D. (1990). Toxic endotelial cell destruction of the cornea after extracapsular cataract surgery. *Arch Ophthalmol,* 1990, 108: 1121-1125. ISSN:0003-9950

Buzard K., Zhang J.R., Thumann G., Stripecke R., & Sunalp M. (2010). Two cases of toxic anterior segment syndrome from generic trypan blue. *J Cataract Refract Surg,* 2010, 36(12): 2195-2199: ISSN 0886-3350

Cakir M., Imamoğlu S., Cekiç O., Bozkurt E., Alagöz N., Oksüz L., & Yilmaz O.F. (2009). An outbreak of early-onset endophthalmitis caused by Fusarium species following cataract surgery. *Curr Eye Res,* 2009, 34(11):988-995. ISSN 0271-3683

CDC. Recommendations for preventing the spread of vancomycin resistance.(1995). *Morb Mort Wkly Rep,* 1995,44(RR-12):1-13. ISSN: 0886-3350

Ciulla T.A., Starr M.B., & Masket S. (2002). Bacterial endophthalmitis prophylaxis for cataract surgery: an evidence-based update. *Ophthalmology,* 2002, 109: 13-24. ISSN: 0161-6420

Cusumano A., Busin M., & Spitznas M. (1994). Bacterial growth is significantly enhanced on foldable intraocular lenses. *Arch Ophthalmol, 1994,* 112: 1.015-1.016. ISSN: 0003-9950

Díez M.R., de la Rosa G., Pascual R., Girón C., & Arteta M. (2009). Prophylaxis of the postoperative endophthalmitis with cefuroxime intracameral: a five years´experience. *Arch Soc Esp Oftalmol,.* 2009, Feb, 84(2):85-89. ISSN: 0365-6691

Driebe W.T., Mandelbaum S., Forster R.K., Schwartz L.K., & Culbertson W.W. (2006). Pseudophakic endophthalmitis. Diagnosis and management *Ophthalmology,* 1986, 93:442–8. ISSN: 0161-6420

Duffy R.E., Brown S.E., Caldwell K.L., Lubniewski A., Anderson N., Edelhauser H., Holley G., Tess A., Divan H., Helmy M., Arduino M., & Jarvis W.R. (2000). An epidemic of corneal destruction caused by plasma gas sterilization; the Toxic Endothelial Cell Destruction syndrome investigate Team. *Arch Ophthalmol,* 2000, 118:1167-1176. ISSN: 0003-9950

Eleftheriadis H., Cheong M., Sanderman S., Syam P.P., Brittain P., Klintworth G.K., Lloyd A., & Liu C. (2002). Corneal toxicity secondary to inadvertent use of benzalkonium chloride preserved viscoelastic material in cataract surgery. *Br J Opthalmol,* 2002, 86: 299-305. ISSN 1468-2079

Eloy R., Parrat D., & Duc T.M. (1993). In vitro evaluation of inflammatory cell response after CF4 plasma surface modification of polymethyl methacrylate intraocular lenses. *J Cataract Refract Surg,* 1993, 19: 364-370. ISSN: 0886-3350

Endophthalmitis Vitrectomy Study Group. (1995). Results of the Endophthalmitis Vitrectomy Study: a randomized trial of immediate vitrectomy and of intravenous antibiotics for the treatment of postoperative bacterial endophthalmitis. *Arch Ophthalmol,* 1995, 113(12):1479-1496. ISSN: 0003-9950

Endophthalmititis Vitrectomy Study Group. (1995). Results of the Endophthalmitis Vitrectomy Study. A randomized trial of immediate vitrectomy and of intravenous antibiotics for the treatment of postoperative bacterial endophthalmitis. *Arch Ophthalmol,* 1995, 113: 1479-1496. ISSN: 0003-9950

ESCRS Endophthalmitis Study Group. (2007). Prophylaxis of postoperative endophthalmitis following cataract surgery: results of the ESCRS multicenter study and identification of risk factors. *J Cataract Refract Surg,* 2007, 33: 978–988. ISSN: 0886-3350

Fernández-Rubio E., Cuesta-Rodriguez T., & Cortés-Valdés C. (2004). Antibioterapia tópica preoperatoria en la cirugía de cataratas. *Arch Soc Esp Oftalmol,* 2004, 79: 213-220. ISSN: 0365-6691

Ferro J.F., De-Pablos M., & Logrono M.J. (1997). Postoperative contamination alter vancomycin and gentamycin during phacoemulsification. *Arch Ophthalmol,* 1997,115:165-170. ISSN: 0003-9950

Feys J.F., Salvanet-Bouccara A., Emond J., & Dublanchet A. (1997). Vancomycin prophylaxis and intraocular contamination during cataract surgery. *J Cataract Refract Surg,* 1997, 23:894-897. ISSN: 0886-3350

Fine I.H., Hoffman R.S., & Oacker M. (2007). Profile of clear corneal cataract incisions demonstrated by ocular coherence tomography. *J Cataract Refract Surg,* 2007, 33(1):94-97. ISSN: 0886-3350

Garat M., Moser C.L., Alonso-Tarrés C., Martín-Baranera M., & Alberdi A. (2005). Intracameral cefazolin to prevent endophthalmitis in cataract surgery:3-year retrospective study. *J Cataract Refract Surg,* 2005, 31(11):2230-4. ISSN: 0886-3350

Garcia-Arumi J., Fonollosa A., Sarasols L., Fina F., Martinez-Castillo V., Boixader A., Zapata M.A., & Campins M. (2007). Topical anestesia: posible risk factor for endophthalmitis alter cataract extraction. *J Cataract Refract Surg,* 2007, 33:989-992. ISSN: 0886-3350

García-Sáenz M.C., Arias-Puente A., Rodríguez-Caravaca G., & Bañuelos J.B. (2010). Effectiveness of intracameral cefuroxime in preventing endophthalmitis after cataract surgery. *J Cataract Refract Surg,* 2010, 36:203-207. ISSN: 0886-3350

Gills J.P (1991). Filters and antibiotics in irrigating solution for cataract surgery [letter]. *J Cataract Refract Surg,* 1991, 17:385. ISSN: 0886-3350.

Gimbel H.V., Sun R., & DeBroff B.M. (1994). Prophylactic intracameral antibiotics during cataract surgery:the incidence of endophthalmitis and corneal endothelial loss. *Eur J Implant refract Surg,* 1994, 6:280-285

Gordon Y.J. (2001). Vancomycin prophylaxis and emerging resistance: Are Ophthalmologists the villains? The heroes? *Am J Ophthalmol,* 2001, 131(3):371-376. ISSN: 0002-9394

Greenbaum S. (2007). Topical anesthesia and postoperative endophthalmitis. *J Cataract Refract Surg,* 2007, 33:2011-2012. ISSN: 0886-3350

Groden L.R., Murphy B., Rodnite J., & Genvert G.I. (1991). Lid flora in blepharitis. *Cornea,* 1991, 10:1:50-53. ISSN: 0277-3740

Gupta M.S., McKee H.D., Saldana M., & Stewart O.G. (2005). Macular thickness after cataract surgery with intracameral cefuroxime. *J Cataract Refract Surg,* 2005, 31:1163–1166. ISSN: 0886-3350

Guzel A.G., Ozekinci T., Ozkan U., Celik Y., Ceviz A., & Belen D. (2009). Evaluation of the skin flora alter clorhexidine and povidone-iodine preparation in neurosurgical practice. *Surgical Neurology,* 2009, 71:207-210. ISSN: 0090-3019

Hellinger W.C., Hasan S.A., Bacalis L.P., Thornblom DM,Beckmann S.C., Blackmore C., Forster T.S., Tirey J.F., Ross M.J., Nilson C.D., Mamalis N., Crook J.E., Bendel R.E., Shetty R., Stewart M.W., Bolling J.P., & Edelhauser H.F. (2006). Outbreak of toxic anterior segment syndrome following cataract surgery associated with impurities in autoclave steam moisture. *Infect Control Hosp Epidemio,l* 2006, 27: 294-298. ISSN: 0899-823X

Hellinger W. C., Bacalis L. P., Edenhauser H. F.,Mamalis M., Milstein B., Masket S. (2007). Recommended practices for cleaning and sterilizing intraocular surgical instruments. *J Cataract Refract Surg,* 2007, 33:1095-1100. ISSN: 0886-3350

Heuermann T., Hartman C., & Anders N. (2002). Long-term endotelial cell loss after phacoemulsification; peribulbar anesthesia versus intracameral lidocaine 1%; prospective, randomized clinical trial. *J Cataract Refract Surg,* 2002, 28:639-643. ISSN: 0886-3350.

Holland S.P., Lee T.L., & Morck D.W. (2007). Update on toxic anterior segment syndrome. *Curr Opin Ophthalmol,* 2007, 18:4-8. ISSN: 1040-8738

Hollander D.A., Vagefi M.R., Seiff S.R., & Stewart J.M. (2006). Bacterial endophthalmitis after resident-performed cataract surgery. *Am J Ophthalmol,* 2006,141 (5):949-51. ISSN: 0002-9394

Hospital Infection Control Practices Advisory Committee (HICPAC). (1995). Recommendations for preventing the spread of vancomycin resistance. *Infect Control Hosp Epidemiol,* 1995, 16:105–113, erratum, 498. ISSN: 0899-823X

Jensen M.K., Fiscella R.G., Moshirfar M., & Mooney B. (2008). Third- and fourth-generation fluoroquinolones: retrospective comparison of endophthalmitis after cataract surgery performed over 10 years. *J Cataract Refract Surg,* 2008, 34:1460–1467. ISSN: 0886-3350

Jun E.J., & Chung S.K. (2010). Toxic anterior segment syndrome after cataract surgery, *J Cataract Refract Surg,* 2010, 36: 344-346. ISSN: 0886-3350.

Kadonoso K., Ito N., Yazama F., Nishide T., Sugita M., Sawada H., & Ohno S. (1998). Effect of intracameral anesthesia on the corneal endotelio. *J Cataract Refract Surg,* 1998, 24:1377-1381. ISSN: 0886-3350.

Kamalarajah S. Ling R., Silvestri G., Sharma N.K., Cole M.D., Cran G., & Best RM. (2007). Presumed infectious endophthalmitis following cataract surgery in the UK: a case-control study of risk factors. *Eye,* 2007, 21(5):577-9. ISSN: 0950-222X

Kelkar A., Kelkar J., Amuaku W., Kelkar U., & Shaikh A. (2008). How to prevent endophthalmitis in cataract surgeries? *Indian J Ophthalmol,* 2008, 56(5):403-7. ISSN: 0301-4738

Khan R.I., Kennedy S., & Barry P. (2005). Incidence of presumed postoperative endophthalmitis in Dublin for a 5-year-period (1997-2001). *J Cataract Refract Surg,* 2005, 31: 1575-1581. ISSN 0886-3350

Kim J.Y., Ali R., Cremers S.L., & Henderson B.A. (2007). Perioperative prophylaxis for postcataract extraction endophthalmitis. *Int Ophthalmol Clin,* 2007, 47(2):1-14. ISSN: 0020-8167

Kowalski R.P., Kowalski B.R., Romanowski E.G., Mah F.S., Thompson P.P., & Gordon Y.J. (2006). The in vitro impact of moxifloxacin and gatifloxacin concentration (0.5% vs 0.3%) and the addition of benzalkonium chloride on antibacterial efficacy. *Am J Ophthalmol,* 2006, 142:730–735. ISSN 0002-9394

Kowalski R.P., Romanowski E.G., Mah F.S., Yates K.A., & Gordon Y.J. (2005). Intracameral vigamox (moxofloxacin 0.5%) is non-toxic and effective in preventing endophthalmitis in a rabbit model. *Am J Ophthalmol,* 2005, 497e1-497e8. ISSN 0002-9394

Kramann C., Pitz S., Schewenn O., Haber M., Hommel G., & Pfeiffer N. (2001). Effects of intraocular cefotaxime on the human corneal endothelium. *J Cataract Refract Surg,* 2001, 27:250-255. ISSN: 0886-3350

Kreisler K.R., Martin S.S., Young C.W., Anderson C.W., & Mamalis N. (1992). Postoperative inflammation following cataract extraction caused by bacterial contamination of the cleaning bath detergent. J Cataract Refract Surg, 1992, 18:106-110. ISSN: 0886-3350.

Kutty P.K, Forster T.S., Wood-Koob C., Thayer N., Nelson R.B., Berke S.J., Pontacolone L., Beardsley T.L., Edelhauser H.F., Arduino M.J., Mamalis N., & Sriinivasan A. (2008). Multistate outbreak of toxic anterior segment síndrome, 2005. *J Cataract Refracr Surg,* 2008, 34:585-590. ISSN: 0886-3350

Lacey R.W. & Catto A. (1993). Action of povidone-iodine against methicillin-sensitive and -resistant cultures of Staphylococcus aureus. *Postgrad Med J*, 1993, 69: S78-S83.

Lane S.S., Osher R.H., Masket S., & Belani S. (2008). Evaluation of the safety of prophylactic intracameral moxifloxacin in cataract surgery. *J Cataract Refract Surg*, 2008, 34:1451–1459. ISSN: 0886-3350

Liesegang T.J.(2001). Use of antimicrobials to prevent postoperative infection in patients with cataracts. *Current Opinion in Ophthalmology*, 2001, 12:68–74. ISSN 1040-8738

Liu H., Routley I., & Teichmann K.D. (2001). Toxic endotelial cell destruction from intraocular benzalkonium chloride. *J Cataract Refract Surg*, 2001, 27: 1746-1750. ISSN: 0886-3350

Mammalis N., Edelhauser H.F., Dawson D.G., Chew J., LeBoyer R.M., & Werner L. (2006). Toxic anterior segment síndrome. *J Cataract Refract Surg*, 2006, 32:324-333. ISSN: 0886-3350

Masket S. (1998). Preventing, diagnosing, and treating endophthalmitis. *J Cataract Refract Surg*, 1998, 24:725—726. ISSN: 0886-3350

Masket S. (2007). Reply: Patching to prevent postoperative endophthalmitis. *J Cataract Refract Surg*, 2007, 33 (10):1673. IOSSN: 0886-3350

Mathys K.C., Cohen K.L., & Bagnell C.R (2008). Ideentification of unknown intraocular material after cataract surgery: evaluation of a potential cause of toxic anterior segment syndrome. *J Cataract Refract Surg*, 2008, 34:465-469. ISSN: 0886-3350

Melo G.B., Bispo P.J., Regatieri C.V., Yu M.C., Pignatari A.C., & Höfling-Lima A.L.. (2010). Incidence of Endophthalmitis after cataract surgery (2002-2008) at a Brazilian university-hospital. *Arq Bras Oftalmol*, 2010, 73(6): 505-507. ISSN: 0004-2749

Mendivil A. & Mendivil M.P. (2000). The effect of topical povidone-iodine, intraocular vanomycin or both in aqueous humorcultures at the time of cataract surgery. *Am J Ophthalmol* 2000, 131: 293-300. ISSN: 0002-9394

Menikoff J.A., Speaker M.G., Marmor M., & Raskin E.M. (1991). A case-control study of risk factors for postoperative endophthalmitis. *Ophthalmology*, 1991, 98:1761–1768. ISSN: 0161-6420

Miller J., Scott I.U., Flynn H.W., Smiddy W.E., Newton J., & Miller D. (2005). Acute–onset Endophthalmitis after cataract surgery 2000-2004: Incidence, clinical settings and visual acuity outcomes after treatment. *Am J Ophthalmol*, 2005, 139(6):983-987. ISSN: 0002-9394

Mills D.M., Bodman M.G., Meyer D.R., & Morton A.D. (2007). 3rd; ASOPRS Dacryocystitis Study Group. The microbiologic spectrum of dacryocystitis: a national study of acute versus chronic infection. *Ophthal Plast Reconstr Surg*, 2007, 23: 302-306. ISSN: 1537-2677

Miño de Kaspar H., Chang R.T., Singh K., Egbert P.R., Blumenkranz M.S., & Ta CN. (2005). Prospective randomized comparison of 2 different methods of 5% povidone-iodine applications for the anterior segment intraocular surgery. *Arch Ophthalmol*, 2005, 123:161-165. ISSN: 0003-9950

Miño de Kaspar H., Shriver E.M., Nguyen E.V., Egbert P.R., Singh K., Blumenkranz M.S., & Ta C.N.(2003). Risk factors for antibiotic-resistant conjunctival bacterial flora in patients undergoing intraocular surgery. *Graefes Arch Clin Exp Ophthalmol*, 2003, 241(9):730-733. Epub 2003 Aug 20. ISSN: 0721-832X

Miño De Kaspar H., Ta C.N., Froehlich S.J., Schaller U.C., Engelbert M., Klauss V., & Kampik A. (2009). Prospective study of risk factors for conjunctival bacterial contamination in patients undergoing intraocular surgery. *Eur J Ophthalmol,* 2009,19(5):717-722. ISSN 1120-6721

Monson M.C., Mamalis N., & Olson R.J. (1992). Toxic anterior segment inflammation following cataract surgery. *J Cataract Refract Surg,* 18, 1992,184-189,ISSN: 0886-3350

Montan P., Montan P., Wejde G., Setterquist, Koranyi G., & Rylander M. (2002). Prophylactic intracameral cefuroxime. Evaluation of safety and kinetics in cataract surgery. *J Cataract Refract Surg,* 2002, 28:982-987. ISSN: 0886-3350

Montan P., Wejde G., Koranyi G., & Rylander M. (2002). Prophylactic intracameral cefuroxime. Efficacy in preventing endophthalmitis after cataract surgery. *J Cataract Refract Surg,* 2002, 28:977-981. ISSN: 0886-3350

Morlet N., Gatus B., & Coroneo M. (1998). Patterns of peri-operative prophylaxis for cataract surgery: a survey of Australian ophthalmologists. *Aust NZ J Ophthalmol,* 1998, 26:5 – 12. ISSN: 0814-9763

Nakata K., Inoue Y., Harada J., Maeda N., Watanabe H., Tano Y., Shimomura Y., Harino S., & Sawa M. (2000). A high incidence of Staphylococcus aureus colonization in the external eyes of patients with atopic dermatitis. *Ophthalmology,* 2000, 107: 2167-2171. ISSN: 0161-6420

Ng E. & Barrett G.D., Baudman R. (1996). In vitro bacterial adherence to hydrogel and PMMA intraocular lenses. *J Cataract Refract Surg,* 1996, 22 (sup 2): 1.331-1.335. ISSN: 0886-3350

O'Brien T.P., Arshinoff S.A., & Mah F.S. (2007). Perspectives on antibiotics for postoperative endophthalmitis prophylaxis: potential role of moxifloxacin. *J Cataract Refract Surg,* 2007, 33:1790–1800. ISSN: 0886-3350

Parikh C, Sippy B.D., Martin D.F., Edelhauser H.F. (2002). Effects of enzymatic sterilization detergents on the corneal endothelium. *Arch Ophthalmol,* 2002, 120: 165-172. ISSN: 0003-9950

Parikh C.H., & Edelhauser H.F. (2003). Ocular surgical pharmacology: corneal endotelial safety and toxicity. *Curr Opin Ophthalmol,* 2003, 14: 178-185. ISSN: 1040-8738

Peck C.M.C., Brubaker J., Clouser S., Danford C., Edelhauser HF., & Mamalis N. (2010). Toxic anterior segment syndrome: common causes. *J Cataract Refract Surg,* 2010, 36: 1073-1080. ISSN: 0886-3350

Pijla B.J., Theelena T., Tilanusa M.A., Rentennaarb R., & Cramaa N. (2010). Acute endophthalmitis after cataract surgery: 250 consecutive cases treated at a tertiary referral center in the Netherlands. *Am J Ophthalmol,* 2010, 149:482-287.e2. ISSN: 0002-9394

Pinna A., Usai D., Sechi L.A., Zanetti S., Jesudasan N.C., Thomas P.A., & Kaliamurthy J. (2009). An outbreak of post-cataract surgery endophthalmitis caused by Pseudomonas aeruginosa. *Ophthalmology,* 2009, 116(12):2321-2326.e1-4. Epub 2009 Oct 7. ISSN: 01616-6420

Romero P., Méndez I., Salvat M., Fernández J., & Almena M. (2006). Intracameral cefazolin as prophylaxis against endophthalmitis in cataract surgery. *J Cataract Refract Surg,* 2006, 32:438–441. ISSN: 0886-3350

Sato T., Emi K., Ikeda T., Bando H., Sato S., Morita S., Oyagi T., & Sawada K. (2010). Severe intraocular inflammation after intravitreal injection of bevacizumab. *Ophthalmology,* 2010, 117(3):512-6, 516.e1-2. Epub 2010 Jan 19. ISSN 0161-6420

Schauersberger J., Amon M., Aichinger D., & Georgopoulos A. (2003). Bacterial adhesion to rigid and foldable posterior chamber intraocular lenses: in vitro study. *J Cataract Refract Surg,* 2003, 29:361-6. ISSN: 0886-3350

Scoper S.V. (2008). Review of third- and fourth-generation fluoroquinolones in ophthalmology: in-vitro and in-vivo efficacy. *Adv Ther,* 2008, 25:979–994

SERV. "Endoftalmitis infecciosa. Guías de Práctica clínica de la SERV". (2011). Available in www.serv.es

Sharify E., Porco T.C., & Naseri A. (2009). Cost-effectiveness analysis of intracameral cefuroxime use for prophylaxis of endophtalmitis after cataract surgery. *Ophthalmology,* 2009, 16:1887-1896. ISSN: 0161-6420

Shaw J., Smith E.F., Deai R.U., Enriquez B., & Schrier A. (2010). Can intraocular lenses deliver antibiotics intracamerally? *J Ocul Pharmacol Ther,* 2010, 26 (6): 587-589. ISSN: 1080-7683

Speaker M.G., Milch F.A., Shah M.K., Eisner W., & Kreiswirth B.N. (1991). Role of external bacterial flora in the pathogenesis of acute postoperative endophthalmitis. *Ophthalmology,* 1991, 98: 639-649. ISSN: 0161-6420

Vasavada A.R., Gajjar D., Raj S.M., Vasavada V., & Vasavada V. (2008). Comparison of 2 moxifloxacin regimens for preoperative prophylaxis: prospective randomized triple-masked trial. Part 2: Residual conjunctival flora. *J Cataract Refrac Surg,* 2008, 34:1383-1388. ISSN 0886-3350.

Wallace E.J., Imrie F., Roxburgh S., Coleiro J., & Ironside J. (2007). Epithelial downgrowth as a complication of toxic anterior segment syndrome. *J Cataract Refract Surg,* 33, 2007, 1976-1977. ISSN: 0886-3350

Werner L., Sher J.H., Taylor J.R., Mamalis N., Nash W.A., Csordas J.E., Green G., Maziarz E.P., & Liu X.M. (2006). Toxic anterior segment syndrome and possible association with ointment in the anterior chamber following cataract surgery. *J Cataract Refract Surg,* 2006, 32:227-235. ISSN: 0886-3350

Yoeruek E., Spitzer M.S., Saygili O., Tatar O., Biedermann T., Yoeruek E., Bartz-Schmidt K.U., & Szurman P. (2008). Comparison of in vitro safety profiles of vancomycin and cefuroxime on human corneal endothelial cells for intracameral use. *J Cataract Refract Surg,* 2008, 34:2139–2145. ISSN: 0886-3350

Yu-Wai-Man P., Morgan S.J., Hildreth A.J., Steel D.H., & Allen D. (2008). Efficacy of intracameral and subconjunctival cefuroxime in preventing endophthalmitis after cataract surgery. *J Cataract Refract Surg,* 2008, 34:447-451. ISSN: 0886-3350

Section 4

Cataract Surgery in Special Situations

23

Cataract Surgery in Retina Patients

Kemal Örnek
Kırıkkale University, School of Medicine, Department of Ophthalmology, Turkey

1. Introduction

Cataract surgery accounts for a significant part of the surgical load of ophthalmologists and it continues to be the commonest surgical procedure on the world. It has a high level of efficacy, has lower rate of complications and is convenient for the patients. Combined with the age-related demographic shift, advances in instrumentation and surgical techniques has led the cataract surgery to become more frequent and easier.

A large portion of cataract patients have coexisting retinal diseases such as diabetic retinopathy, epiretinal membrane and age-related macular degeneration etc. Surgery is necessary for postoperative visual acuity improvement, for a better view of the retina intraoperatively, and for visualization of the retina postoperatively in these patients. Retinal diseases may also influence the cataract surgery including timing of surgery, the surgical technique, the type of intraocular lenses implanted or final visual outcome. In addition, previous vitreoretinal surgery is a risk factor for cataract surgery due to many factors, such as intraocular lens power of a silicone filled eye, abnormal fluctuations in anterior chamber depth, zonular weakness etc.

This chapter will focus mainly on two subjects; cataract surgery in the presence of coexisting retinal diseases and cataract surgery with retinal surgery.

2. Cataract surgery and retinal diseases

Certain retinal diseases like diabetic retinopathy, age-related macular degeneration, epiretinal membrane and retinal vein occlusions may be exacerbated by cataract surgery. Therefore, retinal diseases with the potential for progression should be evaluated and treated prior to cataract surgery. With careful preoperative planning, attention to details during surgery and close postoperative follow up, these eyes may have visual improvement following cataract surgery.

2.1 Age-related macular degeneration

The true risk of progression of age-related macular degeneration following cataract surgery is controversial. Multiple epidemiological studies suggest that cataract surgery accelerates the progression of age-related macular degeneration. The Beaver Dam Eye Study reported an association between cataract surgery and early age-related macular degeneration; Freeman et al found an association between cataract surgery and late age-related macular degeneration (Freeman et al, 2003); the Blue Mountains Eye Study did not find an association between cataract surgery and either early or late age-related macular degeneration and the Rotterdam Study found an association between cataract surgery and early age-related macular degeneration but not wet age-related macular degeneration.

A recent prospective study of 71 patients with non-exudative age-related macular degeneration found that, at 12 months following cataract surgery, the rate of progression to neovascular age-related macular degeneration was not higher than what would have been expected without the surgery (Dong et al, 2009). Another study looked at the 10-year incidence of age-related macular degeneration and its association with both cataract and cataract surgery (Klein et al, 2002). It was found that cataract at baseline was associated with early age-related macular degeneration, but not with late age-related macular degeneration. At 10 years after cataract surgery, there was an increased incidence of late age-related macular degeneration. The authors conclude that cataract surgery increased the risk for late age-related macular degeneration.

Pollack et al. studied a group of patients with bilateral, nonexudative age-related macular degeneration who underwent extracapsular cataract extraction. In these patients, subsequent choroidal neovascular membrane was more prevalent in pseudophakic eyes than in control eyes (Pollack et, 1996). In another report, Van de Schaft et al. showed a higher prevalence of disciform macular degeneration in pseudophakic eyes compared with phakic control eyes by postmortem histopathologic examination (Van de Schaft et al, 1994)). Shuttleworth et al. retrospectively reviewed the charts of 99 patients with age-related macular degeneration who had received cataract surgery. Visual acuity was noted to improve in the postoperative period. Most patients (66%) experienced an improvement in visual acuity postoperatively. Progression of age-related macular degeneration was identified in 10% of patients, while choroidal neovascular membrane was seen in 2.0% (Shuttleworth et al, 1998)).

Prior to cataract extraction, it is very important to examine the macular region in detail to detect the presence of age-related macular degeneration. If cataract surgery is performed in the presence of age-related macular degeneration, special care should be taken to reduce the possibility of inflammation even if it would require immediate use of antiinflammatory drugs. Cystoid macular edema should be aggressively treated, with careful follow-up emphasized. Delaying cataract surgery, until the optical coherence tomography indicates improvement of macular edema and/or subretinal fluid is usually recommended. Cataract surgery should not be performed on the patient with active "wet" macular degeneration until it has been brought to a dry stage. If there is bleeding from a neovascular membrane, cataract surgery should be delayed until at least six months after the blood has completely reabsorbed and there has been no recurrence of the bleeding has been present. In patients with macular scars and dense cataracts, surgical removal of the opacified lens with intraocular lens implantation may be of benefit in recovering some degree of pericentral or peripheral vision. No cataract surgery should be performed unless the cataract is opaque enough so that when it is removed, the patient will probably perceive the benefit of the operation.

In patients with age-related macular degeneration, the Age-related Eye Disease Study (AREDS) report showed that the AREDS nutritional supplement did not affect visual acuity outcomes in patients who had cataract surgery. Improved visual acuity was seen in the group receiving either the AREDS supplement or placebo after surgery. The long-term benefits of the AREDS supplement in patients with age-related macular degeneration are, however, well established, and it is recommended that those who fit the criteria of the AREDS study for risk of age-related macular degeneration progression take these supplements and continue to do so after surgery. Ultraviolet light and sun exposure are commonly thought to be risk factors for age-related macular degeneration. Surgeons may consider a choice of a ultraviolet light-blocking intraocular lens in patients with age-related macular degeneration who are undergoing cataract surgery. It is also important to advise patients to get ultraviolet light protection by wearing glasses and hats on sunny days postoperatively.

2.2 Diabetic retinopathy

Many patients undergoing cataract surgery have preexisting diabetic retinopathy which may put additional stress on the eye and can lead to macular edema, progressive retinopathy and limited vision. Diabetic patients tend to develop cataracts at an earlier age and may be more prone to developing posterior subcapsular cataracts than other patients. It is important to establish that the degree of cataract seen corresponds to the patients' visual acuity and reported visual dysfunction. Diabetics at any stage of retinopathy are susceptible to macular edema, which is one of the main causes of central visual loss in these patients. A detailed dilated fundus examination can reveal many of these pathologies, but additional tests including optical coherence tomography or fluorescein angiography can reveal more subtle lesions.

Significant diabetic ocular pathology should be treated before cataract surgery is considered. This involves argon laser panretinal photocoagulation as the primary treatment for proliferative retinopathy and focal macular laser for clinically significant macular edema. Additional treatment involves intravitreal injection of vascular endothelial growth factor inhibiting medications and steroids (Cheema et al, 2009; Lam et al, 2005). The patient should also achieve a tight control of systemic blood glucose, and this should be demonstrated in the patient's hemoglobin A1c levels (Suto et al, 2006). For patients with significant diabetic retinopathy, it is better to work with a retinal specialist. The anterior segment can also be inversely affected by poorly controlled diabetes. These are neovascularization of the iris and angle, which often leads to neovascular glaucoma. Aggressive treatment of neovascular glaucoma must take priority over cataract treatment because prolonged increase in intraocular pressure can cause permanent damage to the optic nerve and severe visual loss. Working with a retinal colleague may be the best approach in these complicated patients.

Once the diabetic retinopathy is quiescent and the macula is dry, cataract surgery can be planned. Intraocular lens preference should lean to monofocal, toric, or sometimes accommodating intraocular lenses. Multifocal intraocular lenses should be avoided in eyes with a history of macular lesions or the likelihood of developing macular pathology. Acrylic intraocular lenses are preferred for patients who are likely to undergo vitrectomy for proliferative diabetic retinopathy in the future, whereas silicone intraocular lenses may be a reasonable choice in patients with well-controlled diabetes and mild retinopathy. Steps to make cataract surgery less traumatic include minimizing phaco energy, running less fluid through the eye, and avoiding contact with the iris. These complex patients do better when surgery is performed by a more experienced surgeon rather than a novice. Diabetic eyes often have poor pupillary dilation, particularly when active rubeosis iridis or even regressed neovascularization is present. Pupil stretching should be avoided because these vessels can rupture and cause intracameral bleeding. In some cases, intravitreal injection of triamcinolone or vascular endothelial growth factor inhibiting medications is given at the time of or before cataract surgery. For diabetic patients with nonclearing vitreous hemorrhages or tractional retinal detachments, cataract surgery can be combined with a pars plana vitrectomy.

In eyes with advanced diabetic retinopathy, cataract surgery may lead to progression and worsening of retinopathy, which can have detrimental effects on vision (Dowler et al, 1992). In eyes with minimal diabetic changes, cataract surgery is not as likely to cause progression of retinopathy (Wagner et al, 1996; Krepler et al, 2002; Flesner et al, 2002; Kim et al, 2007). Therefore, performing cataract surgery at an earlier stage may be beneficial for diabetic patients because it is associated with fewer complications and better postoperative recovery of vision. Postoperatively, topical steroids and nonsteroidal antiinflammatory drugs are prescribed because they control inflammation and may play a role in the prevention and treatment of macular edema. Macular thickness can be evaluated at serial postoperative visits via optical coherence tomography before the topical medications are stopped. Development of posterior capsular opacification and persistent postoperative inflammation may be more common in diabetics. Consideration should be given to the use of a larger diameter optic in conjunction with a larger capsulotomy for patients with diabetes (Kato et al, 2001).

Despite an uneventful cataract surgery, diabetic retinopathy can become exacerbated in the postoperative period, so patients should be monitored closely with serial dilated funduscopic examinations and referred to retinal colleagues as needed.

2.3 Retinal vein occlusion

Retinal vein occlusion is the second most common retinal vascular disease of the eye after diabetic retinopathy. Many of the patients are elderly and have cataracts, and a common treatment of retinal vein occlusion, an intravitreal steroid injection, increases the risk of cataract formation or progression. Unfortunately, small or resolved branch retinal vein occlusions may go unnoticed and only manifest as unexplained visual loss. A careful preoperative evaluation with close attention to unexplained visual loss (out of proportion to the degree of cataract) is critical to detect deficits that will not improve with cataract surgery and to recognize any cystoid macular edema risk.

Retinal vein occlusions may lower the threshold for blood retina barrier breakdown. Both central retinal vein occlusion and branch retinal vein occlusion are risk factors. Patients with retinal vein occlusion who undergo cataract surgery have an increased risk of postoperative cystoid macular edema. In a large study by Henderson et al conducted between 2001 and 2006, the risk of postoperative cystoid macular edema in uncomplicated cataract surgery was 30 times higher if the operated eye had a history of retinal vein occlusion (Henderson et al, 2007). This risk persisted even in eyes without preoperative macular edema. Intravitreal triamcinolone acetonide and vascular endothelial growth factor inhibiting medications seem to be an effective primary treatment option for macular edema due to retinal vein occlusions and may be given at the time of or before cataract surgery (Jonas et al, 2005, Rensch et al, 2009). Topical nonsteroidal anti-inflammatory drops may be used to prevent the development of cystoid macular edema in patients with retinal vein occlusion (Henderson et al, 2007).

Rare retinal vascular diseases may also increase the risk of cystoid macular edema in cataract patients. These include retinal telangiectasis (Coats' disease, radiation retinopathy, and idiopathic retinal telangiectasia) and several forms of retinal vasculitis (Eales' disease, Behçet's syndrome, sarcoidosis, necrotizing angiitis, multiple sclerosis).

2.4 Epiretinal membrane

It is well known that idiopathic epiretinal membrane occurs typically after posterior vitreous detachment, and gradually progresses with aging. A previous retrospective study suggested that extracapsular cataract extraction is the most common surgical cause of epiretinal membrane (Appiah et al, 1988). A more recent prospective study also showed that the prevalence of idiopathic epiretinal membrane increased from 14.8% preoperatively to 25.3% at 6 months after extracapsular cataract extraction (Jahn et al, 2001). The risk of post-cataract surgery cystoid macular edema is also increased in patients with epiretinal membrane (Henderson et al, 2007).

Idiopathic epiretinal membrane surgery has been reported to improve visual acuity in between 67% and 82% of cases (Margherio et al, 1985). However, subsequent development of progressive nuclear sclerosis occurs in 12.5% to 63% of post vitrectomy patients (Margherio et al, 1985). Ando and associates compared visual outcomes of the combined vitrectomy and cataract procedure to simple vitrectomy in idiopathic epiretinal membrane cases (Ando et al, 1998). Preoperative visual acuities and other patient characteristics were similar in the two study groups. Although more postoperative complications were noted in the combined group with two cases of fibrin formation, one case of macular edema, and four cases of anterior chamber inflammation, the visual outcomes were similar. Post-operatively, both groups showed initial visual improvement; 73% of combined procedure group compared to 88% of the simple vitrectomy group. However, within two years, cataracts formed in 70% of the simple vitrectomy group. The authors recommend the combined procedure for phakic patients older than 55 years undergoing vitrectomy for epiretinal membrane. Alexandrakis et al. described the surgical outcomes of combined cataract surgery and pars plana vitrectomy in eight cases of idiopathic epiretinal membrane formation (Alexandrakis et al, 1999). No intraoperative complications were observed, and at a mean follow-up visit of 22 months, visual acuity had improved in seven patients (88%. Median pre-operative and post-operative visual acuity were 20/200 and 20/50, respectively. Other studies that use the combined procedure to remove epiretinal membranes have reported favorable results as well (Koenig et al, 1992; Demetriades et al, 2003). Cataract surgery seems to be essential in phakic eyes to achieve long-term improvement in visual acuities in eyes with epiretinal membranes and good preoperative acuities.

In a study, the progression of idiopathic epiretinal membrane is not accelerated by small-incision phacoemulsification cataract surgery. Furthermore, visual acuity is not impaired markedly at least for the following year (Hayashi and Hayashi, 2009). However, it is still unclear whether or not a secondary epiretinal membrane progresses after cataract surgery in eyes with other retinal morbidity such as retinal detachment surgery or retinal pathology.

2.5 Peripheral retinal breaks and retinal detachment

The preoperative treatment of the retinal breaks and retinal degenerations has traditionally come into consideration as a possible means of preventing retinal detachments after cataract extraction, especially in myopic eyes. Specifically, flap retinal tears (even when asymptomatic) are usually treated. Round retinal holes, lattice degeneration, white without pressure, and other peripheral retinal abnormalities are typically observed.

There is an increasing tendency to support the concept that retinal detachments generally are associated with recent retinal breaks. Reports supporting the prophylactic treatment of preexisting retinal breaks prior to cataract surgery is lacking. Most of the eyes with lattice degeneration do not detach after small incision cataract extraction even when YAG laser capsulotomy is performed later. Those that do develop a retinal detachment frequently do not detach from retinal breaks adjacent to or within the lattice lesions, but from unrelated areas which previously looked clinically normal. If a patient has a history of retinal detachment in one eye and lattice degeneration with retinal holes in the other eye, cryosurgery or laser surgery is needed to close the holes in the second eye. Usually cryosurgery is required because the cataract may preclude the use of laser. The type of tear present and other factors including the location of the tear and the existence of high myopia would influence the ophthalmologist's judgment in deciding when to treat. Since seven to eight percent of the population has lattice degeneration, it is obvious that not all patients with lattice degeneration should be treated. Regardless of whether the patient is treated prior to cataract surgery, those patients should be followed closely with careful examination of the peripheral retina postoperatively following cataract removal.

Girard and Saade reported a 3.5% incidence of simultaneous primary rhegmatogenous retinal detachment and visually significant cataract (Girard and Sade, 1997). In such cases, they advocate a combined procedure including phacoemulsification, intraocular lens implantation and scleral buckling surgery. Cataract formation is a common occurrence after retinal detachment repair, especially when gas tamponade is employed. For this reason, recurrent retinal detachment may be found in eyes with cataracts, which may make repair more difficult. Options available to the retinal surgeon include cataract surgery followed by pars plana vitrectomy or combined cataract surgery and vitrectomy.

Another study described experiences using the combined procedure to treat 16 cases of recurrent retinal detachments (Chaudhry et al, 2000). Eyes were selected for inclusion in the study based on presence of a dense cataract and a recurrent rhegmatogenous retinal detachment with mild proliferative vitreoretinopathy following primary surgical repair using encircling scleral buckle. In nine eyes (56%), visual acuity improved to 20/200 or better post-operatively. In 13 eyes (81%), the initial reoperation was successful in retinal reattachment. Two additional eyes achieved retinal reattachment with a second pars plana vitrectomy, increasing the anatomic success rate to 94%. The study had a selection bias in that the eyes with more severe proliferative vitreoretinopathy were not found suitable for the combined procedure. However for primary rhegmatogenous retinal detachment and recurrent retinal detachment with mild proliferative vitreoretinopathy, the combined procedure appears to be well tolerated.

2.6 Macular hole

Macular holes are commonly found in older patients. Some eyes have concurrent macular hole and cataract, making internal limiting membrane peeling more difficult during vitrectomy because of blurred media. The incidence of cataract development following macular hole surgery is also extremely high. Thompson et al. reported visually significant cataract formation in 76% of the study eyes following vitrectomy for macular hole (Thompson et al, 1995). Consecutive and combined surgeries for macular hole and cataract extraction are both effective procedures.

Various studies found that the functional and anatomic results of combined surgery were equivalent to consecutive procedures (Theocharis et al, 2005; Simcock and Scalia, 2001; Kotecha et al, 2000; Muselier et al, 2010). Nevertheless, combining cataract surgery with vitrectomy may prevent a second operation to correct post-vitrectomy cataract formation. In the largest series, Lahey and associates described combined procedure to treat 89 cases of macular holes (Lahey et al, 2002). These patients received combined phacoemulsification, implantation of posterior chamber intraocular lens and pars plana vitrectomy. Additionally, to prevent posterior capsule opacification and post-operative vision loss, the authors included a posterior capsulotomy as part of the procedure. Post-operatively, 61 patients (65%) had improved to 20/40 or better. Closure of the macular hole after the initial surgery occurred in 80 patients (89%). Four holes closed with an additional operation. After nine months or more, three patients experienced reopening of the macular hole, which was successfully managed with repeat vitrectomy. Reported complications included eight (9%) post-operative cases of cystoid macular edema, all of which were resolved by topical and sub-Tenon's steroid application. Another eight patients (9%) developed small, segmental synechiae of the anterior capsule iris. Post-operative retinal detachments occurred in only three patients (3%). The combined procedure also allows for a more complete vitrectomy that includes removal of the anterior vitreous without the risk of lens injury. Thus, a better gas fill can be achieved which may provide longer tamponade and an increased closure rate for macular holes (Thompson et al, 1996).

Simcock and Scalia reported the results of combined phacoemulsification cataract removal and vitrectomy in 13 consecutive eyes with full thickness macular holes. Mild preoperative lens opacity was present in all 13 patients. Each eye underwent phacoemulsification followed by pars plana vitrectomy and finally intraocular lens implantation. Twelve of the 13 patients had visual improvement in the postoperative period. None of the eyes developed cystoid macular edema (Simcock and Scalia, 2000). There have been concerns regarding the incidence of cystoid macular edema following combined procedure for macular hole. Sheidow and Gonder reported a 43% incidence of both clinical and angiographical evidence of cystoid macular edema in a study of seven eyes undergoing combined procedure for macular hole (Sheidow and Gonder, 1998). However, other studies have not confirmed this observation and macular hole appears to be an acceptable indication for combined procedure.

In combined surgeries, intraoperative aphakia provided maximum visibility for posterior vitreous peeling and peripheral visualization. Scleral ports could be placed more anteriorly reducing the risk of a retinal tear. The risk of vitrectomy induced cataract was eliminated and a more complete vitrectomy could be performed leading to greater gas fill and therefore a better postoperative tamponade.

2.7 High myopia

Cataract development is more frequent in patients with high myopia than in the general population. Reports have shown that the mean age for cataract surgery in patients with high myopia is 65 years. However, in eyes with an axial length greater than 29mm, the incidence is significant at age 50 years. Nuclear cataract is most typical in high myopia and in its earliest stage, increases the optical power of the lens and thus the optical power of the myopic eye. In these patients, nuclear cataract may be difficult to recognize, because in some cases nuclear sclerosis is the initial step in nuclear cataract development. Middle-aged patients who developed cataract might have had early nuclear sclerosis without evidence of cataract. The earliest manifestation may be an increase in the dioptric correction of myopia (Metge and Pichot de Champfleury, 1994; Wong et al, 2001; Leske et al, 2002; Younan et al, 2002).

Myopic eyes have a higher risk of retinal complications compared with emmetropic eyes. During the preoperative evaluation, a careful examination should be done for any retinal breaks, holes or degenerations, as well as any macular pathology. The highly myopic patients may also have myopic macular degeneration, epiretinal membranes or other significant changes. These may limit the postoperative visual acuity and may influence the development of postoperative complications such as cystoid macular edema. If any posterior segment issues are detected, referral to a vitreoretinal colleague for treatment is recommended before cataract surgery. In addition to the typical cataract evaluation, care must be taken to accurately assess the retinal status and measure the axial length of the eye. Highly myopic eyes often have a posterior staphyloma, which can give an erroneously long axial length when measured with the standard A-scan ultrasound. Using an optical method for measurement tends to be more accurate, as it measures directly at the fovea. The intraocular lens calculation formulae are less accurate at the extremes, and this is particularly true for highly myopic eyes. Of the two-variable formulae, the SRK/T tends to perform particularly well, as do more complex formulae such as the Haigis and Holladay 2 (Wang et al, 2008). The selection of the intraocular lens depends on each patient's ocular status and needs.

The advantage of cataract surgery in myopic patients is the larger anterior chamber depth, which allows more working room during phacoemulsification. However, the infusion pressure from the phaco handpiece can cause over-inflation of the anterior chamber and a tendency to push the entire lens-iris diaphragm posteriorly. To overcome this, the infusion pressure can be decreased by lowering the bottle height; however, this will result in less inflow of fluid and a higher tendency for surge. Another solution is to break the reverse pupillary block by making sure that there is fluid flow under the iris to equalize the anterior and posterior chamber pressures. By neutralizing this pressure gradient, the cataract will not be pushed so deeply within the eye, and adequate infusion pressure can be used. The postoperative refraction in myopes can take time to stabilize due to the variation in effective lens position as the capsular bag shrink-wraps around the intraocular lens. During this period, inflammation can be controlled using topical steroids and nonsteroidal anti inflammatory drugs. During the postoperative period, repeat dilated fundus examinations are mandatory in order to search for possible retinal breaks that may have been created during surgery (Alio et al, 2000; Tosi et al, 2003; Güell et al, 2003).

2.8 Retinoblastoma

Cataract formation is one of the most common ocular complications of external beam radiotherapy for retinoblastoma, which typically occurs in three years following treatment (Schipper et al, 1985; Miller et al 2005). Studies have shown that cataract surgery in patients who have previously received radiation therapy for retinoblastoma is generally not associated with tumor recurrence or spread (Brooks et al, 1990; Portellos and Buckley, 1998).

Controversies in cataract management include the surgical approach, the management of the posterior capsule and anterior vitreous. In the setting of prior treatment for retinoblastoma, these decisions take on even greater importance with the added concern for reactivation or metastasis of the tumor. Both clear corneal and pars plana approaches have been used with success in children undergoing cataract surgery following treatment for retinoblastoma. Although Brooks et al advised against pars plana approachs based on their experience of tumor recurrence, other series have not reported tumor recurrences with pars plana insicions (Brooks et al, 1990). Miller and associates reported a series of 16 eyes, all of which underwent a combined pars plana vitrectomy and cataract extraction, and showed no evidence of tumor recurrence in their series (Miller et al 2005). Payne et al have also shown that limbal approach was not associated with tumor recurrence or metastasis (Payne et al, 2009).

Management of the posterior capsule is controversial in the setting of previous treatment for retinoblastoma. Theoretically, the posterior capsule may act as a barrier to tumor spread if viable tumor cells are present in the eye, therefore, the posterior capsule should be kept intact whenever possible. Nevertheless, it is frequently necessary to perform a primary posterior capsulotomy and anterior vitrectomy in pediatric cataracts, even in the setting of prior treatment for retinoblastoma. Since posterior capsular opacity is common after external beam radiotherapy, it is sometimes necessary to remove the posterior capsule to clear the visual axis. The risks and benefits of primary posterior capsulotomy and anterior vitrectomy should be considered on a case-by-case basis, taking into account the location of the cataract, the age of the patient, the availability of the YAG laser, the length of the quiescent period, and the location and stage of the tumor (Payne et al, 2009).

2.9 Retinitis pigmentosa

Cataract is a well-recognised complication of all types of retinitis pigmentosa. When compared with patients with age related cataract, patients with retinitis pigmentosa develop lens opacities earlier (Pruett, 1983; Fishman et al, 1985; Heckenlively, 1982). In addition, a relatively minor lens opacity may cause significant functional symptoms in these patients. Apart from the general risks of cataract surgery, there are specific additional factors that may result in a poor visual outcome after cataract extraction in the presence of retinitis pigmentosa. These include, retinal atrophy at the macula, macular edema occurring in approximately 10–15% of patients and phototoxic retinal damage in normal patients undergoing cataract extraction (Grover et al, 1997; Spalton et al, 1978; Newsome, 1986; Lee and Sternberg, 1993). The threshold for light damage is probably lower in retinitis pigmentosa, which could adversely affect visual outcome. Posterior capsular opacification and anterior capsular contraction is more aggressive in the presence of retinitis pigmentosa, (Nishi and Nishi, 1993; Hayashi et al, 1998). The reason for the increased cellular proliferation on the capsular remnant in retinal dystrophies is unknown, although the cellular nature of the posterior capsule in retinal dystrophies may account for this (Fishman et al, 1985).

Patients with retinitis pigmentosa benefit from early cataract surgery, and that the vast majority have a subjective improvement in their symptoms of glare. The benefit of surgery for patients with a poor preoperative visual acuity is less marked, usually because of preexisting macular disease, but postoperative macular edema was less common than expected. Patients with retinitis pigmentosa appear to be susceptible to anterior capsule contraction and therefore a small capsulorhexis should be avoided. It would appear to be sensible to avoid silicone intraocular lenses because of the risk of their dislocation if an early capsulotomy is required (Jackson et al, 2001).

2.10 Retinopathy of prematurity

Cataracts occur more commonly in retinopathy of prematurity patients compared to general population. Low birth weight and prematurity are risk factors for both retinopathy of prematurity and cataracts (San Giovanni et al, 2002; Repka et al, 1998). Cataracts develop at a greater frequency over time, as current treatment modalities have preserved vision in eyes that would have otherwise been lost. Transpupillary laser photocoagulation is now the standard treatment for threshold retinopathy of prematurity. However, laser-treated eyes have a higher incidence of secondary cataracts than cryo-treated eyes (Christiansen and Bradford, 1995; Christiansen and Bradford, 1997; Kaiser and Trese, 1995). Lens opacities associated with retinopathy of prematurity appears in three types. First, focal punctuate or vacuolated opacities may occur at the subcapsular level. These are usually transient and visually insignificant. Second, progressive lens opacities may occur in patients without retinal detachment. Most of these eyes have had transpupillary laser treatment or "lens sparing" vitrectomy. These cataracts may progress rapidly or much more slowly, but they almost always eventually obstruct the entire visual axis and require surgery (Alden et al, 1973; Drack et al, 1992).

A visually significant cataract after laser treatment or vitrectomy for retinopathy of prematurity is approached much like childhood cataracts in children without retinopathy of prematurity (Wilson et al, 2005). At times the anterior capsule can be fibrotic, but a vitrectorhexis can still be easily performed. Intraocular lens calculations can be performed using an immersion A-scan ultrasound unit and a portable keratometer in the operating room, after the child is under general anesthesia for cataract surgery. Intraocular lenses are implanted routinely, unless the child is in the early months of life and has microphthalmia. Most commonly, a single-piece hydrophobic acrylic intraocular lens is implanted in children. In anticipation of myopic shift of refraction, the intraocular lens power for a child undergoing cataract surgery should be customized based on many characteristics - especially age, laterality (one eye or both), amblyopia status (mild or severe), likely compliance with glasses, and family history of myopia. For a child with retinopathy of prematurity and cataract, slightly higher hypermetropia may be considered in anticipation of developing more myopia, especially if treated with cryotherapy (Trivedi et al, 2007). A primary posterior capsulectomy and anterior vitrectomy is performed for children who are younger than 6 years ofage. If previous vitrectomy has been performed as part of the retinopathy of prematurity treatment, the surgeon must be aware that the posterior capsule may have been violated during the previous surgery.

The two surgical approaches in stage V retinopathy of prematurity are pars plana lensectomy versus lensectomy via the limbal approach. A pars plana lensectomy can be combined with an attempt to repair retinal pathology. The limbal approach is easier and more consistent, as the pars plana entry may be difficult in these immature eyes with retinal detachment. Even when the anterior chamber is extremely shallow, an anterior corneal entry can usually be made with the assistance of a viscous ophthalmic viscosurgical device.

Although cataract extraction in eyes with regressed retinopathy of prematurity may present challenges, such as high myopia, monocularity, glaucoma, and previous ocular surgery, phacoemulsification in these eyes proved to be relatively safe as well as visually rehabilitating. The surgeon should be aware of the special considerations in this population, alert to potential zonular weakness intraoperatively, and careful of increased postoperative risks, including retinal detachment (Farr et al, 2001).

3. Cataract surgery and retinal surgery

Cataract and vitreoretinal diseases often occur simultaneously. The surgical management of patients with vitreoretinal diseases and cataract has always been a unique situation for vitreoretinal surgeons. The major difficulty is not only visual interference created by lens opacification, but also deciding on a patient-by patient basis whether cataract extraction should be combined or approached as a two-step procedure.

The patient's history is particularly important to determine the onset of symptoms and the development of the cataract. After most pars plana vitrectomy surgeries, cataracts develop slowly, over the course of months or years after retinal surgery, in the form of increased nuclear sclerosis and often posterior subcapsular opacities. The use of intraocular gas or silicone oil as a retinal tamponade may induce cataract changes at a somewhat more rapid rate, but it is still typically months before the patient notices a visual decline. If the patient reports a history of quickly developing a cataract, such as a white cataract, days or weeks after the vitrectomy, then iatrogenic damage to the lens capsule should be suspected. While it is uncommon, it is possible for the pars plana vitrectomy instruments to damage the posterior lens capsule, which can rupture and then cause the lens to opacify very quickly.

Clinical examination should include careful evaluation of the posterior capsule by either slit lamp or ultrasound, if direct visualization is not possible. If the ultrasound shows an abnormally large lens thickness or an out-pouching of the posterior lens surface, a defect in the posterior lens capsule likely exists. Intraocular lens calculations may be somewhat less accurate due to difficulty in estimating the postop effective lens position. The absence of vitreous and possible prior damage to zonules may cause the intraocular lens to sit more posterior than predicted, resulting in a hyperopic surprise. This is why aiming for a mild degree of postop myopia by using a slightly higher-powered intraocular lens tends to give better results. Three-piece monofocal acrylic intraocular lenses in these eyes may have more options for lens fixation, such as in-the-bag, in-the-sulcus and sulcus placement of the haptics with optic capture through the capsulorrhexis. In addition, the acrylic material minimizes condensation on the optic and adhesion to silicone oil if a repeat vitrectomy is needed in the future.

3.1 Cataract surgery and pars plana vitrectomy

Mastering in surgical techniques for cataract extraction and improvements in intraocular lens technology have increased the indications for cataract surgery. Additionally, pars plana vitrectomy is now performed for a wide variety of vitreoretinal diseases. It is widely accepted today that the most effective procedure for lens extraction is sutureless clear corneal phacoemulsification. The common approach for pars plana vitrectomy is transconjunctival small incision sutureless vitrectomy, also known as minimally invasive vitreoretinal surgery (Fujii et al, 2002; Eckardt, 2005).

Combined phacoemulsification and vitrectomy is indicated if the opacified lens interferes with the visualization of the retina, hindering the operation. However, if the cataract allows for good visualization of the posterior pole, the surgeon must decide on the best approach; a combined procedure, clear cornea phacoemulsification and then pars plana vitrectomy, both performed at the same surgical session, or a two-step procedure, pars plana vitrectomy is performed first, and then clear cornea phacoemulsification performed as a secondary procedure during a second surgical session (Pollack et al, 2004).

3.1.1 Combined procedure

A combined approach with minimally invasive vitreoretinal surgery has been rising in popularity among vitreoretinal surgeons, mainly because it has several advantages when compared with the two-step procedure. These include faster visual recovery and patient satisfaction, no suture-related astigmatism, less postoperative inflammation, less conjunctival fibrosis, easier vitreous shaving, better access to the vitreous base, and more effective postoperative tamponade (Koenig et al, 1990; Pollack et al, 2004; Axer-Siegel et al, 2006; Mochizuki et al, 2006; Treumer et al, 2006; Demetriades et al, 2003; Wensheng et al, 2009).

There are three ways to start this procedure. One option is to introduce the vitrectomy trocars, then perform phacoemulsification, complete the vitrectomy via pars plana, and leave intraocular lens implantation as the last step. A second option is to start by performing phacoemulsification and, once this is completed, introduce the vitrectomy transconjunctival trocars. Perform the vitrectomy via pars plana and, once again, leave intraocular lens implantation for the last step. A third option is to perform phacoemulsification with intraocular lens implantation first, and then perform vitreoretinal surgery. After phacoemulsification and intraocular lens implantation, a prophylactic 10-0 nylon suture is placed to avoid anterior chamber collapse, and iris prolapse. It is recommended to leave viscoelastic material in the anterior chamber during the vitrectomy procedure to maintain anterior chamber depth.

3.1.2 Two-step procedure

The vitreous body is semi-solid, thick and viscous in a healthy eye. These properties allow it to help support the cataract during surgery when the patient is supine. This results in a normal anterior chamber depth and a more routine cataract surgery. In an eye that has undergone a prior vitrectomy, saline and aqueous have replaced the vitreous, resulting in a fluid-filled eye that does not provide additional support of the cataract during phacoemulsification. This causes the anterior chamber to be overly deep during cataract surgery. To address this, the infusion pressure can be decreased by lowering the bottle height on the phacoemulsification machine. To compensate for lower infusion, the aspiration flow rate should also be dropped.

Additionally, posterior support can be increased by giving a retrobulbar block because the anesthetic bolus will tend to provide pressure to the back of the eye. If there is reverse pupillary block, caused when the iris makes a tight seal on the anterior lens capsule, this can be solved by tenting up the iris with a second instrument or even by placing a single iris hook. These eyes may also have zonular damage or laxity, which can lead to difficulties during cataract surgery. If there is a posterior capsule rupture, either from the vitrectomy or cataract surgery, the lens nucleus should be brought forward, out of the capsular bag, and viscoelastic should be placed behind it to support it. If any cataract pieces are displaced into the posterior segment, they will rapidly descend onto the retina due to the lack of vitreous. These pieces are best removed by the vitreoretinal surgeon using a pars plana approach.

Patients who undergo cataract surgery after a prior retinal surgery are at higher risk for some postoperative complications. Patients with prior macular surgery are more prone to cystoid macular edema, even after an uncomplicated cataract surgery. These patients should be treated with anti-inflammatory medications for a prolonged period, and their macular status should be monitored at postoperative visits. Patients with prior retinal detachment surgery are at a higher risk for a recurrent detachment after cataract surgery, so their retinal periphery should be checked carefully. In addition, it may take longer for these patients to heal after surgery and to achieve a stable postoperative refraction. Although total intraoperative time is shorter for a two step procedure compared with a combined approach, patients who undergo sequential surgeries may experience increasing discomfort. Another disadvantage is cost; two surgeries cost more than the combined procedure (Grusha et al, 1998; Chang et al, 2002; Ahfat et al, 2003).

There are advantages and disadvantages to each approach, but both are safe and effective. Combined surgery requires a shorter postoperative recovery time, anterior vitreous structures can be removed without risk of touching the lens, visualization of the posterior pole is good during vitrectomy, and it involves only one surgical session, which may reduce patient discomfort and decrease risks and costs. Also, patients with retinal vascular diseases frequently undergo panretinal photocoagulation during the operation, decreasing the risk of developing retinal and iris neovascularization.

However, there are potential disadvantages to combined surgery, such as increased operating time and stress on the surgeon, difficulty visualizing the capsulorrhexis because of an absent or reduced red reflex, cataract wound dehiscence caused by globe manipulation during subsequent vitreous surgery, and intraoperative miosis after cataract extraction. Other disadvantages include bleeding from anterior structures, loss of corneal transparency from corneal edema and Descemet's folds, inadvertent exchange of anterior segment fluids with posterior segment tamponading agents, intraocular lens decentration and iris capture in eyes with gas-air or silicone oil tamponade and prismatic effects and undesirable light reflexes during vitreoretinal surgery caused by intraocular lens before posterior segment procedures.

Postsurgical complications are similar in both approaches. In the two-step procedure, it should be kept in mind that the surgeon is facing complications associated with phacoemulsification and pars plana vitrectomy, just as in the combined procedure, but during separate surgical sessions (Koenig et al, 1990). The most common intraoperative complications associated with phacoemulsification include tears during anterior capsulorrhexis, rupture of the posterior capsule with the phaco tip, and dislocation of nuclear fragments into the vitreous cavity.

3.2 Cataract surgery and scleral buckling surgery

Scleral buckling surgery is associated with a lower rate of cataract formation than pars plana vitrectomy or combined vitrectomy and buckle surgeries. Therefore, scleral buckling may be considered as the primary surgical option in the treatment of uncomplicated rhegmatogenous retinal detachments where the crystalline lens is sufficiently clear.

Haller and Kerrison reported that eyes which have undergone scleral buckling surgery have good visual outcomes after cataract surgery and a low risk of recurrent retinal detachment. The same study showed more intraoperative complications during extracapsular cataract surgery in patients who had undergone vitrectomy for retinal detachment but a low rate of intraoperative complications in patients with previous scleral buckling (Haller and Kerrison, 1997). Smiddy and associates reported no recurrent retinal tears or detachments in patients who underwent extracapsular cataract surgery after previous scleral buckling with an average follow-up period of 24 months (Smiddy et al, 1988). Ruiz and Saatci reported a favorable outcome for extracapsular cataract surgery with intraocular lens implantation in eyes that had undergone successful scleral buckling. In this study however, 3.4% of eyes developed recurrent retinal redetachment 15 months after cataract surgery (Ruiz and Saatçi, 1991) . Eshete et al

demonstrated that phacoemulsification and intraocular lens implantation can be performed safely after scleral buckling surgery and excellent best-corrected visual acuity results can be attained in most eyes without any modification in surgical technique. No eye had retinal redetachment in their study (Eshete et al, 2000).
Combining phacoemulsification with scleral buckling rather than vitrectomy may be a more optimal surgical decision in selected cases. However, proper case selection (fresh rhegmatogenous retinal detachment with minimal proliferative vitreoretinopathy, etc) and familiarity with the surgical techniques is mandatory for achieving higher success rates. Conventional large incision cataract surgeries cannot be combined with scleral buckling because of the instability of the wound and inability to maintain the eyeball contour because of fluctuation in intraocular pressure (Garder et al, 1993). Also, there is an increased risk of vitreous loss and aggravation of retinal pathology. Phacoemulsification provides a better stability of the wound during the procedure because of the small incision size.
Combined scleral buckling for retinal detachment and phacoemulsification was first reported by Lazar and Bracha (Lazar and Bracha, 1977). Girard and Saade reported a case series of 15 patients who underwent a triple procedure; phacoemulsification, intraocular lens implantation and scleral buckling for recurrent rhegmatogenous retinal detachment with a significant cataract (Girard and Sade, 1997). They noted high postoperative intraocular pressure in only one of their cases, which was attributed to the use of viscoelastic. Overall anatomical success rate was 87% and functional success was 54%. They concluded that combined phacoemulsification and scleral buckling was a safe and effective procedure. Tsai and Wu confirmed the effectiveness of cataract surgery together with scleral buckling, with no significant complications. The authors believed that combined cataract surgery and scleral buckling can improve visualization for detection of peripheral retinal holes and can improve the results of the operation (Tsai and Wu, 2004).

3.3 Cataract surgery and pneumatic retinopexy

Pneumatic retinopexy is an alternative to scleral buckling for the surgical repair of selected retinal detachments. A gas bubble is injected into the vitreous cavity, and the patient is positioned so that the bubble closes the retinal break, allowing absorption of the subretinal fluid. Cryotherapy or laser photocoagulation is applied around the retinal break to form a permanent seal. Temporary gas tamponade for pneumatic retinopexy is not associated with permanent changes in lens transparency (Mougharbel et al, 1994).

4. Conclusion

Cataract surgery improves vision in patients with preexisting retinal disease and is necessary for the physician to monitor and treat the underlying pathology. However, surgeons must be cautious about certain retinal diseases and previous retinal surgeries which can make a patient more prone to complications following cataract surgery. Understanding the risk factors and applying certain methods of preventative treatment can minimize both intraoperative and postoperative effects. In addition, working closely with retina specialists in the management of patients whose cataract surgery is complicated by retinal issues may help the cataract surgeon to bring these cases to a more successful outcome.

5. References

Ahfat FG, Yuen CHW & Groenewald CP (2003). Phacoemulsification and intraocular lens implantation following pars plana vitrectomy: a prospective study. *Eye*. 2003; 17:16–20.

Alden ER, Kalina RE & Hodson WA (1973). Transient cataracts in low birth weight infants. *J Pediatr*. 1973;82: 314–8.

Alexandrakis G, Chaudhry NA, Flynn HW Jr & Murray TG (1999). Combined cataract surgery, intraocular lens insertion, and vitrectomy in eyes with pars plana vitrectomy and lens management 141 idiopathic epiretinal membrane. *Ophthalmic Surg Lasers*. 1999; 30:327–328.

Alió JL, de la Hoz F, Ruiz-Moreno JM & Salem TF (2000). Cataract surgery in highly myopic eyes corrected by phakic anterior chamber angle-supported lenses. *J Cataract Refract Surg*. 2000; 26:1303-11.

Ando A, Nishimura T & Uyama M (1998). Surgical outcome on combined procedures of lens extraction, intraocular lens implantation, and vitrectomy during removal of the epiretinal membrane. *Ophthalmic Surg Lasers*. 1998; 29: 974–979.

Appiah AP, Hirose T & Kado M (1988). A review of 324 cases of idiopathic preremacular gliosis. *Am J Ophthalmol* 1988; 106: 533–535.

Axer-Siegel R, Dotan G, Rosenblatt I, Benjamini Y & Weinberger D (2006). Combined pars plana vitrectomy and cataract surgery: outcome of phacoemulsification versus manual extracapsular cataract extraction through a sclerocorneal tunnel. *Ophthalmic Surg Lasers Imaging*. 2006; 37: 94-8.

Brooks HL Jr, Meyer D, Shields JA, Balas AG, Nelson LB & Fontanesi J (1990). Removal of radiation-induced cataracts in patients treated for retinoblastoma. *Arch Ophthalmol* 1990;108: 1701-8.

Chang MA, Parides MK, Chang S & Braunstein RE (2002). Outcome of phacoemulsification after pars plana vitrectomy. *Ophthalmology*. 2002;109:948–954.

Chaudhry NA, Flynn HW Jr, Murray TG, Belfort A & Mello M Jr (2000). Combined cataract surgery and vitrectomy for recurrent retinal detachment. *Retina*. 2000;20: 257–261.

Cheema RA, Al-Mubarak MM, Amin YM & Cheema M (2009). Role of combined cataract surgery and intravitreal bevacizumab injection in preventing progression of diabetic retinopathy: prospective randomized study. *J Cataract Refract Surg*. 2009; 35: 18–25.

Christiansen SP & Bradford JD (1995). Cataract in infants treated with argon laser photocoagulation for threshold retinopathy of prematurity. *Am J Ophthalmol*. 1995;119:175–80.

Christiansen SP & Bradford JD (1997). Cataracts following diode laser photoablation for retinopathy of prematurity. *Arch Ophthamol*. 1997;115:275–6.

Demetriades AM, Gottsch JD, Thomsen R, Azab A, Stark WJ, Campochiaro PA, de Juan E Jr & Haller JA (2003). Combined phacoemulsification, intraocular lens implantation, and vitrectomy for eyes with coexisting cataract and vitreoretinal pathology. *Am J Ophthalmol*. 2003; 135: 291-6.

Dong LM, Stark WJ, Jefferys JL, Al-Hazzaa S, Bressler SB, Solomon SD & Bressler NM (2009). *Arch Ophthalmol* 2009; 127(11):1412–1419.

Dowler JGF, Hykin PG, Lightman SL & Hamilton AM (1992). Visual acuity following extracapsular cataract extraction in patients with diabetes. *Br J Ophthalmol*. 1992;76: 221–224.

Drack AV, Burke JP, Pulido JS & Keech RV (1992). Transient punctuate lenticular opacities as a complication of argon laser photoablation in an infant with retinopathy of prematurity. *Am J Ophthalmol*.1992;113:583–4.

Eckardt C (2005). Transconjunctival sutureless 23-gauge vitrectomy. *Retina*. 2005; 25:208–211.

Eshete A, Bergwerk KL, Masket S & Miller KM (2000). Phacoemulsification and lens implantation after scleral buckling surgery. *Am J Ophthalmol* 2000;129: 286-290.

Farr AK, Stark WJ & Haller JA (2001). Cataract surgery by phacoemulsification in adults with retinopathy of Prematurity. *Am J Ophthalmol*. 2001 Sep;132(3): 306-10.

Flesner P, Sander B, Henning V, Parving HH, Dornonville de la Cour M & Lund-Andersen H (2002). Cataract surgery on diabetic patients. A prospective evaluation of risk factors and complications. *Acta Ophthalmol Scand*. 2002; 80: 19–24.

Fishman GA, Anderson RJ & Loureco P (1985). Prevalence of posterior subcapsular lens opacities in patients with retinitis pigmentosa. *Br J Ophthalmol* 1985; 69: 263–6.

Freeman EE, Munoz B, West SK, Tielsch JM & Schein OD (2003). Is there an association between cataract surgery and age-related macular degeneration? Data from three population-based studies. *Am J Ophthalmol*. 2003;135: 849-856.

Fujii GY, De Juan E Jr, Humayun MS, Chang TS, Pieramici DJ, Barnes A & Kent D (2002). Initial experience using the transconjunctival sutureless vitrectomy system for vitreoretinal surgery. *Ophthalmology*. 2002;109: 1814-1820.

Garder TW, Quillen DA, Blankenship GW & Marshall WK (1993). Intraocular pressure fluctuation during buckling surgery. *Ophthalmology*. 1993;100:1050–4.

Girard P & Saade G (1997). A triple procedure: phacoemulsification, intraocular lens implantation, and scleral buckling surgery. *Retina*. 1997;17(6): 502-6.

Gold RS (1997). Cataracts associated with treatment for retinopathy of prematurity. *J Pediatr Ophthalmol Strabismus*. 1997; 34: 123–4.

Güell JL, Rodriguez-Arenas AF, Gris O, Malecaze F &Velasco F (2003). Phacoemulsification of the crystalline lens and implantation of an intraocular lens for the correction of moderate and high myopia: four-year follow-up. *J Cataract Refract Surg*. 2003;29: 34-8.

Grover S, Fishman GA, Fiscella RG & Adelman AE (1997). Efficacy of dorzolamide hydrochloride in the management of chronic cystoid macular edema in patients with retinitis pigmentosa. *Retina*. 1997;17: 222-31.

Grusha YO, Masket S & Miller KM (1998). Phacoemulsification and lens implantation after pars plana vitrectomy. *Ophthalmology*. 1998;105: 287-94.

Haller JA & Kerrison JB (1997). Cataract extraction after retinal detachment. *Curr Opin Ophthalmol* 1997;8: 39-43.

Hayashi K & Hayashi H (2009). Influence of phacoemulsification surgery on progression of idiopathic epiretinal membrane. *Eye*. 2009; 23, 774–779.

Hayashi K, Hayashi H, Matsuo K, Nakao F & Hayashi F (1998). Anterior capsule contraction and intraocular lens dislocation after implant surgery in eyes with retinitis pigmentosa. *Ophthalmology* 1998;105:1239–43.

Heckenlively J (1982). The frequency of posterior subcapsular cataract in the hereditary retinal degenerations. *Am J Ophthalmol*. 1982;93: 733–8.

Henderson BA, Kim JY, Ament CS, Ferrufino-Ponce ZK, Grabowska A & Cremers SL (2007). Clinical pseudophakic cystoid macular edema. Risk factors for development and duration after treatment. *J Cataract Refract Surg*. 2007; 33:1550-8.

Jackson H, Garway-Heath D, Rosen P, Bird AC & Tuft SJ (2001). Outcome of cataract surgery in patients with retinitis Pigmentosa. *Br J Ophthalmol.* 2001; 85: 936-8.

Jahn CE, Minich V, Moldaschel S, Stahl B, Jedelhauser P, Kremer G & Kron M (2001). Epiretinal membranes after extracapsular cataract surgery. *J Cataract Refract Surg* 2001; 27: 753-760.

Jonas JB, Kreissig I, Budde WM & Degenring RF (2005). Cataract surgery combined with intravitreal injection of triamcinolone acetonide. *Eur J Ophthalmol.* 2005;15: 329-35.

Kaiser RS & Trese MT (1995). Iris atrophy, cataracts, and hypotony following peripheral ablation for threshold retinopathy of prematurity. *Arch Ophthalmol.* 1995;119:615–7.

Kato S, Oshika T, Numaga J, Hayashi Y, Oshiro M, Yuguchi T & Kaiya T (2001). Anterior capsular contraction after cataract surgery in eyes of diabetic patients. *Br J Ophthalmol* 2001; 85: 21–23.

Kim SJ, Equi R & Bressler NM (2007). Analysis of macular edema after cataract surgery in patients with diabetes using optic coherence tomography. *Ophthalmology.* 2007;114: 881–889.

Klein R, Klein BE, Wong TY, Tomany SC & Cruickshanks KJ (2002). *Arch Ophthalmol* 2002; 120:1551–1558.

Koenig SB, Mieler WF, Han DP & Abrams GW (1992). Combined phacoemulsification, pars plana vitrectomy, and posterior chamber intraocular lens insertion. *Arch Ophthalmol.* 1992;110:1101–1104.

Koenig SB, Han DP, Mieler WF, Abrams GW, Jaffe GJ & Burton TC (1990). Combined phacoemulsification and pars plana vitrectomy. *Arch Ophthalmol.* 1990;108:362–364.

Kotecha AV, Sinclair SH, Gupta AK & Tipperman R (2000). Pars plana vitrectomy for macular holes combined with cataract extraction and lens implantation. *Ophthalmic Surg Lasers.* 2000; 31: 387–393.

Krepler K, Biowski R, Schrey S, Jandrasits K & Wedrich A (2002). Cataract surgery in patients with diabetic retinopathy: visual outcome, progression of diabetic retinopathy, and incidence of diabetic macular edema. *Graefes Arch Clin Exp Ophthalmol.* 2002;240:735–738.

Lahey JM, Francis RR, Fong DS, Kearney JJ & Tanaka S (2002). Combining phacoemulsification with vitrectomy for treatment of macular holes. *Br J Ophthalmol.* 2002; 86:876–878.

Lam DS, Chan CK, Mohamed S, Lai TY, Lee VY, Lai WW, Fan DS & Chan WM (2005). Phacoemulsification with intravitreal triamcinolone in patients with cataract and coexisting diabetic macular edema: a 6-month prospective pilot study. *Eye.* 2005;19: 885–890.

Lazar M & Bracha R (1977). Combined phacoemulsification and scleral buckling operation. *Am J Ophthalmol.* 1977; 83: 422–3.

Lee BL & Sternberg JP (1993). Microscope light toxicity. *Sem Ophthalmol* 1993; 8: 151–5.

Leske M C, Wu SY, Nemesure B, Hennis A & Barbados Eye Studies Group (2002). Risk factors for incident nuclear opacities. *Ophthalmology* 109, 1303–1308.

Margherio RR, Cox MS Jr, Trese MT, Murphy PL, Johnson J & Minor LA (1985). Removal of epimacular membranes. *Ophthalmology.* 1985; 92: 1075–1083.

Metge P & Pichot de Champfleury A (1994). La cataracte du myope fort. In: Mondon H, Metge P, eds, *La Myopie Forte*. Paris, Masson, 1994; 447–465.

Miller DM, Murray TG, Cicciarelli NL, Capo H & Markoe AM (2005). Pars plana lensectomy and intraocular lens implantation in pediatric radiation- induced cataracts in retinoblastoma. *Ophthalmology* 2005;112: 1620-24.

Mochizuki Y, Kubota T, Hata Y, Miyazaki M, Suyama Y, Enaida H, Ueno A & Ishibashi T (2006). Surgical results of combined pars plana vitrectomy, phacoemulsification, and intraocular lens implantation. *Eur J Ophthalmol.* 2006; 16: 279-86.

Mougharbel M, Koch FH, Böker T & Spitznas M (1994). No cataract two years after pneumatic retinopexy. *Ophthalmology.* 1994 ; 101:1191-4.

Muselier A, Dugas B, Burelle X, Passemard M, Hubert I, Mathieu B, Berrod JP, Bron AM & Creuzot-Garcher C (2010). Macular hole surgery and cataract extraction: combined vs consecutive surgery. *Am J Ophthalmol.* 2010;150: 387-91.

Newsome DA (1986). Retinal fluorescein leakage in retinitis pigmentosa. *Am J Ophthalmol* 1986;101:354–60.

Nishi O & Nishi N (1993). Intraocular lens encapsulation by shrinkage of the capsulorrhexis opening. *J Cataract Refract Surg* 1993; 19: 544–5.

Payne JF, Hutchinson AK, Hubbard III GB & Lambert SR (2009). Outcomes of cataract surgery following radiation treatment for retinoblastoma. *J AAPOS* 2009;13: 454-458.

Pollack A, Marcovitch A, Bukelman A & Oliver M (1996). Age-related macular degeneration after extra-capsular cataract extraction with intraocular lens implantation. *Ophthalmology* 1996, 103:1546–1556.

Pollack A, Landa G, Kleinman G, Katz H, Hauzer D & Bukelman A (2004). Results of combined surgery by phacoemulsification and vitrectomy. *Isr Med Assoc J.* 2004; 6: 143–146.

Portellos M & Buckley EG (1998). Cataract surgery and intraocular lens implantation in patients with retinoblastoma. *Arch Ophthalmol* 1998; 116: 449-52.

Pruett RC. Retinitis pigmentosa: clinical observations and correlations (1983). *Trans Am Acad Ophthalmol Soc* 1983; 81: 693–735.

Rensch F, Jonas JB & Spandau UH (2009). Early intravitreal bevacizumab for non-ischaemic branch retinal vein occlusion. *Ophthalmologica.* 2009; 223: 124-7.

Repka MX, Summers CG, Palmer EA, Dobson V, Tung B & Davis B (1998). The incidence of ophthalmic interventions in children with birth weights less than 1251 grams. Results through 5 1/2 years. Cryotherapy for Retinopathy of Prematurity Cooperative Group. *Ophthalmology.* 1998;105:1621–7.

Ruiz RS & Saatci OA (1991). Extracapsular cataract extraction with intraocular lens implantation after scleral buckling surgery. *Am J Ophtalmol* 1991;111: 174-178.

SanGiovanni JP, Chew EY, Reed GF, Remaley NA, Bateman JB, Sugimoto TA & Klebanoff MA (2002). Infantile cataract in the collaborative perinatal project: prevalence and risk factors. *Arch Ophthalmol.* 2002;120:1559–65.

Schipper J, Tan KE & van Peperzeel HA (1985). Treatment of retinoblastoma by precision megavoltage radiation therapy. *Radiother Oncol* 1985;3: 117-32.

Sheidow TG & Gonder JR (1998). Cystoid macular edema following combined phacoemulsification and vitrectomy for macular hole. *Retina.* 1998;18:510–514.

Shuttelworth GN, Luhishi BA & Harrad RA (1998). Do patients with age related maculopathy and cataract benefit from cataract surgery? *Br J Ophthalmol* 1998, 82: 611–666.

Simcock PR & Scalia S (2000): Phaco-vitrectomy for full thickness macular holes. *Acta Opthalmol Scand* 2000, 78:684–686.

Simcock PR & Scalia S (2001). Phacovitrectomy without prone posture for full thickness macular holes. *Br J Ophthalmol.* 2001;85: 1316 –1319.

Smiddy WE, Michels RG, Stark WJ & Maumenee AE (1988). Cataract extraction after retinal detachment surgery. *Ophthalmology* 1988;95:3-7.

Spalton DJ, Bird AC & Cleary PE (1978). Retinitis pigmentosa and retinal oedema. *Br J Ophthalmol* 1978;62:174

Suto C, Hori S, Kato S, Muraoka K & Kitano S (2006). Effect of perioperative glycemic control in progression of diabetic retinopathy and maculopathy. *Arch Ophthalmol.* 2006; 124: 38–45.

Thompson JT, Glaser BM, Sjaarda RN & Murphy RP (1995). Progression of nuclear sclerosis and long-term visual results of vitrectomy with transforming growth factor beta-2 for macular holes. *Am J Ophthalmol.* 1995;119:48–54.

Thompson JT, Smiddy WE, Glaser BM, Sjaarda RN & Flynn HW Jr (1996). Intraocular tamponade duration and success of macular hole surgery. *Retina.* 1996;16:373–382.

Theocharis IP, Alexandridou A, Gili NJ & Tomic Z (2005). Combined phacoemulsification and pars plana vitrectomy for macular hole treatment. *Acta Ophthalmol Scand* 2005; 83: 172–175.

Tosi GM, Casprini F, Malandrini A, Balestrazzi A, Quercioli PP & Caporossi A (2003). Phacoemulsification without intraocular lens implantation in patients with high myopia: long-term results. *J Cataract Refract Surg.* 2003;29: 1127-31.

Treumer F, Bunse A, Rudolf M & Roider J (2006). Pars plana vitrectomy, phacoemulsification and intraocular lens implantation. Comparison of clinical complications in a combined versus two-step surgical approach. *Graefes Arch Clin Exp Ophthalmol.* 2006; 244: 808-15.

Trivedi RH, Wilson ME. IOL power calculation for children. In: Garg A, Lin, eds. Mastering Intraocular Lenses. New Delhi: Jaypee Brothers Medical Publishers; Chapter 9, 2007: 84–91.

Tsai TC & Wu WC (2004). Combined phacoemulsification, intraocular lens implantation, and scleral buckling surgery for cataract and retinal detachment. *Ophthalmic Surg Lasers Imaging* 2004; 35:13-15.

Wagner T, Knaflic D, Rauber M & Mester U (1996). Influence of cataract surgery on the diabetic eye: a prospective study. *Ger J Ophthalmol.* 1996; 5: 79–83.

Wang JK, Hu CY & Chang SW (2008). Intraocular lens power calculation using the IOLMaster and various formulas in eyes with long axial length. *J Cataract Refract Surg.* 2008;34: 262-7.

Wensheng L, Wu R, Wang X, Xu M, Sun G & Sun C (2009). Clinical complications of combined phacoemulsification and vitrectomy for eyes with coexisting cataract and vitreoretinal diseases. *Eur J Ophthalmol.* 2009;19:37-45.

Wilson ME, Trivedi RH & Pandey SK, eds (2005). *Pediatric Cataract Surgery: Techniques, Complications, and Management.* Philadelphia, PA: Lippincott Williams and Wilkins 2005:179–83.

Wong TY, Klein BE, Klein R, Tomany SC & Lee KE (2001) Refractive errors and incident cataracts: the Beaver Dam eye study. *Invest. Ophthalmol. Vis. Sci.* 42, 1449–1454.

Van de Schaft TL, Mooy CM, Mulder PGH, Pameyer JH & de Jong PT (1994). Increased prevalence of disciform macular degeneration after cataract extraction with implantation of intraocular lens. *Br J Ophthalmol* 1994, 441–445.

Younan C, Mitchell P, Cumming RG, Rochtchina E & Wang, JJ (2002). Myopia and incident cataract and cataract surgery: the blue mountains eye study. *Inves. Ophthalmol Vis Sc.* 43, 3625–3632.

24

Cataract Surgery and Dry Eye

Ramin Daneshvar
Mashhad University of Medical Sciences
Iran

1. Introduction

The World Health Organization (WHO) estimated the presence of approximately 37 million blind people in the world in 2002 (Resnikoff et al., 2004). This awful figure was expected to double by the year 2020 if appropriate preventive measures were not administered (Frick and Foster, 2003). Cataract, the opacification of the crystalline lens, is the single most important cause of blindness in the world. It is estimated that nearly 18 million people are bilaterally blind from cataract, representing almost 48% of all causes of blindness due to eye disease (Resnikoff et al., 2004). Age related cataract cannot usually be prevented; however, cataract surgery is one of the most cost-effective interventions in the field of medicine, resulting in almost immediate visual rehabilitation (Lansingh et al., 2007). Particularly, phacoemulsification is increasingly applied in the management of cataract patients because of its earlier refractive stabilization, reduced induced astigmatism, and milder postoperative inflammation, all resulting in faster visual rehabilitation. It has been shown that improvement in visual acuity following cataract surgery is accompanied by considerable gains in real life activities, emotional and social life components (Lamoureux et al., 2010). Cataract surgery is comparable in terms of cost-effectiveness to hip arthroplasty, and is generally more cost-effective than either knee arthroplasty or cardiac defibrillator implantation, and is cost-effective when considered in absolute terms (Agarwal and Kumar, 2010).

On the other hand, dry eye is estimated to have a prevalence of 11% to 33% depending on population and parameters studied and its prevalence increases with increasing age (Brewitt and Sistani, 2001; Lee et al., 2002; Moss et al., 2000; Schein et al., 1997a; Shimmura et al., 1999). Current evidence clearly demonstrates that dry eye, as a chronic disease, has significant impacts on quality of life and specifically, dry eye is one of the most important factors influencing quality of life in elderly populations. Reduction in quality of life is inevitable when symptoms of dry eye occur. These symptoms range from mild transient irritation to persistent dryness, burning, itchiness, redness, pain, ocular fatigue and visual disturbance. In the United States alone, approximately 7-10 million Americans require artificial tear preparations, with consumers spending over $100 million/year (Lee et al., 2002). In moderate and severe cases, dry eye can impair the ability of patients to perform activities of daily living, impact work productivity, and influence mood and confidence (Friedman, 2010).

Obviously, a high proportion of cataract patients who are candidates for cataract surgery have dry eye; furthermore, there are overwhelming evidences suggesting aggravation or

initiation of dry eye following cataract surgery (Cohen, 1982; Gharaee et al., 2009; Hardten, 2008; Insler et al., 1985; Jones and Maguire, 1992; Khanal et al., 2008; Ram et al., 2002; Ram et al., 1998; Roberts and Elie, 2007). So even following uneventful cataract extraction and vision improvement the patient could be unsatisfied. A main cause of dissatisfaction in such cases has been shown to be eye fatigue and foreign body sensation due to dry eye syndrome.
With these figures in mind, in this chapter, associations between cataract surgery and dry eye are discussed and probable pathogenic factors are highlighted.

2. The healthy tear film: Anatomy and physiology

A healthy tear film plays four major functions in the human eye, namely washing, lubricating, protecting, and forming a smooth optical surface on the cornea. Tear film constituents (the mucin, aqueous, and lipid components) work in concert to provide these functions and any alterations to the quality or quantity of the tear film threaten this fragile homeostasis.
Detailed discussion of the lacrimal system is out of scope of this chapter; however in brief, goblet cells in the conjunctiva are responsible for the production of the mucin layer, while the aqueous layer is secreted by the main and accessory lacrimal glands. The mucin layer plays a role in producing an even distribution of aqueous layer on the ocular surface. The lipids of the tear film generally originate at the meibomian glands, but also from other sources in the conjunctiva, cornea, and lacrimal glands (Butovich, 2008), and compose an interface between the underlying aqueous and mucin and the external environment. Alterations to the quality or quantity of the lipids in the human tear film may especially affect tear film evaporation. Regulation of tear secretion is through a complex neurohormonal system.

2.1 Sensory innervation of the cornea

Corneal sensation is a function of the long ciliary nerves of the ophthalmic division of the fifth (trigeminal) cranial nerve. It is estimated that there are approximately 7000 sensory receptors per square millimeter in the human corneal epithelium, implying that injuries to individual epithelial cells may be adequate to give a sensation (Muller et al., 2003). Traditionally, it was believed that most sensory nerves enter into the cornea along a transverse meridian (3- and 9-o'clock); this was in accordance with the clinical findings of better corneal sensation and less dry eye symptoms in patients undergoing laser in situ keratomileusis (LASIK) with a nasal hinge (Donnenfeld et al., 2003; Kohlhaas, 1998; Lee and Joo, 2003). However, the current description is that nerve bundles enter the peripheral mid-stromal cornea in a radial fashion, along different meridians and parallel to the corneal surface. Most stromal nerve fibers are located in the anterior third of the stroma; however, thick stromal nerve trunks move from the periphery toward the center below the anterior third of the stroma due to the organization of the collagen lamellae (Muller et al., 2003). Soon after entering the cornea, the main stromal bundles branch repeatedly and dichotomously into smaller fascicles that ascended into progressively more superficial layers of the stroma. Eventually, the stromal nerve fibers abruptly turn 90 degrees, penetrate Bowman's layer, and proceed toward the corneal surface. The nerves penetrate Bowman's layer throughout the peripheral and central cornea (Muller et al., 1996). After penetrating Bowman's layer, the large nerve bundles divide into several smaller ones. Each small nerve bundle then turns abruptly once more at 90 degrees and continues parallel to the corneal surface, between Bowman's layer and the basal epithelial cell layer, forming the sub-basal nerve plexus. Sub-basal fibers subsequently form branches that turn upward and enter the corneal epithelium between the basal cells to reach the wing cells, where they terminate (Muller et al., 1996; Ueda et al., 1989). The exact orientation and the depth of nerve fiber bundles are not known and may vary between patients (Kim and Foulks, 1999; Muller et al., 2003; Muller et al., 1996; Muller et al., 1997).

Intact corneal innervation is mandatory for normal blinking and tearing reflexes, which in turn is essential to maintaining the integrity of the ocular surface. Under normal physiologic conditions, sensory nerves in the cornea transmit an afferent stimulation signal through the ophthalmic division of the trigeminal nerve to the brain stem and then, after a series of interneurons, the efferent signal is transmitted to the lacrimal gland through the parasympathetic and sympathetic nerves that innervate the gland and drive tear production and secretion (Dartt, 2004). Damage to this neural circuit interrupts the normal regulation of lacrimal gland secretion and influences both basal and stimulated tear production. This is one of the major pathogenic pathways in induction of postoperative dry eye in patients undergoing ophthalmic surgeries.

Most surgical procedures that cause denervation of the cornea result in impaired epithelial wound healing, increased epithelial permeability, decreased epithelial metabolic activity and loss of cytoskeletal structures associated with cellular adhesion (Donnenfeld et al., 2003; Kohlhaas, 1998). As mentioned earlier, the normal corneal epithelium has the highest density of sensory nerve endings throughout the human body. These receptors are located between the wing cell layers of the corneal epithelium and are protected from direct environmental stimulation by the overlying tear film and the intact surface epithelial cells. In early stages of dry eye, and in the presence of an unstable tear film and superficial punctate keratopathy, the environmental stimuli have greater access to the sensory nerve endings and this may be a key cause for the marked symptoms of ocular irritation experienced by dry eye patients, even in mild cases.

On the other hand, it has been demonstrated that hyposecretion of tears may lead to pathologic alterations in corneal nerves and a decline in corneal sensitivity which subsequently perpetuate the dry eye state in these patients (Xu et al., 1996). The exposure of nerve endings, in conjunction with tear hyperosmolarity and increased expression of a number of inflammatory cytokines, including interleukin (IL)-1alpha and IL-1beta, IL-6, and tumor necrosis factor-alpha may cause injury to the corneal nerves and incite neural degeneration (Barton et al., 1997; Solomon et al., 2001; Yoon et al., 2007). Meanwhile, many of these inflammatory cytokines can induce synthesis of a number of neurotrophic factors, including nerve growth factors, which stimulate the regeneration of corneal nerves (Dastjerdi and Dana, 2009). Changes in corneal nerves in patients with dry eye encompass a wide range of morphologic changes (such as presence of nerve sprouts, abnormal tortuosity, increased bead-like formation and thinning of nerve fiber bundles) to decreased, or paradoxically increased, number of nerve fibers depending on the stage of dry eye (Benitez del Castillo et al., 2004; Erdelyi et al., 2007; Hosal et al., 2005; Tuominen et al., 2003; Villani et al., 2007; Zhang et al., 2005). This could be an explanation for the discrepancy between dry eye signs and symptoms observed in many patients (Dastjerdi and Dana, 2009; Hay et al., 1998).

In addition, the presence of nerve fibers invaginating corneal epithelial cells and keratocytes suggests that both cell types are directly innervated. Immunocytochemical staining indicates the presence of different neuropeptides within the cell soma and peripheral axonal fibers of corneal neurons, suggesting that they are functionally heterogeneous. Until now, at least 17 different neuropeptides and neurotransmitters have been described in the corneal nerves (Dastjerdi and Dana, 2009). There are evidences that intact corneal nerve fibers exert trophic influences on the corneal epithelium and neuroregulation is responsible for maintenance of the integrity and repair of the ocular surface (Donnenfeld et al., 2003).

The mechanism underlying corneal damage in patients with reduced corneal sensation and dry eye -for instance, following surgery - is thought to be related to reduced levels of neurotransmitters. Peptidergic transmitters in nerve fibers may be involved in neuroimmunomodulation of the cornea (Muller et al., 1996). Enhanced epithelial cell proliferation is strongly believed to be mediated by neurotransmitters and nerve growth factors released from corneal nerve endings (Cavanagh and Colley, 1989). For example, it has been reported that acetylcholine derived from the corneal sensory nerve endings, increases intracellular levels of cyclic guanosine monophosphate (cGMP), which is associated with epithelial mitosis in the cornea and therefore enhances epithelial cell growth (Cavanagh and Colley, 1989). Substance P is a neuropeptide present in corneal nerves and has been found to stimulate DNA synthesis and promote corneal epithelial cell growth; it may also play a role in corneal epithelial wound healing. Calcitonin gene related peptide (CGRP), which often colocalizes with substance P in most ocular nerve fibers, also plays important roles in epithelial renewal and wound repair (Dastjerdi and Dana, 2009; Muller et al., 2003).

3. Dry eye syndrome

In a restructured definition of dry eye and its classifications by the International Dry Eye Workshop, dry eye is defined as a disorder of the lacrimal functional unit (LFU), an integrated system comprising the lacrimal glands, ocular surface (cornea, conjunctiva, and meibomian glands) and lids, and the sensory and motor nerves that connect them (2007). Disease or damage to any component of the LFU (the afferent sensory nerves, the efferent autonomic and motor nerves, and the tear-secreting glands) can destabilize the tear film and lead to ocular surface condition that expresses itself as dry eye.

A vital portion of the LFU is the part played by sensory impulses, which arise from the ocular surface and this is thought to be the main area of possible damage in ophthalmic surgeries involving the cornea.

As discussed earlier, disruption of a sufficient sensory drive from the ocular surface is strongly believed to be associated with the occurrence of dry eye by two exclusive and functionally diverse mechanisms: by decreasing reflex-induced lacrimal secretion (tear deficient dry eye) and by reducing the blink rate and, consequently, increasing evaporative loss (evaporative dry eye) (Bron, 1997; Lemp, 1995).

Corneal nerve alterations, either as a primary reason for tear hyposecretion or just the outcome of dryness of the ocular surface, have crucial effects on the integrated system of the LCU and can compromise various aspects of it, such as blinking, the tear reflex, and trophism of the epithelial cells, thus neatly contributing to the increase of the vicious circle of hypo-tearing leading to inflammation causing cell/nerve damage (Dastjerdi and Dana, 2009).

Different risk factors for dry eye have been identified, including increasing age, various systemic diseases (including diabetes, arthritis, allergy, and so), systemic medications, hormonal changes (menopause), neural alterations, ocular conditions (glaucoma, pterygium, meibomian gland dysfunction, lacrimal duct obstruction, contact lens wear) or environmental influences (climate, cigarette smoking) and many others (Manaviat et al., 2008; Moss et al., 2000; Ousler et al., 2005; Stern et al., 1998; Wolfe and Michaud, 2008).

Most dry-eye symptoms result from an abnormal, nonlubricative ocular surface that increases shear forces under the eyelids and diminishes the ability of the ocular surface to respond to environmental challenges. Dry eye manifestations could be described as visual fatigue, secretion, foreign body sensation, eyelids heaviness, dryness, uncomfortable eyes, pain, tears, blurred vision, itchiness, photophobia, and eye redness.

3.1 Dry eye diagnosis

Dry eye signs tend to agree poorly with patient-reported symptoms (Hay et al., 1998; McCarty et al., 1998; Moss et al., 2000; Schein et al., 1997b; Shimmura et al., 1999). As alleviation of dry eye symptoms is of primary importance in dry eye treatment, identification of dry eye symptoms can be regarded as important as objective dry eye tests are (Bandeen-Roche et al., 1997; Lemp, 1995; Nichols et al., 2000). More recently, the impact of dry eye on quality of life parameters has been suggested as a more valuable tool for assessing the burden of disease as well as response to treatment (Friedman, 2010).

Currently, the majority of clinicians probe into the patient's symptomatology regularly and the clinical tests most routinely used to evaluate severity of dry eye are tear break up time and corneal staining (Smith et al., 2008).

Finally, it is important to remember that diurnal variation is known to occur in symptomatology and clinical signs, and to affect the visual function capabilities of dry eye patients (Abelson et al., 2009; Walker et al., 2010).

3.1.1 Ocular Surface Disease Index (OSDI)

The Ocular Surface Disease Index (OSDI) was developed by the Outcomes Research Group (OSDI®, Allergan, Inc., Irvine, CA, USA) and consists of a 12-item questionnaire designed to provide a rapid assessment of the symptoms of ocular irritation consistent with dry eye disease and their impact on vision-related functioning. The questions are subscaled in three major categories: vision-related function, ocular symptoms, and environmental triggers. The total score of the OSDI ranges from zero to 100, where the higher scores represent a greater disability (Li et al., 2007; Vroman et al., 2005).

3.1.2 Tear Break-up Time (TBUT)

A commercially available fluorescein-impregnated strip wet with non-preserved saline is used in this test and placed in the inferior fornix. Alternatively, sodium fluorescein can be instilled; however, the first method seems to disturb the natural condition of the ocular surface less. The patient is then asked to blink 3 times, and then to look straight ahead without any blink. The tear film is observed using a cobalt blue filter under wide beam illumination at the slit-lamp. The interval between the last blink and the appearance of the first randomly appeared corneal dry spot is measured as TBUT. A value less than 10 seconds is regarded as abnormal (Gharaee et al., 2009; Liu et al., 2008).

Patients with a tear break up time of less than 10 seconds before surgery have been shown to be at significant risk of experiencing tear film instability following phacoemulsification (Liu et al., 2002).
However, there are some concerns that fluorescein itself can reduce the break up time of tear film (Taylor, 1980).

3.1.3 Schirmer's 1 test (S1T)

The test is performed under natural lighting conditions without topical anesthesia. One of several types of commercially available filter paper, standardized for the Schirmer's test, is placed in the lower fornix, over the junction of the middle and lateral thirds of the lower eyelid, and left in place for 5 minutes while the eyes are closed. The distance moistened is directly read off the scale on the paper itself. A reading of less than 10 mm is considered abnormal (Cho and Kim, 2009; Gharaee et al., 2009; Liu et al., 2008). Noticeably, it has been suggested that in patients who are candidates for LASIK surgery, those with S1T less than 20 mm/ 5 min may be more likely to develop chronic dry eye after surgery (Konomi et al., 2008). However, there may be many differences between the incision of LASIK and that of cataract surgery with respect to incision width, depth, and location (Cho and Kim, 2009).

3.1.4 Tear Meniscus Height (TMH)

This value is evaluated by measuring the height of the lacrimal river (tear film meniscus) and reading the scale on slit lamp microscopy without fluorescein. In dry eye patients, the lacrimal river may disappear.

3.1.5 Corneal staining

The cornea fluorescein staining is evaluated by using fluorescein test paper to contact the lower fornix of the eye. After 3 blinks, the subjects are asked to look straight ahead without any blink. The cornea is assessed under the wide beam cobalt blue light of the biomicroscope. Staining in any part of the cornea is considered abnormal. There are various classification schemes for grading the severity of staining.

3.1.6 Ocular surface stress test

Hardten introduced the "ocular surface stress test" as a tool to detect patients most at risk of developing initial or worsening manifestations of dry eye following phacoemulsification. In this test, ophthalmic examinations are performed in the usual manner and after instillation of dilating and anesthetic eye drops, the patient is instructed to sit in the waiting room for 30 - 60 minutes. The patient is then re-examined and the presence of epithelial irregularity or punctate keratopathy after fluorescein staining is regarded as an alarming sign of an ocular surface problem (Hardten, 2008).

3.1.7 Ocular Protection Index (OPI)

The OPI is a binomial parameter incorporating TBUT and blink rate to decipher the level of ocular surface protection provided by the tear film between blinks. The OPI is calculated by dividing TBUT (in seconds) by inter-blink interval (or number of seconds between blinks) (Ousler, III et al., 2008).

4. Dry eye in cataract patients

Multiple studies have demonstrated somewhat less favorable outcomes of cataract surgery in patients with dry eye, especially in those with associated connective tissue disorders (Adenis et al., 1996; Cohen, 1982; Gharaee et al., 2009; Golubovic and Parunovic, 1987; Hirsch, 2003; Insler et al., 1985; Krachmer and Laibson, 1974; Mehra and Elaraoud, 1992; Pfister and Murphy, 1980; Radtke et al., 1978; Ram et al., 2002; Ram et al., 1998; Zabel et al., 1989). In addition, there are several studies, investigating dry eye in healthy patients undergoing cataract surgery and there are evidences that dry eye manifestations such as red eye, foreign body sensation and fatigue will inevitably emerge in most patients after cataract surgery (Cho and Kim, 2009; Gharaee et al., 2009; Li et al., 2007).

Various complications including punctuate epithelial erosions, persistent or recurrent epithelial defects, filamentary keratitis, secondary infections, corneal ulceration, and keratolysis have been reported after cataract surgery in patients with dry eye. Patients with Sjögren's syndrome are predisposed to complications such as suture abscesses, infectious keratitis, peripheral keratolysis, filamentary keratitis, and endophthalmitis following conventional extracapsular cataract extraction (Cohen, 1982; Insler et al., 1985; Jones and Maguire, 1992; Krachmer and Laibson, 1974; Mehra and Elaraoud, 1992; Ormerod et al., 1988; Pfister and Murphy, 1980; Radtke et al., 1978; Ram et al., 2002; Ram et al., 1998). In addition, dry eyes are more susceptible to infection especially with Staphylococci and Streptococci (Dohlman et al., 1970; Jain et al., 1983; Ram et al., 1998; Scott et al., 1996). This could be due to decreased quantities of various protective enzymes such as lysozymes, lactoferrins, beta-lysins, and immunoglobulins in the tear film. (Dohlman et al., 1970; Holly and Lemp, 1977; Scott et al., 1996; Seal et al., 1986).

Various factors play a role in outcomes in the patients with or without dry eye that have surgery. Most important is postoperative corneal desensitization (Lyne, 1982). Conventional extracapsular cataract extraction requires an incision that involves at least 4 to 5 clock hours of the limbus, denervating the superior half of the cornea. Lyne reported that the loss of corneal sensitivity after cataract surgery often persists for more than 2 years and can be permanent (Lyne, 1982). Corneal sensitivity impairment after ocular surface surgery is dependent on the extent of the corneal incision (Lyne, 1982). As mentioned earlier, the sensory denervation interferes with the normal physiology of the corneal epithelium and decreases epithelial cell mitosis, delaying wound healing.

In addition, topical anesthesia and eye drops containing preservatives like benzalkonium chloride are well known to have effects on the corneal epithelium (Walker, 2004). Exposure to light from the operating microscope might also be associated with postoperative dry eye (Cho and Kim, 2009). Furthermore, the use of ultrasound in cataract surgery may damage corneal structures such as the epithelium, stroma, keratocyte, endothelium, and nerve plexuses (Mencucci et al., 2005).

Ocular surface complications are much rarer following small incision phacoemulsification. Phacoemulsification has several advantages compared with extracapsular cataract extraction in patients with dry eye , including a much smaller incision with less corneal denervation, minimal tear-film surfacing problems (Khanal et al., 2008), and absence of sutures and so, smaller risk of infections (Ram et al., 2002). In addition, the shorter duration of phacoemulsification is accompanied by shorter microscope light exposure and the faster visual rehabilitation permits rapid tapering of topical medications.

In a study on dry eye following cataract surgery, my colleagues and I focused on tear film changes after phacoemulsification and the effect of clear corneal incision location on tear film (Gharaee et al., 2009). We enrolled 68 eyes of 68 patients without preoperative dry eye and with senile cataract requiring phacoemulsification in a prospective, cohort study. Basic Tear Secretion Test (BTST), Tear Meniscus Height (TMH) measurement, Tear Break Up Time Test (TBUT) and Schirmer's 1 Test (S1T) were performed in all participants before and three months after surgery. Preoperative keratometry was used to determine the steepest meridian and corresponding location of the clear corneal incision. The cohort included 46 men (67.6%) and 22 women (32.3%), with an age range of 48 to 82 years (mean, 66.9±9.4 years). Phacoemulsification was performed with a temporal clear corneal incision in 36 eyes (52.9%) and with a superotemporal clear corneal incision in 32 eyes (47.1%). All incisions were made using a 3.2mm, single-use surgical knife (MSL 32, Mani Ophthalmic Knife, Japan) and left un-sutured at the conclusion of surgery. Topical chloramphenicol and betamethasone eye drops were administered on a tapering dose for one month postoperatively. There was no statistically significant difference between the results of pre- and post- operative S1T, TMH and BTST. These latter tests were not statistically different between incisions at different locations. However, TBUT results differed significantly in pre- and post-operative examination in both incision location groups ($P<0.001$) - though there was no statistically significant difference in TBUT results comparing incision locations (Gharaee et al., 2009). We had speculated that cutting more sensory nerves on the rich temporal meridians would have more effect on the tear film properties. However, this hypothesis was not confirmed in our study and this is in accordance with the newer description of the corneal nerve distribution described in this chapter (Muller et al, 1996; Ueda et al, 1989). Interestingly, Vroman and colleagues investigated the effect of hinge location on corneal sensation and dry eye after LASIK in a cohort of 47 myopic patients. In their series patient with a nasal hinge had significantly better corneal sensation than those with a superior hinge; however, dry eye occurred with the same frequency in both groups (Vroman et al., 2005).

Cho and associates investigated the effect of incision location and shape on postoperative dry eye in patients undergoing phacoemulsification. Their results suggested that incision location has no effect on dry eye signs in either patients with or without preoperative dry eye; however, with regard to incision shape, a grooved incision was associated with more dry eye signs than single plane incisions in those patients without preoperative dry eye. In addition, there was significant correlation between microscopic light exposure time and dry eye test values. Moreover, corneal suture removal was associated with aggravation of dry eye symptoms in patients with preoperative dry eye (Cho and Kim, 2009).

Khanal and associates investigated post-phacoemulsification changes in corneal sensitivity and tear physiology in a longitudinal, randomized trial on 18 patients (Khanal et al., 2008). They found that deterioration in corneal sensitivity and tear physiology is seen immediately after phacoemulsification. Despite a trend toward full-recovery, corneal sensitivity does not return to preoperative levels until 3 months postoperatively, whereas the tear functions recover within 1 month. In addition, postoperative treatment with tear lubricant was not found to have any effect on the improvement of tear physiology and corneal sensitivity post-surgically. In our study, we evaluated tear film properties 3 months after surgery and similarly we did not found statistically significant changes in tear tests (Gharaee et al., 2009).

In another study, Ram and associates evaluated the outcome of phacoemulsification in 23 patients with dry eye (Ram et al., 2002). Although all patients with dry eye reported more

discomfort and irritation for 3 to 4 weeks following cataract surgery compared to preoperatively, and a minimal detrimental effect on Schirmer's and TBUT tests was also found, they concluded that phacoemulsification was safe and led to minimal complications in patients with age-related dry eye with or without associated systemic disorders.
It is estimated that up to 20% of all cataract surgeries are performed on diabetic patients (Liu et al., 2008) and nearly half of diabetic patients had dry eye in some reports (Manaviat et al., 2008). Liu and coworkers compared 25 diabetic cataract patients with 20 age-matched non-diabetic cataract patients (Liu et al., 2008). They found that tear secretion was reduced in diabetic cataract patients after phacoemulsification, which worsened dry eye symptoms and predisposed those patients to ocular damage. However, in non-diabetics there was no significant, persistent change in tear film. As we found in our study, they also observed a transient increase in S1T in the early postoperative period, which returned to preoperative levels in 180 days.
Li and colleagues investigated pathogenic factors responsible for dry eye in patients after cataract surgery (Li et al., 2007). In their study impression cytology demonstrated that, even 3 months following cataract surgery, goblet cells were reduced in the bulbar conjunctiva along with changes of squamous metaplasia, and this was most marked in the regions covered by the lower lid; these findings suggest that dry eye might be induced by eye drops (Li et al., 2007).The authors stated that dry eye could develop or deteriorate dramatically after cataract surgery if not treated timely and this could happen as early as one week postoperatively and peaks at about one month. Furthermore, misuse of eye drops is one of the major pathogenic factors that causes dry eye after cataract surgery. Other authors had similar findings previously (Lyne, 1982; Zabel et al., 1989); however, the role of eye drops in postoperative dry eye has not been confirmed in all studies (Khanal et al., 2008; Ram et al., 2002).

5. Treatment

Due to the many different causes and pathophysiologies, dry eye treatment continues to present a substantial challenge to the clinician. Dry eye aggravation following cataract surgery, especially with modern microincision phacoemulsification techniques, seems to be self-limited. In patients with preoperative dry eye, augmentation of dry eye treatment may be necessary; however, in those with normal tear status prior to surgery, temporary measures may be adequate. Over-the-counter ocular lubricants remain the mainstay of treatment, and a formulation of cyclosporine A is the only Food and Drug Administration (FDA)-approved ophthalmic solution for dry eye, but its indication is limited to patients who experience inflammation associated with dry eye. Punctal plugs and dissolving inserts placed in the subconjunctival sacs are other treatment options. Nutritional influences on dry eye are well-known and omega-3 and omega-6 fatty acid intake could have beneficial effects on dry eye.

6. Conclusion

Dry eye manifestations appear or are aggravated following cataract surgery in most patients. Before surgery, patients should be informed about the presence of dry eye manifestations and the possible increase in dry eye symptoms. This would decrease the likelihood that patients will blame the cataract surgery per se for "tired eyes" or "fluctuation of vision," which are often signs of ocular surface disease. Increasing awareness helps the patient separate those dry eye symptoms from those of the surgery and makes postoperative care and counseling easier for the staff and physician (Hardten, 2008).

Intraoperative exposure to the operating microscope light should be minimized. The clinician should also be cognizant of the fact that grooved incisions, despite their advantages in other respects, can aggravate dry eye symptoms and signs in eyes that were healthy preoperatively (Cho and Kim, 2009). In addition, it is advised that eye drops should be carefully administered before and after cataract surgery to avoid or reduce the occurrence of dry eye postoperatively.

The use of artificial tears was found not to facilitate recovery of tear physiology following phacoemulsification in all studies. Nevertheless, based on the findings of some studies (Foulks, 2003; Tomlinson et al., 1998; Yazdani et al., 2001), it may still be advisable for patients experiencing postoperative dry eye symptoms to use artificial tears to alleviate the symptoms. In patients with postoperative dry eye, timely effective treatment such as with artificial tears or lacrimal plugs is necessary (Li et al., 2007).

Future research should focus on realistic modifications to the phacoemulsification procedure to achieve a safer approach in patients with ocular surface problems.

7. References

2007, The definition and classification of dry eye disease: report of the Definition and Classification Subcommittee of the International Dry Eye WorkShop (2007): Ocul.Surf., v. 5, no. 2, p. 75-92.

Abelson, M. B., G. W. Ousler, III, and C. Maffei, 2009, Dry eye in 2008: Curr. Opin. Ophthalmol., v. 20, no. 4, p. 282-286.

Adenis, J. P., J. A. Bernard, A. Ducasse, B. Fayet, and J. L. George, 1996, [Dry syndrome and cataract surgery. A case]: J Fr.Ophtalmol., v. 19, no. 3, p. 222-224.

Agarwal, A., and D. A. Kumar, 2010, Cost-effectiveness of cataract surgery: Curr. Opin. Ophthalmol..

Bandeen-Roche, K., B. Munoz, J. M. Tielsch, S. K. West, and O. D. Schein, 1997, Self-reported assessment of dry eye in a population-based setting: Invest Ophthalmol.Vis.Sci., v. 38, no. 12, p. 2469-2475.

Barton, K., D. C. Monroy, A. Nava, and S. C. Pflugfelder, 1997, Inflammatory cytokines in the tears of patients with ocular rosacea: Ophthalmology, v. 104, no. 11, p. 1868-1874.

Benitez del Castillo, J. M., M. A. Wasfy, C. Fernandez, and J. Garcia-Sanchez, 2004, An in vivo confocal masked study on corneal epithelium and subbasal nerves in patients with dry eye: Invest Ophthalmol.Vis.Sci., v. 45, no. 9, p. 3030-3035.

Brewitt, H., and F. Sistani, 2001, Dry eye disease: the scale of the problem: Surv. Ophthalmol., v. 45 Suppl 2, p. S199-S202.

Bron, A. J., 1997, The Doyne Lecture. Reflections on the tears: Eye (Lond), v. 11 (Pt 5), p. 583-602.

Butovich, I. A., 2008, On the lipid composition of human meibum and tears: comparative analysis of nonpolar lipids: Invest Ophthalmol.Vis.Sci., v. 49, no. 9, p. 3779-3789.

Cavanagh, H. D., and A. M. Colley, 1989, The molecular basis of neurotrophic keratitis: Acta Ophthalmol.Suppl, v. 192, p. 115-134.

Cho, Y. K., and M. S. Kim, 2009, Dry eye after cataract surgery and associated intraoperative risk factors: Korean J.Ophthalmol., v. 23, no. 2, p. 65-73.

Cohen, K. L., 1982, Sterile corneal perforation after cataract surgery in Sjogren's syndrome: Br.J.Ophthalmol., v. 66, no. 3, p. 179-182.

Collins, M., R. Seeto, L. Campbell, and M. Ross, 1989, Blinking and corneal sensitivity: Acta Ophthalmol.(Copenh), v. 67, no. 5, p. 525-531.

Dartt, D. A., 2004, Dysfunctional neural regulation of lacrimal gland secretion and its role in the pathogenesis of dry eye syndromes: Ocul.Surf., v. 2, no. 2, p. 76-91.

Dastjerdi, M. H., and R. Dana, 2009, Corneal nerve alterations in dry eye-associated ocular surface disease: Int.Ophthalmol.Clin., v. 49, no. 1, p. 11-20.

Dohlman, C. H., M. A. Lemp, and F. P. English, 1970, Dry eye syndromes: Int. Ophthalmol. Clin., v. 10, no. 2, p. 215-251.

Donnenfeld, E. D., K. Solomon, H. D. Perry, S. J. Doshi, M. Ehrenhaus, R. Solomon, and S. Biser, 2003, The effect of hinge position on corneal sensation and dry eye after LASIK: Ophthalmology, v. 110, no. 5, p. 1023-1029.

Erdelyi, B., R. Kraak, A. Zhivov, R. Guthoff, and J. Nemeth, 2007, In vivo confocal laser scanning microscopy of the cornea in dry eye: Graefes Arch.Clin.Exp.Ophthalmol., v. 245, no. 1, p. 39-44.

Ernest, P., R. Tipperman, R. Eagle, C. Kardasis, K. Lavery, A. Sensoli, and M. Rhem, 1998, Is there a difference in incision healing based on location?: J.Cataract Refract.Surg., v. 24, no. 4, p. 482-486.

Foulks, G. N., 2003, The evolving treatment of dry eye: Ophthalmol.Clin.North Am., v. 16, no. 1, p. 29-35.

Frick, K. D., and A. Foster, 2003, The magnitude and cost of global blindness: an increasing problem that can be alleviated: Am.J Ophthalmol., v. 135, no. 4, p. 471-476.

Friedman, N. J., 2010, Impact of dry eye disease and treatment on quality of life: Curr.Opin.Ophthalmol., v. 21, no. 4, p. 310-316.

Gharaee, H., M. N. Mousavi, R. Daneshvar, M. Hosseini, and S. Sazande, 2009, Effect of Clear Corneal Incision Location on Tear Film following Phacoemulsification Surgery : Iranian Journal of Ophthalmology, v. 21, no. 3, p. 29-34.

Golubovic, S., and A. Parunovic, 1987, Corneal perforation in dry eye patients: Fortschr.Ophthalmol., v. 84, no. 1, p. 33-37.

Hardten, D. R., 2008, Dry eye disease in patients after cataract surgery: Cornea, v. 27, no. 7, p. 855.

Hay, E. M., E. Thomas, B. Pal, A. Hajeer, H. Chambers, and A. J. Silman, 1998, Weak association between subjective symptoms or and objective testing for dry eyes and dry mouth: results from a population based study: Ann.Rheum.Dis., v. 57, no. 1, p. 20-24.

Hirsch, J. D., 2003, Considerations in the pharmacoeconomics of dry eye: Manag.Care, v. 12, no. 12 Suppl, p. 33-38.

Hoffman, R. S., I. H. Fine, and M. Packer, 2005, New phacoemulsification technology: Curr.Opin.Ophthalmol., v. 16, no. 1, p. 38-43.

Holly, F. J., and M. A. Lemp, 1977, Tear physiology and dry eyes: Surv.Ophthalmol., v. 22, no. 2, p. 69-87.

Hosal, B. M., N. Ornek, G. Zilelioglu, and A. H. Elhan, 2005, Morphology of corneal nerves and corneal sensation in dry eye: a preliminary study: Eye (Lond), v. 19, no. 12, p. 1276-1279.

Insler, M. S., G. Boutros, and D. W. Boulware, 1985, Corneal ulceration following cataract surgery in patients with rheumatoid arthritis: J.Am.Intraocul.Implant.Soc., v. 11, no. 6, p. 594-597.

Jain, I. S., A. Gupta, J. Ram, and Dhir SP., 1983, Mima polymorpha: a dangerous opportunist in ocular infections.: J OcularTher Surg, v. 2, p. 143-145.

Jones, R. R., and L. J. Maguire, 1992, Corneal complications after cataract surgery in patients with rheumatoid arthritis: Cornea, v. 11, no. 2, p. 148-150.

Khanal, S., A. Tomlinson, L. Esakowitz, P. Bhatt, D. Jones, S. Nabili, and S. Mukerji, 2008, Changes in corneal sensitivity and tear physiology after phacoemulsification: Ophthalmic Physiol Opt., v. 28, no. 2, p. 127-134.

Kim, J., and G. N. Foulks, 1999, Evaluation of the effect of lissamine green and rose bengal on human corneal epithelial cells: Cornea, v. 18, no. 3, p. 328-332.

Kohlhaas, M., 1998, Corneal sensation after cataract and refractive surgery: J Cataract Refract.Surg, v. 24, no. 10, p. 1399-1409.

Konomi, K., L. L. Chen, R. S. Tarko, A. Scally, D. A. Schaumberg, D. Azar, and D. A. Dartt, 2008, Preoperative characteristics and a potential mechanism of chronic dry eye after LASIK: Invest Ophthalmol.Vis.Sci., v. 49, no. 1, p. 168-174.

Krachmer, J. H., and P. R. Laibson, 1974, Corneal thinning and perforation in Sjogren's syndrome: Am.J.Ophthalmol., v. 78, no. 6, p. 917-920.

Lamoureux, E. L., E. Fenwick, K. Pesudovs, and D. Tan, 2010, The impact of cataract surgery on quality of life: Curr.Opin.Ophthalmol..

Lansingh, V. C., M. J. Carter, and M. Martens, 2007, Global cost-effectiveness of cataract surgery: Ophthalmology, v. 114, no. 9, p. 1670-1678.

Lawrenson, J. G., 1997, Corneal sensitivity in health and disease: Ophthalmic Physiol Opt., v. 17 Suppl 1, p. S17-S22.

Lee, A. J., J. Lee, S. M. Saw, G. Gazzard, D. Koh, D. Widjaja, and D. T. Tan, 2002, Prevalence and risk factors associated with dry eye symptoms: a population based study in Indonesia: Br.J.Ophthalmol., v. 86, no. 12, p. 1347-1351.

Lee, K. W., and C. K. Joo, 2003, Clinical results of laser in situ keratomileusis with superior and nasal hinges: J Cataract Refract.Surg, v. 29, no. 3, p. 457-461.

Lemp, M. A., 1995, Report of the National Eye Institute/Industry workshop on Clinical Trials in Dry Eyes: CLAO J, v. 21, no. 4, p. 221-232.

Li, X. M., L. Hu, J. Hu, and W. Wang, 2007, Investigation of dry eye disease and analysis of the pathogenic factors in patients after cataract surgery: Cornea, v. 26, no. 9 Suppl 1, p. S16-S20.

Liu, X., Y. S. Gu, and Y. S. Xu, 2008, Changes of tear film and tear secretion after phacoemulsification in diabetic patients: J.Zhejiang.Univ Sci.B, v. 9, no. 4, p. 324-328.

Liu, Z. et al., 2002, [Tear film changes after phacoemulsification]: Zhonghua Yan.Ke.Za Zhi., v. 38, no. 5, p. 274-277.

Lyne, A., 1982, Corneal sensitivity after surgery: Trans.Ophthalmol.Soc.U.K., v. 102 (pt 2), p. 302-305.

Manaviat, M. R., M. Rashidi, M. Afkhami-Ardekani, and M. R. Shoja, 2008, Prevalence of dry eye syndrome and diabetic retinopathy in type 2 diabetic patients: BMC.Ophthalmol., v. 8, p. 10.

Mathers, W. D., 2000, Why the eye becomes dry: a cornea and lacrimal gland feedback model: CLAO J., v. 26, no. 3, p. 159-165.

McCarty, C. A., A. K. Bansal, P. M. Livingston, Y. L. Stanislavsky, and H. R. Taylor, 1998, The epidemiology of dry eye in Melbourne, Australia: Ophthalmology, v. 105, no. 6, p. 1114-1119.

McDonnell, P. J., M. Taban, M. Sarayba, B. Rao, J. Zhang, R. Schiffman, and Z. Chen, 2003, Dynamic morphology of clear corneal cataract incisions: Ophthalmology, v. 110, no. 12, p. 2342-2348.

Mehra, K. S., and M. S. Elaraoud, 1992, Total central keratolysis: Ann.Ophthalmol., v. 24, no. 2, p. 54-55.

Mencucci, R., S. Ambrosini, C. Ponchietti, M. Marini, G. B. Vannelli, and U. Menchini, 2005, Ultrasound thermal damage to rabbit corneas after simulated phacoemulsification: J Cataract Refract.Surg, v. 31, no. 11, p. 2180-2186.

Moss, S. E., R. Klein, and B. E. Klein, 2000, Prevalence of and risk factors for dry eye syndrome: Arch.Ophthalmol., v. 118, no. 9, p. 1264-1268.

Muller, L. J., C. F. Marfurt, F. Kruse, and T. M. Tervo, 2003, Corneal nerves: structure, contents and function: Exp.Eye Res., v. 76, no. 5, p. 521-542. Erratum in: Exp Eye Res. 2003 Aug; 77(2):253

Muller, L. J., L. Pels, and G. F. Vrensen, 1996, Ultrastructural organization of human corneal nerves: Invest Ophthalmol.Vis.Sci., v. 37, no. 4, p. 476-488.

Muller, L. J., G. F. Vrensen, L. Pels, B. N. Cardozo, and B. Willekens, 1997, Architecture of human corneal nerves: Invest Ophthalmol.Vis.Sci., v. 38, no. 5, p. 985-994.

Nakamori, K., M. Odawara, T. Nakajima, T. Mizutani, and K. Tsubota, 1997, Blinking is controlled primarily by ocular surface conditions: Am.J.Ophthalmol., v. 124, no. 1, p. 24-30.

Nichols, K. K., J. J. Nichols, and K. Zadnik, 2000, Frequency of dry eye diagnostic test procedures used in various modes of ophthalmic practice: Cornea, v. 19, no. 4, p. 477-482.

Ormerod, L. D., L. P. Fong, and C. S. Foster, 1988, Corneal infection in mucosal scarring disorders and Sjogren's syndrome: Am.J Ophthalmol., v. 105, no. 5, p. 512-518.

Ousler, G. W., P. J. Gomes, D. Welch, and M. B. Abelson, 2005, Methodologies for the study of ocular surface disease: Ocul.Surf., v. 3, no. 3, p. 143-154.

Ousler, G. W., III, K. W. Hagberg, M. Schindelar, D. Welch, and M. B. Abelson, 2008, The Ocular Protection Index: Cornea, v. 27, no. 5, p. 509-513.

Pfister, R. R., and G. E. Murphy, 1980, Corneal ulceration and perforation associated with Sjogren's syndrome: Arch.Ophthalmol., v. 98, no. 1, p. 89-94.

Prause, J. U., and M. Norn, 1987, Relation between blink frequency and break-up time?: Acta Ophthalmol.(Copenh), v. 65, no. 1, p. 19-22.

Radtke, N., S. Meyers, and H. E. Kaufman, 1978, Sterile corneal ulcers after cataract surgery in keratoconjunctivitis sicca: Arch.Ophthalmol., v. 96, no. 1, p. 51-52.

Ram, J., A. Gupta, G. Brar, S. Kaushik, and A. Gupta, 2002, Outcomes of phacoemulsification in patients with dry eye: J.Cataract Refract.Surg., v. 28, no. 8, p. 1386-1389.

Ram, J., A. Sharma, S. S. Pandav, A. Gupta, and P. Bambery, 1998, Cataract surgery in patients with dry eyes: J.Cataract Refract.Surg., v. 24, no. 8, p. 1119-1124.

Resnikoff, S., D. Pascolini, D. Etya'ale, I. Kocur, R. Pararajasegaram, G. P. Pokharel, and S. P. Mariotti, 2004, Global data on visual impairment in the year 2002: Bull.World Health Organ, v. 82, no. 11, p. 844-851.

Roberts, C. W., and E. R. Elie, 2007, Dry eye symptoms following cataract surgery: Insight., v. 32, no. 1, p. 14-21.

Roszkowska, A. M., P. Colosi, F. M. Ferreri, and S. Galasso, 2004, Age-related modifications of corneal sensitivity: Ophthalmologica, v. 218, no. 5, p. 350-355.

Schein, O. D., B. Munoz, J. M. Tielsch, K. Bandeen-Roche, and S. West, 1997a, Prevalence of dry eye among the elderly: Am.J Ophthalmol., v. 124, no. 6, p. 723-728.

Schein, O. D., J. M. Tielsch, B. Munoz, K. Bandeen-Roche, and S. West, 1997b, Relation between signs and symptoms of dry eye in the elderly. A population-based perspective: Ophthalmology, v. 104, no. 9, p. 1395-1401.

Scott, I. U., H. W. Flynn, Jr., W. Feuer, S. C. Pflugfelder, E. C. Alfonso, R. K. Forster, and D. Miller, 1996, Endophthalmitis associated with microbial keratitis: Ophthalmology, v. 103, no. 11, p. 1864-1870.

Seal, D. V., J. I. McGill, I. A. Mackie, G. M. Liakos, P. Jacobs, and N. J. Goulding, 1986, Bacteriology and tear protein profiles of the dry eye: Br.J Ophthalmol., v. 70, no. 2, p. 122-125.

Shimmura, S., J. Shimazaki, and K. Tsubota, 1999, Results of a population-based questionnaire on the symptoms and lifestyles associated with dry eye: Cornea, v. 18, no. 4, p. 408-411.

Smith, J., K. K. Nichols, and E. K. Baldwin, 2008, Current patterns in the use of diagnostic tests in dry eye evaluation: Cornea, v. 27, no. 6, p. 656-662.

Solomon, A., D. Dursun, Z. Liu, Y. Xie, A. Macri, and S. C. Pflugfelder, 2001, Pro- and anti-inflammatory forms of interleukin-1 in the tear fluid and conjunctiva of patients with dry-eye disease: Invest Ophthalmol.Vis.Sci., v. 42, no. 10, p. 2283-2292.

Stern, M. E., R. W. Beuerman, R. I. Fox, J. Gao, A. K. Mircheff, and S. C. Pflugfelder, 1998, The pathology of dry eye: the interaction between the ocular surface and lacrimal glands: Cornea, v. 17, no. 6, p. 584-589.

Taylor, H. R., 1980, Studies on the tear film in climatic droplet keratopathy and pterygium: Arch.Ophthalmol., v. 98, no. 1, p. 86-88.

Tomlinson, A., J. P. Craig, and G. E. Lowther, 1998, The biophysical role in tear regulation: Adv.Exp.Med.Biol., v. 438, p. 371-380.

Tuominen, I. S., Y. T. Konttinen, M. H. Vesaluoma, J. A. Moilanen, M. Helinto, and T. M. Tervo, 2003, Corneal innervation and morphology in primary Sjogren's syndrome: Invest Ophthalmol.Vis.Sci., v. 44, no. 6, p. 2545-2549.

Ueda, S., C. M. del, J. A. LoCascio, and J. V. Aquavella, 1989, Peptidergic and catecholaminergic fibers in the human corneal epithelium. An immunohistochemical and electron microscopic study: Acta Ophthalmol.Suppl, v. 192, p. 80-90.

Villani, E., D. Galimberti, F. Viola, C. Mapelli, and R. Ratiglia, 2007, The cornea in Sjogren's syndrome: an in vivo confocal study: Invest Ophthalmol.Vis.Sci., v. 48, no. 5, p. 2017-2022.

Vroman, D. T., H. P. Sandoval, L. E. Fernandez de Castro, T. J. Kasper, M. P. Holzer, and K. D. Solomon, 2005, Effect of hinge location on corneal sensation and dry eye after laser in situ keratomileusis for myopia: J.Cataract Refract.Surg., v. 31, no. 10, p. 1881-1887.

Walker, P. M., K. J. Lane, G. W. Ousler, III, and M. B. Abelson, 2010, Diurnal variation of visual function and the signs and symptoms of dry eye: Cornea, v. 29, no. 6, p. 607-612.

Walker, T. D., 2004, Benzalkonium toxicity: Clin.Experiment.Ophthalmol., v. 32, no. 6, p. 657.

Wolfe, F., and K. Michaud, 2008, Prevalence, risk, and risk factors for oral and ocular dryness with particular emphasis on rheumatoid arthritis: J Rheumatol., v. 35, no. 6, p. 1023-1030.

Wolkoff, P., J. K. Nojgaard, C. Franck, and P. Skov, 2006, The modern office environment desiccates the eyes?: Indoor.Air, v. 16, no. 4, p. 258-265.

Wolkoff, P., J. K. Nojgaard, P. Troiano, and B. Piccoli, 2005, Eye complaints in the office environment: precorneal tear film integrity influenced by eye blinking efficiency: Occup.Environ.Med., v. 62, no. 1, p. 4-12.

Xu, K. P., Y. Yagi, and K. Tsubota, 1996, Decrease in corneal sensitivity and change in tear function in dry eye: Cornea, v. 15, no. 3, p. 235-239.

Yazdani, C., T. McLaughlin, J. E. Smeeding, and J. Walt, 2001, Prevalence of treated dry eye disease in a managed care population: Clin.Ther., v. 23, no. 10, p. 1672-1682.

Yoon, K. C., I. Y. Jeong, Y. G. Park, and S. Y. Yang, 2007, Interleukin-6 and tumor necrosis factor-alpha levels in tears of patients with dry eye syndrome: Cornea, v. 26, no. 4, p. 431-437.

Zabel, R. W., G. Mintsioulis, I. M. MacDonald, J. Valberg, and S. J. Tuft, 1989, Corneal toxic changes after cataract extraction: Can.J Ophthalmol., v. 24, no. 7, p. 311-316.

Zhang, M., J. Chen, L. Luo, Q. Xiao, M. Sun, and Z. Liu, 2005, Altered corneal nerves in aqueous tear deficiency viewed by in vivo confocal microscopy: Cornea, v. 24, no. 7, p. 818-824.

25

Cataract Surgery in People with a Severe Learning Disorder

Nel T. Tijmes
Bartimeus, Medical Department
The Netherlands

1. Introduction

In nature acquired blindness is a dangerous situation. Blind animals living in herds have difficulties associating with their group. For such animals it is often impossible to live alone. This can result in starvation and death. If intellectually competent humans are going blind they have the possibility to express to others what problems they face living in a society. They have difficulties in work and are, in many situations, dependent on other people. People with learning difficulties, especially the severely intellectually disabled are already care-dependent but they have additional difficulties expressing the problems associated with acquired blindness. Cataract is one of the leading causes of treatable blindness (Vision 2020, 2010). With an aging population the incidence of cataract is growing. Since life expectancy in severely intellectually disabled people has increased in western countries the incidence of cataract will also grow in this group (Bittles et al 2002, Bittles et al 2006).
The intellectually retarded represent a large group of individuals who require better eye and vision care than the general population but who do not always receive it, especially if the mental disability is severe (Bothe et al, 1991, Castane & Peris, 1993, Evenhuis & Nagtzaam, 1997, Goto et al 1995, Warburg, 2001, Van Isterdael et al 2006, Van Isterdael et al, 2008, Van Splunder et al 2004). The prevalence of cataract in intellectually retarded adults is higher than in the age-matched general population (Evenhuis, 1995, Klaver et al 1998, Limburg 2007,). Ophthalmological abnormalities are often found in intellectually retarded people. In the last 15 years much research has been done on this topic. Many studies describe the frequency and cause of eye diseases in this group. However follow-up in these studies is often limited or absent. Little research has been done on the implementation of recommendations for treatment e.g. cataract surgery (Sjoukes, 2008). In this chapter an overview of different published studies is provided. Research has been done into the frequency of cataract in this population and how often the operation takes place as well as the indications for cataract treatment. The particular challenges and results of cataract operations in the severely intellectually retarded are also examined as well as how this population differs from a conventional one. Also described is who is involved in the decision-making after diagnosis for treatment. Special attention is given to the procedure before, during and after the operation. The significance of quality of life measures and cost-effectiveness will be discussed. The outcome data from operations will be provided. Recommendations for diagnosis, treatment and postoperative monitoring are also made.

What is the prevalence of severe intellectual handicap? In the Netherlands in 2008, 60,000 people had a severe mental handicap (Woittiez & Ras, 2010). This was out of a total population for the Netherlands of 16,445,593 (Woittiez & Ras, 2010). This means that the prevalence of severe mental handicap in the Netherlands is 3 per thousand.
This varies from 5 per thousand in younger people to 1 per thousand in people of about 70 years of age. In the period 1998 till 2008 the prevalence increased. This was not due to a greater incidence per se but due to longer life expectancy. Comparison with data from other European countries is difficult because of different methods of registration in these countries. All these people are dependent on care. In younger age groups they sometimes live at home with their parents. As the population of the severe mentally handicapped is becoming older it is usually not possible for their parents to care for them

2. A retrospective study of 5205 intellectually handicapped people

This study focussed on an institutionalised population of 5205 people with an intellectual disability who were referred for visual assessment between 1993 and 2003. The author tried to determine the prevalence of treatable visual impairment and how many times advice for treatment was implemented (van Isterdael et al 2006, 2008).

2.1 Materials and methods

The records of 5205 consecutive people examined by the Visual Advisory Centre of Bartimeus, Zeist, The Netherlands, from 1 January to 31 December 2003, were retrospectively reviewed. Bartimeus is a Dutch institution providing education, care and services to the blind and those with partial sight. The Visual Advisory Centre was started in 1991 to identify the visual problems of people living in institutions with intellectual disability, to provide information and to explore the possibilities for treatment. The Visual Advisory Centre now works at 7 establishments in the Netherlands. The centre works with 15 employers in 119 institutions. In a year around 3000 people are examined.
All subjects were people with an intellectual disability living in institutions and were referred to the Visual Advisory Centre by doctors specialising in their care. Doctors were responsible for selecting those people who could benefit from the centre, for example those who were difficult to assess or had a reduced visual performance.
Trained optometrists and an ophthalmologist examined the participants ophthalmologically according to a standard protocol. Full assessment required 90 minutes. Referring doctors provided personal data, data on limitation of overall physical mobility and the cause of intellectual disability, and a general medical history. Optometrists tested visual performance by assessing visual acuity and visual fields. Visual acuity was assessed with two tests - the Teller or Cardiff tests. The results were expressed in Snellen equivalents. Visual fields were assessed using the confrontation method. Ophthalmic assessment by the ophthalmologist included anterior segment examination, fundoscopy and retinoscopy with mydriasis.
Degree of intellectual disability was defined according to the Diagnostic and Statistical Manual, 4th edition TR classification: mild, IQ 55-70, moderate, IQ 35-55, severe IQ 25-35 and profound IQ<25 (American Psychiatric association, 2000). Visual performance was defined according to the World Health Organization (WHO) criteria: normal vision, visual acuity >0.8 and visual field >50degrees equating with mild vision loss, visual acuity >0.3 and <0.8

and/or visual fields >10 degrees and <30 degrees equating with profound vision loss to near blindness, light perception to visual acuity <0.05 and/or visual fields 10 degrees or less to, blindness, and no light perception. Statistical analyses, demographic data, visual assessment data and causes of intellectual disability, visual disorders and co-morbidity were analysed using SPSS V.10.1 and Microsoft Excel V.2002

2.2 Results

The percentage of men was 52.7 %. The mean age was 38.5 years. The percentage of participants >50 years was 23.5 %. Severe or profound intellectual disability was found in 93% of subjects. Immobility was found in 28.4% of subjects. Moderate vision loss to blindness was present in 43.8%. A specific cause of intellectual disability was reported in 58.4%. Down's syndrome was the most frequent cause of intellectual disability.

The prevalence of cataract in this population and patterns of referral are shown in Table 1. An unoperated cataract with a significant effect on vision was found in 10% of subjects. A visually significant cataract that had not previously been diagnosed before was found in 399 patients. The Visual Advice Centre advised referral to an ophthalmic surgeon unless it was contraindicated for medical reasons. 98% had cataract in both eyes. 219 of 399 (55%) patients were referred to the ophthalmic surgeon of whom 26% had cataract surgery.

No consent for the operation was obtained from the relatives in 14% of cases. In 74% of the referred patients the ophthalmologist performed no cataract surgery. The reason for treatment or non-treatment was not clear. The results of the 119 operated patients (119 out of 119 eyes) were satisfactory. In 117 patients vision improved and there was a very good improvement in living skills and behaviour commensurate with this afterwards. One patient moved to an unknown address so was not followed up and one patient suffered a retinal detachment. Although he received retinal detachment surgery vision was not better than before cataract surgery. After the unexpected hospitalisation for the retinal surgery his behaviour was difficult.

Self-mutilation of the eyes was present in 5% of the study population. This an important observation, because self-mutilation is a high risk factor for severe ocular morbidity. On the other hand is it possible that severe ocular morbidity can result in self-mutilation.

A specific cause of intellectual disability could be established in 58% of people who were studied, compared with 41-88.6 % in the literature (Arvio & Sillanpaa, 2003, Beange & Taplin, 1996, Haugen et al, 1995, Van Splunder, 2006, Warburg, 2001). Down's syndrome was reported in 21% of people, which is consistent with the literature (13.1-29%) (Arvio & Sillanpaa 2003, Haugen et al 1995, Hou et al 1998,Warburg 2001).

The prevalence of cataract in this group is difficult to compare with other studies because in many studies the age of patients is not comparable. Severe or profound intellectual disability was present in 93% of the study population, compared with 55% in the total Dutch institutionalised population with intellectual disability. Combined figures for visual impairment and blindness in institutionalised people with intellectual disability reported in the literature vary between 18.7% and 37% compared with 44% in the study's population (Arvio & Silllanpaa 2003, Van Splunder 2006).

2.3 Challenges in ophthalmic examination and treatment

Most severely intellectually retarded people are diagnosed with an intellectual disability from childhood. These people are more prone to common risk factors for poor health related to diet, weight and physical inactivity as well as impaired vision and hearing, respiratory diseases and dental problems. Up to one third have an associated physical disability which puts them at risk of postural deformities, pulmonary infections, gastrointestinal problems and urinary incontinence (Cooper et al 2004). They are 20 times more likely to have epilepsy.

Determining factors for cataract operation*	No referral (n=180)		No surgery after referral (n=87)		Surgery after referral (n=57)	
Other ophthalmic problems						
corneal	46 (26%)		23 (26%)		17 (30%)	
retinal	61 (34%)		22 (25%)		14 (25%)	
nystagmus	49 (27%)		25 (29%)		16 (29%)	
opticus nerve atrofie	15 (8%)		4 (5%)		2 (4%)	
cerebral visual impairment	30 (17%)		11 (13%)		9 (16%)	
total	137 (76%)		59 (68%)		41 (72%)	
contra-indication						
bad medical condition	11 (6%)		7 (8%)		5 (9%)	
behaviourproblems	32 (18%)		16 (18%)		13 (23%)	
ophthalmological	45 (25%)		14 (16%)		10 (18%)	
total	78 (43%)		33 (38%)		19 (33%)	
Very strong intelectually handicap	68/92 (74%)		32/42 (76%)		20/27 (74%)	
No permission	26 (14%)	†	11 (13%)	‡	0 (0%)	†‡
Bilateral cataract	34 (19%)	†	24 (28%)	‡	39 (68%)	†‡

* multiple determining factors possible
† $p < .05$
‡ $p < .05$

Table 1. Survey of Referral and Operation, n=324.

	better	same	unknown	worse
Vision	98%	1%	1%	0%
Quality of live	98%	0%	1%	1%
Challenging behavour	98%	0%	1%	1%

Table 2. Results of operated patients.

These health needs are often unrecognized or misdiagnosed. Their mental health problems have an even greater likelihood of going unrecognized. Another important issue is the challenging behaviour displayed by about 45% of people with a severe intellectual disorder, including aggressive, destructive, attention-seeking, self-injurious, noisy and hyperactive behaviour which in many cases can be treated by using correct healthcare.

Visual problems go frequently unrecognised. Identifying visual problems in this group is difficult and these people rarely mention them spontaneously. Clinicians need to think of visual problems as part of a differential diagnosis if there is a progressive uncertainty in the thought processes shown by these patients, especially when placed in new situations. Further in cases of self-mutilation and behavioural problems doctors must be alerted to the possibility of visual problems.

Eye examination has to be done in a special way. It can be time-consuming - 90 minutes on average for such patients. In addition it is of significant benefit if the examiner is familiar with this population.

It is not recommended to perform the examination alone. The patients are often very anxious because they do not understand what is being done. Explanation is difficult or impossible. Further they do not like irregular activities. It is very important to discover how near you can get to them before they stop co-operating or even start to hit, kick or bite. It is very important to display an attitude of professional calm. During the examination one has to encourage the patient in a positive way.

Most people in this group of severe intellectual handicapped people cannot read or understand pictures, many of them cannot even talk making communication even more difficult. Assessment of visual acuity in this group therefore requires special strategies. In most cases the vision can be only be measured by detection methods for example with Teller cards or Cardiff test (Clifford-Donaldson et al 2006) (Figure 1)

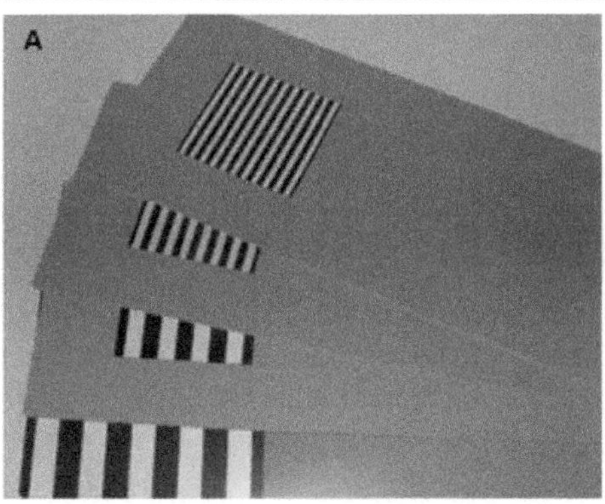

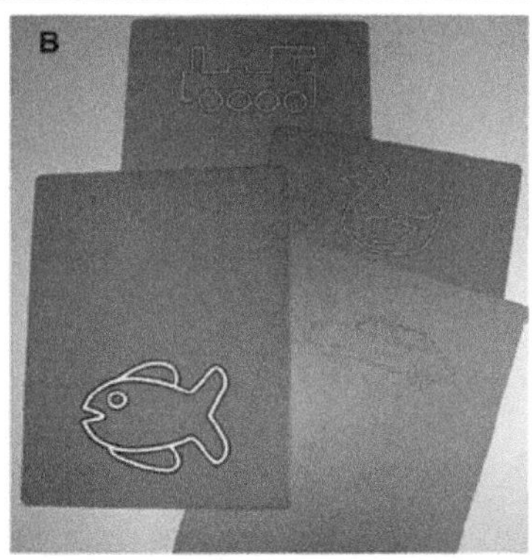

Fig. 1. A. Teller acuity cards, B. Cardiff acuity cards. Both are examples of resolution acuity.

The Teller acuity cards offer eye care practitioners a rapid and reliable method of assessing visual acuity in very young children and non-verbal adults. The set of seventeen cards allows clinicians to measure the ability to resolve black and white striped patterns on the cards. The eye care practitioner judges the patient's visual attention to each series of cards containing stripes of different widths (spatial frequencies). The Cardiff acuity test is also designed for measuring visual acuity in young children and people with intellectual impairment. The test works by preferential looking - that is the patient simply looks towards the target and the examiner watches this eye movement response to determine whether the patient can see the target. If the patient reliably looks at the target, it is assumed in the test that he/she can see it. The principal of the target design is that of the vanishing optotype. The targets are pictures drawn with a white band bordered by two black bands, all on a neutral grey background. The average brightness of the picture is equal to that of the grey background. If the patients detail vision is good enough to resolve the white and black bands, the picture will be visible and the patient can look towards it. If the target lies beyond the acuity limit, the picture merges with the grey background and becomes invisible. The patient cannot look at the picture, because the grey card appears completely black. In the Cardiff test, each picture is located either in the top half or in the bottom half of the card. The examiner, watching the child's eye movements, can judge the position of the target from those eye movements. The pictures are all of the same size, but decrease in width of white and black bands. The visual acuity is scored as the narrowest white band for which the picture is visible. An important feature of the preferential looking technique is that the examiner should not know in advance the position of the target. The Cardiff test includes three cards at each acuity level. The three cards have the same picture, but two are at the top of the card and one at the bottom, or two are at the bottom and one at the top. This means that once one card has been presented the examiner cannot predict the position of the next card. Most of the time visual acuity even in persons with severe intellectual handicap can be measured. Because of physical restrictions and anxiety in the patients the anterior segment can only be examined by a portable handheld slit-lamp. Examination can be very demanding (figure 2).

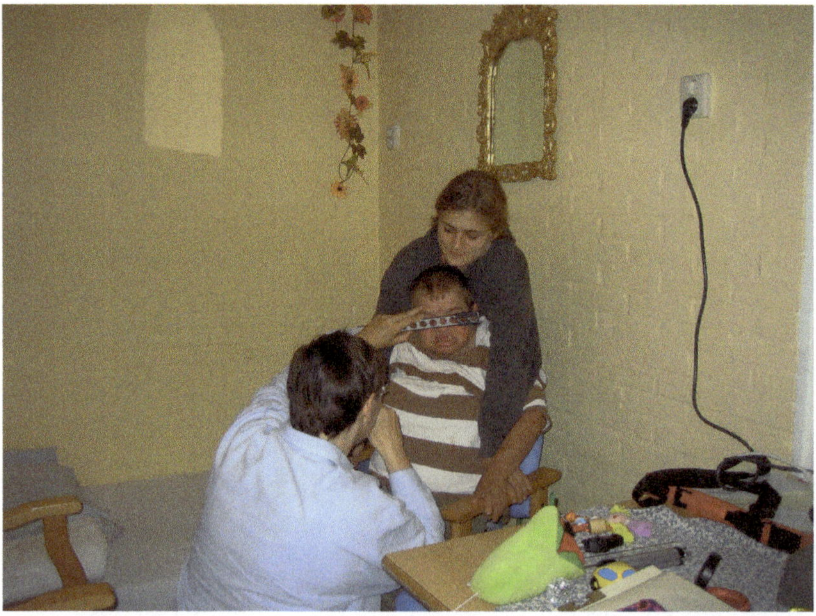

Fig. 2. Eye examinations with severe intellectually disabled people can be very demanding

2.4 Decision-making when considering cataract surgery

If an operable cataract is diagnosed the therapeutic possibilities need to be evaluated. One has to be sure that there is no other ocular pathology responsible for vision loss. As operations in this group can only be performed under general anesthesia a decision has to be made as to whether this risk is acceptable. Cardiac, neurological and other systemic contraindications have to be excluded.

Extensive information is necessary for the decision-making process. Who is involved in the decision-making? The patient themselves, their family, in the Netherlands the curator of the institution, the doctors and nurses who care for the patient on a day to day basis and of course the specialist ophthalmic surgeon all need to decide. The group of patients is incompetent to understand information about the disease and to foresee the consequences of treatment. So other people have to decide and give consent on the part of the patient.

Many relatives are afraid of the impact of changes to their relative's vision and cannot foresee the problems that could arise during and after the operation. It is of great importance to explain the new methods of cataract surgery which allow faster rehabilitation. Examples include the use of smaller incisions than previously, the possibility of follow-up care in the community such as a polyclinic, and the use of new devices and medicines. Nurses and non-specialist doctors also need to be well-informed about the entire pre-, peri- and postoperative period since they are unlikely to be very familiar with care for the patient undergoing eye surgery. Many of them are afraid of the consequences of the visual deterioration in their patients' condition in the period building up to cataract surgery. Therefore it is important to stress that behavioural problems and uncertainty are often caused by visual disturbances and that the patient improves after the operation when his sight is better.

While the ophthalmic surgeon has the surgical experience of managing the patient with visual loss few ophthalmologists have more than basic medical familiarity in caring for people with a severe mental disorder. In the Netherlands there is comparatively little attention paid to these patients during general medical education of doctors. It is very important to inform the ophthalmologist about what to expect from the patient's behaviour in advance. Nowadays data and pictures of the patient can be sent by internet before consultation.

The Visual Advisory Centre developed a protocol for giving preoperative and postoperative instructions. If an ophthalmic surgeon preferred another protocol it was mentioned and included in the instructions. It is very important for intellectually disabled people to recapitulate the procedure several times. The Visual Advisory Centre conducted work using pictograms. Eyes, eye drops and doctors were reproduced on these pictograms.

In most of the operations prophylactic antibiotics were started one day before surgery. Depending on the patient a little sedation was given before surgery, on the day of the operation and afterwards. Cataract surgery was always performed under general anesthesia. Most of the surgeons liked to give a subconjunctival injection with corticosteroids and antibiotics after the operation. The postoperative period was in most patients less difficult than might have been expected. As soon as the patient noticed their better visual acuity they were much more co-operative than expected. Adjustment of eye drops was straightforward. Infections were not present and no patients touched their operated eye in a destructive way.

In the last few years it was noticed that some ophthalmic surgeons developed greater familiarity in operating on this group of patients. They became more eager to perform cataract surgery on these patients. This phenomenon is probably due to positive

reinforcement in this group. In spite of their limitations in expressing themselves this group of patients are satisfied and never complain about the results of surgery. Nurses and doctors are also content because giving care is easier to patients who do not complain.
It would be useful to perform a prospective study on this matter. Such a study has to determine the reason for treatment or no-treatment being decided in people with a severe intellectual handicap. The results of cataract surgery in this group should be compared with a conventional group of patients.
Complaints would need to be evaluated by anamnesis of patients, their families and care givers. Vision before and after operation would have to be compared. Ophthalmological examination of the anterior segment and fundus would be required before and after operations. Problems during anesthesia would also have to be evaluated. Beyond these core requirements trained staff would need to evaluate the quality of life score before and after the cataract operation. This can be done using instruments from the World Health Organisation (WHO) and the Visual Function Questionnaire of the National Eye Institute (National Eye Institute). A prospective study along these lines was organised in the Netherlands. Unfortunately the authors of the above study did not succeed in raising the monetary funds required for this project, partly due to the low priority given to this area by funding bodies and partly as the team split up.

2.5 Cases

Two patients from the group will be described in detail. The first patient AM was born in 1957. She had a severe intellectual handicap because of an inborn error of metabolism. Since the age of 30 she has been living in an institution. At that time her parents could not care for her anymore. In the beginning she was a relatively easy person to care for but in a few years she developed very difficult behaviour. She was aggressive and mutilated herself in a very destructive way. She even removed her right eye. Two persons were needed to cope with her 24 hours a day. The next most important aspect to her care was her regular treatment by a haptonomist. The Visual Advisory Centre was asked to assess her visual acuity. Eye examination revealed that she was blind because of severe cataract in her only eye. The Visual Advisory Centre advised referral to an ophthalmic surgeon. The family did not give permission. They blamed the institution for the change in behaviour. After 10 years of blindness and a lot of problems the curator of the institution gave permission. She was operated on. After the operation the vision improved up to 0.7.
She now lives in her own room, is happy with some simple activities and needs no extra care (Figure 3).
It was not possible to take photographs before the operation.
The second patient PB was a male, born in 1960 who had lived in an institution since the age of 35. His parents died and other family members were not able to care for him. He was an enthusiastic resident of the institution. His daily activity consisted of working in the garden. After some years he was becoming anxious in the morning and evenings when it was dark. He also could not find his chamber. He had bad vision in one eye because of congenital ptosis (Figure 4). The Visual Advisory Centre discovered a mature cataract in the other eye. He was referred to an ophthalmic surgeon with the permission of his curator. The ophthalmic surgeon performed cataract surgery in one eye and ptosis correction in the other eye. It is difficult for severe mentally handicapped people to understand the cause of change in their vision. He thought the eye caps (shield) with holes applied after the operation to protect the eye from damage caused the better vision. He did not want them removed as

would otherwise be routine. Two months later he was still living with the caps on. His vision improved to 0.8 in both eyes.

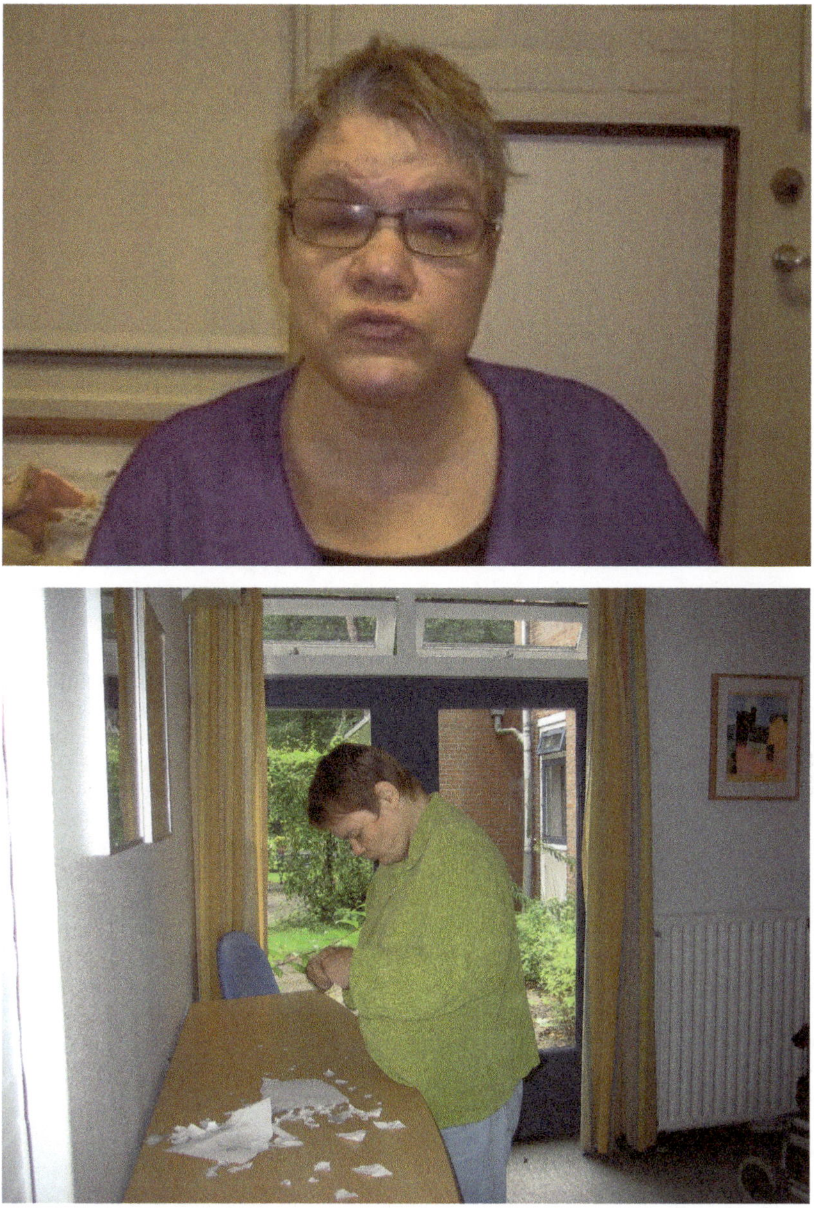

Fig. 3. Patient AM self-caring after the cataract operation. One eye was auto-enucleated.

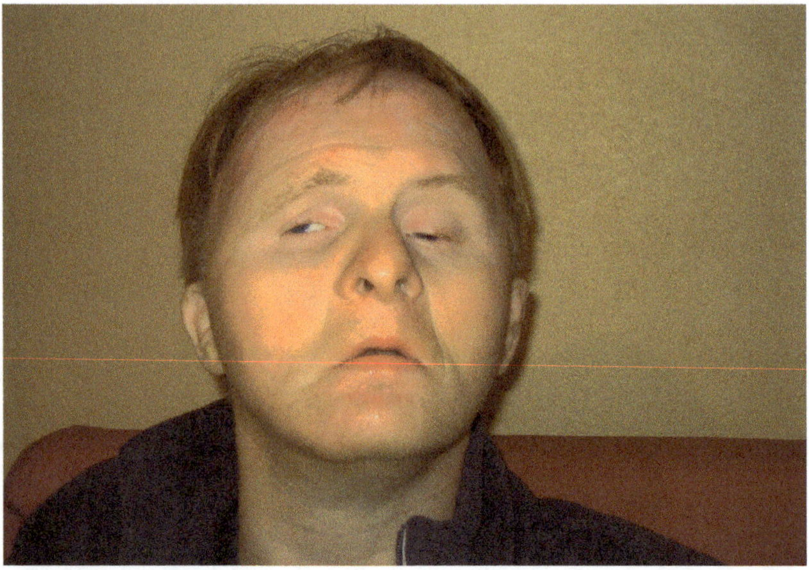

Fig. 4. Patient PB before the cataract operation. Note additionally the squint, ptosis and consequent chin-up posture.

3. Costs of avoidable blindness

In Australia a study examined the costs of blindness for the whole population. The costs of eye diseases in 2004 which accrued in Australian dollars due to suffering and premature death were calculated - 1824 million Australian dollars were incurred in direct medical costs, 1781 million Australian dollars were incurred due to lost earnings for the visually impaired and costs for caregivers (family, friends) were 845 million Australian dollars (Abu Raihan, 2010).

In severely intellectually disabled people the situation is in some ways different. Loss of earnings from visual impairment are not relevant to consider as the sufferers are not considered part of the working population. However costs due to suffering and also from premature death may be incurred. Medical costs are another area. If a person is blind he needs more care especially if behaviour is also disturbed. On the other hand eye examinations in severely intellectual disabled people are time-consuming, as is the operation itself. In the Netherlands health care and health cure have different budgets. This means that if a person is treated because of avoidable blindness, institutions have to pay less but hospitals more. In many institutions dentists are paid for their work by the organisation. They even give general anesthesia to patients. While eye surgery is technically very demanding and intricate it therefore seems feasible in principle for a special (mobile) unit to perform eye operations on these intellectually disabled people, paid for by the care institution.

4. Conclusions

The group of subjects discussed in this chapter with a severe intellectual handicap lived in institutions. In the Netherlands many intellectual handicapped people live in small protected units but for this group, most of them older than 30 years in age and severely handicapped, living in a specialised institution is unfortunately the most appropriate option. The Visual Advisory Centre examined these people in a novel way. A lot of eye diseases were found. Cataract was diagnosed frequently. Despite referral only a small percentage of the patients received cataract surgery. The patients who were operated upon showed good improvement in vision, quality of life and behaviour. Recommendations have been provided for future research and treatment.

5. Acknowledgment

I like to thank Bartimeus for the financial support, the workers from the Visual Advice Centre for their efforts, the care givers for their trust and the ophthalmic surgeons for their courage. Finally I would like to thank Annemarie Sanders for her comments.
Consent was obtained for the photographs.

6. References

American Psychiatric Association (2000) Diagnostic and statistical manual of mental disorders, 4th edn, text revision. Washington, DC : APA, 2000

Arvio & Sillanpaa Prevalence, aetiology and comorbidity of severe and profound intellectual disability in Finland Vol. 47 (2003) pp. 108-12

Beange & Taplin Prevalence of intellectual disability in northern Sydney adults Journal Intellectual disabled Vol. 40 (1996) pp. 191-7

Bittles et al The influence of intellectual disability on life expantacy Journal of Gerontology Vol.57 (2002) pp. 470-72

Bittles et al The four ages of Down syndrome European Journal of Public Health Vol.17 (2006) pp.221-25

Bothe et al Development of impaired vision in mentally handicapped children Klin Monatsbl Augenheilkunde Vol.39 (1991) pp. 509-14

Cooper et al People with intellectual disabilities:their health needs differ and need to be recognised and met British Medical Journal Vol. 329: (2004) PP.414-415

Castane & Peris Visual problems in people with severe mental handicap Journal Intellectual Disability Vol.37 (1993) pp. 469-78

Evenhuis Medical aspects of ageing in a population with intellectual disability Journal Intellectual Disability Vol.39 (1995) pp.19-25

Evenhuis & Nagtzaam Directions for active detection of visual disturbances in people with intellectual disability Nederlands Tijdschrift voor Geneeskunde Vol 143 (1999) pp.187-92

Clifford_Donaldson et al Teller Acuity Card norms with and without use of a testing stage J AAPOS Vol. 10 (2006) pp547-51

Haugen et al Refraction state and correction of refractive errors among mentally retarded adults in a central institution Acta Ophthalmologica Scandinavion Vol.73 (1995) pp. 129-32

Hou et al Anepidemiological and aetiological study of children with intellectual disability in Taiwan Vol 42 (1998) pp.137-43

Klaver et al Age-specific prevalence and causes of blindness and visual impairment in an older population Archives Ophthalmology Vol.16 (1998) pp. 653-8

Limburg, H (2007) Epidemiologie van visuele beperkingen en een demografische verkenning. www.vision2020.nl/contents/InZicht_ rapport.pdf

National Eye Institute. Visual Function Questionnaire-25 www.nei.gov/resources > VFQ-25

Raihan Costs of blindness and poverty alleviation www.thedailystar.net (2010)

Sjoukes L (2008) The impact of visual impairment on adults with an intellectual disability, Kerkhoven, ISBN 978-90-9023384-0, Beilen

Van Isterdael et al 6220 institutionalised people with intellectual disability referred for visual assessment between 1993 and 2003 British journal Ophthalmology Vol.90 (2006) pp. 1297-303

Van Isterdael et al Determining factors for deciding wheter or not to treat refractive errors and cataract in people with a learning disability Nederlands tijdschrift voor Geneeskunde Vol. 152 (2008) pp. 1048-51

Van Splunder et al Prevalence of ocular diagnoses found on screening 1539 adults with intellectual disabilities Ophthalmology Vol.111(2004) pp.1457-63

Van Splunder J (2006)Visual impairment, prevalence and causes of visual impairment in adults with intellectual disabilities, J. Meuwese-Jongejeugd , ISBN 90-8559-203-8, Utrecht

Vision 2020 A compelling case, www.v2020.org (2010)

Warburg Visual impairment in adult people with intellectual disability :literature review Vol.45 (2001) pp. 424-38

Warburg visual impairment in adult people with moderate, severe and profound intellectual disability Acta Ophthalmological Scandinavian Vol 79 (2001) PP. 450-4

Woittiez &Ras (2010) Hoe vaak komt een verstandelijke handicap voor ? nationaal kompas disclaimer (http://www.nationaalkompas.nl/algemeen/menu-rechts)

26

Pseudoexfoliation and Cataract

George K. Andrikopoulos and Sotirios P. Gartaganis
Department of Ophthalmology, Medical School, University of Patras
Greece

1. Introduction

Pseudoexfoliation (PXF) syndrome is a pathologic accumulation of abnormal fibrillar deposits on various ocular structures and extraocular tissues (Figure 1). It is an age-related disorder of the extracellular matrix that may affect up to 20% of people over the age of 60. Although the specific synthesis and pathogenesis of PXF syndrome are still unknown the concept of an elastotic process has recently been established by the finding of the lysyl oxidase-like 1 (LOXL 1) gene as a major risk factor for PXF syndrome and PXF glaucoma (Thorleifsson et al., 2007). It was first described by a Finnish ophthalmologist named John Lindberg, in 1917 in his doctoral thesis. With the aim of a newly developed slit-lamp, he defined the grayish flecks and the changes on the lens and the pupillary margin of the iris in 50% of patients with chronic glaucoma.

The reported prevalence rates vary extensively in different populations like: general population, persons over a certain age, patients with cataract or glaucoma, patients with severe glaucoma. The examiner and the method (mydriasis or not, early stages or not) also play an important role in the prevalence. Its prevalence varies considerably between countries and even within regions or between ethnic groups within many countries. Low rates have been found in Greenland Eskimos (0%), in India (4.2% in patients older than 70 years), in the eastern part of the United States (5% in patients between 75 and 85 years old), in Germany (1.5% in patients 70-79 years of age and 6.3% in those between 80 and 89) and in Britain (2% in 70-79 and 5.4% in 80-89) (Vesti & Kivela, 2000). Also in Australia (2.2% in older than 40), in Japan (1.24% in older than 40) (Ringvold, 1999) and in Austria (1.7%), in Denmark (2%) and in Switzerland (2%) in patients older than 60 years old (Forsius, 1988). On the other hand, high frequencies have been reported in Iceland (31.5%), Finland (>20%), Saudi Arabia (26.5%), Russia (21.4%), Tunisia (19.1%), all in patients older than 70 years old and in Greece (20.1% in ages 70-79 and 46.9% in patients older than 80) (Vesti & Kivela, 2000). Also, in Sweden (18% in ages 65-74), in Norway (16.9% in older than 65) (Ringvold, 1999) and in Turkey (18% in older than 60) (Forsius, 1988). In southwestern Greece in a cross-sectional study of patients admitted at the hospital for cataract surgery we found the prevalence of PXF syndrome to be 27.9% (Andrikopoulos et al., 2009).

Pseudoexfoliation syndrome has been associated with cataract progression, increased intraocular pressure and intraoperative complications like zonular or posterior capsule rupture, poorly dilating pupils, vitreous loss and postoperative fibrinoid reaction or luxation of intraocular lens implants. It is the most common identifiable cause of open-angle glaucoma, the pseudoexfoliation glaucoma. The later is characterized by worse prognosis than primary open angle glaucoma, rapid progression and higher resistance to medical therapy.

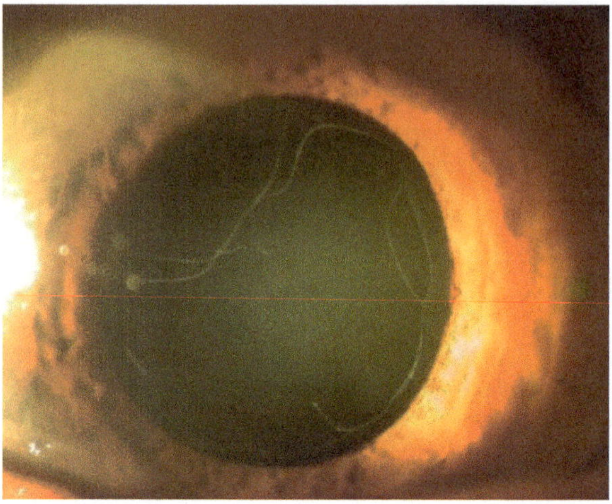

Fig. 1. Pseudoexfoliation material.

The definite clinical diagnosis of PXF deposits can be made only in the last stages of classic PXF (fibers in the two zones) and in the stage of mini-PXF (focal defects in the precapsular layer nasal superiorly). Next to the lens PXF deposits are most prominent to the pupillary border. Additional subtle clinical signs at the slit-lamp examination include loss of melanin from the peripupillary pigment epithelium of the iris, transillumination defects in the sphincter area, insufficient mydriasis, posterior synechiae, zonular instability, melanin deposition and melanin dispersion (on the structures of anterior segment) after pupillary dilation.

It appears that a variety of epithelial and mesenchymal cells may be associated with disordered synthesis of the extracellular fibrillar material in different sites. The intraocular material seems to be produced mainly in the pre-equatorial lens epithelium, the nonpigmented ciliary epithelium and the iris pigment epithelium and secondarily in the corneal endothelium, the trabecular endothelium and by almost all cell types of the iris stroma (Ritch & Schlötzer-Schrehardt, 2001). Secondary distribution by the aqueous humor is responsible for its passive deposition on the other structures of the anterior segment. The extraocular PXF material has been demonstrated electron microscopically in close proximity to fibroblasts, smooth and striated muscle cells, and heart muscle cells (Schlötzer-Schrehardt et al., 1992a; Streeten et al., 1992). These types of cells are probably involved in its production in various visceral organs.

There are two major theories on the pathogenesis of PXF syndrome. The first links the exfoliation fibers to the elastic microfibrils of the elastic system. It describes PXF syndrome as a type of elastosis, an elastic microfibrillopathy with excessive production of elastic fiber components (Garner & Alexander, 1984; Streeten et al., 1986). The second theory considers PXF syndrome to be a generalized disorder of the basement membranes (Dickson & Ramsay, 1975), with a variety of basement membrane components to have been recognized in the PXF material (Eagle et al., 1979; Harnisch et al., 1981; Konstas et al., 1990; Kubota et al., 1998; Schlötzer-Schrehardt et al., 1992b; Tawara et al., 1996). Growth factors (GFs) and particularly Transforming Growth Factor-β1 (TGF-β1), impaired cellular protection system with increased cellular and oxidative stress, an imbalance between Matrix Metalloproteinases (MMPs) and Tissue Inhibitor of Metalloproteinases (TIMPs), ischemia/hypoxia, cross-linking process and aggregation of misfolded stressed proteins appear to be involved in the pathogenetic concept of this fibrotic disorder with accumulation of extracellular material (Gartaganis et al., 2001, 2002, 2005, 2007; Schlötzer-Schrehardt & Naumann, 2006; Schlötzer-Schrehardt, 2009).

The exact chemical composition of PXF material remains unknown. It seems to consist a complex of glycoprotein/proteoglycan with epitopes of the basement membrane and the elastic fiber system. The protein components of PXF material include non-collagenous basement membrane elements (such as laminin, nidogen, and fibronectin), epitopes of elastic fibers (such as elastin, tropoelastin, amyloid P, vitronectin) and components of elastic microfibrils such as fibrillin-1, emilin, microfibril-associated glycoprotein-1, and latent TGF-β binding proteins 1-2) (Ritch & Schlötzer-Schrehardt, 2001). Other proteins are cross-linking enzymes, chaperones, apolipoproteins, glycosaminoglycans, complement proteins, proteolytic enzymes and their inhibitors, and cytokines like TGF-β1. The glycosaminoglycans and proteoglycans include heparan sulfate proteoglycan, chondroitin sulfate proteoglycan, dermatan sulfate proteoglycan, keratan sulfate proteoglycan, and hyaluronan (Fitzsimmons et al., 1997; Harnisch et al., 1981; Schlötzer-Schrehardt et al., 1992b; Tawara et al., 1996). The microfibrillar subunits seem to form a core surrounded by an amorphous matrix, which is suggested to represent glycosaminoglycans on the surface of the exfoliation fibrils.

2. Pseudoexfoliation syndrome and cataract formation

An association between PXF and cataract formation appears to exist. Nuclear cataract and secondarily subcapsular cataract are more frequently found in eyes with PXF than in eyes without PXF. And opposite, PXF has a higher prevalence in eyes with cataract (Hietanen et al., 1992). In a study conducted by the authors the prevalence of cataract in eyes with PXF was found 87.4% and in eyes without PXF 79.9%. And opposite, PXF prevalence in eyes with cataract was found 24.2% and in eyes without cataract 15.5% (Andrikopoulos, 2009). Eyes with PXF have been found with poorer visual acuity and more often lens opacification than clinically uninvolved fellow eyes (Puska, 1994). Cataract formation may be related to ocular ischemia, aqueous hypoxia, reduced protection against ultraviolet radiation, increased growth factor levels and oxidative stress. Ascorbic acid, that plays an important role in protecting the lens from ultraviolet irradiation, has been found reduced in the aqueous humor of patients with PXF deposits (Koliakos et al., 2003).

3. Pseudoexfoliation syndrome and cataract surgery

3.1 Intraocular manifestations of pseudoexfoliation syndrome that predispose to surgical complications

Lens In contrast to the characteristic changes in the anterior capsule which are relatively harmless, the pre-equatorial lens epithelium disorders may be associated with dangers for the intraocular surgeon. In the area corresponding to the proliferative zone of the epithelium and the zone of zonular anchorage, deposits infiltrate and disrupt the lens capsule and the zonular lamella, resulting in separation of the zonules insertion on the capsule surface (Schlötzer-Schrehardt & Naumann, 1994). This peripheral region is the only area with active production of PXF material by the metabolically active epithelium. These changes are hidden behind the iris and thus clinically invisible, but responsible for the instability of the zonular attachment.

Zonules and ciliary body In cases associated with phacodonesis or lens luxation, degeneration of zonular attachment sites is usually observed (Schlötzer-Schrehardt & Naumann, 1994). Areas of weakness and zonular dehiscence include the zonular fibers themselves but also their anchorage sites to the defective basement membranes of the ciliary epithelium and lens. Proteolytic-lysosomal enzymes, that have been found within PXF material, may also be linked with the zonular disintegration. Zonular instability and subsequent laxity of the lens allows anterior lens movement resulting in pupillary or even ciliary block, that predispose to angle closure glaucoma. Attacks of angle closure glaucoma, because of inferior displacement of the lens, can occur, particularly under miotic therapy.

Iris Virtually all iris cell types are involved in PXF material production and deposition. Clinically PXF iris is characteristically rigid with reduced dilating properties. Dispersion of melanin granules, after pharmacological dilation, due to rupture of degenerative posterior pigment epithelial cells, may result in acute rise in IOP. Iris stromal vessels, because of deposition of fibers in the adventitia, may become obliterated resulting in hypoperfusion and iris microneovascularization. Neovascularization may result in microhyphema after pharmacologic dilation. PXF ocular ischemia may play a role in cataract formation too. Iris vasculopathy may be associated with a chronic breakdown in the aqueous barrier, that may manifest as pseudouveitis with posterior synechiae and elevated aqueous flare. Blood-aqueous barrier dysfunction is greater in eyes with PXF compared to eyes without PXF, after intraocular surgery, resulting in a transitory fibrinoid reaction. Posterior synechiae are common in PXF eyes due to adherence of the posterior pigment epithelium to the PXF coated anterior lens capsule or to miotics that inhibit iris movement. A combination of PXF fibers deposition in the stroma and muscle tissue with vascular disorders leads to hypoxia (Repo et al., 1995) and tissue degeneration that result in reduced dilating properties of iris (Asano et al., 1995). Even without mydriatics, the pupil in PXF eyes may be smaller (suggesting a defective dilator muscle or reduced sympathetic innervation).

Trabecular meshwork The deposits of PXF material and probably the melanin pigment throughout the trabeculum and the degenerating changes of the juxtacanalicular tissue beneath the inner wall of Schlemm's canal are the major mechanisms of PXF open-angle glaucoma (Ringvold & Vegge, 1971; Schlötzer-Schrehardt & Naumann, 1995). The pathologic alterations of Schlemm's canal include narrowing, fragmentation and obstruction in advanced cases. Apart from the obstruction to trabecular outflow, increased aqueous protein levels (due to persistent blood-aqueous barrier breakdown), an impaired ocular and retrobulbar perfusion and disorder of elastic tissue of the lamina cribrosa (Netland et al., 1995), have also been proposed. It is well known that PXF is the most common identifiable cause of open-angle glaucoma (Ritch, 1994a). It is also associated with a higher incidence of narrow angles (Herbst, 1976; Ritch, 1994b).

Cornea The corneal endothelium shows focal degeneration, phagocytosis of melanin granules and PXF fibers production. Central corneal thickness has been found greater in eyes with PXF. These changes together with a reduced endothelial cell density may lead to an irregular thickening of the Descement membrane. The dysfunctional endothelium in PXF eyes increases the risk of corneal endothelial decompensation with normal or after moderate rises in intraocular pressure (IOP), for example after mydriasis or after cataract surgery.

3.2 Preoperative considerations

Recognition of PXF material is critical for reducing operative complications. The classic pattern of three distinct zones of PXF material on the anterior lens surface represents a very late stage of the disease. In early stages a diffuse pre-capsular layer of microfibers ("early PXF") can be observed on the entire surface of the anterior lens capsule. Later focal defects in the midperipheral zone usually superonasally ("mini PXF") may alert the ophthalmologist. The importance of a dilated pupil and the comparison with the fellow eye have been emphasized by a number of authors. Iris changes like transillumination defects, melanin pigment liberation associated with pupil dilation, poor mydriasis or asymmetric pupil sizes and circular posterior synechiae are useful signs. Other early clinical signs are: PXF or melanin deposition on the anterior chamber structures (especially the trabecular meshwork), marked asymmetry of IOP or marked IOP rise after pupillary dilation, phacodonesis and atypical cornea guttata. In eyes with mature cataract it is mandatory to look carefully for PXF deposits as they may have the same colour with the grey-white cataract.

The complication rates of cataract extraction in PXF syndrome are higher compared to control. Phacoemulsification in PXF eyes is associated with increasd rates of capsular and zonular tears and vitreous loss (Drolsum et al., 1993; Shingleton et al., 2003). On the other hand, recent studies around the world have shown no statistically significant difference in complication rates during phacoemulsification of PXF eyes (Akinci et al., 2008; Dosso et al., 1997; Hyams et al., 2005) than earlier studies that showed up to a 10-fold increase. Phacoemulsification performed by experienced surgeons, in combination with advanced technologies and devices, have decreased the risks. It is reported, in recent studies, that a thorough cataract consideration is important, in eyes with PXF syndrome, as it can minimize the risk for complications (Belovay et al., 2010; Drolsum et al., 2007; Shingleton et al., 2009; Tanhehco & Chen, 2010).

Zonule weakness The signs of zonular weakness include phacodonesis, lens subluxation, narrow iridocorneal angle, zonule dialysis and iridodonesis. Iridodonesis is best assessed prior to dilation, while phacodonesis, lens subluxation and zonule dialysis after maximum mydriasis. A shallow or hyper-deep anterior chamber may consist an indirect sign of zonule instability and lens displacement. A central anterior chamber depth less than 2.5 mm has been reported to increase the risk for surgical complications 5-fold in PXF eyes (Küchle et al., 2000). An asymmetry in anterior chamber depth or significant differences in refraction between the two eyes may be indicative of a subluxated lens. The increased cataract density, the increasing age and the reduced pupil size are indirect clinical predictors of zonule instability, while the amount of PXF material does not seem to be a predicting factor (Moreno et al., 1993). Ultrasound biomicroscopy can be useful to check the zonule status like infiltration of PXF fibrils, fragmentation or zonule loss. Zonular fragility has been associated with a 3 to 10-fold increased risk of zonular rupture and lens dislocation and a 5-fold increased risk of vitreous loss (Schlötzer-Schrehardt & Naumann, 2006).

Small pupil Poor pupil dilation may limit the size of the capsulorhexis. A small capsulorhexis often leads to increased and traumatic forces on the zonular apparatus and increased risk for capsular tear and postoperative capsule phimosis. The increased difficulty in extracting nuclear material from the capsular bag, due to a small pupil, can also lead to iris trauma and intraoperative bleeding.

It is also important to check carefully the corneal endothelial status, as reduced endothelial cell counts increases the risk of corneal endothelial dysfunction or decompensation.

3.3 Intraoperative considerations

Many surgical approaches have been used to avoid corneal failure and to manage a small pupil and zonular weakness.

Corneal endothelium Dispersive ophthalmic viscosurgical devices are helpful to adhere, coat and protect the cornea. Cohesive ophthalmic viscosurgical devices can help to dilate a small pupil and to maintain the anterior chamber (Shingleton et al., 2009). Overinflating the anterior chamber with viscoelastics should be avoided as it may cause undue stress on the zonules.

Small pupil In phacoemulsification it is not needed to extrude the nucleus through a full dilated pupil as in extracapsular cataract extraction. However, as PXF eyes respond poorly to mydriatics many strategies are frequently required intraoperatively. Pharmacologically, nonsteroid anti-inflammatory drops in combination with mydriatics can help to expand the pupil (Keates & McGowan, 1984). Mechanical enlargement of the pupil includes stretching, cohesive ophthalmic viscosurgical devices, release of posterior synechiae, sphincterotomy as well as iris hooks and pupil dilator rings. Special iris hooks (Figure 2a) can be used to allow visualization of the peripheral capsule and to release posterior synechiae. Bimanual stretching with Y-hooks, the Beehler pupil dilator, iris retractor hooks and pupil dilator polymethyl methacrylate rings have all been shown to be equally effective (Akman et al., 2004). Other pupil expansion devices like the Malyugin ring (Figure 2b), the Perfect pupil expansion device and the Graether pupil expander have also been used. However, pupil stretching and cutting should be avoided in patients predisposed to floppy-iris syndrome (Chang et al., 2008). Also, pupil mechanical dilation may lead to iris injury and hyphema, pigment release, postoperative inflammation and sometimes to a permanently dilated pupil.

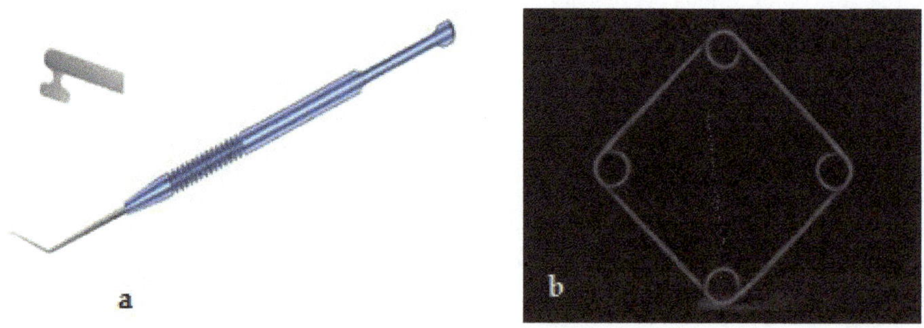

Fig. 2. a. Iris hook, b. Malyugin ring.

Zonule weakness When the zonules are loose a capsule tension ring (CTR) placed within an intact capsular bag may be useful (Figure 3a). It provides capsular bag expansion and supports the part of zonule instability, distributing the zonule tensions from the weakened zonules onto the remaining zonules. In this way it can provide buttress for the entire capsule-zonular apparatus (Menapace et al., 2000). It is reported that a CTR can center a mildly subluxed lens (equal or less than 4 hours zonulopathy and/or mild phacodonesis) (Hasanee & Ahmed, 2006) but does not prevent the progressive zonulopathy and the following decentration in the presence of PXF material (Ahmed et al., 2005a). Also, it should not be used in cases of anterior or posterior capsular tear. Although a CTR can be implanted at any time after performing the capsulorhexis, most surgeons propose delaying implantation. It was found that CTR implantation before nucleus extraction gave increased capsular torque and displacement compared to implantation after the nucleus had been extracted (Ahmed et al., 2005b). Although some surgeons propose the use of a CTR in all PXF cases, regardless of whether zonule instability is present, the implantation can be hazardous and should better be performed only in cases of zonule instability, as it may create capsule and zonule trauma or entrapment of cortex behind it (Ahmed et al., 2005b). Regardless of these limitations, a CTR implantation has been found to reduce intraoperative complications in PXF cases and to decrease postoperative IOL decentration and tilt (D.-H. Lee et al., 2002). Lower rate of intraoperative zonular separation, posterior capsular rupture and increased rate of intraocular lens (IOL) fixation in the capsular bag have also been reported in PXF eyes with CTR implantation compared to controls (standard phacoemulsification) (Bayraktar et al., 2001).

In more advanced cases of profound zonule fragility a modified CTR, with a single or double eyelet for suture fixation to the sclera in areas of weakness, should be considered (Cionni & Osher, 1998) (Figure 3b). Capsule either iris retractors placed at the edge of capsulorhexis can be effective in holding capsulorhexis in place during phacoemulsification. They can also provide support for the capsulozonular complex (V. Lee & Bloom, 1999; Santoro et al., 2003). In advanced cases of profound zonule instability a capsule tension segment (CTS) can be useful (Figure 3c). The capsule tension segment serves as retracting apparatus and supporting stent for the capsular bag during phacoemulsification (Hasanee et al., 2006). It has an eyelet that can be used for suture fixation to the sclera in areas of weakness providing postoperative stability and good centration of the IOL/capsular bag complex. Unlike the larger CTR and modified CTR, the CTS can be positioned atraumatically and safely in the presence of an anterior or posterior capsule tear provided the CTS is not positioned within the tear itself. One or two CTR devices can be used simultaneously too.

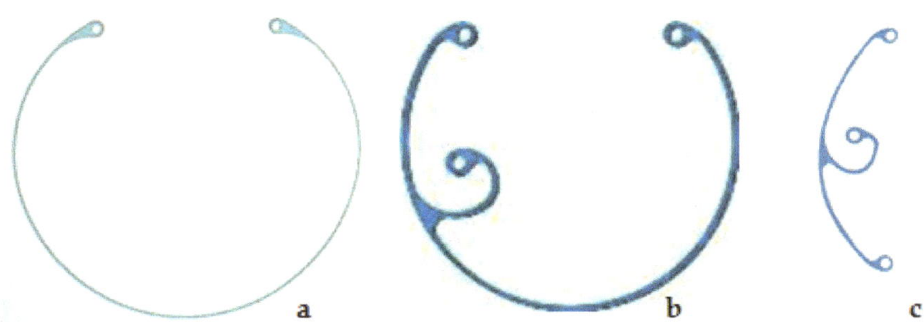

Fig. 3. a. Capsule Tension Ring, b. modified Capsule Tension Ring, c. Capsule Tension Segment.

If despite the use of all the above devices intraoperative subluxation of lens fragment or capsular bag complex occur, the technique should be modified. In these cases most capsule tension devices are contraindicated and the available options include elevating the remaining lens into the anterior chamber for anterior phacoemulsification or conversion to extracapsular or modified intracapsular cataract extraction. If there is a deep vitreous dislocation, pars plana vitrectomy and lensectomy are preferred. Posterior chamber lens may also be placed in the ciliary sulcus, even in the presence of small capsular tears providing sufficient support exists. Otherwise, an angle-supported IOL, an iris-claw IOL or an IOL fixed to the sclera wall may be mandatory (Dick & Augustin, 2001). An angle-supported anterior chamber IOL should probably be avoided in cases of eyes with glaucoma or corneal endothelial cell abnormalities (Drolsum, 2003).

Surgical technique In phacoemulsification the rate of intraoperative complications in PXF eyes is significantly lower than in extracapsular cataract extraction (ECCE) and seems to be related to zonular and not to capsule weakness (Shingleton et al., 2003). Small incision, less tension on the capsule and the zonules, less anterior chamber depth fluctuations are some of the advantages provided by the phocoemulsification, that have increased the safety of cataract surgery. On the other hand, the increased force needed to extrude the lens through a small pupil and the previous can-opener or envelope techniques with the increased risk of posterior capsule rupture may explain the higher frequency of intraoperative complications in ECCE.

When zonule instability is suspected, overinflating the anterior chamber with viscoelastics should be avoided. Also, avoidance of excessive fluctuations in anterior chamber pressure and gentle manipulation of the lens in phacoemulsification are recommended. Maintenance of anterior chamber avoids vitreous prolapse around the capsular bag. Small incision surgery, controlled paracentesis and adequate hydrodissection are some more useful strategies.

The continuous circular capsulorhexis (CCC) should be neither too small, nor too large. The ideal size is 5-5.5mm in diameter. A small CCC may lead to increased stress to a loose zonule during manipulation of the lens and to anterior capsular phimosis. A large CCC may preclude the use of capsule devices and may be suboptimal for IOL fixation. In PXF cases with zonule instability, CCC initiation and spread of the capsular tear may be difficult, as countertraction is decreased. A sharp needle puncture, a CCC forceps or a bimanual technique with a micrograsper and a sharp tipped instrument can help in CCC initiation. Hooks or capsule retractors at the cut edge of the CCC can help address the spread of the capsule tear (Shingleton et al., 2009). Capsule staining (trypan blue) may be helpful allowing for visualization of all capsular layers in cases of capsule-splitting phenomena in which multiple layers of a split capsule may be raised (Jacobs et al., 2006).

Adequate hydrodissection allows unimpeded rotation of the nucleus and facilitates cortex removal (Vasavada et al., 2002). The procedure has to be performed gently as an aggressive injection of fluid may lead to further downward stress and zonular weakness. Alternatively, the entire nucleus should be hydrodissected and luxated anteriorly for supracapsular phacoemulsification (Drolsum et al., 2007). The choice of IOL does not differ much between eyes with PXF and eyes without PXF. So, none of the common IOL materials seem to be superior to the others (Wagoner et al., 2003). Plate-haptic PC IOLs, accommodating IOLs, multifocal IOLs and aspheric IOLs are associated with a higher risk of subluxation or phimosis. Although most foldable PC IOLs are reasonable options in eyes with PXF, the slower unfolding acrylic PC IOLs may provide additional control and minimize zonule stress during insertion (Shingleton et al., 2009). Acrylic IOLs also seem to cause less anterior capsular opacification than silicone ones (Werner et al., 2000).

Despite the advances in phacoemulsification power modulation and fluidics, PXF eyes continue to have an increased risk of capsule injury particularly from the phacoemulsification tip and instruments. Signs of capsular bag collapse include infolding of the peripheral posterior capsule, collapse of the capsule equator or visualization of the capsule fornix (Belovay et al., 2010). Working in the safe central zone of the anterior chamber is proposed. Adequate hydrodissection as well as the use of viscodissection to separate cortex from the capsule facilitate cortex removal (Shingleton et al., 2009).

3.4 Postoperative considerations

After surgery frequent follow-up examinations are important as early and late postoperative complications may occur more frequently in eyes with PXF material. In the early period after cataract surgery the main complications include inflammation, keratopathy and IOP spikes while in the long term posterior capsule opacification, anterior capsule contraction (phimosis) and IOL decentration.

Inflammation On the basis of blood-aqueous barrier dysfunction intense and/or prolonged postoperative inflammation, increased aqueous flare, fibrinoid reaction, posterior synechiae, IOL deposits, anterior capsule contraction and macular edema are more frequent in eyes with PXF. However, advances in phacoemulsification have reduced dramatically the risk of an inflammatory response. PXF eyes with glaucoma have been reported to have increased risk for macular edema after phacoemulsification (Yüksel et al., 2008). Iris trauma, which is more common in PXF eyes, has been associated with higher rates of macular edema too (Gulkilik et al., 2006).

Intraocular pressure The presence of trabecular outflow and blood-aqueous barrier alterations results in an increased risk of early postoperative IOP elevation, particularly in patients with preexisting glaucoma (Pohjalainen et al., 2001; Shingleton et al., 2008). Postoperative IOP spikes should be prevented through careful aspiration of viscoelastic material at the end of the surgery procedure, and meticulous monitor IOP, and use prophylactic ocular hypotensive agents, at least in high-risk patients.

Several studies demonstrate a reduction of IOP in glaucomatous eyes after cataract surgery with IOL implantation (Handa et al., 1987; Shingleton et al., 1999). It has been reported that the IOP reduction is even greater in PXF eyes and it may be explained by a greater outflow improvement, as previously deposited PXF material is expeditiously cleared by the high flow states during phacoemulsification and irrigation/aspiration (Shingleton et al., 2003). Eyes with higher preoperative IOP and/or narrow angles tend to have greater IOP reduction after cataract surgery (Issa et al., 2005; Poley et al., 2008). However, these conclusions have been argued by another study that found no difference in IOP reduction after cataract surgery between non-glaucomatous eyes with and without PXF (Pohjalainen et al., 2001).

Keratopathy The endothelial cell count is reduced and mean endothelial cell area enlarged in exfoliative eyes, predisposing some of them to develop early corneal endothelial decompensation even with only moderate rises in IOP or after cataract surgery (Naumann & Schlötzer-Schrehardt, 2000). PXF is reported to have a negative influence on endothelial cell loss during cataract surgery (Kaljurand & Teesalu, 2007). Working in a safe distance from the cornea and adequate viscoelastic can help to protect the endothelial cells during surgical maneuvers.

Late intraocular lens problems Secondary cataract has been found increased significantly in PXF eyes than in controls (Küchle et al., 1997). This increase may be related to a persistent breakdown in the blood-aqueous barrier, hypoxia of the anterior chamber, cortical remnants and a compromised capsule-zonular complex leading to posterior capsular folds with subsequent facilitated migration of lens epithelial cells (Drolsum et al., 2007). Now that phacoemulsification is a standard procedure and IOL material is improved, postoperative posterior capsule opacification, corneal decompensation and inflammation, even in PXF eyes, are rare.

Even with uneventful phacoemulsification late in-the-bag IOL tilt or dislocation may occur many years postoperatively. Age, capsule contraction/phimosis, instability of the blood-aqueous barrier, surgical trauma to the zonules or postoperative trauma and progressive zonular disintegration have been proposed to contribute to the process (Gimbel et al., 2005; Gross et al., 2004; Jehan et al., 2001; Kato et al., 2002). PXF syndrome has been reported in >50% of all late in-the-bag IOL dislocations (Breyer et al., 1999). The mean time of the late subluxation of the IOL-capsular bag complex was 8+ years (range 9 months to 17 years) (Jehan et al., 2001). If the IOL optic remains in the pupillary area any intervention can be postponed. However, it is usually preferable to intervene surgically as long as an anterior approach is still possible. The options are to either reposition or exchange the IOL. We can reposition and suture the IOL to the sclera or to the iris. Otherwise, we have to exchange the IOL with an angle-supported anterior chamber (AC) IOL (Drolsum et al., 2007). If a dislocation far posteriorly of the IOL-capsule complex occurs, a vitreoretinal approach should be combined.

Anterior capsule contraction/phimosis can lead to postoperative IOL subluxation and dislocation (Hayashi et al., 1998). Age, blood-aqueous disorder, PXF material, retained cortex, IOL material, zonular weakness and a small CCC can lead to increased capsular shrinkage (Gimbel et al., 2005; Kato et al., 2002; Kimura et al., 1998; Werner et al., 2000). A neodymium: YAG laser radial anterior capsulotomy or a surgical release of the centripetal traction of the anterior capsule and zonules should be performed to treat phimosis.

We studied retrospectively nine patients (ten eyes) with PXF syndrome and late spontaneous dislocation of the bag-IOL complex. All patients had undergone uncomplicated cataract extraction with posterior chamber IOL implantation 4 to 17 years ago (mean 8.5) by the same surgeon (SPG). In one patient IOL dislocation occurred in both eyes approximately four months apart. Five surgeries had been performed by the extracapsular cataract extraction while in five cases a standardized surgical technique for phacoemulsification had been used. A CCC measuring approximately 5.0 to 5.5 mm in diameter had been made using forceps. In all cases surgical management included dislocated IOL removal and anterior chamber IOL implantation. Five cases underwent 3-port pars plana vitrectomy and five underwent anterior vitrectomy. Of the ten explanted IOLs, two were found to be one-piece polymethylmethacrylate (PMMA) posterior IOLs, one a three-piece PMMA IOL with polypropylene haptics, four were three-piece acrylic IOLs, two three-piece acrylic IOLs and one a silicone lens; the IOLs' overall length was 13.0 mm. The explanted IOLs underwent microscopic examination and were found to be intact, encased in the capsular bag. In six eyes visual acuity improved, in three eyes remained stable, and in one eye was found to be deteriorated after 24 months of follow-up, due to the development of age related macular disease. In our series, we observed that in five cases where an anterior CCC had been performed, a circumferential anterior capsular overlap of the optic edge was found to be at least for 1 mm wide of the 6.0 mm optic zone of the dislocated IOL. Conversely, in cases where a can-opener capsulotomy had been made, the edge of the anterior capsule remnant was localized outside the edge of the optic part of the IOL. When comparing the cases of capsulorhexis to the cases of capsulotomy with regard to the interval between cataract surgery and IOL dislocation, we observed that in four cases of can-opener capsulotomy dislocation occurred much later (10-17 years) than in the cases of CCC (4-7 years). The earlier (4 years) IOL dislocation in an eye with a can-opener capsulotomy may be attributed to the co-existence of retinitis pigmentosa and PXF in the same patient that may accumulatively have contributed to zonular instability. In the can-opener capsulotomy patients both loops of the one-piece PMMA lenses may suggest that the retentive memory of the haptics provide stronger resistance to capsule contraction. The long-term dislocation in patients with one-piece PMMA IOLs could demonstrate that this type of IOL may also function as a capsular tension ring that stabilizes the capsular bag via a centrifugal tension on the capsular fornices.

The aforementioned considerations related to cataract surgery in PXF eyes are summarized in Table 1.

Intraoperative	**Postoperative**
Corneal endotheliopathy	Fibrinoid reaction
Small pupil	Aqueous flare
Zonule weakness	Posterior synechiae
Anterior chamber depth disorders	IOL deposits
Posterior capsule dehiscence	Macular edema
Vitreous prolapse	Postoperative pressure spikes
	Corneal edema
	Anterior capsule contraction (phimosis)
	Secondary cataract
	IOL subluxation/dislocation

Table 1. Intraoperative and postoperative considerations in cataract surgery in PXF eyes.

4. Conclusion

PXF syndrome may cause a spectrum of serious ocular and surgical complications. The problems related to cataract surgery are mainly initiated by zonular instability and, to some degree, by insufficient pupillary dilation. Awareness of the structural and functional features of this disorder may help avoid or minimize most of them. The early recognition of the syndrome in addition to advanced phacoemulsification techniques and associated surgical devices have increased the percentage of operative success. Through careful consideration with preoperative preparation, surgical awareness and postoperative follow up favorable outcomes can be achieved in cataract surgery.

5. References

Ahmed, I.I.K., Chen, S.H., Kranemann, C., & Wong, D.T. (2005a). Surgical repositioning of dislocated capsular tension rings. *Ophthalmology*, Vol.112, No.10, (October 2005), pp. 1725–1733.

Ahmed, I.I.K., Cionni, R.J., Kranemann, C., & Crandall, A.S. (2005b). Optimal timing of capsular tension ring implantation: Miyake-Apple video analysis. *Journal of Cataract & Refractive Surgery*, Vol.31, No.9, (September 2005), pp.1809–1813.

Akinci, A., Batman, C., & Zilelioglu, O. (2008). Phacoemulsification in pseudoexfoliation syndrome. *Ophthalmologica*, Vol.222, No.2, (February 2008), pp. 112–116.

Akman, A., Yilmaz, G., Oto, S., & Akova, Y.A. (2004). Comparison of various pupil dilatation methods for phacoemulsification in eyes with a small pupil secondary to pseudoexfoliation. *Ophthalmology*, Vol.111, No.9, (September 2004), pp. 1693-1698.

Andrikopoulos, G.K., Mela, E.K., Georgakopoulos, C.D., Papadopoulos, G.E., Damelou, A.N., Alexopoulos, D.K., & Gartaganis, S.P. (2009). Pseudoexfoliation syndrome prevalence in Greek patients with cataract and its association to glaucoma and coronary artery disease. *Eye*, Vol.23, No.2, (February 2009), pp. 442-447.

Andrikopoulos, G.K. (2009). *Pseudoexfoliation and coronary artery disease* [dissertation (in Greek)], University of Patras, Patras, Greece.

Asano, N., Schlötzer -Schrehardt, U.M., & Naumann, G.O.H. (1995). A histopathologic study of iris changes in pseudoexfoliation syndrome. *Ophthalmology*, Vol.102, No.9, (September 1995), pp. 1279-1290.

Bayraktar, S., Altan, T., Küçüksümer, Y., & Yılmaz, Ö.F. (2001). Capsular tension ring implantation after capsulorhexis in phacoemulsification of cataracts associated with pseudoexfoliation syndrome : intraoperative complications and early postoperative findings. *Journal of Cataract & Refractive Surgery*, Vol.27, No.10, (October 2001), pp. 1620–1628.

Belovay, G.W., Varma, D.K., & Ahmed, I.I.K. (2010). Cataract surgery in pseudoexfoliation syndrome. *Current Opinion in Ophthalmology*, Vol.21, No.1, (January 2010), pp. 25-34.

Breyer, D.R., Hermeking, H., & Gerke, E. (1999). Late dislocation of the capsular bag after phacoemulsification with endocapsular IOL in pseudoexfoliation syndrome. *Ophthalmologe*, Vol.96, No.4, (April 1999), pp. 248–251.

Chang, D.F., Braga-Mele, R., Mamalis, N., Masket, S., Miller, K.M., Nichamin, L.D., Packard, R.B., & Packer, M. (2008). ASCRS White Paper: Clinical review of intraoperative floppy-iris syndrome. *Journal of Cataract & Refractive Surgery*, Vol.34, No.12, (December 2008), pp. 2153–2162.

Cionni, R.J., & Osher, R.H. (1998). Management of profound zonular dialysis or weakness with a new endocapsular ring designed for scleral fixation. *Journal of Cataract & Refractive Surgery*, Vol.24, No.10, (October 1998), pp. 1299–1306.

Dick, H.B., & Augustin, A.J. (2001). Lens implant selection with absence of capsular support. *Current Opinion in Ophthalmology*, Vol.12, No.1, (February 2001), pp. 47–57.

Dickson, D.H., & Ramsay, M.S. (1975). Fibrillopathia epitheliocapsularis (pseudoexfoliation): a clinical and electron microscope study. *Canadian Journal of Ophthalmology*, Vol.10, No.2, (April 1975), pp. 148-161.

Dosso, A.A., Bonvin, E.R., & Leuenberger, P.M. (1997). Exfoliation syndrome and phacoemulsification. *Journal of Cataract & Refractive Surgery*, Vol.23, No. 1, (January - February 1997), pp. 122–125.

Drolsum, L., Haaskjold, E., & Davanger, M. (1993). Results and complications after extracapsular cataract extraction in eyes with pseudoexfoliation syndrome. *Acta Ophthalmologica*, Vol.71, No.6, (December 1993), pp. 771–776.

Drolsum, L. (2003). Longterm follow-up of secondary flexible, open-loop, anterior chamber intraocular lenses. *Journal of Cataract & Refractive Surgery*, Vol.29, No.3, (March 2003), pp. 498–503.

Drolsum, L., Ringvold, A., & Nicolaissen, B. (2007). Cataract and glaucoma surgery in pseudoexfoliation syndrome: a review. *Acta Ophthalmologica Scandinavica*, Vol.85, No.8, (December 2007), pp. 810–821.

Eagle Jr., R.C., Font, R.L., & Fine, B.S. (1979). The basement membrane exfoliation syndrome. *Archives of Ophthalmology*, Vol.97, No.3, (March 1979), pp. 510-515.

Fitzsimmons, T.D., Fagerholm, P., & Wallin, O. (1997). Hyaluronan in the exfoliation syndrome. *Acta Ophthalmologica Scandinavica*, Vol.75, No.3, (June 1997), pp. 257-260.

Forsius, H. (1988). Exfoliation syndrome in various ethnic populations. *Acta Ophthalmologica*, Vol.66 (Suppl 184), (March 1988), pp. 71-85.

Garner, A., & Alexander, R.A. (1984). Pseudoexfoliative disease: histochemical evidence of an affinity with zonular fibres. *British Journal of Ophthalmology*, Vol.68, No.8, (August 1984), pp. 574-580.

Gartaganis, S.P., Georgakopoulos, C.D., Exarchou, A.M., Mela, E.K., Lamari, F., & Karamanos, N.K. (2001). Increased aqueous humor basic fibroblast growth factor and hyaluronan levels in relation to the exfoliation syndrome and exfoliative glaucoma. *Acta Ophthalmologica Scandinavica*, Vol.79, No.6, (December 2001), pp. 572-575.

Gartaganis, S.P., Georgakopoulos, C.D., Mela, E.K., Exarchou, A., Ziouti, N., Assouti, M., & Vynios, D.H. (2002). Matrix metalloproteinases and their inhibitors in exfoliation syndrome. *Ophthalmic Research*, Vol.34, No.3, (May-June 2002), pp. 165-171.

Gartaganis, S.P., Georgakopoulos, C.D., Patsoukis, N.E., Gotsis, S.S., Gartaganis, V.S., & Georgiou, C.D. (2005). Glutathione and lipid peroxide changes in pseudoexfoliation syndrome. *Current Eye Research*, Vol.30, No.8, (January 2005), pp. 647-651.

Gartaganis, S.P., Patsoukis, N.E., Nikolopoulos, D.K., & Georgiou, C.D. (2007). Evidence for oxidative stress in lens epithelial cells in pseudoexfoliation syndrome. *Eye*, Vol.21, No.11, (November 2007), pp. 1406-1411.

Gimbel, H.V., Condon, G.P., Kohnen, T., Olson, R.J., & Halkiadakis, I. (2005). Late in-the-bag intraocular lens dislocation: incidence, prevention, and management. *Journal of Cataract & Refractive Surgery*, Vol.31, No.11, (November 2005), pp. 2193–2204.

Gross, J.G., Kokame, G.T., & Weinberg, D.V. (2004). In-the-bag intraocular lens dislocation. *American Journal of Ophthalmology*, Vol.137, No.4, (April 2004), pp. 630–635.

Gulkilik, G., Kocabora, S., Taskapili, M., & Engin, G. (2006). Cystoid macular edema after phacoemulsification: risk factors and effect on visual acuity. *Canadian Journal of Ophthalmology*, Vol.41, No.6, (December 2006), pp. 699–703.

Handa, J., Henry, J.C., Krupin, T., & Keates, E. (1987). Extracapsular cataract extraction with posterior chamber lens implantation in patients with glaucoma. *Archives of Ophthalmology*, Vol.105, No.6, (June 1987), pp. 765–769.

Harnisch, J.P., Barrach, H.J., Hassell, J.R., & Sinha, P.K. (1981). Identification of a basement membrane proteoglycan in exfoliation material. *Graefe's Archives for Clinical and Experimental Ophthalmology*, Vol.215, No.4, (January 1981), pp. 273-278.

Hasanee, K., & Ahmed, I.I.K. (2006). Capsular tension rings: update on endocapsular support devices. *Ophthalmology Clinics of North America*, Vol.19, No.4, (December 2006), pp. 507–519.

Hasanee, K., Butler, M., & Ahmed, I.I.K. (2006). Capsular tension rings and related devices: current concepts. *Current Opinion in Ophthalmology*, Vol.17, No.1, (February 2006), pp. 31–41.

Hayashi, H., Hayashi, K., Nakao, F., & Hayashi, F. (1998). Anterior capsule contraction and intraocular lens dislocation in eyes with pseudoexfoliation syndrome. *British Journal of Ophthalmology*, Vol.82, No.12, (December 1998), pp. 1429–1432.

Herbst, R.W. (1976). Angle closure glaucoma in a patient with pseudoexfoliation of the lens capsule. *Annals of Ophthalmology*, Vol.8, No.7, (July 1976), pp. 853–856.

Hietanen, J., Kivela, T., Vesti, E., & Tarkkanen, A. (1992). Exfoliation syndrome in patients scheduled for cataract surgery. *Acta Ophthalmologica (Copenh)*, Vol.70, No.4, (August 1992), pp. 440-446.

Hyams, M., Mathalone, N., Herskovitz, M., Hod, Y., Israeli, D., & Geyer, O. (2005). Intraoperative complications of phacoemulsification in eyes with and without pseudoexfoliation. *Journal of Cataract & Refractive Surgery*, Vol.31, (May 2005), pp. 1002–1005.

Issa, S.A., Pacheco, J., Mahmood, U., Nolan, J., & Beatty, S. (2005). A novel index for predicting intraocular pressure reduction following cataract surgery. *British Journal of Ophthalmology*, Vol.89, No.5, (May 2005), pp. 543–546.

Jacobs, D.S., Cox, T.A., Wagoner, M.D., Ariyasu, R.G., & Karp, C.L. (2006). Capsule staining as an adjunct to cataract surgery; a report from the American Academy of Ophthalmology (Ophthalmic Technology Assessment). *Ophthalmology*, Vol.113, No.4, (April 2006), pp. 703–713.

Jehan, F.S., Mamalis, N., & Crandall, A.S. (2001). Spontaneous late dislocation of intraocular lens within the capsular bag in pseudoexfoliation patients. *Ophthalmology*, Vol.108, No.10, (October 2001), pp. 1727–1731.

Kaljurand, K., & Teesalu, P. (2007). Exfoliation syndrome as a risk factor for corneal endothelial cell loss in cataract surgery. *Annals of Ophthalmology*, Vol.39, No.4, (December 2007), pp. 327–333.

Kato, S., Suzuki, T., Hayashi, Y., Numaga, J., Hattori, T., Yuguchi, T., Kaiya, T., & Oshika, T. (2002). Risk factors for contraction of the anterior capsule opening after cataract surgery. *Journal of Cataract & Refractive Surgery*, Vol.28, No.1, (January 2002), pp. 109–112.

Keates, R.H., & McGowan, K.A. (1984). The effect of topical indomethacin ophthalmic solution in maintaining mydriasis during cataract surgery. *Annals of Ophthalmology*, Vol.16, No.12, (December 1984), pp. 1116-1121.

Kimura, W., Yamanishi, S., Kimura, T., Sawada, T., & Ohte, A. (1998). Measuring the anterior capsule opening after cataract surgery to assess capsule shrinkage. *Journal of Cataract & Refractive Surgery*, Vol.24, No.9, (September 1998), pp. 1235–1238.

Koliakos, G.G., Konstas, A.G.P., Schlötzer-Schrehardt, U., Hollo, G., Katsimbris, I.E., Georgiadis, N., & Ritch, R. (2003). 8-Isoprostaglandin F2a and ascorbic acid concentration in the aqueous humour of patients with exfoliation syndrome. *British Journal of Ophthalmology*, Vol.87, No.3, (March 2003), pp. 353-356.

Konstas, A.G., Marshall, G.E., & Lee, W.R. (1990). Immunogold localisation of laminin in normal and exfoliative iris. *British Journal of Ophthalmology*, Vol.74, No.8, (August 1990), pp. 450-457.

Kubota, T., Khalil, A., Tawara, A., Zhang, X., & Inomata, H. (1998). Double staining of proteoglycans and the HNK-1 carbohydrate epitope in pseudoexfoliation material. *Current Eye Research*, Vol.17, No.1, (January 1998), pp. 60-64.

Küchle, M., Amberg, A., Martus, P., Nguyen, N.X., & Naumann, G.O.H. (1997). Pseudoexfoliation syndrome and secondary cataract. *British Journal of Ophthalmology*, Vol.81, No.10, (October 1997), pp.862–866.

Küchle, M., Viestenz, A., Martus, P., Handel, A., Junemann, A., & Naumann, G.O.H. (2000). Anterior chamber depth and complications during cataract surgery in eyes with pseudoexfoliation syndrome. *American Journal of Ophthalmology*, Vol.129, No.3, (March 2000), pp. 281-285.

Lee, V., & Bloom, P. (1999). Microhook capsule stabilization for phacoemulsification in eyes with pseudoexfoliation-syndrome-induced lens instability. *Journal of Cataract & Refractive Surgery*, Vol.25, No.12, (December 1999), pp. 1567–1570.

Lee, D.-H., Shin, S.-C., & Joo, C.-K. (2002). Effect of a capsular tension ring on intraocular lens decentration and tilting after cataract surgery. *Journal of Cataract & Refractive Surgery*, Vol.28, No.5, (May 2002), pp. 843–846.

Menapace, R., Findl, O., Georgopoulos, M., Rainer, G., Vass, C., & Schmetterer, K. (2000). The capsular tension ring: designs, applications, and techniques. *Journal of Cataract & Refractive Surgery*, Vol.26, No.6, (June 2000), pp. 898–912.

Moreno, J., Duch, S., & Lajara, J. (1993). Pseudoexfoliation syndrome: clinical factors related to capsular rupture in cataract surgery. *Acta Ophthalmologica*, Vol.71, No.2, (April 1993), pp. 181-184.

Naumann, G.O.H., & Schlötzer-Schrehardt, U. (2000). Keratopathy in pseudoexfoliation syndrome as a cause of corneal endothelial decompensation. A clinicopathologic study. *Ophthalmology*, Vol.107, No.6, (June 2000), pp. 1111–1124.

Netland, P.A., Ye, H., Streeten, B.W., & Hernandez, M.R. (1995). Elastosis of the lamina cribrosa in pseudoexfoliation syndrome with glaucoma. *Ophthalmology*, Vol.102, No.6, (June 1995), pp. 878-886.

Pohjalainen, T., Vesti, E., Uusitalo, R.J., & Laatikainen, L. (2001). Intraocular pressure after phacoemulsification and intraocular lens implantation in nonglaucomatous eyes with and without exfoliation. *Journal of Cataract & Refractive Surgery*, Vol.27, No.3, (March 2001), pp. 426–431.

Poley, B.J., Lindstrom, R.L., & Samuelson, T.W. (2008). Long-term effects of phacoemulsification with intraocular lens implantation in normotensive and ocular hypertensive eyes. *Journal of Cataract & Refractive Surgery*, Vol.34, No.5, (May 2008), pp. 735–742.

Puska, P. (1994). Lens opacity in unilateral exfoliation syndrome with or without glaucoma. *Acta Ophthalmologica*, Vol.72, No.3, (June 1994), pp. 290-296

Repo, L.P., Suhonen, M.T., Terasvirta, M.E., & Koivisto, K.J. (1995). Color Doppler imaging of the ophthalmic artery blood flow spectra of patients who have had a transient ischemic attack: Correlations with generalized iris transluminance and pseudoexfoliation syndrome. *Ophthalmology*, Vol.102, No.8, (August 1995), pp. 1199-1205.

Ringvold, A., & Vegge, T. (1971). Electron microscopy of the trabecular meshwork in eyes with exfoliation syndrome (pseudoexfoliation of the lens capsule). *Virchows Archiv Abteilung A Pathologische Anatomie*, Vol.353, No.2, (June 1971), pp. 110-127.

Ringvold, A. (1999). Epidemiology of the pseudoexfoliation syndrome. A review. *Acta Ophthalmolodica Scandinavica*, Vol.77, No.4, (August 1999), pp. 371-375.

Ritch, R. (1994a). Exfoliation syndrome—the most common identifiable cause of open-angle glaucoma. *Journal of Glaucoma*, Vol.3, No.2, (Summer 1994), pp. 176–178

Ritch, R. (1994b). Exfoliation syndrome and occludable angles. *Transactions of the American Ophthalmological Society*, Vol.92, pp. 845–944.

Ritch, R., & Schlötzer-Schrehardt, U. (2001). Exfoliation syndrome. *Survey of Ophthalmology*, Vol.45, No.4, (January 2001), pp. 265-315.

Santoro, S., Sannace, C., Cascella, M.C., & Lavermicocca, N. (2003). Subluxated lens: phacoemulsification with iris hooks. *Journal of Cataract & Refractive Surgery*, Vol.29, No.12, (December 2003), pp. 2269–2273.

Schlötzer-Schrehardt, U.M., Koca, M.R., Naumann, G.O.H., & Volkholz, H. (1992a). Pseudoexfoliation syndrome. Ocular manifestation of a systemic disorder? *Archives of Ophthalmology*, Vol.110, No.12, (December 1992), pp. 1752-1756.

Schlötzer-Schrehardt, U., Dorfler, S., & Naumann, G.O.H. (1992b). Immunohistochemical localization of basement membrane components in pseudoexfoliation material of the lens capsule. *Current Eye Research*, Vol.11, No.4, (April 1992), pp. 343-355.

Schlötzer-Schrehardt, U.M., & Naumann, G.O. (1994). A histopathologic study of zonular instability in pseudoexfoliation syndrome. *American Journal of Ophthalmology*, Vol.118, No.6, (December 1994), pp. 730-743.

Schlötzer-Schrehardt, U.M., & Naumann, G.O.H. (1995). Trabecular meshwork in pseudoexfoliation syndrome with and without open-angle glaucoma. A morphometric, ultrastructural study. *Investigative Ophthalmology and Visual Science*, Vol.36, No.9, (August 1995), pp. 1750-1764.

Schlötzer-Schrehardt, U.M., & Naumann, G.O.H. (2006). Ocular and systemic pseudoexfoliation syndrome. *American Journal of Ophthalmology*, Vol.141, No. 5 (May 2006), pp. 921-937.

Schlötzer-Schrehardt, U. (2009). Molecular pathology of pseudoexfoliation syndrome/ glaucoma - New insights from LOXL1 gene associations. *Experimental Eye Research*, Vol.88, No.4, (April 2009), pp. 776-785.

Shingleton, B.J., Gamell, L.S., O'Donoghue, M.W., Baylus, S.L., & King, R. (1999). Long-term changes in intraocular pressure after clear corneal phacoemulsification: normal

patients versus glaucoma suspect and glaucoma patients. *Journal of Cataract & Refractive Surgery*, Vol.25, No.7, (July 1999), pp. 885–890.
Shingleton, B.J., Heltzer, J., & O'Donoghue, M.W. (2003). Outcomes of phacoemulsification in patients with and without pseudoexfoliation syndrome. *Journal of Cataract & Refractive Surgery*, Vol.29, No.6, (June 2003), pp. 1080–1086.
Shingleton, B.J., Laul, A., Nagao, K., Wolff, B., O'Donoghue, M., Eagan, E., Flattem, N., & Desai-Bartoli, S. (2008). Effect of phacoemulsification on intraocular pressure in eyes with pseudoexfoliation: single-surgeon series. *Journal of Cataract & Refractive Surgery*, Vol.34, No.11, (November 2008), pp. 1834–1841.
Shingleton, B.J., Crandall, A.S., & Ahmed, I.I.K. (2009). Pseudoexfoliation and the cataract surgeon: Preoperative, intraoperative, and postoperative issues related to intraocular pressure, cataract, and intraocular lenses. *Journal of Cataract & Refractive Surgery*, Vol.35, No.6, (June 2009), pp. 1101–1120.
Streeten, B.W., Gibson, S.A., & Dark, A.J. (1986). Pseudoexfoliative material contains an elastic microfibrillar-associated glycoprotein. *Transactions of the American Ophthalmological Society*, Vol.84, pp. 304-317.
Streeten, B.W., Li, Z.Y., Wallace, R.N., Eagle, R.C., & Keshgegian, A.A. (1992). Pseudoexfoliative fibrillopathy in visceral organs of a patient with pseudoexfoliation syndrome. *Archives of Ophthalmology*, Vol.110, No.12, (December 1992), pp. 1757-1762.
Tanhehco, T., & Chen, S.H. (2010). Pseudoexfoliation syndrome and cataract surgery. *International Ophthalmology Clinics*, Vol.50, No.1, (Winter 2010), pp. 81-93.
Tawara, A., Fujisawa, K., Kiyosawa, R., & Inomata, H. (1996). Distribution and characterization of proteoglycans associated with exfoliation material. *Current Eye Research*, Vol.15, No.11, (November 1996), pp. 1101-1111.
Thorleifsson, G., Magnusson, K.P., Sulem, P., Walters, G.B., Gudbjartsson, D.F., Stefansson, H., Jonsson, T., Jonasdottir, A., Jonasdottir, A., Stefansdottir, G., Masson, G., Hardarson, G.A., Petursson, H., Arnarsson, A., Motallebipour, M., Wallerman, O., Wadelius, C., Gulcher, J.R., Thorsteinsdottir, U., Kong, A., Jonasson, F., & Stefansson, K. (2007). Common sequence variants in the LOXL1 gene confer susceptibility to exfoliation glaucoma. *Science*, Vol.317, No.5843, (September 2007), pp. 1397-1400.
Vasavada, A.R., Singh, R., Apple, D.J., Trivedi, R.H., Pandey, S.K., & Werner, L. (2002). Effect of hydrodissection on intraoperative performance: randomized study. *Journal of Cataract & Refractive Surgery*, Vol.28, No.9, (September 2002), pp. 1623–1628.
Vesti, E., & Kivelä, T. (2000). Exfoliation syndrome and exfoliation glaucoma. *Progress in Retinal and Eye Research*, Vol.19, No.3, (May 2000), pp. 345-368.
Wagoner, M.D., Cox, T.A., Ariyasu, R.G., Jacobs, D.S., & Karp, C.L. (2003). Intraocular lens implantation in the absence of capsular support; a report by the American Academy of Ophthalmology. *Ophthalmology*, Vol.110, No.4, (April 2003), pp. 840–859.
Werner, L., Pandey, S.K., Escobar-Gomez, M., Visessook, N., Peng, Q., & Apple, D.J. (2000). Anterior capsule opacification: a histopathological study comparing different IOL styles. *Ophthalmology*, Vol.107, No.3, (March 2000), pp. 463–471.

Yüksel, N., Doğu, B., Karabaş, V.L., & Çağlar, Y. (2008). Foveal thickness after phacoemulsification in patients with pseudoexfoliation syndrome, pseudoexfoliation glaucoma, or primary open-angle glaucoma. *Journal of Cataract & Refractive Surgery*, Vol.34, No.11, (November 2008), pp. 1953–1957.

27

Cataract Surgery in Patients with a History of Retinoblastoma and Melanoma

A.C. Schefler and T.G. Murray
Bascom Palmer Eye Institute, Department of Ophthalmology, University of Miami Miller School of Medicine
USA

1. Introduction

Both pediatric and adult malignant intraocular ocular tumors are often treated with external beam radiation or brachytherapy. Because the lens is the most radiosensitive ocular structure, cataracts are a common occurrence after such treatments. Some studies report up to an 87% occurrence of cataracts within 3 years in retinoblastoma patients treated with external beam radiation (Blach et al., 1996; Fontanesi et al., 1996). In the Collaborative Ocular Melanoma Study, the largest multicenter prospective randomized trial ever performed for uveal melanoma patients, 83% of patients had developed cataracts by 5 years post-treatment (Collaborative Ocular Melanoma Study Group, 2007). Because many patients treated for intraocular tumors survive for extended periods and have the capacity for excellent vision, cataract surgery is an important part of the treatment algorithm for these patients. However, this group of patients poses a unique set of surgical challenges not present in standard cataract patients. In this chapter, we will review the incidence, surgical techniques, visual and anatomic outcomes, and complications for this unique group of patients.

2. Cataracts in retinoblastoma patients

2.1 Epidemiology

2.1.1 Incidence

Cataract is a well-known complication after radiation to the eye after all forms of radiation. Many studies have indicated that after external beam radiation therapy, cataracts can develop after doses as low as 2 Gy (Dynlacht, 2006; Gordon, 1995). For over 100 years, external beam radiation has been used to treat retinoblastoma because in certain cases, it can achieve tumor control and enable retention of vision when other treatment modalities have failed (Chodick et al., 2009). Although other treatment modalities such as chemotherapy and laser are more commonly used for retinoblastoma patients at the present time, external beam radiation is still used as salvage therapy in advanced cases. Furthermore, many patients who received external beam radiation in the past are still under the care of ophthalmic oncologists and are currently in need of or will need cataract surgery in the future. Chodick et al. examined the records of a series of 753 patients who were diagnosed with retinoblastoma from 1914 to 1984. Only one patient who had not had radiotherapy had cataract surgery while 51 cataract surgeries were performed in patients who had had radiation. Overall, Kaplan-Meier analysis demonstrated that after 40 years of follow-up, 77% of eyes with 2 or 3 radiotherapy treatments underwent cataract surgery. The estimated survival time to cataract surgery in eyes that did not undergo radiation was 71.7 years compared to 50.8 years and 31.6 years for eyes treated with one and 2 or 3 radiotherapy treatments, respectively. Of note, many patients in this study underwent older forms of treatment with more radiation scatter such as orthovoltage radiation and cobalt plaques. Nonetheless, the incidence of cataracts requiring cataract surgery in retinoblastoma survivors was high and underscored the necessity for ongoing ophthalmic follow-up in these patients.

2.1.2 Risk factors

In the study by Chodick et al., the clinical risk factors that contributed to cataract development requiring cataract surgery were: increased number of external beam radiation treatments, diagnosis of retinoblastoma after the first year of life (versus earlier), and radiation dose. No other studies published up until this point have had extended follow-up or enough power to assess the risk factors for cataract development adequately.

2.2 Visual and anatomic results

2.2.1 Visual results

There have been several studies examining the visual outcomes in retinoblastoma survivors who have undergone cataract surgery (Table 1).

The data from Table 1 suggests that visual outcomes in these patients can be surprisingly excellent. In particular, the studies by Miller et al. (2005), Payne et al. (2008), and Hoehn et al. (2010) reported good visual results and no major complications. Patients in this population have many other reasons to have poor visual outcomes including tumor involvement of the macula, radiation retinopathy, progressive retinal scarring from laser or cryotherapy treatments, and amblyopia.

2.3 Surgical approach and complications

Controversies in pediatric cataract management include the surgical approach, management of the posterior capsule and anterior vitreous, and IOL implantation. Table 1 demonstrates that there has been a wide range of approaches to these controversies in retinoblastoma patients. Our group, Miller et al. (2005) reported good visual and anatomic results in 16 patients after ECCE/PPV/PCIOL. Payne et al. (2008) also reported good results with an ECCE approach with a capsulotomy, anterior vitrectomy, and IOL placed only in some patients. In contrast, Hoehn et al. (2010) reported outstanding results with only a lens aspiration and IOL with no posterior capsulotomy, deferring this procedure to a later EUA when needed.

The major concern for patients undergoing any intraocular procedure who have a history of retinoblastoma is tumor recurrence or the development of metastatic disease as a result of the surgery. Recurrences have been reported in series by Brooks et al. (1990), Honovar et al. (2005), Moshfeghi et al. (2005), and Osman et al. (2011). All of these series included patients who had short quiescent intervals from the time of attainment of local control of the retinoblastoma and cataract surgery, sometimes as short as 3 months. It seems that a longer quiescent interval is the only identifiable risk factor for this devastating complication. In patients with a short quiescent interval whose fundus cannot be visualized due to a dense cataract, we strongly recommend enucleation rather than performing cataract surgery with its associated risk of tumor recurrence which may or may not be able to be adequately treated.

Author, Year	**No. of eyes**	**Median Quiescent interval (Range)**	**Procedure (No. of eyes)**	**Median follow up, mos (range)**	**No. of RB recur-ences**	**Visual outcome (No. of eyes)**
Monge et al., 1986	2	30 mos (72 mos)	Asp ± PPV	(24-78)	0	6/18 (2)
Brooks et al., 1990	42	29 mos (17-144)	Asp or PPL	72 (6-178)	3	20/20-20/50 (19) 20/80-CF (12)
Portellos & Buckley, 1998	11	55 mos (16-88)	ECCE + caps+Ant Vtx + PCIOL	Mean 20 (6-39	0	20/20-20/30 (6) 20/50-20/250 (5)
Madreperla et al., 2000	3	34 mos (9-40 mos)	Asp	(60-189)	0	20/60 (2); HM (1)
Bhattacharjee et al., 2003	1	84 mos	ECCE+Caps+ PCIOL	144	0	20/30
Shanmugam et al., 2004	5	Minimum 24 mos	Phaco+caps+ Ant Vtx+PCIOL	NA	0	>6/9 (4) at 6 wks
Sinha et al., 2004	9	Minimum 12 mos	Asp	(24-42)	0	"No improvement"
Miller et al., 2005	16	Minimum 18 mos	ECCE+PPV+P CIOL	Mean 66 (30-94)	0	20/20-20/40 (11) 20/200-20/400 (5)
Honovar et al., 2005	34	16 mos (3-54 mos)	ICCE; ECCE; PPL	72 (12-360)	5	>20/200 (12)
Moshfeghi et al., 2005	4	89 mos (12-172 mos)	NA	Mean 184 (60-339)	1	20/30; CF; HM; Enuc
Payne et al., 2008	12	35 mos (17-240)	ECCE ± caps ± Ant Vtx ± PCIOL	72 (13-148)	0	20/20-20/60 (6) 20/70-20/200 (2) CF (2) HM (2)
Hoehn et al., 2010	19	NA	Asp + IOL	Mean 58 (19-105)	0	20/20-20/60 (3) 20/70-20/200 (4) 20/400 (4) CF (5) HM (1) F+F (1) Enuc (1)
Osman et al., 2011	21	21.5 ms (3-164 mos)	ECCE or Asp ± caps ± Ant Vtx ± IOL	Mean 90 ± 69	3	20/20 (4) 20/20-20/200 (9) <20/200 (2) NLP (3) NA (3)

Table 1. Reports of cataract surgery in patients with a history of retinoblastoma. Modified and adapted from Payne et al. (2009). NA, Data not reported; Ant Vtx, anterior vitrectomy; ECCE, extracapsular cataract extraction; ICCE, intracapsular cataract extraction; IOL, posterior chamber intraocular lens; Phaco, phacoemulsification; PPL, pars plana lensectomy; NLP, no light perception; HM, hand motion; CF, count fingers.

3. Cataracts in uveal melanoma patients

3.1 Epidemiology

3.1.1 Incidence

There have been several studies examining the incidence and risk factors for the development of cataracts after Iodine 125 brachytherapy, the most commonly employed treatment for uveal melanoma in the United States (Table 1). Taking these studies as a group, approximately 40% of all patients have been reported to develop cataracts with most studies having a follow-up period of 5 years. Among these studies, however, the Collaborative Ocular Melanoma Study trial was the only prospective, multicenter trial and the rate of cataract development in this study was much higher, 83% by 5 years.

Author, Year	No. of patients at risk/No. of cataracts	Rate of cataract development	Follow-up time Median (Range)	Time to cataract development Median (Range)	Risk factors for cataract development
Garretson et al., 1987	26/3	NA	Mean 45 mos (≥ 2 yrs)	NA	NA
Bosworth et al., 1988	58/13	NA	Mean 48.7 (23-112)	NA	NA
Lean et al., 1990	56/20	NA	Mean 39 mos (20-57)	NA	NA
Mameghan et al., 1992	53/4	NA	NA	NA	NA
Quivey et al., 1993	239/33	25-50% by 5 yrs	NA, (2-10 yrs)	9-81 mos	NA
Shields et al., 2002	270/NA	2% at 2 yrs, 6% at 5 yrs	NA	NA	NA
Bechrakis et al., 2002	152/5	28%	33 mos	NA	NA
Fontanesi et al., 1993	144/43	NA	46 mos (25-90)	3-53 mos	Tumor location
Puusari et al., 2004	96/65	2% by 2 yrs	NA	Median 18 mos	Dose to lens, age, diabetes
Puusari et al., 2004	89/57	69% by 3 yrs	3.5 yrs (0.3-10.4)	<1-8 yrs	NA
Lumbroso-Le Rouic et al., 2004	NA	21% by 2 yrs, 50% by 5 yrs	NA	NA	Gender, age, diameter
Stack et al., 2005	92/9	11%	31 mos (4-86)	NA	NA
COMS, 2007	538/362	83% by 5 yrs	NA (data not provided in this format)	2.5 yrs (6 mos-5 yrs)	Age, Baseline tumor size, Dose to lens
Meta-analysis	1543/614	40%	-	-	-

Table 2. Rates of Cataract Development after Cataract from Iodine 125 Brachytherapy for Uveal Melanoma. Updated and Adapted from Collaborative Ocular Melanoma Study Group (2007). NA, Data not reported.

3.1.2 Risk factors

The number of studies reporting risk factors for cataract development after Iodine 125 brachytherapy is limited. Overall, a review of the literature indicates that cataractogenesis is likely a function of tumor size, tumor location, radiation dose, and patient age. There appears to be no obvious advantage to any particular form of radiation (i.e. Cobalt 60, Ruthenium 106, proton beam therapy) (Collaborative Ocular Melanoma Study, 2007).

3.2 Visual and anatomic results

3.2.1 Visual results

Several studies have reported on visual acuity results after cataract surgery. In the Collaborative Ocular Melanoma Study, in patients with medium-sized tumors undergoing cataract surgery, the median best corrected visual acuity at baseline was 20/25 (Collaborative Ocular Melanoma Study Group, 2007). In the group that underwent cataract surgery, the median visual acuity before surgery was 20/125 (range 20/25< 20/1600) and median visual acuity at the study visit immediately after cataract surgery was 20/50 (range 20/20-20/1600). In the study, 32 of the 48 eyes (66%) had improved vision of greater than or equal to 2 lines, 13 eyes (27%) remained stable, and 3 (6%) had decreased vision of greater than or equal to 2 lines at final follow-up. Figure 1 demonstrates the change in visual acuity in the 3 months after cataract surgery in patients in the Collaborative Ocular Melanoma Study.

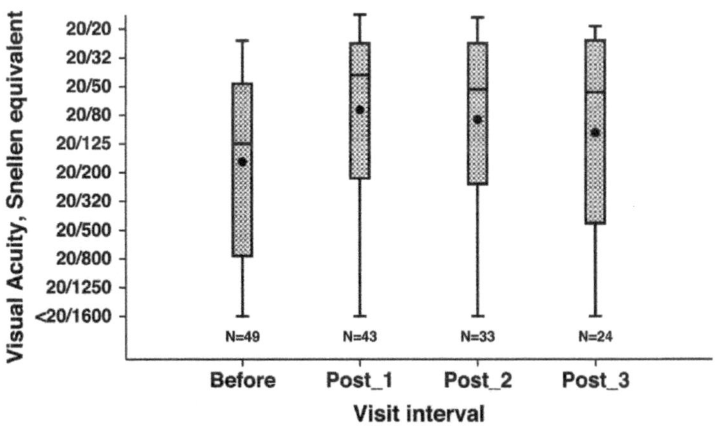

Fig. 1. Patients' visual acuity before and in the 3 visits after cataract surgery in the Collaborative Ocular Melanoma Study. The dot represents the mean of the box and the range of the box extends from the 25th percentile to the 75th percentile. The whiskers extend up to 1.5 times with interquartile range from each end of the box. Reproduced with permission from Collaborative Ocular Melanoma Study (2007).

Our group investigated visual acuity outcomes in patients undergoing cataract surgery with injection of intravitreal triamcinolone injection (Cebulla et al., 2008). In this study, 51 eyes of 49 patients with a history of choroidal nevi or uveal melanoma underwent cataract surgery with injection of intravitreal triamcinolone (IVTA) during surgery. There were 30 patients who had had a history of melanoma treated with Iodine-125 brachytherapy in the cohort. Among the melanoma patients, the visual acuity at 6 months after surgery was worse in 2 patients (11%), stable in 2 patients (11%), and better in 14 patients (78%). At the final follow-up, vision was worse in 3 patients (10%), stable in 7 patients (24%), and better in 19 patients (66%). The mean number of Snellen lines gained after surgery was 3.9 ± 3.8 (SD) at 6 months and 3.1 ± 3.8 at last follow up (both $p<0.001$). This data compares favorably to the data outlined above and from Gragoudas et al. (1992), the largest study published to date in patients undergoing proton beam radiotherapy (Figures 2A-2G).

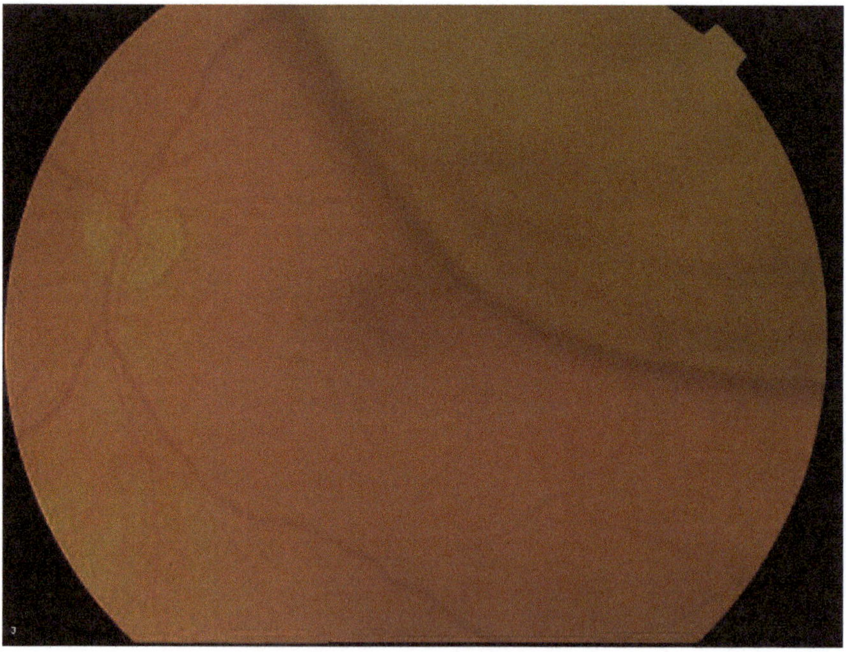

Fig. 2A. Patient with uveal melanoma at the time of diagnosis. Visual acuity was 20/40.

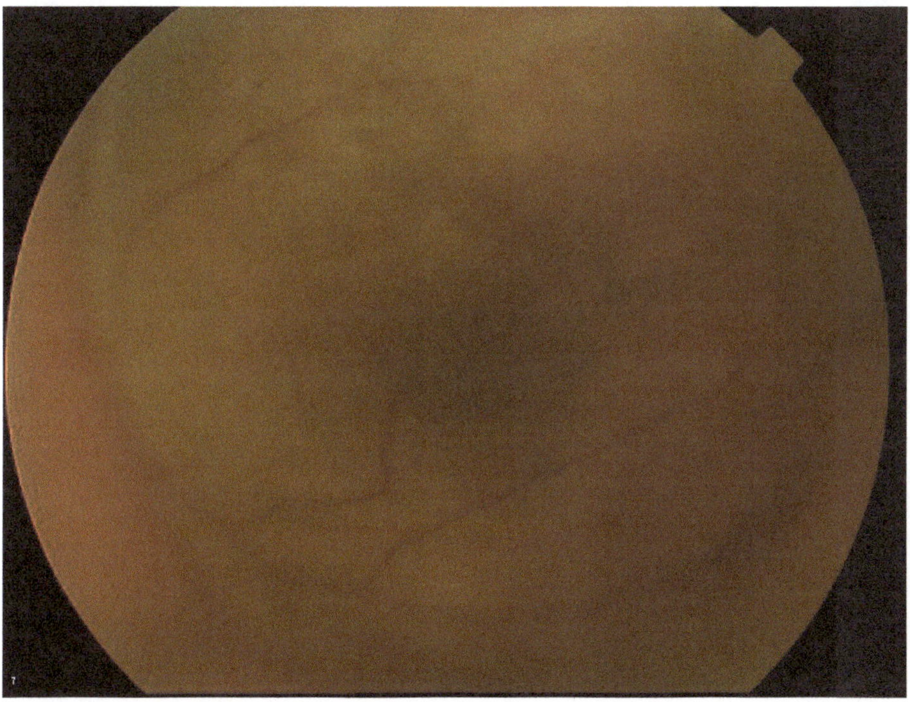

Fig. 2B. Photo of tumor apex of patient in Figure 2A at diagnosis.

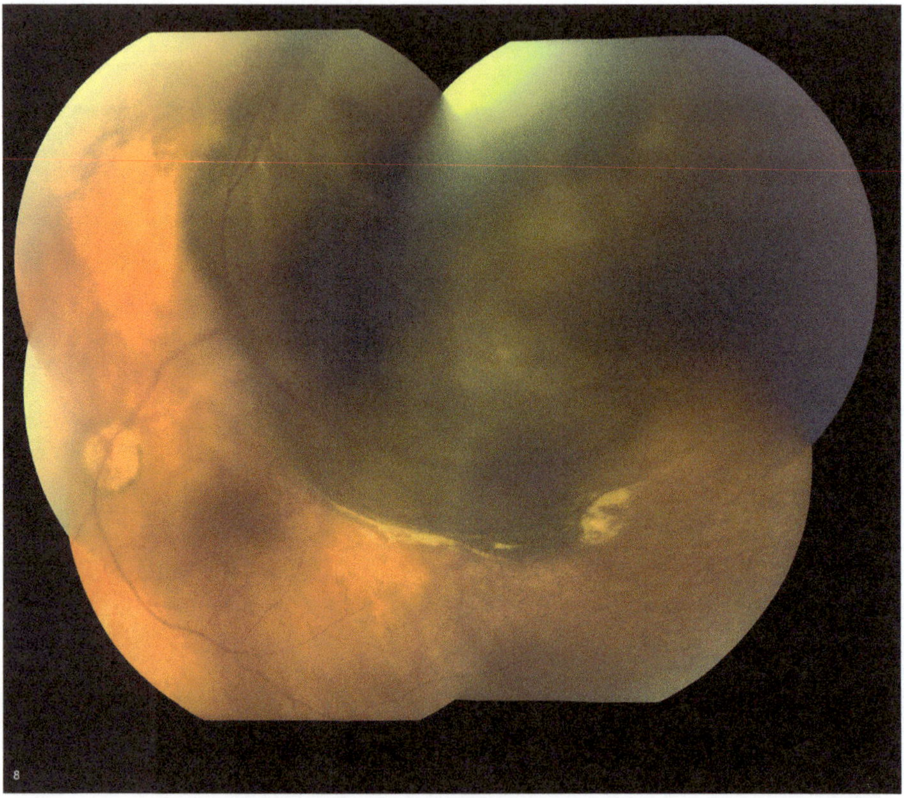

Fig. 2C. Patient in Figure 2A, 21 months after diagnosis. Note the yellow hue of the photograph and inability to visual the macula and optic nerve well to assess radiation retinopathy. The vision was 20/80. The patient subsequently underwent cataract surgery with intravitreal triamcinolone acetonide.

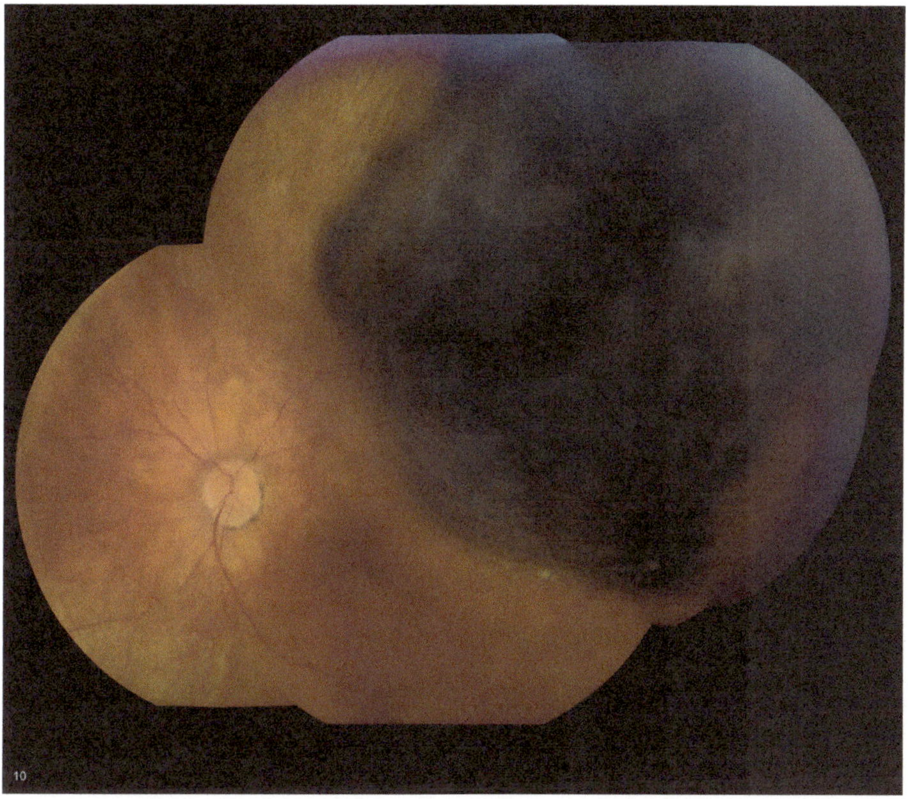

Fig. 2D. Patient in Figure 2C after cataract surgery. Note the increased ability to visualize the macula and optic nerve. The patient's best corrected vision improved to 20/60.

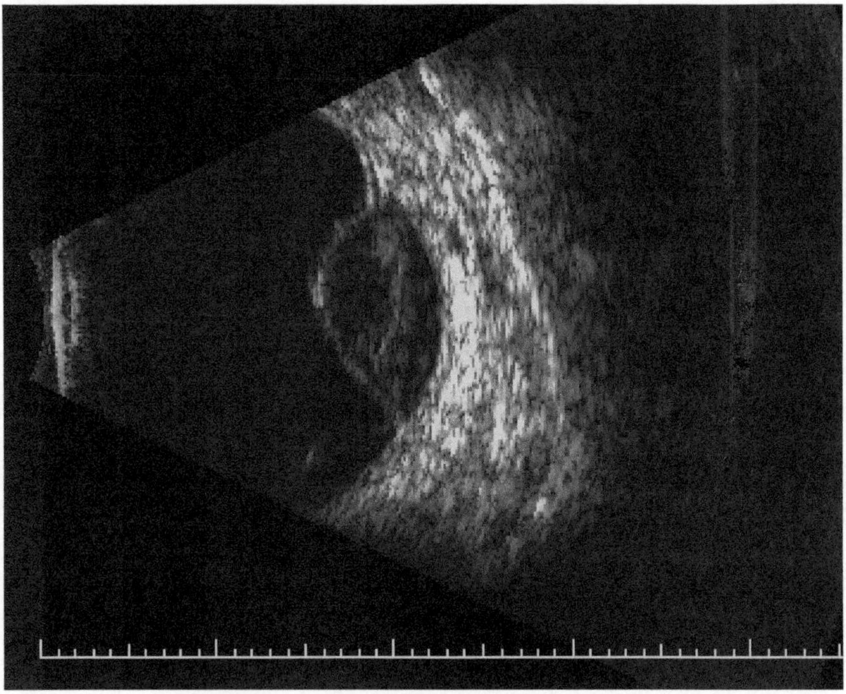

Fig. 2E. B-scan ultrasound of the tumor in Figure 2A at diagnosis with an apical height of 7.5 mm.

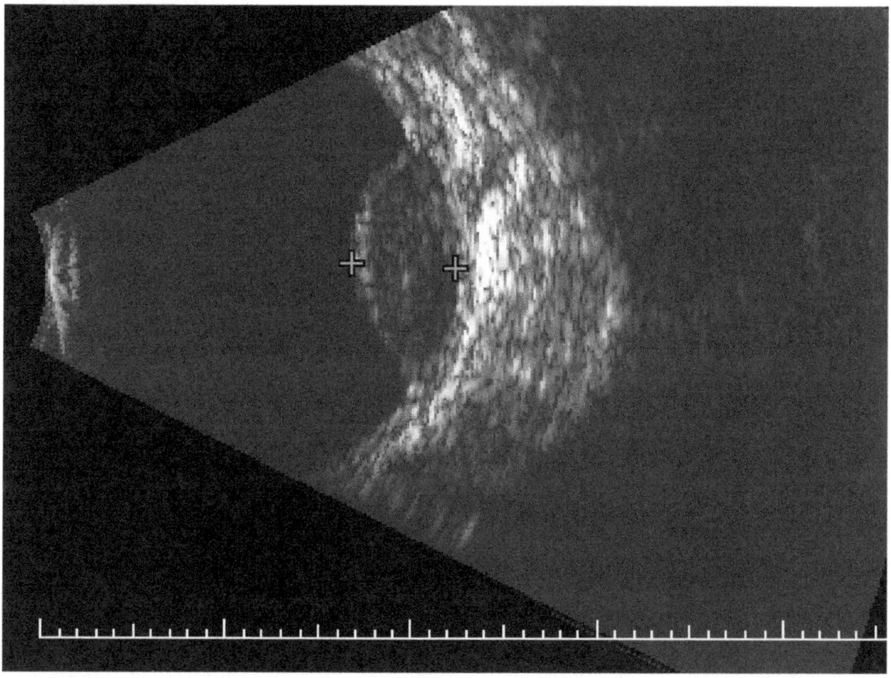

Fig. 2F. B-scan ultrasound of the tumor in Figure 2E after plaque surgery just before cataract surgery with an apical height of 5.8 mm.

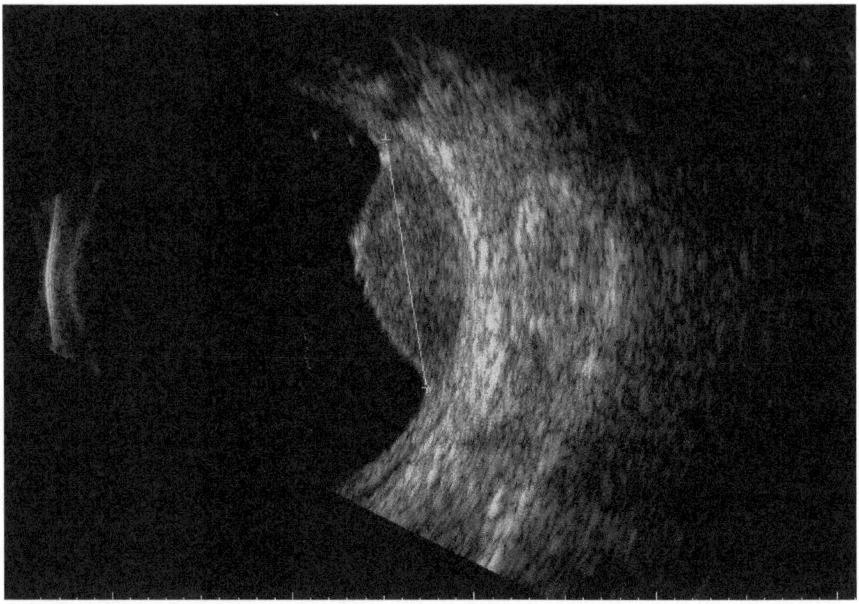

Fig. 2G. B-scan ultrasound of the tumor in Figure 2E eight months after cataract surgery. The tumor's apical height has decreased further to 5.6 mm.

3.2.2 Anatomic outcomes

The study by our group published in 2008 is the only study to our knowledge which has addressed the issue of anatomic changes induced in the treated melanoma as a result of cataract surgery (Cebulla et al., 2008). In this study, cataract surgery was combined with intravitreal triamcinolone (IVTA) at the time of surgery. Triamcinolone was chosen because it has been demonstrated to inhibit angiogenesis and to have direct antineoplastic activity (DiSorbo et al., 1986; Ebrahem et al., 2006). Furthermore, triamcinolone acetonide has been used to decrease radiation retinopathy and optic neuropathy in eyes with uveal melanoma treated with plaque therapy (Shields et al., 2006). In the study, echographic measurements of patients' tumors were followed in melanoma patients after cataract surgery-IVTA. This analysis demonstrated that 12 (46%) of 26 melanomas diminished in size over a median follow-up period of 11.8 months (range, 1-26 months). Regression analysis demonstrated a shallow but statistically significant ($p=0.039$) negative slope in tumor height after cataract surgery-IVTA. Tumor growth did not occur in any patients. It was difficult to determine if this effect was due to a continuing effect from previous brachytherapy, although the median interval between plaque therapy and cataract surgery was 34 months (range 7-114 months), and the majority of the decrease in tumor height typically occurs within the first 2.5 years of tumor treatment. Ultimately, in long-term follow-up, the rate of tumor recurrence in this population may be lower than the published rates of 2.0% to 19.4% (Gragoudas et al., 1992; Wachtlin et al., 2000) due to the additional antitumoral effect from the IVTA approach. Further prospective studies are needed to address this question.

3.3 Complications

The complications reported in large studies of patients undergoing cataract surgery after plaque therapy for uveal melanoma are listed in Table 3.

Author	Complication	Incidence
Cebulla et al., 2008	Tumor recurrence	0 (0%)
	Posterior capsular opacity	8 (27%)
	Cystoid macular edema	1 (3%)
COMS et al., 2007	Cystoid macular edema	13 (27%)
	Neovascular glaucoma	6 (12%)
	Retinal detachment	1 (2%)
Wachtlin et al., 2000	Enucleation required for tumor recurrence, scleral necrosis, or pain	7 (10%)
	Dislocated IOL	1 (1.4%)
	Posterior capsular opacity	8 (11%)
	Vitreous hemorrhage	4 (6%)
	Retinal detachment	2 (3%)
Gragoudas et al., 1992	Tumor recurrence	2 (3%)
	Retinal detachment	2 (3%)
	Vitreous hemorrhage	1 (1%)
	Chronic wound leak	1 (1%)
	Neovascular glaucoma	3 (4%)
	Enucleation for retinal detachment, neovascular glaucoma, pain, tumor recurrence	5 (6%)

Table 3. Complications observed after cataract surgery in patients with a history of uveal melanoma after plaque brachytherapy or proton beam radiotherapy.

Complication profiles seem to have improved over the past 20 years, likely due to the modernization of phacoemulsification techniques such as small incisions, and of the more judicious use of cataract surgery, reserving the procedure only for patients with preoperative visual potential and no pre-existing neovascular glaucoma secondary to radiation vasculopathy.

4. Conclusion

In summary, cataract surgery has been safely performed in patients with a history of both retinoblastoma and melanoma. Controversy still exists regarding the best technique in patients with a history of retinoblastoma, but we have had success with no tumor recurrences in a series of patients with long-term follow-up using a ECCE/PPV/IOL approach. Tumor recurrence is a known risk of this surgery, and patients should demonstrate a quiescent interval of at least 18 months before surgery. Visual results are largely dependent on side effects from the primary tumor. In uveal melanoma patients, cataracts are common after plaque therapy and occur on average 2.5 years after initial treatment. Most patients regain vision and vision is typically limited by radiation retinopathy, cystoid macular edema, and neovascular glaucoma. Surgical adjuncts such as IVTA may help in decreasing the inflammatory nature of these tumors and contribute to tumor regression. Further prospective studies are needed.

5. References

Blach, L. et al. (1996). External beam radiation therapy and retinoblastoma: long term results in the comparison of two techniques. *International Journal of Radiation Oncology, Biology, and Physics*, Vol. 35, pp. 45-51.

Bechrakis, N. et al. (2002). Iodine 125 plaque brachytherapy versus transcleral tumor resection in the treatment of large uveal melanomas. *Ophthalmology*, Vol. 109, pp. 1855-1861.

Bhatterjee, H. et al. Cataract surgery and intraocular lens implantation in a retinoblastoma case treated by external-beam radiation therapy. *Journal of Cataract and Refractive Surgery*, Vol. 29, 1837-1841.

Brooks, H. et al. (1990). Removal of radiation-induced cataracts in patients treated for retinoblastoma. *Archives of Ophthalmology*, Vol. 108, pp. 1701-1708.

Bosworth, J. et al. (1988). Choroidal melanoma: I-125 plaque therapy. *Radiology*, Vol. 169, 169, pp. 249-251.

Cebulla, C. et al. Tumor voume reduction with intravitreal triamcinolone. *Journal of cataract and Refractive Surgery*, Vol. 34, pp. 1669-1673.

Chodick, G. et al. (2009). Risk of cataract extraction among adult retinoblastoma survivors. *Archives of Ophthalmology, Vol. 127*, pp. 1500-1504.

Collaborative Ocular Melanoma Study Group (2007). Incidence of cataract and outcomes after cataract surgery in the first 5 years after Iodine 125 brachytherapy in the collaborative ocular melanoma study. COMS Report No. 27. *Ophthalmology*, Vol. 114, pp. 1363-1371.

DiSorbo, D. et al. (1986). Effect of triamcinolone acetonide on the growth of NEL-M1 human melanoma cells cultured in the presence and absence of growth stimulatory agents. *Cancer Research*, Vol. 46, 1986, pp. 3964-3968.

Dynlacht, J. et al. (2006). Effect of estrogen on radiation-induced cataractogenesis. *Radiation Research*, Vol. 165, pp. 9-15.

Ebrahem, Q et al. (2006). Triamcinolone acetonide inhibits IL-6 and VEGF-induced angiogenesis downstream of the IL-t and VEGF receptors. *Investigative Ophthalmology and Visual Sciences*, Vol. 46, 4935-4941.

Fontanesi, J. et al. (1993). Treatment of choroidal melanoma with I-125 plaque. *International Journal of Radiation Oncology, Biology, and Physics.* Vol. 26, pp. 619-623.

Fontanesi, J. et al. (1996). Treatment outcome and dose-response relationship in infants younger than 1 year treated for retinoblastoma with primary irradiation. *Medical and Pediatric Oncology*, Vol.26, pp. 297-304.

Garretson, B. et al. (1987). Choroidal melanoma treatment with iodine 125 brachytherapy. *Archives of Ophthalmology*, Vol. 105, pp. 1394-1397.

Gordon, K. (1995). Late effects of radiation on the eye and ocular adnexa. *International Journal of Radiation Oncology, Biology, and Physics*, Vol. 31, pp. 1123-1139.

Gragoudas, E. et al. (1992). Cataract extraction after proton beam irradiation for malignant melanoma of the eye. *Archives of Ophthalmology*, Vol. 110, pp. 475-479.

Hoehn, M. et al. (2010). Outcomes after cataract extraction in young children with radiation-induced cataracts and retinoblastoma. *Journal of AAPOS*, Vol. 14, pp. 232-234.

Honovar, S. et al. (2001) Intraocular surgery after treatment of retinoblastoma. *Archives of Ophthalmology*, Vol. 119, pp. 1613-1621.

Lean, E. et al. (1990). Episcleral radioactive plaque therapy: initial clinical experience in 56 patients. *American Journal of Clinical Oncology*, Vol, 13, pp. 185-190.

Lumbroso-Le Rouic, L. (2004). I125 plaque brachytherapy for anterior uveal melanomas. *Eye*. Vol. 18, pp. 911-916.

Madreperla, S. et al. (2000). Repair of late retinal detachment after successful treatment of retinoblastoma. *Retina*, Vol. 20, pp. 28-32.

Mameghan, H. et al. (1992). Iodine-125 irradiation of choroidal melanoma: clinical experience from the Prince of Wales and Sydney Eye Hospitals. *Australas Radiology*, Vol. 36, pp. 249-252.

Miller, D. et al. (2005). Pars plana lensectomy and intraocular lens implantation in pediatric radiation-induced cataracts in retinoblastoma. *Ophthalmology*, Vol. 112, pp. 1620-1624.

Monge, O. et al. (1986). Sightsaving therapy in retinoblastoma: Experience with external megavoltage radiotherapy. *Acta Ophthalmologica*, Vol. 64, pp. 414-420.

Moshfeghi, D. et al. (2005). Intraocular surgery after treatment of germline retinoblastoma. *Archives of Ophthalmology*, Vol. 123, pp. 1008-1012.

Osman, I. et al. (2011) Modern cataract surgery for radiation-induced cataracts in retinoblastoma. *British Journal of Ophthalmology*. Vol. 95, pp. 227-230.

Payne, J. et al. (2009). Outcomes of cataract surgery following radiation treatment for retinoblastoma. *Journal of AAPOS*, Vol. 13, pp. 454-458.

Portellos M. & Buckley, E. (1998) Cataract surgery and intraocular lens implantation in patients with retinoblastoma. *Archives of Ophthalmology*, Vol. 116, 449-452.

Puusari, I. et al. (2004). Effect of radiation dose on ocular complications after iodine brachytherapy for large uveal melanoma: empirical data and simulating information of collimating plaques. *Investigative Ophthalmology and Visual Sciences*, Vol. 45, pp. 3425-3434.

Puusari, I. et al. (2004). Ocular complications after iodine brachytherapy for large uveal melanoma. *Ophthalmology*, Vol. 111, pp. 1768-1777.

Quivey, J. et al. (1993). High intensity 125-iodine (I125) plaque treatment of uveal melanoma. *International Journal of Radiation Oncology, Biology, and Physics*, Vol. 26, pp. 613-618.

Shanmugan, M. (2004). Cataract surgery and intraocular lens implantation in retinoblastoma. *Journal of Cataract and Refractive Surgery*, Vol. 30, 1825-1826.

Shields, C. et al. (2002). Combined plaque radiotherapy and transpupillary thermotherapy for choroidal melanoma: tumor control and treatment complications in 270 consecutive patients. *Archives of Ophthalmology*, Vol. 120, pp. 933-940.

Shields, C. et al. (2006). Intravitreal triamcinolone acetonide for acute radiation papillopathy. *Retina*, Vol. 26, pp. 537-544.

Sinha, R. et al. (2004). Management of radiotherapy-induced cataracts in eyes with retinoblastoma. *Journal of Cararact and Refractive Surgery*, Vol. 30, pp. 1145-1146.

Stack, R. et al. (2005) New Zealand experience of I125 brachytherapy for choroidal melanoma. *Clinical and Experimental Ophthalmology*, Vol. 33, pp. 490-494.

Wachtlin, J. et al. (2000) Phacoemulsification following treatment of choroidal melanoma. *Graefes Archives of Clinical and Experimental Ophthalmology*, Vol. 34, pp. 942-948.

28

The Management of Age Related Cataract in Sub-Saharan Africa

Lawan Abdu
Department of Ophthalmology, Faculty of Medicine, Bayero University Kano Nigeria

1. Introduction

Cataract simply means opacity of the crystalline lens. The human lens is essentially an ectodermal structure and develops from the lens placode about the fifth week of gestation. The lens has a capsule formed early in the gestation period. This makes lens protein isolated from the human immune system ab-initio. The lens grows through out life from about 90 grams at birth to 250 grams in weight at the age of sixty years. The equatorial diameter is 9 to 10mm in adults. It is an avascular structure and obtains nutrition from surrounding vitreous and aqueous humor. Metabolic processes include the hexose monophosphate, the pyrubic and the aldose reductase pathway which produce sorbitol. The active substance produced by the numerous pathways is glucose 6 phosphates essential for generating energy for the lens metabolism. Fluid movement in the lens is mediated by Na^+/K ATpase. The lens structure consists of a nucleus with two "Y" shaped sutures, erect anteriorly and inverted posteriorly. This is surrounded by the cortex. The epithelium lies under the capsule except posteriorly. The lens function includes accommodation and contributes one third of the refractive power of the human eye being second to the cornea in this role. Cataract formation is an age related change that occurs from about the age of forty years. Various mechanisms have been advocated as the cause of this opacification notably oxidative damage by free radicals generated during normal metabolic activity and 300 to 400nm radiation present in the natural human environment. There are lens enzymes that function to protect against free radical damage such glutathione peroxidase, catalase and superoxide dismutase. The level of these enzymes is reduced in the lens of patients who develop age related cataracts. There are various morphological types of age related cataracts. The location of the opacity defines the morphological appearance and this may be nuclear, sutural, cortical sub capsular (anterior or posterior), and or, capsular. Cataract can be described as immature, mature or hyper mature based on the density of the opacification. The location of the cataract has a role in determining the extent, type and severity of the symptoms. A cataract causes painless progressive loss of vision. Ordinary, it is expected that the symptoms parallel the degree of loss of lens transparency. This is not entirely true as even a smaller opacity on the visual axis particularly when close to the nodal point of the eye as seen in posterior sub capsular cataract can cause significant visual disability irrespective of extent of opacification. The nature of day to day life of the individual and occupational demands can contribute to the patient's awareness of visual limitation even at an early stage. Age related cataract is one of the leading causes of avoidable or curable blindness worldwide and affect half of the estimated forty five million world's population who are blind. It also causes visual impairment in many others. There is no gender predilection. In developing countries of Africa south of the Sahara, the problem is more severe and the impact on the life of the people is tremendous. Many factors contribute to the large burden of cataract blindness in this part of the World. There is a huge underserved population. Ophthalmologists are very few in numbers with their ratio to the general population are about one to a million. The eye care workers largely concentrate in urban areas whereas seventy percent of the population lives in the rural areas. Most of the trained eye care professionals are not in public service and only the rich can afford to pay for private eye care. There is high level of poverty in this part of the world. Most of the populations are small scale farmers who toil during the rainy season to harvest food that can barely feed the large families. Blindness thus contributes to loss of productivity. In the event of a family member becoming blind the younger children are made to leave school and serve as guide to the disabled adult. This further perpetuates illiteracy, poverty and deprivation. There is cost attached to treatment in the cities for the few who eventually make it there. This is about three times the cost of a bag of corn that families eat over several months. Most public eye hospitals have a waiting list and there is need for improvement in the professionalism of some providers and quality of the services provided. Outreach services are infrequent, poorly sustained and often defend on Non Governmental Organizations (NGO's) based in other countries. Where eye camp services are provided initial evaluation and monitoring at follow up are inadequate. Quacks who masquerade as traditional eye care practitioners abound. Their role is to compound and limit the success of the few hard working trained and registered eye care providers. The trade mark of the traditional eye healers (TEH) is sale to unsuspecting, unassuming, desperate and gullible public of traditional eye medicine (TEM), the nature, content, dosage and ill effects of which is not known even to the vendors of these concoctions. TEM can cause corneal damage and thus blindness and severe visual impairment. Harmful traditional eye practices such as couching results in severe ocular inflammation, hypheama, secondary glaucoma, endophthalmitis and retinal detachment. The activities of TEH are unregulated and they often enjoy patronage of government health departments particularly at district level. Their "successes" in plying their trade may not be unrelated to financial understanding with district health officials in some countries. In this chapter, the practice of cataract surgery in this part of the world is described to further the understanding of surgeons from other parts of the world who may wish to compare to that widely used in sub-Saharan Africa as described in this chapter.

2. Pre operative management of patient with age related cataract

The commonest symptom of age related cataract is painless progressive visual loss. Vision is often described by patients as "smoky" or "hazy" and likened to the environment as it appears during the harmattan season when cold dusty winds blow southwards across the Sahara Desert. Patient evaluation is the most essential step in offering quality eye care. A careful history should include duration and possible interventions tried by the patient.

Presence of other symptoms such as pain may indicate that cataract is associated with other co existing ocular morbidity. Intermittent blurring of vision, seeing rainbow like colors may indicate associated glaucoma co existing or as a differential diagnosis. A history of application of harmful traditional eye medications or traditional eye surgery is important as this may influence the treatment option to be offered. Likewise there is need to ask of history of any medical illnesses particularly diabetes mellitus and hypertension. It is important to know duration of these diseases and treatment offered including compliance with medication as retinal complications of diabetes mellitus are partly time related. Assessment of the patient includes basic eye examination notably, unaided and pin hole visual acuity. A fully matured cataract usually cause blindness or visual impairment without improvement in pin hole vision. It is not unusual to see patients with bilateral cataracts. The cornea is usually clear in patients with cataract despite the prevalence trachoma presence of opacity is a hall mark of possible attempted couching. The anterior chamber is usually deep and quite. Presence of activity may denote reaction to application of TEM or other cause of inflammation in the anterior segment which may be lens related. Brisk pupil reactions indicate possible absence of gross retinal and optic nerve disease. Poor or absent pupillary reaction to both direct and consensual stimuli should alert the clinician to other causes of vision loss apart from age related cataract. All patients with cataract must have intra ocular pressure measured preferably with an applanation tonometer which is the gold standard. Raised intra ocular pressure (IOP) may indicate co existing glaucoma and thus patient need to have the optic disc evaluated with indirect ophthalmoscope to obtain a clear fundal view after pupil dilation, gonioscopy and also assessment of the contra lateral eye for possible evidence of glaucoma. Various ways of grossly assessing the retina includes the four quadrants light projection test, two-point light discrimination test at, 5, 7 and 12 centimeters from the eye for patients with light perception, hand motion and counting finger vision, respectively. Ophthalmic B mode ultrasound scan can be performed when there is suspicion of retinal detachment. Laser interferometry through selected areas of the cataract to assess retinal function can be applied where such facilities are available. Routine blood pressure measurement, full blood count and fasting blood sugar are advised for all patients in this part of the world. Biometry is performed to determine the power of intra ocular lens required to achieve target post operative visual acuity. To prepare patient for surgery there is need to administer and obtain an informed consent. Preoperative trimming of eye lashes and administration of 500mg of systemic acetazolamide is desirable by ophthalmologist in this part of the world. The surgery of choice in most centers is extra capsular cataract extraction with posterior chamber intra ocular lens implantation (ECCE + PCIOL).

3. Indication for cataract surgery

Poor vision is the commonest indication for removal of cataract. Cataract is the most cost effective surgical intervention. Successful cataract surgery almost gives instantaneous results and restores the patient back to his normal life style. Other reasons for performing cataract surgery are when the presence of the cataract is impeding the health of the eye such as in anteriorly dislocated cataract, intumescent cataract and phacolytic glaucoma. Cataract removal may be required to visualize the posterior segment. Rarely a white cataract is removed in otherwise blind eye to restore black pupil.

4. Anesthesia for cataract surgery

Both general and regional anesthetic block can be used in patients with age related cataracts. However, most cataract operations are performed under local anesthesia. The aim is to provide pain relief for the patients comfort and compliance during the procedure. Akinesia help ophthalmologist to perform the surgery. There are various ways of ensuring lid akinesia. The O'Brien technique blocks the facial nerve around the neck of the mandible. Van Lint's block is of the nerve under the periusteum at the lateral orbital rim and Atkinson's block is applied mid way between these two. The commonly used anesthetic is Lignocaine (xylocaine) mixed with adrenaline (1:100000 dilutions). The anesthetic agent can be injected into the muscle cone behind the globe. The technique is termed the retro-bulbar retro-ocular block though carry a higher risk of globe penetration. This risk is reduced with other para-bulbar techniques relying on injecting relevant areas such as para-bulbar or sub-Tenon's block. Topical anesthesia is rarely practiced in sub-Saharan Africa as most patients tend to have a low pain threshold. The advantage of using lignocaine with adrenaline is that it causes local vasoconstriction ensuring greater effect of the anesthesia and limiting systemic absorption. It can be used alone or with hyaluronidase (healon) to further aid in local distribution and absorption. Xylocaine effect lasts up to two hours and may be mixed with mupivacaine (marcaine heavy) the effect of the later starting within two hours and lasting longer. 2 to 3.5 milliliters can be injected into the retro bulbar space and 5 milliliters is used for facial nerve block. There is need for caution as large quantities can raise the intra orbital pressure (and thus the intra ocular pressure) which makes it more difficult to handle the globe during surgery. The choice of type of regional block partly defends on the circumstances, the patient and the choice of the ophthalmologist. Retro-bulbar injection is not risk free and there are complications in addition to accidental perforation of the globe. Orbital hemorrhage can cause instantaneous proptosis warranting deferral of surgery and may require urgent orbital decompression. Lignocaine used in this procedure can enter the sub arachnoids space and track to the base of the brain interfering with the function of the cardiovascular control mechanism giving raise to fall in systemic blood pressure and hypovolaemic shock. There is need for caution in this procedure and vigilance to ensure prompt intervention when any complications arise. Patients must fast overnight and should not eat on the day of the surgery so that conversion from local to general anesthesia can safely be effected should there be a need to do so. Patients on treatment for other systemic diseases such as diabetic and systemic hypertension must have there medications continued or adjusted in collaboration with the relevant physician.

4.1 Intra capsular cataract extraction with correction of aphakia

In the early part of the nineteenth century Duvial introduced intra capsular cataract extraction (ICCE) using the ab interno limbal incision approach. The aim is to extract the opaque lens with its capsule intact and remove it from the eye. This relatively simple procedure has been practiced in most countries of sub \Saharan Africa until conversion to extra capsular cataract extraction with posterior chamber intra ocular lens became more wide spread in the mid 1990. This procedure is performed under complete asepsis. After regional anesthetic block, the operation site is cleaned and draped. A speculum is applied to open the lids. A superior rectus bridle suture is applied to stabilize the eye ball. A number 15 or 11 surgical blade is used to make a 180 degrees superior limbal incision. Peripheral iridectomy is done routinely to avert some of the complications associated with this procedure. The lens is delivered using vectis loop applied to the proximal lip of the limbal wound and a muscle hook gently applied to the sclera at 6 o' clock position to maneuver the lens through the open wound site. The limbal wound is the closed with interrupted 8/0 silk sutures. The anterior chamber reformed with normal saline or Ringer's solution. Sub conjunctival steroid and antibiotic injection is then administered. Intra operative Atropine 1% eye drop is applied and the eye padded.

4.2 Intra operative complications of intra capsular cataract extraction

Vitreous loss: This complication is relatively common with ICCE and warrants vitrectomy. An anterior vitrector may be used, assisted by administration of intra-ocular triamcenolone. Alternatively, if not available the anterior vitreous surface is lifted with a cell sponge and cut with de Wecker scissors possibly aided Vannas scissors. Poorly managed vitreous loss can lead to retinal detachment, and also an up drawn pupil thus reducing the efficacy of any aphakic correction given to the patient later. Often an inferior sphinterotomy is performed to keep the pupil central. The anterior chamber can be reformed with sterile air to keep the vitreous back. The air is eventually absorbed in a day or two.

Intra operative hypheama**:** Bleeding into the anterior chamber during surgery can easily track down into the vitreous as there is no posterior capsule to serve as a barrier. Blood in the vitreous compromise the visual outcome. Significant amounts of blood in the vitreous can take up to a year to be absorbed and can be a source of fibrous tissue reaction. It can warrant pars plana vitrectomy if a retinal break cannot be excluded on fundoscopy. Any hyphema is immediately and promptly aspirated and the cause of the hemorrhage identified and treated.

Lens dislocation into the vitreous: Occasionally the lens can dislocate into the vitreous as the zonules are weak with age. Caution is necessary as the lens is carefully extracted from the eye.

Other complications: This includes corneal decompensation, descemet membrane stripping and expulsive choroidal hemorrhage.

4.3 Post operative complications of ICCE

Wound dehiscence: This is characterized by shallow anterior chamber and a positive Seidel's test. Padding and bandaging with a contact lens can aid sealing of small opening. Secondary wound closure may be necessary when there is significant wound break down.

Secondary Glaucoma: Secondary glaucoma can occur after intra capsular cataract extraction. Malignant glaucoma arises when aqueous humor track behind the vitreous, pushes the vitreous forward resulting in shallow anterior chamber with raised intra ocular pressure. The condition is treated with oral or intra venous acetazolamide. Patient may require vitrectomy to alter the misdirected aqueous humor. Phacolytic glaucoma is said to arise with the natural immune system react to leaked lens protein. This can occur when there is rapture of the lens capsule or when there is previous exposure of lens matter in the contra lateral eye. Treatment involves the use of topical steroids and anti glaucoma medication. Dislocation of the lens into the anterior chamber for any reason can lead to elevation in the intra ocular pressure and warrants immediate surgery to remove the lens.

Postoperative bacterial endophthalmitis: This is rare but a cause of great concern to ophthalmologists. Sterile endophthalmitis such as toxic anterior segment syndrome can be noticed within 24 hours after surgery and could be caused by the irritating substance in the surgeon's gloves. True bacterial endophthalmitis is seen within 24 to 72 hours after surgery. It is characterized by reduction in vision and pain. The lid appears swollen and the eye is injected. There is reduction in the post operative visual acuity. Most often it is caused by Staphlococcus epidermidis and Staphylococcus aureus though pseudomonas and proteus species have also been implicated. If unattended the condition can rapidly deteriorate leading to panophthalmitis warranting evisceration of the eye. Management includes prompt diagnosis and commencement of relevant topical and systemic antibiotics. Identification of the causative agent requires aqueous and vitreous aspirate for gram stain, culture and sensitivity tests. Intra vitreal antibiotic injections in standard dilutions are administered. Initial choice of antibiotic is modified based on final culture results. Some of the antibiotics used include gentamycin, amikacin, and vancomycin in standardized dilutions for intra vitreal and intra cameral administration. Systemic antibiotics are also administered such as intravenous ceftazidine and oral ciprofloxacin. Periocular antibiotic injections can also be administered. Adjuvant treatment includes cycloplegia and analgesia. Topical steroids may be introduced at a certain stage when infection is control. Steroids are given to reduce severity of the post inflammatory healing process as scars in the visual axis can also hinder the patient's vision.

Cystoid macula edema: This is otherwise called Irvine-Gass syndrome. Although the exact mechanism is unclear vascular incompetence and inflammation is a possible cause. CMO can be a complication of both ICCE and ECCE. Prophylactic administration of prostaglandin synthesases inhibitor such as indomethacin is said to reduce the risk.

Suture related complications: Epithelial in growth to the anterior chamber through the suture track can occur. Sutures can fragment or general fibrosis along its track. Meticulous wound handling is important in reducing such complications.

Retinal detachment: ICCE is associated with aphakic retinal detachment in up to 2% of cases. When there is vitreous loss the risk of retinal detachment is about 10%. The presence of lattice degeneration, vitreous degeneration and pre existing high myopia are predisposing factors. Aphakic detachment requires identification of retinal breaks and vitrectomy or performing a buckling procedure, sealing of all retinal breaks and drainage of sub retinal fluid.

4.4 Correction of aphakia after intra capsular cataract extraction

Correction of aphakia is as important as removing the cataract. There are various ways of correcting aphakia; however the commonest method is by using spectacles. Spectacles for aphakic correction are available and affordable in most countries of the region. Disadvantage of spectacles include weigh, discomfort and the various spherical and chromatic aberrations resulting in poor compliance. High plus lenses causes scotoma which result in the 'Jack in the box' phenomenon. Pincushion distortion causes difficulty in the patient's general mobility particularly through doorways. With advancing age and confusion patients need to be educated on the use of such glasses to prevent falls and injuries. Glasses can be misplaced or loss, they get scratch marks and break. Aphakic spectacle lenses are not suitable for correction of uni-ocular aphakia. They cause a 25% image magnification beyond the 5% image differential which the brain can tolerate to ensure binocular single vision. These untoward effects warrant consideration of other methods of correcting aphakia. Contact lenses (CL) can be used for uni-ocular aphakia. CL is not affordable and unavailable in the rural settings. Their use requires high level of patient education and most of those who need it are semi literate at best. Soft extended wear CLs are rarely affordable and are effectively unavailable in rural settings. Soft extended ware CLs are very expensive and so their cleaning solutions. The living environment is dry and dusty further increasing the risk of corneal abrasion and secondary microbial infection that can result in cornel ulcer. For these reasons a contact lens will usually be a poor choice for correction for a farmer in the rural areas of sub Saharan Africa due to the numerous problems associated with their use. Secondary intraocular lens (IOL) procedures may be considered. Secondary anterior IOL implantation can be performed. Secondary posterior chamber (PC) IOL implantation tends to be more difficult to perform. Often surgeons avoid secondary IOL procedures particularly in patients with aphakia due to couching due to the high risk of retinal detachment. Photo refractive surgery such as epikeratopia (epikeratopia) and keratomileusis are rarely practiced. The skill and equipment required for LASIK and related modern procedures are simply unavailable. Gradually in the last decade or so extra capsular cataract extraction with PC IOL has largely replace ICCE.

4.5 Extra capsular cataract extraction with posterior chamber intra ocular lens implantation

The need to obtain quality post operative vision necessitates the conversion from ICCE to ECCE PCIOL. The IOL implant is within the eye and close to the nodal point hence simulating the role of the crystalline lens. Harold Ridley introduced the use of IOL in 1946 in United Kingdom after the Second World War. The IOL is widely accepted and is the gold standard of correcting aphakia in age related cataracts. The following steps are often observed in performing this procedure in sub-Sahara. The eye lashes are trimmed, 500mg of oral acetazolamide is given at least an hour before surgery to reduce the intraocular pressure and topical Atropine 1% administered to dilate the pupil. Patients require biometry consisting of an ultrasound A scan and Keratometer to determine the power of the intra ocular lens required to give the desired post operative visual acuity. The target post operative visual acuity by most surgeons' is 6/6 (20/20). The surgery is performed under complete aseptic condition. The steps involved in performing this procedure include cleaning with povidone iodine and draping. The lids are opened with a speculum wire. Superior rectus suture is placed to stabilize the eye. Fornix based conjunctiva flap raised.

4.6 Techniques of approach into the anterior chamber

Corneo scleral incision: From time immemorial surgeons are known to make limbal incision superiorly to gain access into the anterior chamber. This approach is quite simple and requires minimal tissue manipulation. Conventionally it is usually located between 10 o'clock and 2 o'clock position but may be modified in the presence of a filtering bleb.

Scleral incision: This is located 2-3mm from the limbus. In the early days before minimal incision cataract surgery these incisions tended to be wide enough to allow the lens to be extracted during intra capsular cataract extraction. The size is relatively smaller in ECCE and even more so in small incision cataract surgery. The advantage is that it causes less post operative astigmatism than a corneoscleral incision. However it tends to bleed more than the former. With advances in cataract surgery scleral tunnel incision is the norm in most minimal access procedures in sub-Saharan Africa. In manual small incision cataract surgeries the opening is 3 to 4 mm and can be even less with phacoemulsification surgery and insertion of foldable intraocular lenses. Sclera tunnel incision give rise to less post operative astigmatism and do not require use of sutures to close the wound.

Corneal incision: This is performed at the superior corneal periphery using a razor blade fragment. The incision is beveled by design to offer a self sealing access though sutures are inserted at the end of the procedure. Corneal incisions can be performed in the presence of a filtering bleb. They cause no significant bleeding, but can lead to more post operative astigmatism particularly with less experienced surgeons. Wound closure can be by interrupted or continuous suture and the stump is buried in the corneal stroma to reduce irritation. The scar is small, parallel to the limbus and hardly noticeable as it is covered by the upper eye lid. The corneal incision has complications such as descemet stripping and can predispose to corneal decompensation. After gaining access into the anterior chamber (AC), viscoelastic material is injected to maintain the AC and protect the corneal endothelium from abrading by the surgeon's instruments.

Anterior capsulotomy: There are various techniques of performing capsulotomy, but the common practice is Can opener capsulotomy. Under visco elastic an angulated insulin needle is used to make small and continuous "v" shaped incisions on the peripheral lens capsule. The anterior capsule is then gently pickup with a capsule or Macpherson's forceps and removed through the wound site thus allowing for vectis nucleus delivery by counter pressure. Other modality includes continuous curvilinear capsulorheisis. The capsule is opened at one position and the torn in round and systematic manner till it is completely peeled off. There are various modifications such as envelope technique whereby the opening is shaped like an envelope. The aim is to provide access for removing the lens cortex and allowing for clean up of cortical matter.

Delivery of the nucleus: In ECCE after anterior capsulotomy, a vectis loop is applied to the proximal scleral side of the limbal wound and a squint muscle hook applied to the sclera at the 6 o'clock position. Gentle counter-pressure is applied to push the nucleus out through the wound edge. This technique is slightly modified in small incision cataract surgery. The symcoe aspiration-irrigation double canula is used to suck out as much cortex as possible using the vacuum in the handheld syringe; the nucleus is maneuvered into the anterior chamber before delivery through the wound site. Should the nucleus appear too large for the wound site, then it is fragmented with Macpherson's forceps into two in the anterior chamber before extrusion from the globe. Irrespective of the technique used, once the nucleus id delivered, the cortical matter is aspirated with irrigation-aspiration canula. This is performed with minimal disturbance to the iris as doing so can provoke more post operative inflammation.

Insertion and positioning of the posterior chamber intra ocular lens: The anterior chamber is reformed with visco elastic material. A lens introducer is used to hold the IOL after the sterile lens pack is opened. The lens is introduced into the eye with the lower haptic pointing to the left of the surgeon. The lower haptic is inserted into the lower portion of the capsule (in the bag) or into the ciliary sulcus behind the iris. The upper haptic is then picked with Macpherson's forceps and gently pushed under the upper iris-pupil border associated with clockwise rotation thus slotting the lens into position. The IOL can then be rotated further by applying the dialer into the dialing hole at the periphery of the lens optic and rotating till the pupil is round and centered indicating that the IOL is properly positioned. The wound can then be closed with interrupted 9/0 or 10/0 silk sutures. The bite depth is two third the thickness of the cornea, the length of the scleral side of the suture is four time that of the corneal side. The sutures are radially oriented and evenly spaced to reduce post operative astigmatism. In small incision cataract surgery the scleral tunnel incision site is not sutured. Any remaining visco elastic material is aspirated from the anterior chamber. Subconjunctival injection consisting of gentamycin 20 mg and dexamethasone 4 mg is given to gently balloon the proximal end of the fornix based flap. Intra operative Tropicamide drop is administered and the eye is padded.

5. Postoperative care of the pseudophakic eye

Cataract surgery can be performed as a day case procedure. Mobile units such as are used in parts of India are not very common in sub-Saharan Africa. A significant proportion of patients come to the hospital from distant and remote places thus there is need for admission for a day or so. Postoperative care involves assessment of the visual acuity unaided and then with pin hole. Visual improvement usually is noted even from the first post operative day. Improvement with pin hole is unpredictable as the effect of cycloplegia is present a day after surgery. The wound site is inspected for any gaping in the wound. The cornea is inspected with the slip lamp. There may be edema and striate keratopathy. The anterior chamber may show flare and cells due to postoperative inflammation. Fundoscopy is performed- the fundus is usually normal though even then the view may appear blurred owing to corneal edema. Intra ocular pressure may be normal or elevated. Postoperative medication consists of topical steroids and antibiotics. Patients are followed up routinely and refraction performed after four weeks.

5.1 Complications of extra capsular cataract extraction with posterior chamber intra ocular lens implantation

A number of complications can occur which can pose special problems in the absence of nearby ophthalmic surgeon with one ophthalmologist to a million population in sub-Saharan Africa.

5.2 Intra operative complications

Posterior capsular tear: A tear or rent in the posterior capsule can occur. The posterior capsule serves as a scaffold upon which the PCIOL rests- a tear in the posterior capsule can alter the procedure. A small rent in the posterior capsule does not preclude insertion of the IOL which can be inserted in the capsular bag if there is enough support or in the ciliary sulcus. Large tears can necessitate more significant modification of the procedure, either non-insertion of the IOL or use of anterior chamber lens possibly as a secondary procedure. Large capsular rent can result in use of anterior chamber rather than posterior chamber intra ocular lens. High intra-orbital pressure which is transmitted to the intraocular pressure can make the ocular tissues more difficult to handle during surgery predisposing to posterior capsular tear. When surgery is performed under regional anesthesia, a restless and uncooperative patient is more likely to have a capsular rent than a more calm and cooperative one. Care of the posterior capsule is of paramount importance in providing a stable scaffold for the PCIOL.

Stripping of the descemet membrane: Occasionally the descemet is peeled usually from the lip of the limbal wound towards the center of the cornea. Visco elastic material can be injected from the center of the anterior chamber towards the stripped edge aiding its re positioning.

Intra operative hypheama: Bleeding into the anterior chamber can occur during surgery from tear in the iris root or anomalous blood vessel, often obscuring the operating view for the surgeon. A platelet plug promptly seal bleeding vessels, the blood is aspirated with Symcoe canula and procedure continued. It is rare for massive bleeding to occur which will warrant more drastic intervention.

Corneal decompensation: The cornea can suddenly become cloudy particularly with diseased endothelium such as guttata. It is therefore mandatory to examine the endothelium carefully before surgery. Care in avoiding contact between the endothelium and the operating instruments are mandatory in all patients.

Choroidal hemorrhage: Expulsive supra choroidal hemorrhage arises from rapture of the long or short posterior ciliary arteries and outcome unless action is immediately taken is expulsion of the contents of the eye. Many factors are associated with suprachoroidal bleeding including sudden fall in intraocular pressure, patient moving like coughing causing damage from instruments, vasalva maneuver, possible changes in blood pressure and use of retrobulbar anesthesia. Treatment includes mandatory immediate closure of the wound with firm sutures to tamponade the intraocular bleeding and some clinicians advocate immediate posterior sclerostomy. The latter can however compound the situation. After wound closure the patients is given one to two weeks before draining the accumulated blood. Some patients may require vitrectomy and air fluid exchange.

5.3 Postoperative complications

Wound leakage: Wound failure is one of the early complications in cataract surgery. It is easily detected by presence of excessive fluid (and may be noticed by the patients as excess tears) associated with the operated eye; the anterior chamber is shallow or may even be flat defending on the extent. Wound leak can be confirmed by applying fluorescein to the eye and examining with the cobalt blue light under slip lamp-the leakage site appears green as the fluorescein is diluted by leaked aqueous humor. Flourescein-impregnated strips can also be used. This use of flourescein is called Seidel's Test. Slight leakage can be sealed by bandage contact lens and if not available padding with firm bandage is used in sub-Saharan Africa. Huge leaks require secondary wound suturing.

Iris prolapse: This can arise from poor wound closure and needs to be reposition and the wound closed properly. It can result in poor wound healing, postoperative astigmatism and increases the possibility of post operative endophthalmitis

Striate keratopathy: Is characterized by corneal edema and folds in the Descemet's membrane. Striate keratopathy is caused by damage to the corneal endothelium by inserted operating instruments. Care must be exercised during surgery to prevent endothelial cell loss. Viscoelastic material is used to protect the endothelium.

Postoperative inflammation (uveitis) and endophthalmitis: Sometimes the inflammatory response after surgery can be marked with fibrin formation. Minimal tissue manipulation results in less severe postoperative reaction. The severity is assessed with slit lamp examination. Medications consisting of anti-inflammatory, cycloplegics and intraocular pressure (IOP) lowering agents are prescribed. In some instances subconjunctival dexamethasone is administered. Patients require close monitoring till the process is fully controlled. Alternatively, endophthalmitis can occur, which demands intravitreal and possibly anterior chamber antibiotics to be administered as an emergency.

Raised intra ocular pressure: All patients must have the intra ocular pressure (IOP) measured postoperatively as the inflammation mentioned above can be associated with elevation in IOP. IOP-lowering drugs are administered when the need arise.

Residual cortex: Meticulous cortical clean-up is desirable though sometimes missed lens matter appears a day or two after surgery. This can cause more inflammation and the threshold for intervention by aspiration should be low.

Malposition of the intra ocular lens: Malposition lead to tilting of the lens from the most optimal position-this can lead to post operative astigmatism and lead to reduction in the patient's visual acuity. Malposition can result in distortion of the pupil which can appear decentered. Conservative management includes use of miotics. Occasionally, the lens has to be redialed into position.

Posterior capsular opacity (PCO): This is the most important long-term complication of ECCE with PCIOL. The cause can be primary opacification due to posterior capsular plague, or proliferation of lens epithelium on the capsule (Elschnig's pearls) or arise from capsular fibrosis. The patient presents with painless progressive loss of vision. Clinical examination demonstrates reduction in visual acuity and the opacity is visible under slit lamp examination. Capsulotomy is indicated when there is reduction in vision, PCO obscure fundal view preventing diagnosis of posterior segment disease or when PCO is causing monoocular diplopia. The neodymium: ytrrium-aluminium-garnet laser (Nd: YAG) laser capsulotomy is the treatment of choice. Because of the post-laser elevation of intra ocular pressure, a drop of apraclonidine 1% is prophylactically applied before commencing the procedure. The procedure is explained to the patient, consent is obtained, the patient is positioned and topical anesthetic drop is applied. A laser contact lens designed for the procedure is placed on the cornea, the laser settings are adjusted, the aiming beam is targeted on the posterior capsule and shots fired at 30° angle to reduce astigmatism. A series of shorts in cruciate form are applied avoiding damage to the intraocular lens. An opening of 3 mm is adequate to improve the patient's vision. Complications include elevation of intraocular pressure. Various reasons have been adduced as to the cause such as blockage of the anterior chamber angle by the fragmented debris and possible inflammation following the procedure. However, the pressure elevation tends to be transient and can be control with anti-glaucoma medications. Retinal detachment is another complication which occurs when Nd: YAG capsulotomy is performed early. Early treatment may not be necessary in most instances as PCO tend to occur from two years after surgery, though this is highly influenced by choice of IOL. Ophthalmologists in sub-Saharan Africa generally avoid doing a Nd: YAG capsulotomy earlier than six months after the cataract surgery.

6. Factors favoring good outcome of surgery

The proficiency, experience and commitment of the surgeon can partly determine the outcome of surgery. A good surgeon will assess the individual patient, prepare the patient effectively, organize good support services and ensure adequate postoperative care. Thus, selection of suitable patient with appropriate preoperative management is crucial in obtaining good visual outcome. Assessment of the patient involves clinical evaluation for any ocular co-morbidity, or systemic disease that can affect the outcome of surgery. Systemic diseases such as diabetes mellitus and hypertension are known to have retinal and optic nerve complications. Eye diseases such as glaucoma unless detected and without patients being appropriately informed during consent about a possible guarded visual prognosis can be a cause of poor outcome of surgery, dissatisfaction to the patient and a cause of great concern to the ophthalmologist. Silent dacryocystitis can predispose to postoperative endophthalmitis and must where possible be treated before cataract surgery. Patient education is important in reducing harmful eye practices such as application of traditional eye medications after surgery. Postoperative refraction to detect and treat any residual refractive errors is essential in achieving complete rehabilitation of the patient after surgery.

There is need for monitoring of outcome in order to determine causes of poor postoperative vision with the aim of finding ways to prevent them. Better resource allocation and utilization is essential in planning eye care, implementation and evaluation of services to ensure underserved areas are treated -an important part in the path of eradicating avoidable blindness in Africa south of the Sahara.

7. References

[1] Abdu L, Foster A. Assessment of resource utilization for the delivery of cataract surgical services Nig J Basic Clin Sci 2005; 2 (1): 1-2

[2] Abdu L. Results of cataract outreach services in a state of Nigeria TAF Prev Med Bull 2010; 9: 225-228

[3] Akinsete E.O; Efficient surgical services for cataracts in Nigeria. Nig J Ophthalmol 1993. 2; 4-5.

[4] American Academy of Ophthalmology. Basic and Clinical Science Course. Section 2: Fundamentals and Principles of Ophthalmology. San Francisco California. 1993-1994 pp 167-174

[5] Ayanniyi AA, Taoheed AA. Fulfilling human resource development goal in West Africa: can the training of ophthalmologist diplomats be improved? West Afr J Med 2009 May; 28 (3): 177-81

[6] Briesen S, Geneau R, Roberts H, Opiyo J, Courtright P. understanding why patients with cataract refuse free surgery: the influence of rumors in Kenya. Trop Med Int Health 2010: 15 (5): 534-9

[7] Courtright P, Murenzi J, Mathenge W, Munana J, Muller A. reaching rural Africans with eye services: findings from primary eye care approaches in Rubavu District, Rwanda. Trop Med Int Health 2010 Jun; 15 (6): 692-6

[8] Dean WH, Patel D, Sherwin JC, Metcalfe NH> follow up survey of cataract surgical coverage and barriers to cataract surgery at Nkhoma, Malawi. Ophthalmic Epidemiol 2011 Aug; 18 (4): 171-8

[9] Egbert PR, Buchanan M. Results of extra capsular cataract surgery and intraocular lens implantation in Ghana. Arch Ophthalmol 1991 Dec; 109 (12): 1764-8

[10] Fine BS, Yanoff M: Ocular Histology, ed 2. Hagerstown, MD. Harper & Row publishers Inc 1979, pp 149-159

[11] Foster A. who will operate Africa's 3 million curably blind people? Lancet 1991 May; 337 (8752): 1267-9

[12] Frick KD, Foster A, Bah M, Faal H. Analysis of cost and benefits of the Gambian Eye Care Program. Arch OIphthalmol 2005 Feb; 123 (2): 239-43

[13] Frimpong-Boateng A, Rufer F, Fiadoyor S, Nkrumah-Mills J, Mensah-Tetteh F, Kudoadzi N, Roider J. [ophthalmological screening via a hospital boat: field study for planning future health care services in remote village at the Volta Lake in Ghana]. Ophthalmologie.2009 Sep; 106 (9): 819-25

[14] Gilbert C, Raman U, Francis V. World Blindness and its prevention. International Agency for Prevention of Blindness. 2005; 7: 67-72

[15] Kyari F, Murthy VSG, Sivsubramaniam S, Gilbert CE, Abdull MM, et al. Prevalence of blindness and visual impairment in Nigeria: The National Blindness and Visual Impairment survey. Invest Ophthalmol Vis Sci 2009; 50 (5): 2033-2039

[16] Limburg H, Foster A, Gilbert C, Johnson GJ, Kyndt M. routine monitoring of visual outcome of cataract surgery. Part 1: Development of an instrument. Br J Ophthalmol 2005 Jan; 89 (1): 45-9

[17] Manual of International Statistical classification if diseases injuries and causes of death. Geneva. WHO. 1997; 53-58.

[18] Ntim-Amponsah CT. Traditional methods of treatment of cataract seen at Korle-Bu Teaching Hospital. West Afr Med J 1995 Apr-Jun; 14 (2): 82-7

[19] Odusote K. human resource development for the prevention of blindness in Anglophone West Africa. West Afr J Med 1998 Jan-Mar; 17 (1): 1-8

[20] Onakpoya OH, Adegbehingbe BO, Adeoye AO, Adewara BA. Ophthalmic admissions in a tertiary hospital in Nigeria. Afri Health Sci 2010 Mar; 10 (1): 54-7

[21] Rabiu MM, Mohammed N. rapid assessment of cataract surgical services in Birnin-Kebbi local government area of Kebbi State, Nigeria. Ophthalmic Epidemiol 2008 Nov-Dec; 15 (6): 359-65

[22] Schemann JF, Bakayoko S, Coulibaly S. traditional couching is not an effective alternative procedure for cataract surgery in Mali. Ophthalmic Epidemiol 2000 Dec; 7(4): 271-83

[23] Thylefors B. The WHO program for the prevention of blindness and cataract in developing countries. Doc Ophthalmol 1992; 81 (3): 339-44

Permissions

The contributors of this book come from diverse backgrounds, making this book a truly international effort. This book will bring forth new frontiers with its revolutionizing research information and detailed analysis of the nascent developments around the world.

We would like to thank Farhan Husain Zaidi, for lending his expertise to make the book truly unique. He has played a crucial role in the development of this book. Without his invaluable contribution this book wouldn't have been possible. He has made vital efforts to compile up to date information on the varied aspects of this subject to make this book a valuable addition to the collection of many professionals and students.

This book was conceptualized with the vision of imparting up-to-date information and advanced data in this field. To ensure the same, a matchless editorial board was set up. Every individual on the board went through rigorous rounds of assessment to prove their worth. After which they invested a large part of their time researching and compiling the most relevant data for our readers. Conferences and sessions were held from time to time between the editorial board and the contributing authors to present the data in the most comprehensible form. The editorial team has worked tirelessly to provide valuable and valid information to help people across the globe.

Every chapter published in this book has been scrutinized by our experts. Their significance has been extensively debated. The topics covered herein carry significant findings which will fuel the growth of the discipline. They may even be implemented as practical applications or may be referred to as a beginning point for another development. Chapters in this book were first published by InTech; hereby published with permission under the Creative Commons Attribution License or equivalent.

The editorial board has been involved in producing this book since its inception. They have spent rigorous hours researching and exploring the diverse topics which have resulted in the successful publishing of this book. They have passed on their knowledge of decades through this book. To expedite this challenging task, the publisher supported the team at every step. A small team of assistant editors was also appointed to further simplify the editing procedure and attain best results for the readers.

Our editorial team has been hand-picked from every corner of the world. Their multi-ethnicity adds dynamic inputs to the discussions which result in innovative outcomes. These outcomes are then further discussed with the researchers and contributors who give their valuable feedback and opinion regarding the same. The feedback is then collaborated with the researches and they are edited in a comprehensive manner to aid the understanding of the subject.

Apart from the editorial board, the designing team has also invested a significant amount of their time in understanding the subject and creating the most relevant covers. They scrutinized every image to scout for the most suitable representation of the subject and create an appropriate cover for the book.

The publishing team has been involved in this book since its early stages. They were actively engaged in every process, be it collecting the data, connecting with the contributors or procuring relevant information. The team has been an ardent support to the editorial, designing and production team. Their endless efforts to recruit the best for this project, has resulted in the accomplishment of this book. They are a veteran in the field of academics and their pool of knowledge is as vast as their experience in printing. Their expertise and guidance has proved useful at every step. Their uncompromising quality standards have made this book an exceptional effort. Their encouragement from time to time has been an inspiration for everyone.

The publisher and the editorial board hope that this book will prove to be a valuable piece of knowledge for researchers, students, practitioners and scholars across the globe.

List of Contributors

Mammie Motiang
University of Limpopo (Medunsa Campus), South Africa

Matthew A. Cantrell and Heather R. Bream-Rouwenhorst
University of Iowa College of Pharmacy, Department of Pharmacy Practice and Science, Iowa City, Iowa, USA

Christopher Watts and Thomas A. Oetting
University of Iowa Carver College of Medicine, Iowa City, Iowa, USA

James A. Davison
Wolfe Eye Clinic, Iowa, USA

Alparslan Apan
Department of Anaesthesiology and Reanimation, Kirikkale University Faculty of Medicine, Turkey

Hiroshi Kobayashi
Department of Ophthalmology, Kanmon Medical Center, Shimonoseki, Japan

F.J. Ascaso
University of Zaragoza, Spain

V. Huerva
University of Lleida, Spain

Farhan Husain Zaidi
Consultant Ophthalmic Surgeon, Maidstone and Tunbridge Wells NHS Trust, Kent, Honorary Fellow, Moorfields Eye Hospital, London, UK

Takao Tanaka, Maiko Hirose, Shigemitu Ishii and Satoshi Fujita
Hachioji Medical Center, Tokyo Medical University Hospital, Hachioji Tokyo, Japan

Keisuke Kimura
Department of Ophthalmology, Tokyo Medical University, Tokyo, Japan

Allan Storr-Paulsen
Department of Ophthalmology, Cataract Outpatient Surgery Unit, Frederiksberg University Hospital, Frederiksberg, Denmark

Radin Tahvildari, Hanieh Fattahi and Ahmad Amjadi
Sharif University of Technology, Iran

Radin Tahvildari
University of Ottawa, Canada

Hanieh Fattahi
Max Planck Institute of Quantum Optics, Germany

Yury Spirochkin
Engineering Centre of Nuclear Equipment Strength (ENES), Russia

Anders Behndig, Björn Lundberg and Gunnie Bäckström
Department of Clinical Sciences, Ophthalmology, Umeå University, Umeå, Sweden

Anselmo G. De Oliveira
State of Sao Paulo University-UNESP, School of Pharmaceutical Sciences, Department of Pharmaceutics, Araraquara, SP, Brazil

José A. Cardillo, Fernando Paganelli and Acácio A. S. Lima-Filho
Federal University of Sao Paulo-UNIFESP, Department of Ophthalmology, São Paulo, SP, Brazil

José A. Cardillo and Fernando Paganelli
Eye Hospital of Araraquara, Rua Padre Duarte, Araraquara, SP, Brazil

Arnóbio A. Da Silva-Júnior
Federal University of Rio Grande do Norte-UFRN, Health Sciences Centre, Natal, RN, Brazil

Taiji Sakamoto
Department of Ophthalmology, Kagoshima University Graduate School of Medical and Dental Sciences, Kagoshima, Japan

Toshio Hisatomi
Department of Ophthalmology, Kyushu University Graduate School of Medicine, Fukuoka, Japan

Atilla Bayer
Gulhane Medical Academy, Medical School, Turkey

Rehab Ismail
University of Aberdeen, Health Services Research Unit, Aberdeen, UK

Ahmed Sallam
Gloucestershire Hospitals NHS Foundation Trust, Gloucestershire, UK

Baseer U. Ahmad and Igor Estrovich
Department of Ophthalmology, Cole Eye Institute, Cleveland Clinic Foundation, Cleveland, Ohio, USA

Thomas Steinemann
Department of Ophthalmology, MetroHealth Medical Center, Cleveland, Ohio, USA

Emin Kurt
Department of Ophthalmology, Celal Bayar University, Manisa, Turkey

Hüseyin Mayali
Eye Clinic, Buca Gynaecology and Paediatric Hospital, İzmir, Turkey

Elvis Ojaimi and David T. Wong
University of Toronto, Vitreoretinal Department, St Michael's Hospital, Canada

Avinash Pathengay, Stephen G. Schwartz, Harry W. Flynn Jr. and Darlene Miller
Department of Ophthalmology, Bascom Palmer Eye Institute, University of Miami, Miller School of Medicine, Miami, Florida, USA

Miltiadis K Tsilimbaris, Chrysanthi Tsika, Vasilios Diakonis, Aleksandra Karavitaki and Ioannis Pallikaris
University of Crete Medical School, Department of Ophthalmology, Greece

Rosario Díez, Lourdes Jordano and César Hita
Hospital Universitario de Getafe, Spain

Kemal Örnek
Kirikkale University, School of Medicine, Department of Ophthalmology, Turkey

Ramin Daneshvar
Mashhad University of Medical Sciences, Iran

Nel T. Tijmes
Bartimeus, Medical Department, The Netherlands

George K. Andrikopoulos and Sotirios P. Gartaganis
Department of Ophthalmology, Medical School, University of Patras, Greece

A.C. Schefler and T.G. Murray
Bascom Palmer Eye Institute, Department of Ophthalmology, University of Miami Miller School of Medicine, USA

Lawan Abdu
Department of Ophthalmology, Faculty of Medicine, Bayero University Kano, Nigeria